a LANGE medical book

This book is due for return on or before the last date shown below

Obstetric
Anesthesia

- -

Notice

Medicine is an ever-changing science. As new research and clinical experience broaden our knowledge, changes in treatment and drug therapy are required. The authors and the publisher of this work have checked with sources believed to be reliable in their efforts to provide information that is complete and generally in accord with the standards accepted at the time of publication. However, in view of the possibility of human error or changes in medical sciences, neither the authors nor the publisher nor any other party who has been involved in the preparation or publication of this work warrants that the information contained herein is in every respect accurate or complete, and they disclaim all responsibility for any errors or omissions or for the results obtained from use of the information contained in this work. Readers are encouraged to confirm the information contained herein with other sources. For example and in particular, readers are advised to check the product information sheet included in the package of each drug they plan to administer to be certain that the information contained in this work is accurate and that changes have not been made in the recommended dose or in the contraindications for administration. This recommendation is of particular importance in connection with new or infrequently used drugs.

a LANGE medical book

Obstetric Anesthesia

Alan C. Santos, MD, MPH
Professor of Anesthesiology
Texas Tech University Health Sciences Center
Lubbock, Texas

Jonathan N. Epstein, MD, MA
Assistant Professor of Anesthesiology
Icahn School of Medicine at Mount Sinai
Fellowship Director, Obstetric Anesthesiology
Mount Sinai Roosevelt Hospital
New York, New York

Kallol Chaudhuri, MD, PhD
Professor and Vice Chair (Academics)
Director of Obstetric Anesthesia
Department of Anesthesiology
Texas Tech University Health Sciences Center
Lubbock, Texas

New York   Chicago   San Francisco   Athens   London   Madrid   Mexico City
Milan   New Delhi   Singapore   Sydney   Toronto

Obstetric Anesthesia

1 2 3 4 5 6 7 8 9 0   DOC/DOC   19 18 17 16 15

ISBN 978-0-07-178613-3
MHID 0-07-178613-9

This book was set in Adobe Garamond by Cenveo® Publisher Services.
The editors were Brian Belval and Robert Pancotti.
The production supervisor was Catherine H. Saggese.
Project management was provided by Raghavi Khullar, Cenveo Publisher Services.
Cover Image Credit: Science Picture Co. Caption: Pregnant Woman with Fetus
RR Donnelley was the printer and binder.

This book is printed on acid-free paper.

Library of Congress Cataloging-in-Publication Data

　　Obstetric anesthesia (Santos)
　Obstetric anesthesia / editors, Alan C. Santos, Jonathan N. Epstein, Kallol Chaudhuri.
　　　p. ; cm.— (A Lange medical book)
　Includes bibliographical references and index.
　ISBN 978-0-07-178613-3 (paperback : alk. paper) — ISBN 0-07-178613-9 (paperback : alk. paper)
　I. Santos, Alan C., editor.   II. Epstein, Jonathan N., editor.   III. Chaudhuri, Kallol, editor.
IV. Title. V. Series: Lange medical book.
　　[DNLM:　1. Anesthesia, Obstetrical.　2. Delivery, Obstetric.　3. Fetus—physiology.　4. Pregnancy—physiology.　5. Pregnancy Complications.　WO 450]
　RG732
　617.9′682—dc23   2014027206

Dedicated to my family, particularly my spouse Mike, my son Rondel, and to all the residents, fellows, and staff members with whom I have served.

Alan C. Santos, MD, MPH

To my parents, Ahuva and Gary, who taught me who I am and from where I come.
To my wife, Nina, whose love and devotion have been constant.
And to my wonderful daughters, Abby, Arielle, and Tikva, whom I have adored from the time they were smaller than the model gracing the cover of this book.

Jonathan N. Epstein, MD, MA

Dedicated to my mother and father, Lalima and Jatis Chaudhuri—their love and sacrifices have made all my achievements possible.

Kallol Chaudhuri, MD, PhD

Contents

Contributors

Thomas E. Bate, MBChB, FRCA *(Chapter 11)*
East Sussex Healthcare NHS Trust
    England

Jeanette Bauchat, MD *(Chapter 6)*
Department of Anesthesiology
Northwestern University Feinberg
    School of Medicine
Chicago, Illinois

Yaakov Beilin, MD *(Chapter 12)*
Professor of Anesthesiology and Obstetrics
    Gynecology and Reproductive Sciences
Icahn School of Medicine at Mount Sinai
Director, Obstetric Anesthesiology
Vice Chair for Quality
The Mount Sinai Hospital
New York, New York

Howard H. Bernstein, MD *(Chapter 1)*
Associate Professor, Clinical Anesthesia (retired)
Icahn School of Medicine
The Mount Sinai Hospital
New York, New York

Jessica L. Booth, MD *(Chapter 26)*
Assistant Professor of Obstetric Anesthesiology
Wake Forest University School of Medicine
Winston Salem, North Carolina

James P.R. Brown, MBChB *(Chapter 18)*
Consultant Anesthesiologist
British Columbia Women's Hospital
Clinical Instructor
University of British Columbia
Vancouver, British Columbia, Canada

Ingrid Browne, FFARCSI *(Chapter 8)*
Consultant Anaesthetist
Director of Anaesthesia
National Maternity Hospital
Dublin, Ireland

Brenda A. Bucklin, MD *(Chapter 5)*
Professor of Anesthesiology
Assistant Dean, Clinical Core Curriculum
University of Colorado School of Medicine
Aurora, Colorado

Laura Y. Chang, MD *(Chapter 19)*
Instructor of Anesthesiology
Harvard Medical School
Brigham and Women's Hospital
Boston, Massachusetts

Kallol Chaudhuri, MD, PhD *(Chapter 17)*
Professor and Vice Chair (Academics)
Director of Obstetric Anesthesia
Department of Anesthesiology
Texas Tech University Health Sciences
    Center
Lubbock, Texas

Lorraine Chow, MD, FRCP(C) *(Chapter 24)*
Clinical Assistant Professor, Department of
    Anesthesia
Cumming School of Medicine, University of
    Calgary
Director of Obstetric Anesthesia
Foothills Medical Center
Calgary, Alberta, Canada

Christopher G. Ciliberto, MD *(Chapter 20)*
Assistant Professor of Anesthesiology and
    Pain Medicine
University of Washington School of
    Medicine
Director of OB Anesthesia Fellowship Pro-
gram & Interim Director of Obstetric
    Anesthesia
University of Washington Medical Center
    (UWMC)
Seattle, Washington

Allison Clark, MD *(Chapter 27)*
Obstetric Anesthesiologist
Ochsner Hospital
New Orleans, Louisiana

Christina M. Coleman, MD *(Chapter 3)*
Obstetric Anesthesiology Fellow
Department of Anesthesia and Perioperative
    Care
The University of California
San Francisco, California

Joanne Douglas, MD, FRCPC *(Chapter 18)*
Clinical Emeritus Professor and Consultant
  Anesthesiologist
Department of Anesthesiology, Pharmacology,
  and Therapeutics
University of British Columbia and B.C.
  Women's Hospital
Vancouver, British Columbia, Canada

Jonathan N. Epstein, MD, MA *(Chapters 15 and 16)*
Assistant Professor of Anesthesiology
Icahn School of Medicine at Mount Sinai
Fellowship Director, Obstetric Anesthesiology
Mount Sinai Roosevelt Hospital
New York, New York

Michaela K. Farber, MD, MS *(Chapter 24)*
Instructor of Anesthesia
Harvard Medical School
Fellowship Program Director, Obstetric
  Anesthesia
Brigham and Women's Hospital
Boston, Massachusetts

Pamela Flood, MD *(Chapter 3)*
Professor of Anesthesia and Perioperative
  Care
Professor of Obstetrics, Gynecology, and
  Reproductive Medicine
The University of California
San Francisco, California

Jacqueline Geier, MD *(Chapter 15)*
Obstetric Anesthesiology Fellow
Mount Sinai Roosevelt Hospital
New York, New York

Erica N. Grant, MD, MSCS *(Chapter 29)*
Assistant Professor of Anesthesiology
University of Texas Southwestern
Interim Chief of Obstetric Anesthesia
Parkland Health and Hospital Systems
Dallas, Texas

Oren Guttman, MD, MBA *(Chapter 29)*
Assistant Professor of Anesthesiology
Co-Director Anesthesia Patient Safety
  Simulation Team
University of Texas Southwestern Medical
  Center
Dallas, Texas

Anjali Fedson Hack, MD, PhD *(Chapter 23)*
New York, New York

Elsje Harker, MD *(Chapter 21)*
Assistant Professor of Anesthesiology
University of North Carolina School of
  Medicine
Chapel Hill, North Carolina

Stuart Hart, MD *(Chapter 27)*
Anesthesiologist
Vice Chair of Quality Management
Ochsner Hospital
New Orleans, Louisiana

Dimitrios Kassapidis, DO *(Chapter 22)*
Instructor Clinical Anesthesiology
Icahn School of Medicine
Mount Sinai Roosevelt Hospital
New York, New York

Kamal Kumar, MD *(Chapter 7)*
Assistant Professor
Schulich School of Medicine, Western
  University
Obstetric Anesthesia, Victoria Hospital
London Health Sciences
London, Ontario, Canada

Ruth Landau, MD *(Chapter 20)*
Professor of Anesthesiology
Associate Director of Obstetric Anesthesia
Columbia University Medical Center
Center for Precision Medicine, Department
  of Anesthesiology
Columbia University College of Physicians &
  Surgeons
New York, New York

Natesan Manimekalai, MD *(Chapter 25)*
Director of Obstetric Anesthesiology
Obstetric Anesthesiology Fellowship Program
  Director
University of Florida College of Medicine
Jacksonville, Florida

Andrea McCown, MD *(Chapter 30)*
Resident in Anesthesiology
University of Kansas-Wichita
Wichita, Kansas

Robert S.F. McKay, MD *(Chapter 30)*
Professor and Chair Department of
   Anesthesiology
University of Kansas-Wichita
Wichita, Kansas

Barbara Orlando, MD *(Chapter 16)*
Assistant Professor Clinical Anesthesiology
Icahn School of Medicine
Mount Sinai Roosevelt Hospital
New York, New York

Joana Panni, MD, PhD *(Chapter 25)*
Director of Research of Anesthesiology
Assistant Professor of Anesthesiology
University of Mississippi Medical Center
Jackson, Mississippi

Moeen Panni, MD, PhD *(Chapter 25)*
Professor and Chair of Anesthesiology
Professor of Obstetrics and Gynecology
Chief of Perioperative Services
University of Mississippi Medical Center
Jackson, Mississippi

Estee A. Piehl, MD *(Chapter 5)*
Assistant Professor of Anesthesiology
University of Colorado School of Medicine
University of Colorado Hospital
Aurora, Colorado

J. Sudharma Ranasinghe, MD, FFARCSI
(Chapter 10)
Professor of Anesthesiology
University of Miami Miller School of Medicine
Director of Obstetric Anesthesia
Jackson Memorial Hospital
Miami, Florida

Barak M. Rosenn, MD *(Chapter 4)*
Professor of Obstetrics, Gynecology,
   and Reproductive Science
Icahn School of Medicine at Mount Sinai
Director of Obstetrics and Maternal-Fetal
   Medicine
Mount Sinai Roosevelt Hospital
New York, New York

Melissa B. Russo, MD *(Chapter 27)*
Obstetric Anesthesiologist
Director of Obstetric Anesthesia
Obstetric Anesthesiology Fellowship Director
Ochsner Hospital
New Orleans, Louisiana

Migdalia H. Saloum, MD
(Chapters 22 and 28)
Assistant Professor Clinical Anesthesiology
Icahn School of Medicine
Mount Sinai Roosevelt Hospital
New York, New York

Alan C. Santos, MD, MPH *(Chapter 28)*
Professor of Anesthesiology
Texas Tech University Health Sciences Center
Lubbock, Texas

Scott Segal, MD, MHCM *(Chapter 14)*
Professor and Chair of Anesthesiology
Tufts University School of Medicine
Boston, Massachusetts

Richard Smiley, MD, PhD *(Chapter 21)*
Virginia Apgar M.D. Professor
   of Anesthesiology
Columbia University College of Physicians
   and Surgeons
Chief, Obstetric Anesthesia
Columbia University Medical Center
New York, New York

Mieke A. Soens, MD *(Chapter 13)*
Instructor in Anaesthesia, Harvard Medical
   School
Department of Anesthesiology, Perioperative
   and Pain Medicine
Brigham and Women's Hospital
Boston, Massachusetts

Deborah J. Stein, MD *(Chapter 11)*
Assistant Professor of Anesthesiology
Icahn School of Medicine at Mount Sinai
Director of Obstetric Anesthesia
Mount Sinai Roosevelt Hospital
New York, New York

Weike Tao, MD *(Chapter 29)*
Associate Professor of Anesthesiology
Director, Obstetric Anesthesiology Fellowship
    Program
University of Texas Southwestern Medical
    Center
Dallas, Texas

Paloma Toledo, MD, MPH
Assistant Professor
Department of Anesthesiology
Northwestern University Feinberg School of
    Medicine
Chicago, Illinois

Ashley M. Tonidandel, MD, MS *(Chapter 26)*
Assistant Professor of Obstetric Anesthesiology
Wake Forest University School of Medicine
Winston Salem, North Carolina

Lawrence C. Tsen, MD *(Chapter 13)*
Associate Professor in Anaesthesia
Harvard Medical School
Director, Anesthesia for the Center for
    Reproductive Medicine,
Vice Chair, Faculty Development and
    Education, Department of Anesthesiology,
    Perioperative and Pain Medicine
Brigham and Women's Hospital
Boston, Massachusetts

Timothy P. Turkstra, MD, FRCPC
(Chapter 7)
Associate Professor
Schulich School of Medicine, Western
    University
University Hospital, London Health Sciences
London, Ontario, Canada

Pascal H. Vuilleumier, MD *(Chapter 20)*
Obstetric Anesthesiology Fellow
University of Washington Medical Center
    (UWMC)
Seattle, Washington

Cynthia A. Wong, MD *(Chapter 6)*
Professor of Anesthesiology
Northwestern University Feinberg School of
    Medicine
Vice Chair and Section Chief of Obstetric
    Anesthesiology
Northwestern Memorial Hospital
Chicago, Illinois

Francine Yudkowitz, MD, FAAP *(Chapter 2)*
Professor of Anesthesiology and Pediatrics
Icahn School of Medicine at Mount Sinai
Director, Pediatric Anesthesia
The Mount Sinai Hospital
New York, New York

Preface

The specialty of obstetric anesthesia has seen enormous growth over the past three decades. In part, this is related to greater expectations from women, as well as the need for anesthetic care that goes beyond routine analgesia for labor or anesthesia for cesarean delivery. More and more, women of reproductive age, with sometimes serious comorbidities, are now able to conceive and carry a pregnancy to term, which often results in the need for complicated obstetric and anesthetic interventions. As such, obstetric anesthesiology has become a truly multidisciplinary specialty, with a focus not only on anesthesiology but also on obstetrics, perinatology, critical care, neonatology, and nursing.

With these new expectations comes an increased requirement for education and training. Indeed, the Accreditation Council on Graduate Medical Education has recently recognized obstetric anesthesiology as its own separate medical specialty— one that entails a distinct body of knowledge and uniform training requirements. In addition to the need for education of subspecialists as consultants, it is likely that most anesthesiologists will be called on to provide obstetric anesthesia care in the evolving environment alluded to earlier. This book was born out of the need to provide anesthesiologists, and particularly trainees, with a simple and easy reference guide for managing the basics of obstetric anesthesiology and information about the most common obstetric and comorbid conditions.

The contents of this book follow the structure of a comprehensive textbook, with 30 chapters grouped into 6 sections, with a focus on what is clinically expedient. The role of obstetric anesthesiologists has begun to involve the comprehensive care of women during the puerperium; thus two relevant chapters have been included: Trauma During Pregnancy and Anaphylaxis During Pregnancy. In addition, the usefulness of ultrasound in facilitating neuraxial anesthesia has prompted us to include a chapter dedicated to the use of that technology in obstetric anesthesia. In zone instances, related to clinical frequency, core studies have also been prevented.

We would like to express our appreciation to our contributors, who have devoted their time and shared their extensive knowledge and experience to make this book possible. The contributing authors of this book are all practicing obstetric anesthesiologists, and also well-regarded academic and clinical anesthesiologists. This group of academic clinicians has helped us attain our goal of highlighting the principles of basic management at the point of clinical care. If readers seek additional knowledge, they are directed to any number of comprehensive specialty textbooks, which may be used to provide supplemental medical knowledge in obstetric anesthesiology that may be beyond the scope of this book.

We hope that this book provides our colleagues and trainees with the relevant information, comprehensive knowledge, and sincere motivation necessary to maintain the best standards of care for women and their children.

Section **1**

Pregnancy

Physiologic Changes in Pregnancy

Howard H. Bernstein

CARDIOVASCULAR ADAPTATION

Changes in Hemodynamic Values

$$\text{Cardiac Output} = \text{Heart Rate} \times \text{Stroke Volume}$$

The maternal cardiovascular adaptation to pregnancy is characterized by a marked increase in intravascular volume, with expansion of both plasma and red blood cell volume. Heart rate, stroke volume, and cardiac output also increase, with a decrease in systemic vascular resistance. These changes begin by about 6 weeks of gestation, during the embryonic period of development.

The circulation of early pregnancy is characterized by a high flow–low resistance state.[1] By 6 weeks, there is an increase in heart rate, with no change in cardiac output. The cardiac output is unchanged as the result of a significant drop in brachial systolic and diastolic blood pressure as well as central systolic pressure along with a drop in peripheral vascular resistance[2] and renal vascular resistance. These physiologic changes lead to an increase in renal plasma flow and glomerular filtration rate.[3]

Peripheral vasodilation occurs prior to full placentation accompanied by activation of the renin-angiotensin-aldosterone system (RAAS),[3] as evidenced by an increase in nitric oxide concentration, plasma renin activity, and plasma aldosterone level. By 8 weeks a significant rise in end-diastolic volume, stroke volume, and cardiac output has been observed.[4] At term, cardiac output has increased by 43%, with a 17% increase in pulse rate, 21% decrease in systemic vascular resistance

Table 1-1. Central Hemodynamic Changes at 36 to 38 Weeks Gestational Age[a]

HR	↑ 17%
SVR	↓ 21%
PVR	↓
COP	↓ 14%
CO	↑ 43%
PCWP	No change
CVP	No change
MAP	No change

Abbreviations: CO, cardiac output; COP, colloid oncotic pressure; CVP, central venous pressure; HR, heart rate; MAP, mean arterial pressure; PCWP, pulmonary capillary wedge pressure; PVR, pulmonary vascular resistance; SVR, systemic vascular resistance.
[a]From Clark, SL Cotton DB, Lee W, et al.[5]

and a 14% decrease in colloid oncotic pressure and a return of blood pressure to prepregnancy level[3,5] (Table 1-1).

Change in Intravascular Volume

A 30% increase in blood volume, about 1200 mL, occurs between the 8th and 32nd weeks of pregnancy,[6] with the majority of the increase occurring by 24 weeks' gestation. Only a slight increase is seen between the 24th and 32nd weeks, with a slight decline thereafter. The timing to peak volume and in absolute increase varies by individual; however, percentage changes are consistent (Figures 1-1 and 1-2).

Total hemoglobin levels increase 10% between the 8th and 24th weeks of gestation. After 24 weeks' gestation, the levels were noted to drop continuously, due to the dilutional effect of increased blood volume.[6]

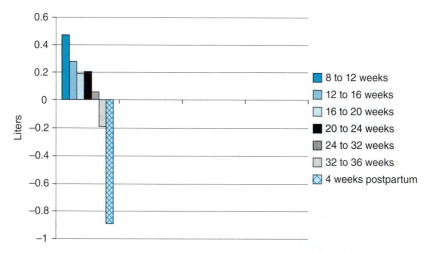

Figure 1-1. Change in liters over time in maternal blood volume from 8 weeks' gestation to 4 weeks' postpartum. (Adapted from Gemzell CA, Robbe H, Sjostrand T.)[6]

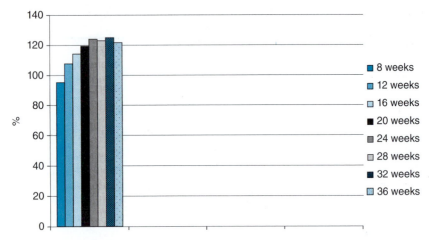

Figure 1-2. Total blood volume as a percentage of the 4 weeks' postpartum value (Adapted from Gemzell CA, Robbe H, Sjostrand T.)[6]

Regulation of Plasma Volume

REGULATION OF PLASMA VOLUME IN THE NONPREGNANT WOMAN

In the nonpregnant state, hypovolemia leads to activation of the volume-sensitive stretch receptors in the atria, carotid sinuses, aortic arch, and kidneys.[7] Stretch receptor activation stimulates sympathetic activity, resulting in an increase in vascular resistance, chronotropy, inotropy, and renally mediated retention of sodium and water via activation of the RAAS, thereby restoring intravascular volume and cardiac output. Angiotensin II is a potent vasoconstrictor and causes sodium retention directly and indirectly by stimulating adrenocortical release of aldosterone. In addition, hyperosmolarity and volume reduction stimulate carotid receptors, inducing posterior pituitary release of antidiuretic hormone and thus promoting renal water retention.

Volume expansion leads to atrial release of atrial natriuretic hormone (ANP). ANP increases glomerular filtration rate and decreases sodium retention, thereby acting as a RAAS antagonist.

REGULATION OF PLASMA VOLUME IN THE PREGNANT WOMAN

Normal pregnancy mimics a state of hypovolemia, activating volume-conserving mechanisms.[1] Deceased vascular sensitivity to angiotensin II and norepinephrine and increased production of nitric oxide and prostacyclin lead to a vasodilated state, decreased systemic vascular resistance, and blood pressure. This leads to activation of the compensatory mechanisms discussed above.[7] Increase in plasma renin activity and aldosterone concentration lead to an increase in water retention and an increase in plasma volume, preload, and cardiac output (Figure 1-3).

The effect of maternal posture on the normal cardiovascular changes of pregnancy has been well documented. The relationship between hypotension and the

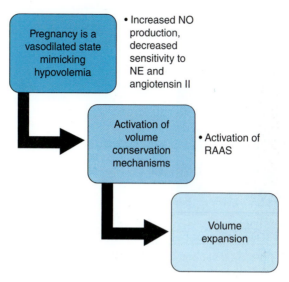

Figure 1-3. Volume regulation during pregnancy. NE, norepinephrine; NO, nitric oxide; RAAS, renin-angiotensin-aldosterone system.

supine position was first described in 1942.[8] In the supine position, there may be obstruction to the aorta and inferior vena cava, leading to significant decrease in venous return, preload, stroke volume, cardiac output, and blood pressure.[9] About 11% to 17% of women will demonstrate a significant decline in blood pressure within a few minutes of assuming the supine position, with rapid return to normal when moved to the lateral position or with left uterine displacement.[10-12]

Cardiovascular Changes During Labor

During the first stage of labor, maternal cardiac output increases between and during contractions by about 11% and 34%, respectively.[13,14] The primary cause of the increase in cardiac output is due to an autotransfusion of about 300 to 500 mL of blood from the uterus to the general circulation with each contraction. As a result of pushing efforts, the second stage of labor will lead to a 50% increase in cardiac output and immediately after delivery, a 60% to 80% increase in cardiac output will occur. The immediate postpartum cardiac output begins to decline within 10 minutes of delivery and is no longer elevated by 24 hours postpartum (Figure 1-4).

UTERINE BLOOD FLOW

Flow is perfusion pressure divided by resistance:

$$\text{Flow} = \text{Perfusion Pressure/Resistance} = \frac{\text{Arterial Pressure} - \text{Venous Pressure}}{\text{Arterial Resistance}}$$

Arterial pressure promotes forward flow. Venous pressure and vascular resistance resist forward flow. In an autoregulated system, flow remains constant over a range of blood pressures as a result of varying arterial resistance.

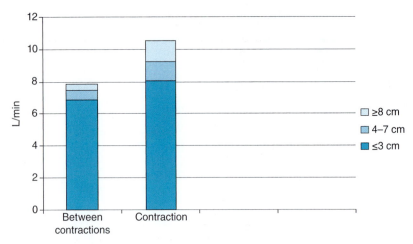

Figure 1-4. Changes in cardiac output between and with contractions as labor progresses. (Adapted from Robson SC, Dunlop W, Boys RJ, Hunter S.)[13]

Uterine blood flow is not autoregulated,[15] because the uterine arteries are maximally vasodilated.

$$\text{Uterine Blood Flow} = \frac{\text{Uterine Artery Pressure} - \text{Uterine Venous Pressure}}{\text{Uterine Artery Vascular Resistance}}$$

In the basal state, uterine venous pressure is low and the uterine artery resistance is at its lowest; therefore, uterine blood flow is directly proportional to maternal blood pressure. Any cause of maternal hypotension, such as supine hypotension, will lead to a decrease in uterine blood flow and oxygen delivery to the fetus. By term, uterine blood flow reaches a mean of 500 to 700 mL/min.

RESPIRATORY SYSTEM CHANGES

$$\text{Minute Ventilation} = \text{Respiratory Rate} \times \text{Tidal Volume}$$

During pregnancy, hyperventilation is the norm, leading to a chronic respiratory alkalosis. The increase in minute ventilation is primarily secondary to a 45% increase in tidal volume. The increase in minute ventilation is initially stimulated by a rise in progesterone levels[16] and then further increased by fetal CO_2 passage across the placenta into the maternal circulation.

There is also change in some of the static lung volumes during pregnancy. Although there is an upward displacement of the diaphragm by the gravid uterus, there is no significant change in total lung capacity due to a widening of the anteroposterior and transverse diameter of the chest during pregnancy. Vital capacity, the sum of the tidal volume (TV), inspiratory reserve volume (IRV), and expiratory reserve volume (ERV) is unchanged during gestation. There is a marked increase in TV, up to 40%[17] and a significant decrease in ERV of 25%, but no significant

Table 1-2. Lung Volumes in the Pregnant and Nonpregnant Woman[a,b]

	TV	IRV	ERV	RV	FRC	VC	TLC
Nonpregnant	450	2050	700	1000	1700	3200	4200
Pregnant	600	2050	550	800	1350	3200	4000

Abbreviations: ERV, expiratory reserve volume; FRC, functional residual capacity; IRV, inspiratory reserve volume; RV, residual volume; TLC, total lung capacity; TV, tidal volume; VC, vital capacity.
[a]From O'Day MP.[17]
[b]All values in milliliters.

change in IRV. In addition, the residual volume (RV) is also decreased by 15%. This leads to a marked decrease in the functional residual capacity (FRC), the sum of the ERV and RV, the pulmonary reserve, by about 21% of the prepregnancy value. For this reason, acute or chronic pulmonary disease during pregnancy may not be well tolerated by the mother (Table 1-2).

Closing volume (CV) is the lung volume at which small airway closure begins to occur. Closing capacity (CC), the lung volume at which the dependent lung zones cease to ventilate due to airway closure, is equal to CV plus RV. Both CV and CC are unchanged during normal pregnancy. Due to a decrease in FRC during pregnancy, the difference between FRC and CC is decreased. This becomes important when the decreased FRC becomes less than the closing capacity, small airway closure will occur during tidal ventilation. This is of particular concern during pregnancies complicated by obesity, multiple gestation, polyhydramnios, chronic or acute lung disease, or during general anesthesia, because airway closure may occur during TV breathing, leading to ventilation-perfusion mismatch and a drop in P_aO_2. In the supine position, the FRC-CC difference is decreased as compared to the sitting position. This is particularly important in the obese patient, the patient with chronic or acute lung disease, and during general anesthesia, when airway closure may occur during TV breathing.

Arterial blood gas values change during pregnancy.[18,19] The state of chronic hyperventilation leads to a fall in measured P_aCO_2, leading to a rise in P_aO_2, as predicted by the alveolar gas equation (Table 1-3). The average P_aO_2 is above 100 mm Hg throughout pregnancy; it is highest in the first trimester and shows a small decrease by term gestation. There is no measured change in alveolar-arterial gradient or

Table 1-3. Alveolar Gas Equation[a]

T
$P_AO_2 = FIO_2(P_B - P_{H2O}) - PACO_2[FIO_2 + (1 - FIO_2)/R]$
$P_AO_2 = FIO_2(713) - 1.2(PaCO_2)$
$P_AO_2 = 0.21(713) - 1.2(30)$
$P_AO_2 = 114$ mm Hg

[a]Assuming 21% oxygen and a $PaCO_2$ of 30 mm Hg.

Table 1-4. Arterial Blood Gas Measured During Each Trimester and at Term[a]

Gestational Age	12 Weeks	24 Weeks	32 Weeks	38 Weeks
pH	7.46	7.44	7.44	7.43
P_aO_2 (mm Hg)	106.4	103.1	102.4	101.8
P_aCO_2 (mm Hg)	29.4	29.5	30.3	30.4
Base excess	−2.1	−2.8	−2.7	−3.1
HCO_3^-				21.7

[a]Adapted from Templeton A, Kelman GR.[18]

in calculated physiologic shunt. Due to the physiologic shunt the maternal PaO_2 is always less than the PAO_2. The degree of respiratory alkalosis remains stable throughout pregnancy and is accompanied by a mild compensatory metabolic acidosis, via renal excretion of bicarbonate (Table 1-4).

GASTROINTESTINAL SYSTEM CHANGES

The Mendelson Syndrome

Aspiration of gastric contents was first described by Dr. Curtis L. Mendelson,[20] an obstetrician at Cornell University Medical College. As an obstetrician, he practiced at a time when many laboring women received inhalation anesthesia, by mask, for delivery. At The New York Lying-In Hospital, the incidence of aspiration of gastric contents during delivery was approximately 0.15% (66/44,016). After noting the disastrous sequelae of aspiration, he studied the aspiration of hydrochloric acid in laboratory animals. After aspiration, these animals developed "bronchiolar spasm, peribronchiolar exudation and congestion, which frequently culminated in pulmonary edema,"[21] similar to humans after aspiration of gastric contents. He recommended antacid prophylaxis to alkalinize stomach contents during labor, increased use of local anesthesia for delivery, administration of general anesthesia *by trained personnel,* and the use of a clear mask. No recommendation for endotracheal intubation with a cuffed tube was made. This article was deemed so important that an abstract was published, that same year, in the journal *Anesthesiology.*[22]

Gastric Emptying During Pregnancy and Gastric pH

Measurement of paracetamol absorption shows delayed gastric emptying by 8 weeks gestation.[23] In nonpregnant women, ultrasound evaluation of gastric contents has shown that the stomach will be empty 4 hours after a standardized meal.[24] Using ultrasound evaluation, these investigators[24] demonstrated that pregnant women who are not in labor have an empty stomach after an overnight fast and 4 hours after eating. However, during labor, there is marked delay in gastric emptying of solids irrespective of the time interval after eating. They found solid food in the stomach up to 24 hours after eating. In addition, the addition of bolus narcotics, fentanyl or meperidine, has been shown to cause a further delay in gastric emptying time. Whereas, fentanyl in amounts less than 100 micrograms has not been determined to slow gastric emptying.[25,26]

The evaluation of gastric emptying of liquids has been studied using both ultrasound and acetaminophen absorption in both obese and nonobese pregnant women.[27,28] In both obese and normal weight patients there was no delay in gastric emptying of liquids whether or not the woman was in labor.

Reflux During Pregnancy

Symptoms of reflux occur in up to 70% of pregnant women.[29] Incompetence of the lower esophageal sphincter, due to the smooth muscle relaxant effect of progesterone, is the most likely cause.[30] Although gastric pressure increases during pregnancy, this has not been proven to result in reflux. Gastric pH, which does not change during pregnancy,[31] is also unrelated to the degree of symptoms. Reflux symptoms will markedly improve within several hours of delivery.

At our institution, nothing by mouth status for elective scheduled cesarean section is no different than for the nonpregnant patient. Patients should refrain from solid food for 8 hours prior to scheduled surgery (2 hours for clear liquids). For patients in labor, clear liquids are allowed, but solids should not be taken.

Liver Physiology

Liver function is not impaired during pregnancy. Liver histology shows only mild nonspecific changes.[32] However, some liver function tests increase or decrease during pregnancy, whereas others remain unchanged. When interpreting liver function during pregnancy, it is critical to understand the changes in liver function testing before making a diagnosis of a liver disease.

There is a consistent rise in alkaline phosphatase during pregnancy, especially in the third trimester,[32,33] due to placental production; this does not represent hepatic dysfunction. Serum protein levels, in particular albumin, fall throughout pregnancy, in part due to hemodilution, secondary to the increase in plasma volume.[32,33] Although there are inconsistencies between laboratory results, serum aspartate transaminase, alanine transaminase, total bile acid concentrations, γ-glutamyl transpeptidase, and serum bilirubin all remain below upper normal limits of the nonpregnant woman[32-34] (Table 1-5).

COAGULATION CHANGES

During Pregnancy

Coagulation is a balanced system of opposing forces: procoagulant, anticoagulant, *fibrinolytic*, and antifibrinolytic; these ultimately come together to ensure vascular patency and integrity. During pregnancy, this balance shifts toward hypercoagulability, as evidenced by both laboratory[35] and clinical[36] findings. This is to ensure placental integrity, thereby maximizing fetal nutrition and oxygenation and to protect against maternal hemorrhage antepartum, intrapartum, and postpartum.

The incidence of venous thromboembolism (VTE) increases during pregnancy and the immediate puerperium and then decreases after the first week postpartum. The absolute risk of VTE during pregnancy has been shown to increase

Table 1-5. Liver Function Tests in Third Trimester as Compared to Nonpregnant Levels[a]

	Albumin (g/L)	Alkaline Phosphatase (IU/L)	Serum Alanine Transaminase (IU/L)	γ-Glutamyl Transpeptidase (IU/L)	Total Bilirubin (μmol/L)	Serum Aspartate Transaminase (IU/L)
Nonpregnant	47.7	34.7	6.3	10.4	6.0	7.7
Pregnant	38.8*	71.4*	7.6	6.5*	2.9*	7.4

*Significant difference from nonpregnant value.
[a]Data from Bacq Y, Zarka O, Brechot J-F, et al.[33]

from 4.1/10,000 pregnant women-years during the first trimester to 59/10,000 pregnant women-years at week 40. In the early puerperal period, the risk increases to 60/10,000 pregnant women-years and then declines to 48.3/10,000 pregnant women-years by 2 weeks after delivery and to 2.1/10,000 pregnant women-years by 12 weeks' postpartum.[36] The relative risk of VTE in pregnant women using oral contraceptives, as compared to nonpregnant women not using oral contraceptives, increases to 1.5 times in the first trimester and rises to 21 times by term. The relative risk falls after the first week postpartum and is no longer elevated after about 3 months postpartum. There is no correlation with the risk of VTE and maternal age.[36]

Global measurements of coagulation are consistent with increased coagulability. The activated partial thromboplastin time (aPTT) and the prothrombin time (PT) as well as the international normalized ratio (INR) are all shortened during pregnancy.[37,38] The INR is decreased to less than 1 by 20 weeks gestational age.[38] The generation of thrombin is the result of multiple reactions occurring in both the initiating and propagation phases of coagulation. Hence, the measurement of thrombin-generating capacity affords a global view of coagulation. Tissue factor–dependent thrombin generation increases over the course of pregnancy with a return to prepregnancy values postpartum.[39] Thromboelastography, another global test of coagulation, also demonstrates increased coagulability[38,40] and decreased fibrinolysis.[40]

Levels and activity of the coagulation factors are altered during normal pregnancy. Fibrinogen, factor I, level rises beginning in the first trimester and peaks at about 500 mg/dl.[41] Levels of PT (factor II) as well as factors VII, VIII, IX, X, and XII rise during pregnancy.[41,42] In addition, the activity of factors V, VIII, IX, X, and XII have been shown to increase during normal pregnancy.[43] Factor XI level and activity show a slight decline over pregnancy.[42,43] Factor XIII levels start to decrease in the first trimester and decline by about 50%.[44] The platelet count remains within normal limits during pregnancy but may decrease at term.[38] Von Willebrand factor levels rise progressively throughout pregnancy[43] (Table 1-6).

A regulatory system exists that limits coagulation to the site of vascular injury. This includes antithrombin III (AT III), thrombomodulin, proteins C and S, and tissue factor pathway inhibitor (TFPI). AT III binds to endogenous heparin to inhibit thrombin and other activated factors. Thrombomodulin complexes with thrombin and activates protein C. Activated protein C and its cofactor protein S inhibit the action of the cofactors V and VIII. TFPI inhibits the action of activated factor VII–tissue factor complex and activated factor X, thereby inhibiting thrombin formation.

Levels of antithrombin do not increase during pregnancy.[43] Thrombomodulin levels are elevated but decrease over the course of pregnancy.[37] Protein C levels do not change, but protein C resistance has been demonstrated.[43,45] Protein S levels fall throughout pregnancy.[43] TFPI levels are increased antepartum but decrease during labor.

Regulation of coagulation also occurs via fibrinolysis and antifibrinolysis. Plasminogen is activated by endothelial-derived tissue plasminogen activator

Table 1-6. Factor Levels and Activity During Pregnancy[a]

	Factor Level	Factor Activity
Fibrinogen	↑↑↑	
Prothrombin	↑	
Factor VII	↑	
Factor VIII	↑	↑
Factor V		↑
Factor IX	↑	↑
Factor X	↑	↑
Factor XII	↑	↑
Factor XI	↓	↓
Factor XIII	↓↓	
Von Willibrand Factor	↑↑↑	
Platelet Count	→ or ↓ at term	

[a]See references 40, 43-46.

(tPA) to form plasmin. Plasmin then cleaves fibrin complex to fibrin degradation products and D-dimer. Fibrinolysis is regulated by tissue plasminogen activator inhibitor (TPAI), endothelial-derived TPAI-1 and placental-derived TPAI-2, and antiplasmin. The tPA inhibitors decrease the production of plasmin by inhibiting plasminogen activator, and antiplasmin inhibits metabolism of fibrin by plasmin.

Alterations to the fibrinolytic/antifibrinolytic system during pregnancy show both enhancement and inhibition of fibrinolysis. Plasminogen level is increased by 50% to 60% by the third trimester[46] as well as the amount of plasminogen activator of both endothelial and renal origin.[42] These changes to the fibrinolytic system in conjunction with the increased level of fibrinogen and enhanced coagulation ultimately result in a 3- to 5-fold increase in D-dimer with a peak in the third trimester.[47] Control of fibrinolysis is simultaneously enhanced. TPAI-1 levels increase after the 20th week of pregnancy and TPAI-2 levels increase by 25 times as compared to nonpregnant levels.[46] By the third trimester, the balance between fibrinolysis and antifibrinolysis favors the later leading to overall down regulation of fibrinolysis by term.[37]

During the Puerperium

The postpartum state is characterized by a marked increase in coagulability. From a teleologic perspective, enhancement of coagulability along with involution of the uterus minimizes the risk of postpartum hemorrhage. On the downside is a marked increase in the risk of postpartum thromboembolism above that of the antepartum state.[48,49] All measures of coagulation are enhanced in the puerperium.[50] This includes shortening of PT and aPTT, elevation of fibrinogen and platelet levels, as well as changes in global tests of coagulation such as thromboelastography consistent with enhanced coagulation. These changes, and the risk of thromboembolism, will remain about 2 to 3 weeks postpartum before falling to predelivery values.[50]

ENDOCRINE SYSTEM CHANGES

Adrenal Gland

The production of cortisol, a glucocorticoid produced by the adrenal cortex, is under the control of the hypothalamic pituitary axis. Corticotropin-releasing hormone (CRH) stimulates the anterior pituitary gland to release adrenocorticotropic hormone (ACTH). ACTH stimulates the adrenal cortex to ultimately secrete cortisol. Cortisol then self-regulates via a negative feedback loop inhibiting ACTH and CRH production. The secretion of ACTH is pulsatile and also diurnal, greatest in the morning.

During pregnancy CRH levels rise gradually beginning at about 16 weeks gestation peaking with a 60-fold rise by term.[51] The CRH is primarily placental in origin.[52] Humans have a CRH–binding protein (CRH-BP). The level of CRH-BP remains normal during the first two trimesters and falls during the third trimester.[53] The majority of CRH produced during pregnancy is bound to and inactivated by CRH-BP. ACTH levels also increase, but only slightly, during late pregnancy.[51] In addition there is a doubling in the production of corticosteroid-binding globulin. This leads to a 2- to 3-fold increase in both free and bound cortisol.[52]

To summarize, pregnancy is characterized by a gradual increase in CRH, ACTH, and cortisol levels with a marked increase during labor and delivery followed by a rapid decline to prepregnancy levels postpartum. Diurnal variation in ACTH production is unchanged during pregnancy.

Thyroid Gland

With pregnancy there are marked changes in the measurement of thyroid function. T4 and T3 are bound by thyroid-binding globulin (TBG). In response to increased estrogen production during pregnancy, there is an increase in TBG levels, peaking at midpregnancy at 2.5-fold higher than in the nonpregnant woman. These levels remain steady throughout the remainder of pregnancy.[54] In response to the increased TBG level, there is a fall in free thyroid hormone levels. This is adjusted through a rise in thyroid-stimulating hormone (TSH) stimulation of the thyroid and increased production of thyroid hormone. The rise in total T4 and T3 peaks during midgestation. A new steady state is reached; thereafter, the daily production of thyroid hormone is no different than prior to pregnancy.[54] Free T4 and T3 levels have shown a decrease by term but remain in the range of nonpregnant women.[54] Despite this small drop, pregnancy is considered a euthyroid state.

TSH levels have been reported to decrease during the first trimester.[54,55] This has been shown to be due to the increased human chorionic gonadotropin (hCG) levels of pregnancy. The actual level of TSH is inversely proportional to the rise in hCG concentration.[56] In some women, with very high hCG levels, the TSH concentration may become undetectable. As hCG exerts a TSH-like effect on the thyroid, despite the decrease in TSH concentration, there is an increase in thyroid hormone production as TBG levels increase[56] (Table 1-7).

Table 1-7. Changes in Thyroid Function Tests During Pregnancy[a]

10% increase in gland size
Fall in thyroid-stimulating hormone (TSH) level, especially during first trimester, due to human chorionic gonadotropin (hCG) production
hCG exerts a TSH-like effect
Doubling of thyroid-binding globulin level by 20 weeks' gestation
50% increase in both T4 and T3 production
Normal to slightly decrease free T4 level
Euthyroid state

[a]See text for references.

Glucose Metabolism

Pregnancy is a diabetogenic state characterized by insulin resistance. During the oral glucose tolerance test, there is an increased insulin-to-glucose ratio, a 3.5-fold increase in insulin secretion, and a 56% decrease in insulin sensitivity.[57] The insulin resistance is induced by the change in the hormonal profile of pregnancy: increased levels of cortisol, human placental lactogen, and prolactin. Cortisol increases hepatic glucose production and decreases insulin sensitivity. Human placental lactogen and prolactin both play a role in insulin resistance.[58] Women who are genetically predisposed to developing type 2 diabetes mellitus are more likely to develop gestational diabetes mellitus.[59]

REFERENCES

1. Duvekot JJ, Cheriex EC, Pieters FA, Menheere PP, Peeters LH. Early pregnancy changes in hemodynamics and volume homeostasis are consecutive adjustments triggered by a primary fall in systemic vascular tone. *Am J Obstet Gynecol.* 1993;169:1382-1392.

2. Mahendru AA, Everett TR, Wilkinson IB, et al. Maternal cardiovascular changes from pre-pregnancy to very early pregnancy. *J Hypertens.* 2012; 30(11):2168-2172.

3. Chapman AB, Abraham WT, Zamudio S, et al. Temporal relationships between hormonal and hemodynamic changes in early human pregnancy. *Kidney Int.* 1998;54:2056-2063.

4. Capeless EL, Clapp JF. Cardiovascular changes in the early phase of pregnancy. *Am J Obstet Gynecol.* 1989;161:1449-1452.

5. Clark, SL Cotton DB, Lee W. Central hemodynamic assessment of normal term pregnancy. *Am J Obstet Gynecol.* 1989;161:1439-1442.

6. Gemzell CA, Robbe H, Sjostrand T. Blood volume and total amount of haemoglobin in normal pregnancy and the puerperium. *Acta Obstet Gynecol Scand.* 1954:33:289-302.

7. Ganzevoort W, Rep A, Bonsel GJ, de Vries JI, Wolf H. Plasma volume and blood pressure regulation in hypertensive pregnancy. *J Hypertens.* 2004;22:1235-1242.

8. Hansen R. Ohnmacht und Schwangerschaft. *Klin Wonchschr.* 1941;21:241-245.

9. Marx GF. Aortocaval compression syndrome: its 50-year history. *Int J Obstet Anesth.* 1992;1:60-64.

10. McRoberts WA. Postural shock in pregnancy. *Am J Obstet Gynecol.* 1951;62:627-632.

11. Howard BK, Goodson JH, Mengert WF. Supine hypotensive syndrome in late pregnancy. *Obstet Gynecol.* 1953;1:371-377.

12. Kennedy RL, Friedman DL, Katchka DM, et al. Hypotension during obstetrical anesthesia. *Anesthesiology.* 1959;20:153-155.

13. Robson SC, Dunlop W, Boys RJ, Hunter S. Cardiac output during labor. *Br Med J (Clin Res Ed).* 1987; 295:1167-1172.

14. Ouzounian JG, Elkayam U. Physiologic changes during normal pregnancy and delivery. *Cardiol Clin.* 2012;30:317-329.

15. Birnbach DJ, Browne IM. Anesthesia for obstetrics. In: Miller RD, Eriksson LI, Fleisher LA, Wiener-Kronish JP, Young WL. *Miller's Anesthesia.* 7th ed. Philadelphia, PA: Churchill Livingstone: 2009; 2203-2240.

16. Milne JA. The respiratory response to pregnancy. *Postgrad Med J.* 1979;55:318-324.

17. O'Day MP. Cardio-respiratory physiological adaptation of pregnancy. *Semin Perinatol.* 1997;21: 268-275.

18. Templeton A, Kelman GR. Maternal Blood-Gases, $(P_AO_2\text{-}P_aO_2)$, Physiological Shunt and VD/VT in normal pregnancy. *Br J Anaesth.* 1976;48:1001-1004.

19. McAuliffe F, Kametas N, Krampl E, Ernsting J, Nicolaides K. Blood gases in pregnancy at sea level and at high altitude. *BJOG.* 2001;108:980-985.

20. Mendelson CL. Aspiration of stomach contents into the lungs during obstetric anesthesia. *Am J Obstet Gynecol.* 1946;52:191-205.

21. Mendelson CL. This week's citation classic: the aspiration of stomach contents into the lungs during obstetric anesthesia. *Curr Cont.* 1983;27:24.

22. Mendelson CL. The aspiration of stomach contents into the lungs during obstetric anesthesia. *Anesthesiology.* 1946;7:694-695.

23. Levy DM, Williams OA, Magides AD, Reilly CS. Gastric emptying is delayed at 8-12 weeks gestation. *Br J Anaesth.* 1994;73:237-238.

24. Carp H, Jayaram A, Stoll M. Ultrasound examination of the stomach contents of parturients. *Anesth Analg.* 1992;74:683-687.

25. Wright PM, Allen RW, Moore J, Donnelly JP. Gastric emptying during lumbar extradural analgesia in labour: effect of fentanyl supplementation. *Br J Anaesth.* 1992;68:248-251.

26. Nimmo WS, Wilson J, Prescott LF. Narcotic analgesics and delayed gastric emptying during labour. *Lancet.* 1975;1(7912):890-893.

27. Wong CA, Loffredi M, Ganchiff JN. Gastric empting of water in term pregnancy. *Anesthesiology.* 2002;96:1395-1400.

28. Wong CA, McCarthy RJ, Fitzgerald PC, Raikoff K, Avram MJ. Gastric emptying of water in obese pregnant women at term. *Anesth Analg.* 2007;105:761-765.

29. Hart DM. Heartburn in pregnancy. *J Int Med Res.* 1978;6(suppl 1):1-5.

30. Richter JE. Review article: the management of heartburn in pregnancy. *Aliment Pharmacol Ther.* 2005;22:749-757.

31. Ngwingtin L, Hardy F, Hamer R, Glomaud D. Changes in the pH and volume of gastric contents during pregnancy and labor. *Cah Anesthesiol.* 1987;35:607-609.

32. Carter J. Liver Function in normal pregnancy. *Aust N Z J Obstet Gynaecol.* 1990;30:296-302.

33. Bacq Y, Zarka O, Brechot JF, et al. Liver function tests in normal pregnancy: a prospective study of 103 pregnant women and 103 matched controls. *Hepatology.* 1996;23:1030-1034.

34. Bacq Y, Zarka O. Liver in normal pregnancy. *Gastroenterol Clin Biol.* 1994;18:767-774.

35. Hellgren M. Hemostasis during normal pregnancy. *Semin Thromb Hemost.* 2003;29:125-130.

36. Virkus RA, Løkkegaard ECL, Bergholt T, et al. Venous thromboembolism in pregnant and puerperal women in Denmark 1995-2005. *Thromb Haemost.* 2011;106:304-309.

37. Hui C, Lili M, Libin C, et al. Changes in coagulation and hemodynamics during pregnancy: a prospective longitudinal study of 58 cases. *Arch Gynecol Obstet.* 2012;285:1231-1236.

38. Karlsson O, Sporrong T, Hillarp A, Jeppsson A, Hellgren M. Prospective longitudinal study of thromboelastography and standard hemostatic laboratory tests in healthy women during normal pregnancy. *Anesth Analg.* 2012;115:890-898.

39. McLean KC, Bernstein IM, Brummel-Ziedins KE. Tissue factor dependent thrombin generation across pregnancy. *Am J Obstet Gynecol.* 2012;207:135.e1-135.e6.

40. Othman M, Falcòn BJ, Kadir R. Global hemostasis in pregnancy: are we using thromboelastography to its full potential? *Semin Thromb Hemost.* 2010;36:738-746.

41. Hale SA, Sobel B, Benvenuto A, et al. Coagulation and fibrinolytic system protein profiles in women with normal pregnancies and pregnancies complicated by hypertension. *Pregnancy Hypertens.* 2012;2:152-157.

42. O'Riordan MN, Higgins JR. Haemostasis in normal and abnormal pregnancy. *Best Pract Res Clin Obstet Gynaecol.* 2003;17:385-396.

43. Clark P, Brennand J, Conkie JA, et al. Activated protein C sensitivity, protein C, protein S and coagulation in normal pregnancy. *Thromb Haemost.* 1998;79:1166-1170.

44. Muszbek L, Bereczky Z, Bagoly Z, et al. Factor XIII: a coagulation factor with multiple plasmatic and cellular functions. *Physiol Rev.* 2011;91:931-972.

45. Schlit AF, Col-De Beys C, Moriau M, Lavenne-Pardonge E. Acquired activated protein C resistance in pregnancy. *Thromb Res.* 1996;84:203-206.

46. Bonnar J, Daly I, Sheppard BL. Changes in the fibrinolytic system during pregnancy. Semin Thromb Hemost. 1990;16:221-229.

47. Eichinger S, Weltermann A, Philipp K, et al. Prospective evaluation of hemostatic system activation and thrombin potential in healthy pregnant women with and without factor V Leiden. *Thromb Haemost.* 1999;82:1232-1236.

48. Simpson EL, Lawrenson RA, Nightingale AL, Farmer RD. Venous thromboembolism in pregnancy and the puerperium: incidence and additional risk factors from a London perinatal database. *BJOG.* 2001;108:56-60.

49. Ray JG, Chan WS. Deep vein thrombosis during pregnancy and the puerperium: a meta-analysis of the period of risk and the leg of presentation. *Obstet Gynecol Surv.* 1999;54:265-271.

50. Saha P, Stott D, Atalla R. Haemostatic changes in the puerperium '6 weeks postpartum' (HIP Study)—implication for maternal thromboembolism. *BJOG.* 2009;116:1602-1612.

51. Laatikainen T, Virtanen T, Raisanen I, Salminen K. Immunoreactive corticotropin-releasing factor and corticotropin during pregnancy, labor and puerperium. *Neuropeptides.* 1987;10:343-353.

52. Mastorakos G, Ilias I. Maternal hypothalamic-pituitary-adrenal axis in pregnancy and the postpartum period. *Ann N Y Acad Sci.* 2003;997:136-149.

53. Linton EA, Perkins AV, Woods RJ, et al. Corticotropin releasing hormone-binding protein (CRH-BP): plasma levels decrease during the third trimester of normal human pregnancy. *J Clin Endocrinol Metab.* 1993;76:260-262.

54. Glinoer D. The regulation of thyroid function in pregnancy: pathways of endocrine adaptation from physiology to pathology. *Endocr Rev.* 1997;28:404-433.

55. Stagnaro-Green A, Abalovich M, Alexander E, et al. Guidelines of the American Thyroid Association for the diagnosis and management of thyroid disease during pregnancy and postpartum. *Thyroid.* 2011;21:1081-1125.

56. Glinoer D, de Nayer P, Bourdoux P, et al. Regulation of maternal thyroid during pregnancy. *J Clin Endocrinol Metab.* 1990;71:276-287.

57. Catalano PM, Tyzbir ED, Roman NM, Amini SB, Sims EA. Longitudinal changes in insulin release and insulin resistance in nonobese pregnant women. *Am J Obstet Gynecol.* 1991;165:1667-1672.

58. Yamashita H, Shao J, Friedman JE. Physiologic and molecular alterations in carbohydrate metabolism during pregnancy and gestational diabetes mellitus. *Clin Obstet Gynecol.* 2000;43:87-98.

59. Catalano PM, Tyzbir ED, Wolfe RR, et al. Carbohydrate metabolism during pregnancy in control subjects and women with gestational diabetes. *Am J Physiol.* 1993;264:E60-E67.

Fetal-Neonatal Physiology and Circulation

2

Francine S. Yudkowitz

At birth, a number of interrelated circulatory and pulmonary changes must occur in order for there to be a smooth transition from the fetal to transitional neonatal circulation. If any of these changes do not occur, the result will be a neonate who is hypoxic and may not have adequate pulmonary and systemic perfusion.

FETAL CIRCULATION (FIGURE 2-1)

Fetal circulation functions as a parallel circuit, where both the right and left sides of the heart provide systemic blood flow. Thus, cardiac output (450 mL/kg/min) in the fetus is the sum of both the right and left ventricular outputs. In utero, the right ventricle contributes approximately 67% and the left ventricle approximately 33% of the total cardiac output. This is in contrast to the extrauterine (adult) circulation that functions in series, where the right side of the heart provides pulmonary blood flow and the left side of the heart provides systemic blood flow. Total cardiac output in adult circulation is determined by each ventricle, and, at birth, approximately 350 mL/kg/min is needed to meet the high metabolic demands of the newborn.

Blood leaving the placenta enters the fetus via the umbilical vein. Approximately 40% to 60% of this blood bypasses the liver via the ductus venosus.[1] On entering the right atrium, one-third of this blood will preferentially flow across the foramen ovale (FO) to the left atrium because of deflection by the crista dividens. This blood will then pass through the left ventricle and exit to the ascending aorta supplying the coronary and cerebral circulation and the upper body of the fetus. Blood

17

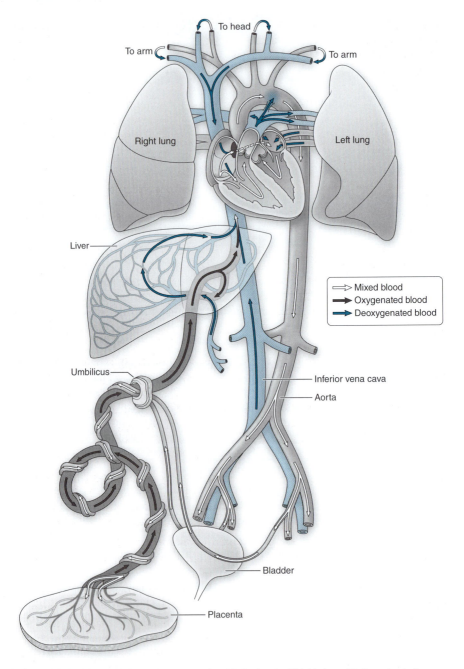

Figure 2-1. Fetal circulation. From Greeley WJ, Berkowitz DH, Nathan AT. Anesthesia for pediatric cardiac surgery. In: Miller RD, Eriksson LI, Fleisher LA, et al. *Miller's Anesthesia.* 7th ed. Philadelphia, PA: Elsevier; 2011.

returning from the cerebral circulation via the superior vena cava enters the right atrium and is preferentially directed toward the right ventricle. Approximately 90% of the blood exiting the right ventricle will be shunted across the ductus arteriosus (DA), while the remaining 10% of the blood will enter the pulmonary circulation providing nutrients for growth. Shunting across the DA occurs because the pulmonary vascular resistance (PVR) is high secondary to pulmonary vasoconstriction and the systemic vascular resistance (SVR) is low secondary to the low-resistance placenta and large-caliber DA.[2] Blood shunted across the DA enters the aorta just before the left subclavian artery and provides nutrients to the lower body of the fetus. From the descending aorta, blood flows to the internal iliac arteries and then umbilical arteries to the placenta.

In the fetus, gas exchange occurs in the placenta. The partial pressure of oxygen (pO_2) of maternal blood in the placenta is 30 to 35 mm Hg (oxygen saturation 65%), much like mixed venous blood. However, once this blood passes into the fetus the oxygen saturation increases to 80% because of the presence of fetal hemoglobin (hemoglobin F; HbF), which has a higher affinity for oxygen than does adult hemoglobin (hemoglobin A; HbA). The blood that enters the fetus from the mother has the highest oxygen saturation to which the fetus will be exposed. As described above, blood from the placenta is preferentially shunted across the FO and supplies the cerebral and coronary circulations, thereby providing essential organs with the greatest amount of oxygen (Figure 2-2).

In contrast, blood returning from the brain with relatively low oxygen saturation (40%) mixes with atrial blood that will increase the oxygen saturation. This blood is preferentially directed to the right ventricle and ultimately to the systemic circulation via the DA, perfusing the lower part of the fetal body. Thus, nonessential organs are perfused with relatively low oxygenated (55%) blood.

FETAL HEMOGLOBIN

The predominant hemoglobin in the fetus is HbF, which is characterized by having a higher affinity for oxygen when compared with HbA. The affinity of hemoglobin to oxygen is described by the oxygen level at which hemoglobin is 50% saturated (P_{50}). The P_{50} of HbF is 20 mm Hg, whereas for HbA it is 27 mm Hg. The higher affinity of HbF is attributed to its low affinity for 2,3-diphosphoglycerate (2,3-DPG). A low level of 2,3-DPG in fetal blood contributes to this as well[3] (Table 2-1).

In utero, HbF, as compared to HbA, is more efficient in the delivery of oxygen to the fetal tissues (Figure 2-3), because at the relatively low oxygen levels present in fetal tissue, HbF will release oxygen more readily than HbA. However, the converse is true after birth, when oxygen tissue levels increase. At these levels, HbA is more efficient in delivering oxygen to the tissues than HbF. To meet the increased metabolic demands of the neonate, the cardiac output is relatively high. However, in addition to cardiac output, hemoglobin is a main determinant of oxygen delivery. Therefore, after birth, it may be necessary to maintain higher hemoglobin levels to compensate for the decrease in tissue oxygen delivery by HbF. As HbF levels decrease and HbA levels increase, the transfusion threshold will decrease

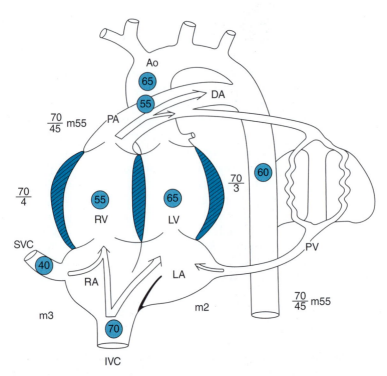

Figure 2-2. Fetal circulation in the lamb. Human neonatal data is extrapolated from studies in fetal lambs. Circled numbers reflect the oxygen saturation at various points in the circulation. Pressure values are outside of the chamber to which they refer. Ao, aorta; DA, ductus arteriosus; IVC, inferior vena cava; LA, left atrium; LV, left ventricle; m, mean pressure; PA, pulmonary artery; PV, pulmonary vein; RA, right atrium; RV, right ventricle; SVC, superior vena cava. Used with permission from Rudolph, AM. (2009). *The Fetal Circulation, in Congenital Diseases of the Heart: Clinical-Physiological Considerations,* 3rd. Edition. Wiley-Blackwell, Oxford, UK. doi: 10.1002/9781444311822.ch1.

depending on the presence of comorbidities. The preterm infant who has received multiple transfusions may have converted to a predominance of HbA. In this situation, lower hemoglobin levels may be well tolerated. However, comorbidities such as respiratory or cardiac pathologies may still dictate higher hemoglobin levels for adequate tissue delivery of oxygen.

Table 2-1. Comparison of Hemoglobin F to Hemoglobin A

	Hemoglobin	pO_2	Oxygen Saturation	P_{50}
Fetal	F	35	80%	20
Maternal	A	35	65%	27

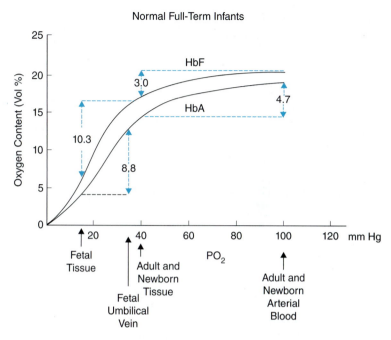

Figure 2-3. Hemoglobin F versus hemoglobin A. Used with permission from Schieber RA. Cardiovascular physiology of the fetus and newborn. In: Cook DR, Marcy JH. *Neonatal Anesthesia.* Pasadena, CA: Appleton-Davies; 1988:2, fig 1-1B.

TRANSITIONAL NEONATAL CIRCULATION

During birth, interrelated changes occur in the respiratory and circulatory systems. When the neonate takes a breath, the lungs expand with air, thereby increasing alveolar pO_2, decreasing alveolar partial pressure of carbon dioxide (pCO_2), and increasing functional residual capacity. These three changes result in a significant decrease in PVR[4] that allows for right ventricular output to now enter the pulmonary circulation easily, thereby now increasing the blood volume returning to the left atrium. Concurrently, the umbilical cord is clamped, removing the low resistance placenta from the circulation. Both these actions, clamping the cord and removing the placenta, result in an increase in neonatal SVR. The increase in blood volume and pressure in the left atrium results in functional closure of the foramen ovale. The DA will functionally close as the arterial pO_2 increases. The ductus venosus closes secondary to removal of the placenta from the circulation (Table 2-2).

The key event that must occur at birth is the decrease in PVR. If PVR does not decrease to levels below SVR, the changes described above will not occur and right-to-left shunting at the atrial level (FO) and extracardiac level (DA) will continue; the neonate will be hypoxic (Figure 2-4). This circulation was once referred to as

Table 2-2. Circulatory Changes After Birth

Decrease in pulmonary vascular resistance
    Expansion of lungs
    Increased pO_2
Increase in systemic vascular resistance
    Clamping umbilical cord
    Removal of placenta from circulation
Closure of ductus arteriosus
    Increased pO_2
    Prostaglandins
Closure of foramen ovale
    Increased pulmonary blood flow
    Increased blood return to left atrium
Closure of ductus venosus
    Removal of placenta

persistent fetal circulation but is now known as persistent pulmonary hypertension, which reflects the underlying pathophysiology that exists.

The circulation at birth is referred to as transitional because the changes that occur at birth are reversible; the two major shunts are functionally and not anatomically closed. Adverse events such as hypoxia, hypercarbia, acidosis, or hypothermia will result in reopening of the two shunts and a conversion back to a fetal pattern.[5] The DA may take 10 to 15 hours to fully functionally close, with complete anatomic closure occurring in 2 to 3 weeks[6] of postnatal life; the vestigial organ remaining is the ligamentum arteriosum. The DA will "reopen" if hypoxia is present. The relationship between PVR and SVR will determine the direction of the shunt across the DA. If PVR is greater than SVR, then right-to-left shunting will occur and worsen hypoxia in the neonate.

The FO closes by a flaplike valve located in the atrial septum on the left side secondary to increased left atrial pressure as compared to right-sided pressures. In 25% to 30% of adults, the FO remains anatomically probe patent.[7] If PVR remains high or increases, this will create a higher pressure on the right side of

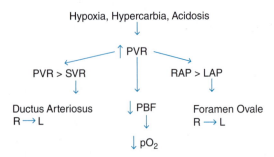

Figure 2-4. Effects of increased pulmonary vascular resistance in the newborn.

the heart, opening the flaplike valve; this results in a patent FO and right-to-left shunting will occur.

Initial management of the neonate in the delivery room should be aimed at ensuring a smooth transition from fetal to transitional circulation. Factors that may adversely affect the decrease in PVR must be avoided. These include hypoxia, hypercarbia, acidosis, and hypothermia. Delivery room management strategies and neonatal resuscitation are discussed in detail in Chapter 11.

SUMMARY

The smooth transition from fetal to transitional circulation is dependent on an appropriate decrease in PVR. Ensuring and maintaining adequate oxygenation, ventilation, and temperature is important to guarantee that the neonate is successful in making this transition and does not revert back to the fetal circulation.

REFERENCES

1. Rudolph AM. The changes in circulation after birth: their importance in congenital heart disease. *Circulation.* 1970;41:343-359.
2. Lyrene RK, Philips JB. Control of pulmonary vascular resistance in the fetus and newborn. *Clin Perinatol.* 1984;11:551.
3. Lister G, Moreau G, Moss M, et al. Effects of alterations of oxygen transport on the neonate. *Semin Perinatol.* 1984;8:192-204.
4. Enhorning G, Adams FH, Norman A. Effect of lung expansion on the fetal lamb circulation. *Acta Pediatr Scand.* 1966;55:441.
5. Haworth SG, Reid LR. Persistent fetal circulation—newly recognized structural features. *J Pediatr.* 1976;88:614.
6. Clyman RI, Mauray F, Roman C, et al. Factors determining the loss of ductus arteriosus responsiveness to prostaglandin E. *Circulation.* 1983;68:433-436.
7. Hagen PT, Scholz DG, Edwards WD. Incidence and size of patent foramen ovale during the first 10 decades of life: an autopsy study of 965 normal hearts. *Mayo Clin Proc.* 1984;59:17-20.

Progress of Labor and Delivery

3

Christina M. Coleman and Pamela Flood

TOPICS

PHYSIOLOGY OF LABOR

Labor is defined as repeated uterine contractions that result in the dilation and effacement of the uterine cervix causing the fetus to be expelled. The mechanisms that initiate labor are not completely known. However, it is clear that preparation for labor begins long before with changes in the cervix that include ingrowth of C-type pain fibers[1,2] and infiltration of inflammatory cells, including neutrophils and macrophages.[3] These inflammatory cells release cytokines that result in softening of the cervix in preparation for labor.

Corticotropin-releasing hormone (CRH) may play a role in the initiation of labor. As the placenta matures, it produces increasing maternal levels of CRH, which peak at the time of delivery. The increase in CRH contributes to a feed-forward cycle in which increasing concentrations of CRH stimulate the pituitary to produce corticotropin, which induces cortisol production in the adrenal glands of both mother and fetus. Cortisol then enhances expression of the *CRH* gene, resulting in increased expression of CRH.[4] Indeed, elaboration of CRH at an unusually high rate is an independent predictor of preterm birth.[5]

Uterine muscle or myometrium is a specialized type of smooth muscle that exhibits a positive feedback loop in response to pressure on the uterine cervix. Activation of sensory neurons in the cervix enhances the release of oxytocin from the posterior pituitary, which increases contractility. Increasing estrogen and progesterone during pregnancy cause an up-regulation of oxytocin receptors in uterine muscle. At term, there is functional progesterone withdrawal that is mediated by

increasing expression of type A progesterone receptor relative to the type B progesterone receptor, which suppresses progesterone responsiveness.[6]

Labor has classically been separated into three stages. The first stage of labor
includes the change of the uterine cervix from a thick closed tube approximately
3 cm long to an opening of approximately 10 cm through which the fetus can be
expelled. The second stage of labor is the expulsion of the fetus through that opening. The third stage is the expulsion of the placenta. The time course of the first
stage of labor was first studied by Emanuel Friedman, who described the course of
labor as sigmoidal (Figure 3-1).[7] Friedman separated the first stage of labor into
a latent phase, an active phase, and a deceleration phase. The sigmoidal nature of
the relationship has since been challenged; there is little evidence for a deceleration
phase as the cervix approaches complete dilation (10 cm).[8,9] However, the separation of the first stage of labor into an early slow phase, called latent labor, and a
more rapid phase of active labor has withstood the test of time.[8,9]

Labor may be abnormal on the basis of having an unusually slow latent labor,
arrest in the active phase, or arrest of descent (failure of stage 2). Abnormal labor
is termed dystocia and may be a result of abnormality in any of the 3 Ps—power,
pelvis, and passenger. Normal labor requires strong, repetitive uterine contractions
(power), a skeletal structure wide enough to accommodate the fetus (pelvis), and
proper fetal size and position (passenger).[10] The diagnosis of dystocia is based on
deviation from normal values derived from populations, and because of that, there
is significant variability between individual women. Friedman defined abnormal
labor progress in the active phase as cervical dilation less than 1.2 cm per hour in
nulliparous women and less than 1.5 cm per hour in multiparous women. The
World Health Organization (WHO) has constructed a "partogram" that is used
extensively in the Third World to diagnose dystocia. It assumes dilation of 1 cm

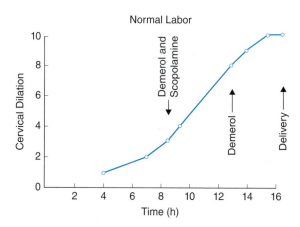

Figure 3-1. Representative tracing of the course of cervical dilation in the labor of
a nulliparous patient. Estimates of cervical dilation (vertical axis) have been plotted
against elapsed time in labor (horizontal axis). The sigmoid curve is characteristic of all
normal labors. Reproduced by permission from Friedman EA.[7]

per hour, after dilation of 3 cm, to be normal. Currently, no appreciable change in cervical dilation in the presence of adequate uterine contractions for more than 2 hours is considered active phase arrest.

The Montevideo unit is traditionally used by obstetricians to assess the adequacy of uterine contractions or power. This unit is defined as the intensity of contractions (in mm Hg measured with an intrauterine catheter) multiplied by the number of contractions that occur in 10 minutes. Generally, 200 or more Montevideo units are considered adequate for labor progress.

MODERN METHODS OF MEASUREMENT OF LABOR PROGRESS

World Health Organization Partogram

Whereas Friedman conceptualized the partograph, or a graphical representation of normal labor progress in a population, the use of the partograph to prevent maternal and fetal morbidity and mortality by identifying and treating dystocia was institutionalized by the WHO.[11] The WHO partograph allows up to 8 hours of a latent phase with an active phase beginning when the cervix is dilated to 3 cm. During the active phase there are alerts and action able items placed 4 hours apart, designed to indicate when a woman's progress of labor has sufficiently deviated from the normal population values to merit concern (alert line) and treatment (action line) (Figure 3-2).

In 1994, the WHO partogram was developed and tested in a population of 35,484 women in southeast Asia. Its application, along with a structured management protocol, was assessed. The structured management protocol would be considered similar to "active management of labor" algorithms today. It included rupture of membranes in the active phase, consideration of oxytocin augmentation, cesarean section, and supportive treatment when the action line was crossed in the active phase of labor. A progress of 1 cm per hour in cervical dilation was expected during active labor (after 3 cm). In the initial study, despite a reduction in the use of oxytocin, the duration of labor was slightly reduced. The incidence of normal spontaneous deliveries was increased by 6%, and emergency cesarean section was reduced by 3%.[11] Since that time, the WHO partograph has been used with variable success in many countries, most commonly in locations with reduced access to maternity care.

Zhang Method

Zhang and colleagues, working at the National Institute of Child Health and Human Development, have devised a different method of modeling labor progress. Rather than assume any correlation in the relationship between time and cervical dilation, they have used a statistical method called repeated measures regression that in very simple terms acts to "connect the dots" created by measuring the average time required for a centimeter change in cervical dilation in a large population of parturients. In 2002, they found that active labor was substantially slower than predicted by the Friedman curve, and they identified no deceleration

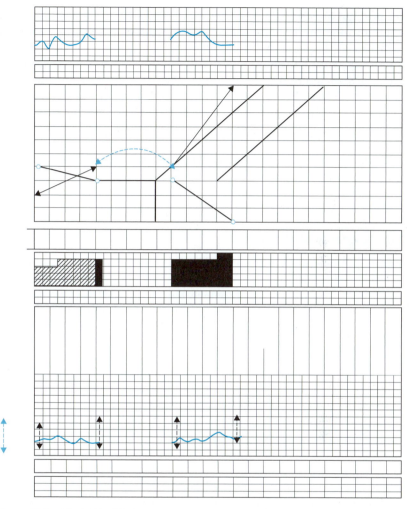

Figure 3-2. World Health Organization partograph. The progress of labor is recorded on the graph of cervical dilation against time (four hourly observations), with space to record all fetal and maternal observations. The illustration shows a woman admitted at 2-cm dilation (latent phase), who progressed to 4 cm at the next vaginal examination. This observation in the active phase is transferred onto the Alert line (1 cm/h—the lower limit of normal progress—and the time scale for all subsequent maternal and fetal observations is shifted to the right accordingly. Full dilation (10 cm) occurred at the next vaginal examination, with delivery 10 minutes later. From Kwast BE, et al.[11]

phase near full dilation.[12] In 2010, the same methods were used to assess labor progress in a large contemporary cohort of parturients enrolled in the Consortium on Safe Labor. All subjects had a singleton gestation, spontaneous onset of labor, and vertex presentation, and they were delivered by normal spontaneous vaginal delivery and had normal neonatal outcome. The researchers found a much slower course of active labor in this contemporary cohort of women, with labor taking more than 6 hours to progress from 4- to 5-cm dilation and more than 3 hours to progress from 5- to 6-cm dilation.[13] From this analysis, they created their own partogram with 95% confidence intervals that serve the same function as the alert and action lines from the WHO partogram. Zhang and coworkers hypothesized that allowing labor to continue for a longer period prior to 6-cm dilation might reduce the rate of intrapartum and repeat cesarean delivery. This partogram has not yet been tested for this purpose in an independent cohort.

Labor Progress Calculator

The aforementioned approaches to a graphical representation of normal labor have several limitations. First, they can only demonstrate norms for a population and cannot speak to expected variability among women. Second, they are constructed from retrospective observation and cannot be used to predict future labor progress or the risk of cesarean delivery. Flood and colleagues have developed an alternative model that is similar to the Friedman model in that it assumes a latent phase of labor, an active phase of labor, and a cervical dilation rate that transitions between the two phases. This model was originally derived from the labor patterns of 500 nulliparous parturients with term singleton vertex gestations who reached full cervical dilation. A biexponential model was used as the best representation of labor progress.[8] This model is unique in that it can address the labor course of an individual parturient in addition to a population. It uses individual variability to identify factors such as obesity, maternal age, and genetic factors, which all may have an impact on labor progress.[8,14,15] Another difference in this model is that it does not assume that a woman's active labor starts at any particular cervical dilation. In fact, the cervical dilation at which active labor begins is an experimental variable that is fit for each woman in addition to a time constant for latent labor and a time constant for active labor (Figure 3-3). This model can be used to predict future labor progress and is available as a computer application.

FACTORS THAT INFLUENCE LABOR PROGRESS

Multiple demographic and genetic factors have been associated with variability in labor progress.[8,9,13-16] Multiparity has been consistently associated with faster labor,[13] whereas larger maternal weight, older age, and large fetal size have been associated with slower labor.[8,14,17] Chorioamnionitis, non-African American ethnicity, and grand multiparity are associated with a prolonged second stage of labor. There is also evidence that heredity may play a role in labor progress.[18,19] Specifically, β_2-adrenergic and oxytocin receptor polymorphisms have been implicated in mediating variability during labor.[14-16] In theory, alterations in receptors

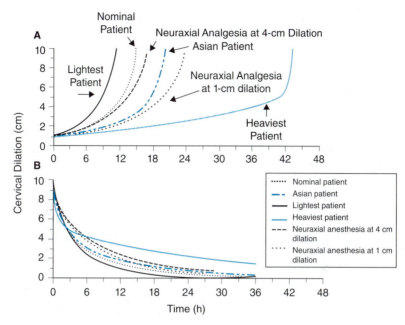

Figure 3-3. Effect of individual factors on labor progress. A, Forward simulations from the labor progression model of the time course required for cervical dilation from 1 to 10 cm for a "nominal" patient (non-Asian patient of median weight without epidural analgesia), lightest patient (a 48-kg non-Asian patient), heaviest patient (a 171-kg non-Asian patient), and a patient (non-Asian, median weight) with epidural analgesia initiated at 1 cm of cervical dilation or at 4 cm of cervical dilation. The x-axis is hours of labor beginning at 1 cm of cervical dilation. B, Predictions from the labor progression model from full cervical dilation (10 cm) through time as actually fit by the model. The x-axis is time before full cervical dilation. Used with permission from Debiec J, Conell-Price J, Evansmith J, Shafer S, Flood P.[8]

may lead to a poor response to intrinsic or extrinsic oxytocin, leading to abnormal contractility as would abnormally strong response to catecholamines.

Many observational studies have suggested that epidural analgesia is associated with slower labor progress.[14,20] This association has been repeatedly found in observational trials but has not been replicated in prospective randomized trials[21,22] or trials in which labor progress was assessed before and after the initiation of an epidural anesthesia service.[23] As such, it does not appear that epidural analgesia directly *causes* slower labor progress. There are a number of confounding variables that could contribute to this association. Clearly, women with more severe pain would be more likely to request analgesia and to request it earlier, both of which may be associated with dystocia. The absence of an association between epidural analgesia and labor progress or risk of cesarean section in these trials makes sense because uterine smooth muscle is not innervated by motor nerves that are blocked by epidural analgesia. There is no known physiologic mechanism by which blockade of sensory transduction or systemic local anesthetic activity that is present during neuraxial anesthesia would impede uterine contractility. In contrast, several prospective trials have suggested that neuraxial anesthesia may cause a modest prolongation of the second stage of labor. This may occur because the expulsion of the fetus normally requires the recruitment of abdominal skeletal muscle and a decrease motor nerve transmission together with a lack of sensory feedback from the perineum can impede coordinated pushing.[21,22] Changes can be made to reduce local anesthetic dose in the second stage if blockade is too dense to allow for coordinated expulsion efforts. When the parturient is comfortable, in the face of epidural analgesia, there is greater tolerance for a longer second stage and to allow uterine contractions to lower fetal station before active efforts at expulsion begin.[24]

METHODS FOR INDUCTION AND AUGMENTATION OF LABOR

When spontaneous labor is not initiated or progressing appropriately, labor may be induced or augmented with pharmacologic and/or physical methods.[25] Induction of labor applies to the exogenous stimulation of uterine contractions before the onset of spontaneous labor to accomplish vaginal delivery. Augmentation of labor refers to increasing the frequency and intensity of existing uterine contractions in a woman in whom labor is not progressing adequately. Induction of labor may be indicated for complications of pregnancy in the mother (ie, preeclampsia, diabetes) or the fetal-placental unit (rupture of membranes, placental insufficiency, intrauterine growth restriction) or may be done by maternal request.

Oxytocin is the most widely used medication for augmentation of labor. By activating the oxytocin receptor, which is G-protein linked, it stimulates strong, concerted uterine contractions that act to induce cervical dilation. Oxytocin is degraded by the gastrointestinal tract so it can only be administered intravenously or by nasal spray. Cochran review of randomized clinical trials comparing oxytocin infusion to expectant management/placebo revealed a greater success in achieving vaginal delivery within 24 hours with a number needed to treat (NNT) of 3.[26] However, oxytocin use can be associated with tachysystole (defined as more than five contractions in 10 minutes averaged over 30 minutes); this may result in placental insufficiency, often manifested by fetal heart rate changes. Oxytocin overuse may result in maternal hypotension with a decrease in mean arterial pressure of 30% or more that can also lead to inadequate perfusion of the fetus. There are rare reports of uterine rupture with oxytocin use, although most patients in whom uterine rupture occurred had previous cesarean sections or myomectomies. Oxytocin is structurally similar to vasopressin and can bind to the vasopressin receptor, resulting in water retention and possible water intoxication if given in large quantities for prolonged periods.[10] The benefit of oxytocin over other medications that enhance uterine contractility is that its short half-life of 3 to 6 minutes allows it to be turned off in the event of fetal or maternal distress. Multiple studies have shown that oxytocin is less effective as an induction agent with an unfavorable cervix. Compared to vaginal prostaglandins, oxytocin failed to achieve vaginal delivery within 24 hours (73/132 versus 40/128; relative risk [RR] 1.77; 95% confidence interval [CI] 1.31 to 2.38; number needed to harm [NNH] 5).[25]

Prostaglandins bind to prostaglandin receptors in myometrial cells causing uterine contractions as well as dissolution of collagen bundles and increased submucosal water content of the cervix (cervical ripening). Prostaglandin E2 has been used since 1979 for induction of labor. There are two formulations, approved by Food and Drug Administration (FDA), for use in cervical ripening. Prepidil contains 0.5 mg dinoprostone in 2.5 mL of gel for intracervical administration. Cervidil is a timed-release vaginal insert containing 10 mg dinoprostone. Both formulations are equally effective in achieving vaginal delivery compared to placebo. There is no increased risk in the rate of cesarean delivery. But a review of 1259 women receiving prostaglandins reported tachysystole with fetal heart rate changes associated with use of intravaginal prostaglandin E2 as compared to control (28/642 versus 3/617; RR 4.14; 95% CI 1.93 to 8.90; NNH 65).[25] These drugs also have the disadvantage of being expensive and require refrigeration.

Misoprostol (prostaglandin E1) can be given orally or vaginally for the induction of labor. Although it is not FDA-approved for use as a cervical ripening agent, the American College of Obstetricians and Gynecologists supports its "off-label" use. A review of misoprostol use has shown a decrease in the number of participants with an unfavorable or unchanged cervix after 12 to 24 hours with an NNT of 2 compared to placebo. Misoprostol is either equal to or superior to other vaginal prostaglandins.[27] Twenty-two trials involving 5229 women comparing vaginal misoprostol with other vaginal prostaglandins found that fewer women receiving misoprostol failed to be delivered within 24 hours (920/2550 versus 1179/2679; RR 0.77; 95% CI 0.66 to 0.89; NNT 10) and were less likely to require oxytocin augmentation.[27] Oral and vaginal misoprostol are equally effective, but studies suggest fewer systemic side effects with oral administration.

Mechanical Techniques to Induce/Augment Labor

Mechanical forms of induction of labor stimulate the release of intrinsic prostaglandins. For instance, amniotomy (artificial rupture of membranes), sweeping of membranes, and cervical dilation with Foley balloon or other cervical devices are widely used in hospitals across the country. There are numerous homeopathic forms of labor induction. Each method of induction is associated with strengths and weaknesses, which are listed in Table 3-1.

SUMMARY

Labor is a complex process that begins with changing the cervix from a closed tube to a 10-cm dilated opening, followed by repetitive uterine contractions and ends with the expulsion of the fetus and placenta from the uterus. This process involves the ingrowth of C-type pain fibers and inflammatory cells into the uterus, up-regulation of oxytocin receptors, and cortisol stimulation. But the actual mechanism that initiates labor is not yet known. Labor is classically divided into three stages: cervical dilation, expulsion of the fetus, and expulsion

Table 3-1. Methods of Induction: Quality of Evidence and Grades of Recommendation[a]

Method	Quality of Evidence	Balance of Benefits/Harms	Grade of Recommendation
Vaginal prostaglandin E2	Moderate	Trade-offs	Strong
Cervical prostaglandin E2	Moderate	Net benefits	Strong
Intravenous oxytocin	Moderate	Trade-offs	Strong
Amniotomy	Moderate	Uncertain trade-offs	Weak
Intravenous oxytocin plus amniotomy	Moderate	Trade-offs	Strong
Vaginal misoprostol	Moderate	Trade-offs	Strong
Oral misoprostol	Moderate	Trade-offs	Strong
Mechanical methods	Moderate	Trade-offs	Weak
Membrane sweeping	Moderate	Net benefits	Strong
Extra-amniotic prostaglandins	Moderate	No net benefit	Strong (against)
Intravenous prostaglandins	Moderate	Net harms	Strong (against)
Oral prostaglandins	Moderate	Net harms	Strong (against)
Mifepristone	Moderate	Net harms	Weak
Estrogens	Very low	Uncertain trade-offs	Weak
Corticosteroids	Very low	Uncertain trade-offs	Weak
Relaxin	Moderate	Uncertain trade-offs	Weak
Hyaluronidase	Very low	Uncertain trade-offs	Weak
Castor oil	Very low	Net harms	Strong (against)
Acupuncture	Moderate	No net benefit	Weak
Breast stimulation	Moderate	Uncertain trade-offs	Weak
Sexual intercourse	Very low	Uncertain trade-offs	Weak
Homeopathic methods	Very low	Uncertain trade-offs	Weak
Isosorbide mononitrate	Moderate	Uncertain trade-offs	Weak
Buccal or sublingual misoprostol	Moderate	Trade-offs	Strong
Hypnosis	Very low	No net benefit	Weak

[a]From Mozurkewich, EL, et al.[25]

of the placenta. The first stage of labor is divided into an early (latent) phase followed by an active phase. Friedman was the first to describe the normal progress of labor. Friedman's labor curves are still used today but have been modified by Zhang, the WHO, and most recently Flood. Maternal factors that influence the progress of labor include multiparity, ethnicity, obesity, and age. Genetic factors have also been linked to variations in normal labor progress. Normal labor requires the 3 Ps—adequate power of uterine contractions; a pelvis that accommodates the fetal size; and a fetus, or passenger, which must be sized and positioned properly. When labor progress is abnormal (dystocia), it can be augmented with oxytocin, amniotomy, and other methods to increase the frequency and strength of uterine contractions. If spontaneous labor does not occur, labor can be induced similarly. Vaginal or cervical prostaglandins are the commonly used medications for induction of labor to soften and dilate the cervix.

Regardless of the method used, the goal is to have a successful vaginal delivery while maintaining the health of both mother and fetus. More studies are needed to fully understand the physiology of labor and identify novel, safer and more efficacious methods to help mothers to achieve a vaginal delivery.

REFERENCES

1. Collins JJ, Usip S, McCarson KE, Papka RE. Sensory nerves and neuropeptides in uterine cervical ripening. *Peptides*. 2002;23(1):167-183.
2. Tong C, Conklin D, Clyne BB, Stanislaus JD, Eisenach JC. Uterine cervical afferents in thoracolumbar dorsal root ganglia express transient receptor potential vanilloid type 1 channel and calcitonin gene-related peptide, but not P2X3 receptor and somatostatin. *Anesthesiology*. 2006;104(4):651-657.
3. Norman JE, Bollapragada S, Yuan M, Nelson SM. Inflammatory pathways in the mechanism of parturition. *BMC Pregnancy Childbirth*. 2007;7(suppl 1):S7.
4. Emanuel RL, Robinson BG, Seely EW, et al. Corticotropin releasing hormone levels in human plasma and amniotic fluid during gestation. *Clin Endocrinol (Oxf)*. 1994;40(2):257-262.
5. Smith R. Parturition. *N Engl J Med*. 2007;356(3):271-283.
6. Mesiano S, Chan EC, Fitter JT, Kwek K, Yeo G, Smith R. Progesterone withdrawal and estrogen activation in human parturition are coordinated by progesterone receptor A expression in the myometrium. *J Clin Endocrinol Metab*. 2002;87(6):2924-2930.
7. Friedman E. The graphic analysis of labor. *Am J Obstet Gynecol*. 1954;68(6):1568-1575.
8. Debiec J, Conell-Price J, Evansmith J, Shafer S, Flood P. Mathematical modeling of the pain and progress of the first stage of nulliparous labor. *Anesthesiology*. 2009;111(5):1093-1110.
9. Laughon SK, Branch DW, Beaver J, Zhang J. Changes in labor patterns over 50 years. *Am J Obstet Gynecol*. 2012;206(5):419 e1-9.
10. Kilpatrick S, Garrison E. Normal labor and delivery. In: Gabbe SG, Niebyl JR, Galan HL, et al. *Obstetrics: Normal and Problem Pregnancies*. 6th ed. Philadelphia, PA; Elsevier; 2012:267-286.
11. Kwast BE, Lenox CE, Farley TMM, et al. World Health Organization partograph in management of labour. *Lancet*. 1994;343(8910):1399-1404.
12. Zhang J, Troendle JF, Yancey MK. Reassessing the labor curve in nulliparous women. *Am J Obstet Gynecol*. 2002;187(4):824-828.
13. Zhang J, Landy HJ, Branch DW, et al. Contemporary patterns of spontaneous labor with normal neonatal outcomes. *Obstet Gynecol*. 2010;116(6):1281-1287.
14. Reitman E, Conell-Price J, Evansmith J, et al. β2-adrenergic receptor genotype and other variables that contribute to labor pain and progress. *Anesthesiology*. 2011;114(4):927-939.
15. Terkawi AS, Jackson WM, Thiet MP, Hansoti S, Tabassum R, Flood P. Oxytocin and catechol-O-methyltransferase receptor genotype predict the length of the first stage of labor. *Am J Obstet Gynecol*. 2012;207(3):184 e1-8.
16. Miller RS, Smiley RM, Daniel D, et al. Beta-2 adrenoceptor genotype and progress in term and late preterm active labor. *Am J Obstet Gynecol*. 2011;205(2):137 e1-7.
17. Vahratian A, Zhang J, Troendle JF, Savitz DA, Siega-Riz AM. Maternal prepregnancy overweight and obesity and the pattern of labor progression in term nulliparous women. *Obstet Gynecol*. 2004;104(5 pt 1):943-951.
18. Algovik M, Nilsson E, Cnattingius S, Lichtenstein P, Nordenskjöld A, Westgren M. Genetic influence on dystocia. *Acta Obstet Gynecol Scand*. 2004;83(9):832-837.
19. Algovik M, Kivinen K, Peterson H, Westgren M, Kere J. Genetic evidence of multiple loci in dystocia—difficult labour. *BMC Med Gen*. 2010;11:105.
20. Thorp JA, Eckert LO, Ang MS, Johnston DA, Peaceman AM, Parisi VM. Epidural analgesia and cesarean section for dystocia: risk factors in nulliparas. *Am J Perinatol*. 1991;8(6):402-410.
21. Wong CA, McCarthy RJ, Sullivan JT, Scavone BM, Gerber SE, Yaghmour EA. Early compared with late neuraxial analgesia in nulliparous labor induction: a randomized controlled trial. *Obstet Gynecol*. 2009;113(5):1066-1074.

22. Wang F, Shen X, Guo X, Peng Y, Gu X; Labor Analgesia Examining Group. Epidural analgesia in the latent phase of labor and the risk of cesarean delivery: a five-year randomized controlled trial. *Anesthesiology.* 2009;111(4):871-880.

23. Zhang J, Klebanoff MA, DerSimonian R. Epidural analgesia in association with duration of labor and mode of delivery: a quantitative review. *Am J Obstet Gynecol.* 1999;180(4):970-977.

24. Gillesby E, Burns S, Dempsey A, et al. Comparison of delayed versus immediate pushing during second stage of labor for nulliparous women with epidural anesthesia. *J Obstet Gynecol Neonatal Nurs.* 2010;39(6):635-644.

25. Mozurkewich EL, Chilimigras JL, Berman DR, et al. Methods of induction of labour: a systematic review. *BMC Pregnancy Childbirth.* 2011;11:84.

26. Alfirevic Z, Kelly AJ, Dowswell T. Intravenous oxytocin alone for cervical ripening and induction of labour. *Cochrane Database Syst Rev.* 2009;(4):CD003246.

27. Hofmeyr GJ, Gulmezoglu AM, Pileggi C. Vaginal misoprostol for cervical ripening and induction of labour. *Cochrane Database Syst Rev.* 2010;(10):CD000941.

Intrapartum Fetal Monitoring

Barak M. Rosenn

Electronic fetal (heart rate) monitoring (EFM) was developed and introduced into clinical practice during the second half of the 20th century, with the expectation that it would provide information on the well-being of the fetus during labor. The hope was that changes in the fetal heart rate (FHR) pattern resulting from fetal hypoxia would alert the clinician to the impending danger of fetal asphyxia and acidosis and would allow timely intervention before permanent damage occurred. Unfortunately, EFM was widely and rapidly adopted throughout the world, and it has become an integral part of modern obstetrics without ever undergoing the necessary scientific scrutiny to validate its merit.[1] Indeed, studies have shown that EFM provides no long-term benefit to infants when compared to intermittent auscultation in labor and actually may cause harm by increasing the rate of operative delivery.[2] Nevertheless, given its widespread use and perceived merits, EFM is unlikely to be subjected to randomized clinical trials in the foreseeable future. Also, despite its limitations, it provides valuable information on the physiologic and pathophysiologic changes that some fetuses experience during labor.

EQUIPMENT

EFM consists of continuous recordings of the FHR and the tone of the uterine muscle. Both these recordings are obtained simultaneously and are recorded graphically on a strip of paper that (in the United States) runs at a standard rate of 3 cm/min (Figure 4-1). These signals can be obtained either externally (from the maternal abdominal surface) or internally (from the fetus and the intrauterine cavity). The external transducer that records the FHR is an ultrasound Doppler transmitter-receiver that receives signals reflected off the moving fetal heart (Figure 4-2). The device calculates the FHR based on the time interval between consecutive movements of the moving part being recorded. The FHR is continuously calculated from beat to beat and recorded graphically as a running line on the paper strip or on an electronic screen. Internal monitoring of the FHR can be achieved if the mother's cervix is dilated and the membranes have been ruptured. A metal spiral electrode (Figure 4-3) is attached transvaginally to the fetal scalp and connected to the monitoring device. The electrode picks up the fetal electrocardiographic signal and calculates the heart rate based on the R-R intervals.

External monitoring of uterine activity is achieved by placing a pressure transducer (tocodynamometer) on the maternal abdomen (Figure 4-2). During a uterine contraction, the curvature of the abdomen changes and creates pressure on the transducer that is reflected as a rise in pressure that is recorded on the moving strip of paper (or the screen). The recorded change in pressure does not reflect the true intrauterine pressure change, because actual pressures are not being measured. Rather, the graph provides information on the timing of contractions, their duration and regularity, and their relative strength. In order to obtain a true measure of the uterine tone and the intensity of contractions, an intrauterine pressure catheter is inserted transvaginally into the uterine cavity. This catheter has a transducer embedded within that provides continuous information on the intrauterine pressure, both between contractions (resting tone) and during contractions. This information is transmitted to the monitoring device and displayed continuously on the paper strip or the screen.

PHYSIOLOGY

As in the adult heart, the FHR is determined by the intrinsic pacemaker in the sinoatrial node. The heart rate is modulated by input from the fetal autonomic nervous system; the parasympathetic system acts to slow the heart rate via impulses transmitted through the vagus nerve, and the sympathetic nerves that innervate the cardiac muscle act to increase heart rate and contractility via secretion of norepinephrine. Adequate oxygenation of the fetal central nervous system is reflected in the normal interaction between the sympathetic and parasympathetic systems, resulting in noticeable variability of the heart rate from beat to beat and FHR accelerations in response to certain stimuli. When fetal oxygenation is compromised, hypoxia of the central nervous system may affect its ability to preserve the normal interplay between the sympathetic and parasympathetic systems with loss of normal beat-to-beat variability. Additionally, in the presence of fetal hypoxemia (decreased level of oxygen in the blood) and hypoxia (decreased level of oxygen in tissues), peripheral chemoreceptors located in the aortic arch and the carotid sinus as well as central chemoreceptors activate the parasympathetic system that slows the FHR via the vagus nerve. Other receptors located in the aortic arch and in the

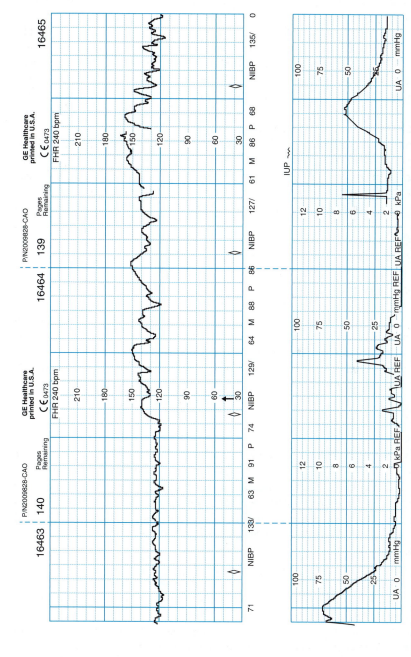

Figure 4-1. Recording of fetal heart rate and uterine activity. The top panel records the fetal heart rate, and the bottom panel records uterine contractions.

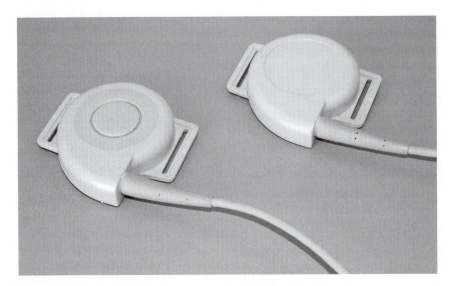

Figure 4-2. External fetal heart rate transducer and tocodynamometer.

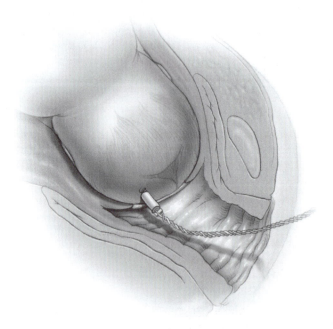

Figure 4-3. Internal fetal heart rate transducer attached to fetal scalp. From Intrapartum assessment. In: Cunningham F, Leveno L, Bloom S, Hauth J, Rause, D, Spong. *Williams Obstetrics.* 23rd ed. New York, NY: McGraw-Hill; 2010.

carotid sinus are sensitive to blood pressure (baroreceptors). When blood pressure rises, they activate the parasympathetic system via the vagus nerve to slow the heart rate as a protective mechanism against the rising blood pressure.

Adequate fetal oxygenation depends on the adequacy of maternal oxygenation, maternal blood flow to the placenta, transfer of oxygen across the placenta to the fetus, blood flow from the placenta to the fetus, and delivery to fetal organs and tissues. Anything that compromises this process may lead to fetal hypoxia and ultimately to fetal acidosis. During normal labor, the uterus contracts regularly every few minutes, usually for 40 to 60 seconds at a time. During each contraction, the flow of maternal blood reaching the placenta through the many spiral arteries that traverse the uterine muscle is temporarily compromised due to the contracting muscle. Thus, with each contraction, there is a temporary decline in the delivery of oxygen to the fetus. However, if the contractions are limited in their frequency and duration, the placenta is basically normal and functions well, the mother is not anemic and is well oxygenated, and perfusion of the uterus and the placenta are normal, then the fetus is able to tolerate the temporary decline in oxygenation that occurs during each contraction. The fetus replenishes its supply of oxygen between the contractions and progresses through labor without being compromised. But when the contractions are too frequent (tachysystole) or when they are prolonged, the fetus may not have the chance to recover and may develop hypoxia. Similarly, if placental function is compromised to begin with (eg, due to poor development or preexisting maternal vascular disease), then the added stress of uterine contractions may compromise placental function further and lead to fetal hypoxia. Thus, fetuses that on ultrasound evaluation are found to be small-for-gestational age (SGA) are at a higher risk of manifesting abnormal FHR tracings during labor, because placental dysfunction is one of the major causes of SGA.

THE ROLE OF ELECTRONIC FETAL MONITORING IN PREVENTING FETAL DAMAGE

The original thought that spurred the development of EFM was that it would identify the hypoxic fetus and prompt its delivery before brain damage occurs. In fact, an abnormal FHR tracing is a very poor predictor of fetal brain damage. Furthermore, randomized trials have not evaluated EFM in comparison to other forms of fetal monitoring, except intermittent auscultation, and most of these trials included only low-risk patients. A recent meta-analysis that included 13 randomized trials comparing continuous EFM to intermittent auscultation in both low-risk and high-risk pregnancies found that using EFM increases the rate of delivery by cesarean section (C-section) and operative vaginal delivery but does not decrease the risk of perinatal mortality, cerebral palsy, cord blood acidosis, hypoxic ischemic encephalopathy, neurodevelopmental impairment, low Apgar scores, or admission to a neonatal intensive care unit.[2] In fact, the positive predictive value of a nonreassuring FHR pattern to predict cerebral palsy among singleton infants weighing 2500 g or more is only 0.14%. In other words, in more than 99% of cases that have a nonreassuring FHR tracing, the infant will not develop cerebral palsy. Therefore, it is no surprise that introduction of EFM has not been associated with a decrease in the incidence of cerebral palsy, because intrapartum events are to blame for only 4% of cases with encephalopathy and the majority of cerebral palsy cases are attributable to events that occurred prior to the onset of labor.[3,4]

Despite these observations that suggest no clear benefit from the use of EFM over intermittent auscultation in low-risk pregnancies, the latter may not be practical in the setting of a normal labor and delivery unit. Furthermore, no data suggest the optimal time intervals for intermittent auscultation. Clearly, in pregnancies with maternal or fetal risk factors for adverse outcome, EFM should be used to identify those fetuses who cannot tolerate the additional stress they are faced with during labor.

NOMENCLATURE

Under most circumstances, EFM tracings are visually interpreted by the clinicians caring for the woman who is in labor. Clear definitions of the various components in the FHR tracing have been provided by the American College of Obstetrics and Gynecology (Table 4-1).[5] However, interpretation of FHR tracings is notoriously subject to intraobserver and interobserver variability.[6,7] In an attempt to aid in the task of standardizing interpretation, computerized programs for automatic interpretation of FHR tracings have been developed and tested,[8] but these are not currently in wide use. Interpretation of the FHR tracing is an ongoing and dynamic process; its purpose is to determine whether at any given time the fetus is well oxygenated or whether there is evidence to suggest the possibility that it is hypoxic and in danger of becoming acidotic.

Baseline Rate

The baseline rate is visually determined by examining a 10-minute segment and determining the mean FHR rounded to increments of 5 beats/min (bpm). It must be possible to define the baseline for a minimum of 2 minutes; otherwise it is undeterminable for that 10-minute segment. Decelerations, accelerations, and periods of marked variability (> 25 bpm) are excluded. The normal baseline FHR is 110 to 160 bpm; a baseline greater than 160 bpm is defined as tachycardia, and a baseline less than 110 bpm is defined as bradycardia.

In some fetuses, a baseline rate of less than 110 bpm represents an extreme of the normal variation and does not reflect fetal compromise. In others, fetal bradycardia may reflect congenital heart block in a well-oxygenated fetus. However, onset of bradycardia in labor may reflect profound vagal stimulation resulting from fetal hypoxia. The cause of hypoxia could be maternal hypotension, placental abruption, uterine rupture, amniotic fluid embolism, or umbilical cord prolapse. Whatever the presumed cause, sudden onset of fetal bradycardia in labor should prompt a search for the cause, while instituting immediate resuscitative measures and preparing for prompt emergency delivery.

Although fetal tachycardia may be a sign of fetal hypoxia, it is most commonly associated with maternal fever and chorioamnionitis. Steps should be taken to decrease the maternal temperature to a normal range (by cooling and administering antipyretics) and to administer antibiotics in case of suspected infection.

Table 4-1. Electronic Fetal Monitoring Definitions[a]

Pattern	Definition
Baseline	The mean FHR rounded to increments of 5 bpm during a 10-minute segment, excluding: • Periodic or episodic changes • Periods of marked FHR variability • Segments of baseline that differ by more than 25 bpm The baseline must be for a minimum of 2 minutes in any 10-minute segment, or the baseline for that time period is indeterminate. In this case, one may refer to the prior 10-minute window for determination of baseline. Normal FHR baseline: 110-160 bpm Tachycardia: FHR baseline ≥ 160 bpm Bradycardia: FHR baseline < 110 bpm
Baseline variability	Fluctuations in the baseline FHR that are irregular in amplitude and frequency Variability is visually quantitated as the amplitude of peak-to-trough in bpm • Absent: amplitude range undetectable • Minimal: amplitude range detectable but ≤ 5 bpm • Moderate (normal): amplitude range 6-25 bpm • Marked: amplitude range > 25 bpm
Acceleration	A visually apparent abrupt increase (onset to peak in < 30 seconds) in the FHR At 32 weeks of gestation and beyond, acceleration has a peak of 15 bpm or more above baseline, with duration of 15 seconds or more but less than 2 minutes from onset to return. Before 32 weeks of gestation, an acceleration has a peak of 10 bpm or more above baseline, with a duration of 10 seconds or more but less than 2 minutes from onset to return. Prolonged acceleration lasts 2 minutes or more but less than 10 minutes in duration. If an acceleration lasts 10 minutes or longer, it is a baseline change.
Early deceleration	Visually apparent usually symmetrical gradual decrease and return of the FHR associated with a uterine contraction A gradual FHR decrease is defined as from the onset to the FHR nadir of 30 seconds or more. The decrease in FHR is calculated from the onset to the nadir of the deceleration. The nadir of the deceleration occurs at the same time as the peak of the contraction. In most cases the onset, nadir, and recovery of the deceleration are coincident with the beginning, peak, and ending of the contraction, respectively.

Abbreviation: bpm, beats per minute; FHR, fetal heart rate.
[a]Used with permission from American College of Obstetricians and Gynecologists (ACOG).[5]

Other causes of fetal tachycardia include maternal administration of beta-mimetic medications and illicit use of cocaine or methamphetamines.

Baseline Variability

In a healthy fetus with a well-oxygenated central nervous system, the interaction between the sympathetic and parasympathetic systems results in irregular fluctuations of the baseline FHR upward and downward. Distinctions made in the past between short-term and long-term variability are no longer considered relevant.

The amplitude (in bpm) from peak to trough is the measure used for classifying variability as either absent, minimal (up to 5 bpm; Figure 4-4), moderate (6-25 bpm; Figure 4-5), or marked (> 25 bpm; Figure 4-6). Moderate variability (6-25 bpm) is considered normal and suggests a nonhypoxic fetus.[9] The significance of marked variability is not entirely clear, but absent variability is a worrisome finding that requires attention, because it may reflect fetal hypoxia. Other causes of decreased variability should be considered, such as a transient fetal sleep cycle, maternal use of medications, or preexisting neurologic damage. The distinction between absent and minimal variability is often difficult and prone to interobserver variability, and some have suggested to relate to minimal and absent variability as one.[10]

Accelerations

An acceleration is an abrupt (< 30 seconds from onset to peak) increase in the FHR of at least 15 bpm above baseline and lasting for at least 15 seconds. A prolonged acceleration is one that lasts for 2 to 10 minutes. Before 32 weeks' gestation, the definition of acceleration includes a rise of 10 bpm or more above baseline lasting for 10 seconds or longer.

Decelerations

Decelerations are visually apparent decreases in the FHR below baseline. Decelerations are defined based on their shape, depth, and duration, as well as their association with uterine contractions.

VARIABLE DECELERATIONS

These are the most common type of decelerations, occurring at some point in the vast majority of FHR tracings during labor. The decrease in the FHR is abrupt (< 30 seconds from onset to nadir), is at least 15 bpm in depth, and lasts at least 15 seconds but no longer than 2 minutes (Figures 4-7 and 4-8). Variable decelerations are usually associated with uterine contractions, but their onset, depth, duration, and overall shape vary from contraction to contraction (hence the term *variable deceleration*). A prolonged deceleration is one that lasts 2 minutes or more but less than 10 minutes (Figure 4-9). A deceleration lasting 10 minutes or more is considered a baseline change—namely, bradycardia. Variable decelerations may be further classified as severe or significant if they meet the "rule of 60s": these are decelerations that last more than 60 seconds and, in addition, have an amplitude of at least 60 bpm below baseline or a trough that reaches 60 bpm or less.[10]

Variable decelerations are thought to result from compression of the umbilical cord during a contraction (eg, between the uterine wall and the fetal head). As a result, the pressure rises abruptly in the fetal vasculature, and the baroreceptors (located in the aortic arch and carotid bodies) activate a vagal response that slows the heart. Thus, the deceleration occurs at the time of a contraction, is abrupt, and resolves abruptly as the contraction resolves and releases the pressure from the umbilical cord. Variable decelerations are not indicative of fetal hypoxia; however, because repetitive variable decelerations reflect repetitive interruptions in the flow

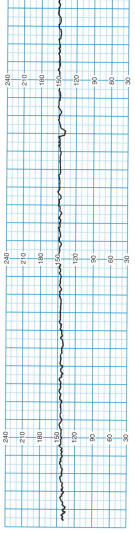

Figure 4-4. Minimal variability. From x Intrapartum assessment. In: Cunningham F, Leveno L, Bloom S, Hauth J, Rause D, Spong C. *Williams Obstetrics*. 23rd ed. New York, NY: McGraw-Hill; 2010.

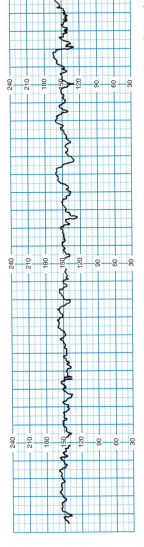

Figure 4-5. **Moderate variability.** From Intrapartum assessment. In: Cunningham F, Leveno L, Bloom S, Hauth J, Rause D, Spong C. *Williams Obstetrics.* 23rd ed. New York, NY: McGraw-Hill; 2010.

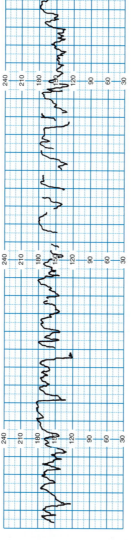

Figure 4-6. **Marked variability.** From Intrapartum assessment. In: Cunningham F, Leveno L, Bloom S, Hauth J, Rause D, Spong C. *Williams Obstetrics.* 23rd ed. New York, NY: McGraw-Hill; 2010.

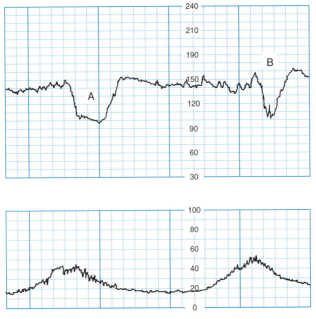

Figure 4-7. Variable decelerations. From Intrapartum assessment. In: Cunningham F, Leveno L, Bloom S, Hauth J, Rause D, Spong C. *Williams Obstetrics.* 23rd ed. New York, NY: McGraw-Hill; 2010.

of oxygenated blood to the fetus, continuous and repetitive variable decelerations may eventually take their toll on the fetus. The longer and deeper the decelerations, and the longer they persist, the more likely the fetus is to develop a deficit in oxygen and demonstrate signs suggestive of hypoxia.

LATE DECELERATIONS

These decelerations are associated with contractions, but differently from the variable decelerations, they appear to lag after the contraction; the onset, nadir, and recovery lag after the onset, peak, and resolution of the associated contraction, respectively (Figure 4-10). Because it is not always easy to pinpoint the exact onset of the deceleration and of the contraction, the most important criterion for defining a late deceleration is that its nadir appears clearly after the peak of the associated contraction. The decelerations are usually symmetrical and the decrease in FHR is gradual (lasting 30 seconds or more from onset to nadir).

Late decelerations are believed to reflect the vagal response activated by the chemoreceptors in the aortic arch and in the carotid sinus in response to hypoxia and hypercapnia. During a contraction, maternal blood flow to the placenta is temporarily interrupted, as is the delivery of oxygen to the fetal blood. The deoxygenated blood flows through the umbilical cord and eventually reaches the chemoreceptors, activating the vagal response that slows the heart rate. Thus, the slowing of the FHR lags behind the onset of the contraction, creating the late deceleration.

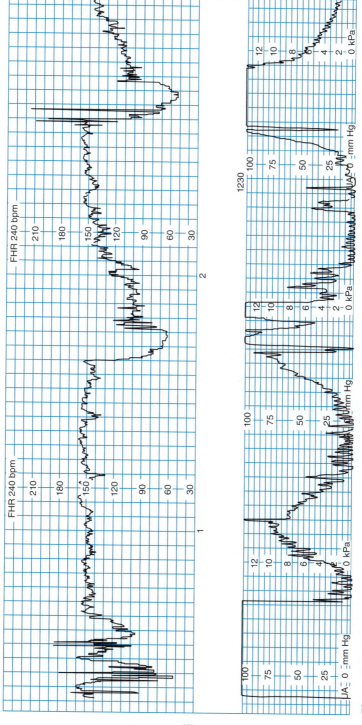

Figure 4-8. Severe variable decelerations.

47

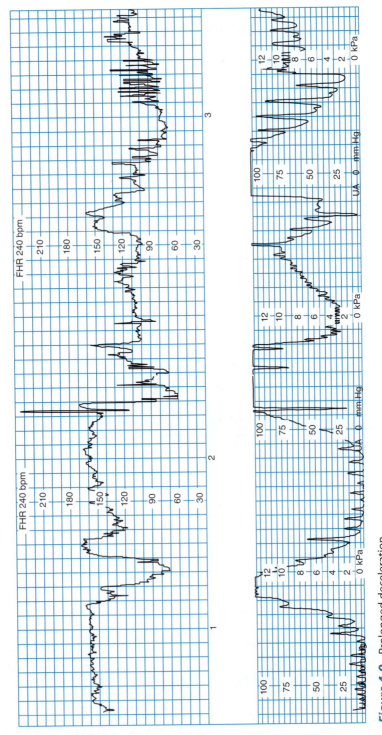

Figure 4-9. Prolonged deceleration.

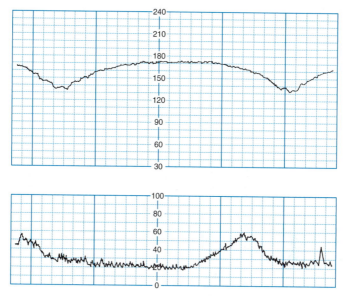

Figure 4-10. Late decelerations with baseline tachycardia and minimal variability. From Intrapartum assessment. In: Cunningham F, Leveno L, Bloom S, Hauth J, Rause D, Spong C. *Williams Obstetrics*. 23rd ed. New York, NY: McGraw-Hill; 2010.

In addition to the reflex vagal response, with persistent and worsening fetal hypoxia, late decelerations reflect direct myocardial depression. In the presence of repetitive late decelerations (decelerations occurring with 50% or more of contractions over 30 minutes), and particularly in combination with minimal or absent baseline variability, there is substantial suspicion of fetal hypoxia and steps should be taken to expedite delivery.

EARLY DECELERATIONS

An early deceleration is a symmetrical and gradual (30 seconds or more from onset to nadir) decrease in the FHR that occurs simultaneously with a contraction and appears as a mirror image of the contraction. The significance of these decelerations is poorly understood, but they are believed to reflect a fetal vagal response from pressure of the maternal pelvic floor on the fetal head during a contractions and do not reflect fetal compromise.

Sinusoidal Pattern

This is a smooth, sine wave–like undulating pattern of the FHR baseline with a cycle frequency of three to five cycles per minute that lasts 20 minutes or longer (Figure 4-11). This pattern may follow the administration of alphaprodine[11] or butorphanol[12] but has also been associated with severe fetal anemia (such as can occur with significant fetomaternal hemorrhage or fetal hemolytic disease). A sinusoidal FHR pattern should prompt close surveillance and evaluation, and the

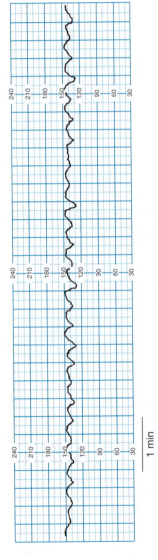

Figure 4-11. Sinusoidal fetal heart rate pattern. From Intrapartum assessment. In: Cunningham F, Leveno L, Bloom S, Hauth J, Rause D, Spong C. *Williams Obstetrics.* 23rd ed. New York, NY: McGraw-Hill; 2010.

1 min

pediatrician should be alerted to the possibility that the newborn infant will require immediate blood transfusion.

THREE-TIER CATEGORIZATION OF FETAL HEART RATE PATTERNS

In 2008, The National Institutes of Child Health and Human Development convened a workshop to review the current published literature dealing with definitions, interpretation, and research guidelines pertaining to EFM.[13] The workshop recommended the adoption of a three-tier system, categorizing FHR patterns into one of three categories (Table 4-2).

Category 1

These are normal FHR patterns that are strongly predictive of a well-oxygenated fetus with a normal acid-base status.

Table 4-2. Three-Tiered Fetal Heart Rate Interpretation System[a]

Category I	Category I FHR tracings include all of the following:
	    Baseline rate: 110-160 bpm
	    Baseline FHR variability: moderate
	    Late or variable decelerations: absent
	    Early decelerations: present or absent
	    Accelerations: present or absent

Category II	Category II FHR tracings include all FHR tracings not categorized as category I or category III. Examples of category II FHR tracings include any of the following:
	    Baseline rate
	        -Bradycardia not accompanied by absent baseline variability
	        -Tachycardia
	    Baseline FHR variability
	        -Minimal baseline variability
	        -Absent baseline variability with no recurrent decelerations
	        -Marked baseline variability
	    Accelerations
	        -Absence of induced accelerations after fetal stimulation
	    Periodic or episodic decelerations
	        -Recurrent variable decelerations accompanied by minimal or moderate baseline variability
	        -Prolonged deceleration > 2 minutes but < 10 minutes
	        -Recurrent late decelerations with moderate baseline variability
	        -Variable decelerations with other characteristics such as slow return to baseline, overshoots, or shoulders

Category III	Category III FHR tracings include either
	    Absent baseline FHR variability and any of the following:
	        -Recurrent late decelerations
	        -Recurrent variable decelerations
	        -Bradycardia
	    Sinusoidal pattern

[a]Used with permission from American College of Obstetricians and Gynecologists (ACOG).[5]

Category 3

These are abnormal FHR tracings that are associated with abnormal fetal acid-base status at the time they are observed.

Category 2

These are indeterminate FHR tracings that do not fall into either category 1 or category 3. They are not predictive of abnormal fetal acid-base status but require continued observation and reevaluation.

Use of the Three-Tier System

In terms of management, the response to the normal category 1 and abnormal category 3 FHR tracings is straightforward: category 1 tracings are normal and require no specific intervention or action, whereas category 3 tracings are abnormal and require prompt evaluation and intervention to either resolve the abnormal FHR pattern or proceed to delivery. The problem lies with the category 2 FHR tracings; a very broad spectrum of FHR tracings fall into this category, and there is no clear guidance to distinguish between (1) tracings that may rapidly deteriorate and represent a fetus in jeopardy of asphyxia and/or acidosis and (2) tracings that represent a well-compensated fetus that currently is not hypoxic. Indeed, the majority of intrapartum FHR tracings do, at some point, fall into category 2. During the last 2 hours of labor, parous and nulliparous women spend 35% and 45% of the time, respectively, with category 2 FHR tracings.[14]

A recently published algorithm suggested by a panel of experts in the field of fetal monitoring attempts to aid clinicians in evaluating the wide spectrum of category 2 FHR tracings based on the presence or absence of reassuring components (moderate FHR variability or accelerations), the persistence of significant decelerations, and the progress of labor.[10] Other algorithms and classification systems have been proposed or adopted by various professional societies.[8,15-17] The purpose of all these systems is to identify the fetus in jeopardy while avoiding unnecessary intervention due to the high false-positive rate of abnormal FHR tracings in predicting fetal acidosis.

RESUSCITATIVE MEASURES

As outlined previously (see Physiology), several factors can contribute to compromise of oxygen delivery to the fetus. Accordingly, when changes in the FHR tracing suggest the possibility of impending or existing fetal hypoxia, several steps can be taken in attempt to alleviate the situation.

Maternal Hydration

Because delivery of oxygen to the placenta is dependent on adequate maternal blood flow to the placenta (at a rate of approximately 400 mL/min), rapid intravenous hydration with a bolus of fluid may improve fetal oxygenation.[18]

Maternal Positioning

Shifting the mother from lying on her back to laying on her right or left side alleviates the pressure on the inferior vena cava and improves cardiac return. Consequently, it improves cardiac output and placental perfusion.[18]

Oxygen Supplementation

Delivery of high concentration supplemental oxygen to the mother, particularly with a nonrebreather mask, can improve fetal oxygenation. The improvement is specifically apparent in fetuses with decreased oxygen saturation as measured by fetal pulse oximetry.[18,19]

Uterine Relaxation

Because maternal blood flow to the placenta is compromised during uterine contractions, it is important to allow the fetus to recover between contractions. Indeed, fetal oxygen saturation is inversely related to the frequency of uterine contractions.[20] Thus, uterine tachysystole (more than five contractions in 10 minutes), baseline uterine hypertonus, and prolonged contractions can all lead to oxygen deficit in the fetus. If the mother is receiving oxytocin, the infusion may be stopped or the rate decreased, or the mother may be given a short-acting tocolytic agent (such as 0.25-mg subcutaneous terbutaline).

Amnioinfusion

Cord compression is presumed to be the cause of variable decelerations. In the presence of severe and repetitive variable decelerations, a catheter that is usually used to measure the intrauterine pressure can be used to infuse a bolus of fluid into the uterine cavity, often alleviating the pressure on the cord with resolution of the decelerations. A meta-analysis of 19 studies showed that amnioinfusion is associated with a significant decrease in persistent decelerations, C-section rate, operative vaginal delivery or C-section for "fetal distress," and low Apgar scores.[21]

EFFECTS OF MEDICATIONS ON FETAL HEART RATE PATTERNS

Several medications that are often used or encountered during the course of labor may affect the FHR pattern. It is important to be familiar with these effects in order to avoid misinterpretation of FHR tracings and unnecessary intervention.

Magnesium Sulfate

Magnesium sulfate ($MgSO_4$) is commonly used in obstetric practice. Often used as a tocolytic agent in women with preterm labor, it is routinely used for seizure prophylaxis in women with preeclampsia and has recently been adopted as antenatal treatment in women with preterm labor for neuroprotection of the fetus that is less than 33 weeks gestational age. Although some studies have found that $MgSO_4$

administration is associated with a decrease in FHR variability,[22] others have not.[23] A well-designed randomized study in nonlaboring pregnant women demonstrated that intravenous administration of $MgSO_4$ was associated with significant decreases in FHR baseline values, variability, and number of accelerations. The magnitude of these changes, however, was small, and the authors questioned their clinical significance.[24] Therefore, decreased FHR variability observed in patients receiving $MgSO_4$ treatment should be addressed with prudence, without necessarily attributing it to the effect of the medication.

Narcotics

Not all women in labor are candidates for regional anesthesia. For example, thrombocytopenia or a bleeding diathesis, anticoagulation therapy, a spinal deformity, or previous spinal surgery may preclude administration of epidural or spinal anesthesia. Additionally, women in the latent phase of labor may require some form of analgesia, particularly when the latent phase is prolonged. Parenterally administered narcotics are often used in these situations. All narcotics administered to the mother rapidly cross the placenta and have similar effects on the FHR; they are associated with a decrease in FHR variability and the frequency of accelerations. This is true for morphine, which was commonly used up to the mid-20th century[25]; meperidine, which replaced the use of morphine for labor analgesia and is currently widely used all over the world[26-28]; fentanyl[29]; nalbuphine[30]; diamorphine[31]; and methadone.[32]

Cocaine

Cocaine use has been associated with decreased FHR variability,[33] a decrease in FHR accelerations,[34] and the appearance of late decelerations.[35] The latter phenomenon may be due to a vasoconstrictive effect on the uterine arteries and appears to be transient, resolving once the effect of cocaine wears off.[36]

Steroids

Steroids are routinely administered to women in preterm labor at 34 weeks' gestation or less. Betamethasone or dexamethasone is administered in split doses over 48 hours to accelerate fetal lung maturation and decrease other risks associated with prematurity. Some authors have found that both medications affect components of the FHR tracing,[37] whereas others have found changes with the use of betamethasone but not with dexamethasone.[38] Steroids are associated with a decrease in FHR baseline, accelerations, and variability,[37] with return to baseline characteristics within 4 to 7 days of initial treatment.

EFFECT OF NEURAXIAL ANALGESIA ON FETAL HEART RATE

Changes in the FHR are often observed after initiation of neuraxial analgesia during labor. Sympathetic blockade resulting in vasodilation of the maternal venous and arterial vascular beds may lead to maternal hypotension, decreased placental perfusion, and subsequent changes in the FHR.[39] Prophylactic intravenous fluid preloading is commonly practiced to address this problem, based on the premise that it may decrease the risk of maternal hypotension and FHR abnormalities.[40] A systematic review of the literature concluded that preloading with intravenous fluid decreases the risks of maternal hypotension and FHR abnormalities in women receiving high-dose epidural analgesia, but the evidence for such a benefit is limited in women receiving low-dose epidural or combined spinal-epidural (CSE) anesthesia.[41]

Several investigators have noted abnormalities in the FHR following spinal administration of opioids despite the absence of maternal hypotension. Indeed, a meta-analysis of 24 clinical trials including 3513 women concluded that the use of intrathecal opioids for labor analgesia was associated with an odds ratio of 1.8 (confidence interval 1.04-3.14) for FHR abnormalities. This, however, was not associated with an increased risk of operative delivery or low Apgar scores in the newborn infants.[42] Furthermore, there appears to be a dose-response effect of intrathecal opioids on the FHR. In a randomized trial, a spinal dose of 7.5 μg of sufentanil produced twice as many FHR changes (bradycardia or late decelerations) compared to 1.5 μg sufentanil (combined with bupivacaine) or conventional epidural analgesia. Conversely, severe maternal hypotension requiring administration of ephedrine was highest among the women receiving low-dose intrathecal sufentanil with bupivacaine (29%) compared to those receiving high-dose intrathecal sufentanil (12%) or epidural analgesia (7%).[43]

Why the administration of spinal or CSE analgesia should cause abnormal changes in the FHR remains a matter of some controversy. Intrathecal opioids appear to be associated with increased uterine activity and increased tonus. It has been suggested that the rapid spread of opioids administered through this route has a central effect on the release of oxytocin, causing uterine hyperactivity and subsequent changes in the FHR.[44] The more commonly accepted hypothesis states that the rapid onset of pain relief associated with spinal or CSE administration of opioids is associated with a rapid decline in the concentration of maternal epinephrine, creating a temporary imbalance between epinephrine and norepinephrine in the maternal circulation. Because epinephrine has a β-sympathomimetic relaxant effect on the myometrium whereas norepinephrine has uterotonic effects, the relative excess of the latter following intrathecal analgesia is associated with a transient increase in uterine tone and activity, leading to abnormal changes in the FHR.[45] Indeed, in women who were randomized to CSE or epidural analgesia in labor, the incidence of uterine hypertonus and FHR abnormalities was significantly increased after CSE, particularly in those women with rapidly advancing, painful labors. Furthermore, the decrease in pain scores immediately after analgesia was positively correlated with the probability of hypertonus and abnormal FHR, supporting the epinephrine/norepinephrine imbalance hypothesis.

Regardless of the cause of FHR changes following the administration of neuraxial analgesia, these changes are usually transient and respond well to resuscitative measures. Administration of ephedrine to increase maternal blood pressure, administration of oxygen, discontinuing oxytocin, administration of a tocolytic agent, maternal repositioning, and administration of intravenous fluids, either singularly or in combination, usually leads to rapid resolution of the abnormal FHR tracing.

SUMMARY

Intrapartum EFM is a universally common practice that is used to monitor fetal well-being during labor. Although the benefits of this practice are subject to continued debate, several characteristics of the FHR tracing can provide reassurance of fetal well-being, whereas others may indicate impending jeopardy. A thorough understanding of the various components of the FHR and their interpretation, as well as familiarity with the effects of medications and interventions to improve fetal oxygenation are essential to optimize the use of this methodology to manage labor safely and effectively.

REFERENCES

1. Grimes DA, Peipert JF. Electronic fetal monitoring as a public health screening program: the arithmetic of failure. *Obstet Gynecol*. 2010;116(6):1397-1400.
2. Alfirevic Z, Devane D, Gyte GM. Continuous cardiotocography (CTG) as a form of electronic fetal monitoring (EFM) for fetal assessment during labour. *Cochrane Database Syst Rev*. May 2013.
3. Hankins GD, Speer M. Defining the pathogenesis and pathophysiology of neonatal encephalopathy and cerebral palsy. *Obstet Gynecol*. 2003;102:628-636.
4. Badawi N, Kurinczuk JJ, Keogh JM, et al. Antepartum risk factors for newborn encephalopathy: the Western Australian case control study. *BMJ*. 1999;317:1549-1553.
5. American College of Obstetricians and Gynecologists (ACOG). Intrapartum fetal heart rate monitoring: nomenclature, interpretation, and general management principles. ACOG Practice Bulletin 106, July 2009.
6. Nielsen PV, Stigsby B, Nickelsen C, Nim J. Intra- and inter-observer variability in the assessment of intrapartum cardiotocograms. *Acta Obstet Gynecol Scand*. 1987;66:421-424.
7. Lotgering FK, Wallenburg HC, Schouten HJ. Interobserver and intraobserver variation in the assessment of antepartum cardiotocograms. *Am J Obstet Gynecol*. 1982;144:701-705.
8. Elliott C, Warrick PA, Graham E, Hamilton EF. Graded classification of fetal heart rate tracings: association with neonatal metabolic acidosis and neurologic morbidity. *Am J Obstet Gynecol*. 2009;202:258. e1-8.
9. Parer JT, King T, Flanders S, Fox M, Kilpatrick SJ. Fetal acidemia and electronic fetal heart rate patterns: is there evidence of an association? *J Matern Fetal Neonatal Med*. 2006;19:289-294.
10. Clarke SL, Nageotte MP, Garite TJ, et al. Intrapartum management of category II fetal heart rate tracings: towards standardization of care. *Am J Obstet Gynecol*. 2013;209(2):89-97.
11. Veren D, Boehm FH, Killam AP. The clinical significance of a sinusoidal fetal heart rate pattern associated with alphaprodine administration. *J Reprod Med*. 1982;27(7):411-414.
12. Hatjis CG, Meis PJ. Sinusoidal fetal heart rate pattern associated with butorphanol administration. *Obstet Gynecol*. 1986;67:377-380.
13. Macones GA, Hankins GDV, Spong CY, Hauth J, Moore T. The 2008 National Institute of Child Health and Human Development Workshop Report on Electronic Fetal Monitoring. Update on definitions, interpretation, and research guidelines. *Obstet Gynecol*. 2008;112:661-666.
14. Jackson M, Holmgren CM, Esplin S, Henry E, Varner MW. Frequency of fetal heart rate categories and short-term neonatal outcome. *Obstet Gynecol*. 2011;118:803-808.
15. Parer JT, Ikeda T. A framework for standardized management of intrapartum fetal heart rate patterns. *Am J Obstet Gynecol*. 2007;197:26.e1-6.
16. Liston R, Sawchuck D, Young D; Society of Obstetrics and Gynaecologists of Canada; British Columbia Perinatal Health Program. Fetal health surveillance: antepartum and intrapartum consensus guideline. *J Obstet Gynaecol Can*. 2007; 29(9 suppl 4):S3-56. Erratum in *J Obstet Gynaecol Can*. 2007;29:909.

17. Royal College of Obstetricians and Gynecologists. Electronic fetal monitoring: the use and interpretation of cardiotocography in intrapartum fetal surveillance. Evidence-based guideline no. 8. http://guidance.nice.org.uk/CGC.

18. Simpson KR, James DC. Efficacy of intrauterine resuscitation techniques in improving fetal oxygen status during labor. *Obstet Gynecol.* 2005;105:1362-1368.

19. Haydon ML, Gorenberg DM, Nageotte MP, et al. The effect of maternal oxygen administration on fetal pulse oximetry during labor in fetuses with nonreassuring fetal heart rate patterns. *Am J Obstet Gynecol.* 2006;195:735-738.

20. Simpson KR, James DC. Effects of oxytocin-induced uterine hyperstimulation during labor on fetal oxygen status and fetal heart rate patterns. *Am J Obstet Gynecol.* 2008;199:34.e1-e5.

21. Hofmeyr GJ, Lawrie TA. Amnioinfusion for potential or suspected umbilical cord compression in labour. *Cochrane Database Syst Rev.* 2012;18:1.

22. Atkinson MW, Belfort MA, Saade GR, Moise KJ Jr. The relation between magnesium sulfate therapy and fetal heart rate variability. *Obstet Gynecol.* 1994;83:967-970.

23. Stallworth JC, Yeh SY, Petrie RH. The effect of magnesium sulfate on fetal heart rate variability and uterine activity. *Am J Obstet Gynecol.* 1981;140:702-706.

24. Hallak M, Martinez-Poyer J, Kruger ML, Hassan S, Blackwell SC, Sorokin Y. The effect of magnesium sulfate on fetal heart rate parameters: a randomized, placebo-controlled trial. *Am J Obstet Gynecol.* 1999;181:1122-1127.

25. Kopecky EA, Ryan ML, Barrett JF, et al. Fetal response to maternally administered morphine. *Am J Obstet Gynecol.* 2000;183:424-430.

26. Hill JB, Alexander JM, Sharma SK, McIntire DD, Leveno KJ. A comparison of the effects of epidural and meperidine analgesia during labor on fetal heart rate. *Obstet Gynecol.* 2003;102:333-337.

27. Sekhavat L, Behdad S. The effects of meperidine analgesia during labor on fetal heart rate. *Int J Biomed Sci.* 2009;5(1):59-62.

28. James BH, James MA, Sharma SK, et al. Comparison of the effects of epidural and meperidine analgesia during labor on fetal heart rate. *Obstet Gynecol.* 2003;102:333-337.

29. Rayburn W, Rathke A, Leuschen MP, Chleborad J, Weidner W. Fentanyl citrate analgesia during labor. *Am J Obstet Gynecol.* 1989;161:202-206.

30. Nicolle E, Devillier P, Delanoy B, Durand C, Bessard G. Therapeutic monitoring of nalbuphine: transplacental transfer and estimated pharmacokinetics in the neonate. *Eur J Clin Pharmacol.* 1996;49:485-489.

31. Farrell T, Owen P, Harrold A. Fetal movements following intrapartum maternal opiate administration. *Clin Exp Obstet Gynecol.* 1996;23:144-146.

32. Jansson LM, Dipietro J, Elko A. Fetal response to maternal methadone administration. *Am J Obstet Gynecol.* 2005;193:611-617.

33. Chazotte C, Forman L, Gandhi J. Heart rate patterns in fetuses exposed to cocaine. *Obstet Gynecol.* 1991;78:323-325.

34. Tabor BL, Soffici AR, Smith-Wallace T, et al. The effect of maternal cocaine use on the fetus: changes in antepartum fetal heart rate tracings. *Am J Obstet Gynecol.* 1991;165:1278-1281.

35. George K, Smith JF, Curet LB. Doppler velocimetry and fetal heart rate pattern observations in acute cocaine intoxication: a case report. *J Reprod Med.* 1995;40:65-67.

36. Perlow JH, Schlossberg DL, Strassner HT. Intrapartum cocaine use: a case report. *J Reprod Med.* 1990;35:978-980.

37. Rotmensch S, Liberati M, Vishne TH, Celentano C, Ben-Rafael Z, Bellati U. The effect of betamethasone and dexamethasone on fetal heart rate patterns and biophysical activities. A prospective randomized trial. *Acta Obstet Gynecol Scand.* 1999;78:493-500.

38. Senat MV, Minoui S, Multon O, Fernandez H, Frydman R, Ville Y. Effect of dexamethasone and betamethasone on fetal heart rate variability in preterm labour: a randomized study. *Br J Obstet Gynaecol.* 1998;105:749-755.

39. Umstad MP, Ross A, Rushford DD, Permezel M. Epidural analgesia and fetal heart rate abnormalities. *Aust N Z J Obstet Gynaecol.* 1993;33:269-272.

40. Ramanathan S, Masih A, Rock I, Chalon J, Turndorf H. Maternal and fetal effects of prophylactic hydration with crystalloids or colloids before epidural anaesthesia. *Anesth Analg.* 1983;62:673-678.

41. Hofmeyr GJ, Cyna AM, Middleton P. Prophylactic intravenous preloading for regional analgesia in labour. *Cochrane Database Syst Rev.* 2004;18(4):CD000175.

42. Mardirosoff C, Dumontb L, Boulvainc M, Trame MR. Fetal bradycardia due to intrathecal opioids for labour analgesia: a systematic review. *BJOG.* 2002;109:274-281.

43. Van de Velde M, Teunkens A, Hanssens M, Vandermeersch E, Verhaeghe J. Intrathecal sufentanil and fetal heart rate abnormalities: a double-blind, double placebo-controlled trial comparing two forms of combined spinal epidural analgesia with epidural analgesia in labor. *Anesth Analg.* 2004;98(4):1153-1159.

44. Van de Velde M. Neuraxial analgesia and fetal bradycardia. *Anesth Analg.* 2005;8:253-256.

45. Segall S, Csavoy AN, Datta S. The tocolytic effect of catecholamines in the gravid rat uterus. *Anesth Analg.* 1998;87:864-869.

Section 2

Providing Anesthesia

Drugs Commonly Used in Obstetric Anesthesia

5

Estee Piehl and Brenda A. Bucklin

INTRODUCTION

A variety of medications are used in obstetric practice by both obstetricians and anesthesiologists. These medications may differ from those used in the surgical operating room. This chapter reviews the medications commonly used in obstetrics.

TOCOLYTIC MEDICATIONS

Tocolytics are used by obstetricians to treat preterm labor in an attempt to prevent premature birth. Preterm birth is the leading cause of perinatal morbidity and mortality and complicates approximately 12% of pregnancies in the United States.[1] Recent Cochrane meta-analyses of tocolytic agents determined that calcium channel blockers and oxytocin antagonists can delay delivery by 2 to 7 days,[2] that β-mimetic drugs delay delivery by 48 hours but carry greater side effects,[3] that there is insufficient evidence regarding cyclooxygenase (COX) inhibitors,[4] and that magnesium sulfate is ineffective.[5] Anesthesiologists may be more involved with other uses of these drugs, including in the treatment of uterine tetany, uterine inversion, retained placenta, and fetal head entrapment.

Magnesium Sulfate

INDICATIONS

Magnesium sulfate has been used for suppression of preterm labor and for seizure prophylaxis in patients with severe preeclampsia. However, it is no longer used as a tocolytic agent because it has not been shown to be more effective than placebo in preventing preterm labor and delivery.[6] Although the primary indication for magnesium sulfate administration remains prevention of seizure activity in patients with severe preeclampsia, a newer use of magnesium administration during preterm labor involves benefit to the brain of the unborn fetus. Studies have demonstrated that premature infants as young as 23 weeks, born to mothers treated with magnesium sulfate, have improved developmental outcomes.[7]

MECHANISM OF ACTION

The systemic effects of magnesium sulfate administration are widespread and require the need for careful monitoring. Magnesium crosses the blood-brain barrier and decreases irritability of the central nervous system (CNS) and decrease N-methyl-D-aspartate activity. These effects likely account for the anticonvulsant and brain protection properties. Magnesium also competes with calcium for binding sites on the sarcoplasmic reticulum, reducing intracellular calcium levels and reducing the force and frequency of muscle contraction in both skeletal and smooth muscle.[8] Magnesium decreases the presynaptic release of acetylcholine, thereby reducing activity at the neuromuscular junction and decreases sensitivity of postjunctional membranes to acetylcholine. In addition, magnesium increases endothelial production of prostaglandin I_2 (PGI_2), increases cyclic guanosine monophosphate (GMP) production, and decreases angiotensin-converting enzyme levels, actions that all promote smooth muscle relaxation and vasodilation,[8] with concomitant increased uterine blood flow.

DOSING

Magnesium sulfate is usually administered as a 4-g IV bolus over 30 minutes, followed by an infusion of 1 g per hour.[9] Therapeutic levels range between 4 and 9 mEq/L. Plasma levels and deep tendon reflexes must be followed rigorously to avoid overdose and complications associated with magnesium toxicity. The effects of increasing magnesium levels are listed in Table 5-1, and the treatment of magnesium toxicity is reviewed in Table 5-2. Because magnesium is excreted by the kidneys, it must be carefully titrated and monitored in patients with renal impairment.

ADVERSE EFFECTS

Maternal side effects range from mild to severe and occur in up to 60% of exposed women. They include flushing, nausea, blurry vision, headache, and lethargy.

Table 5-1. Effects of Increasing Magnesium Levels

Effect	Plasma Level (mg/dL)
Normal	1.5-2.0
Therapeutic	4.0-8.0
Loss of deep tendon reflexes	10-12
Sinoatrial and atrioventricular block	15
Respiratory arrest	15-20
Asystole	> 25

Table 5-2. Treatment of Magnesium Toxicity

Administer:
-Intravenous calcium gluconate 1 g or
-Intravenous calcium chloride 300 mg
Airway management:
-Discontinue magnesium immediately

Besides the side effects and complications associated with magnesium toxicity, there are other important considerations when caring for patients who are receiving magnesium sulfate therapy. These are (1) decreased systemic vascular resistance and pronounced hypotension with neuraxial and general anesthesia, (2) increased risk of postpartum hemorrhage during vaginal or cesarean delivery, (3) reduction in minimum alveolar concentration of volatile anesthetics, (4) increased sensitivity of nondepolarizing neuromuscular blockers, (5) generalized muscle weakness, and (6) increased risk of pulmonary edema. All of these effects may occur at therapeutic levels of magnesium sulfate treatment and should be anticipated when magnesium sulfate is used in the peripartum course.[10-12]

Beta-Mimetic Medications (Ritodrine and Terbutaline)

INDICATIONS

β-Agonists are used to treat preterm labor and uterine tetany. However, β-agonists only prolong pregnancy by 24 to 48 hours, and depending on the gestational age, neonatal morbidity is not decreased.[3] In addition, side effects can seriously limit the use of this class of drugs for treatment of preterm labor. For this reason, calcium channel blockers (CCBs) have replaced the use of β-mimetics to treat preterm labor in many cases. In modern-day practice, β-agonists are now more often used to treat uterine hypertonus and nonreassuring fetal status, especially following the initiation of neuraxial anesthesia. When used in these circumstances, plasma concentrations of epinephrine are increased during labor and produce tocolysis through β-agonist activity. On initiation of a combined spinal-epidural anesthetic, the rapid onset of analgesia causes an equally rapid decrease in catecholamine levels, resulting in unopposed oxytocin-induced uterine tetany and decreased placental perfusion. The β-mimetic properties of terbutaline (0.25 mg intravenously) can treat uterine hypertonus quickly and safely, but because it reaches peak effect in 1 to 2 hours can have the undesired consequence of adversely affecting a woman's contraction pattern and labor curve.

MECHANISM OF ACTION

Uterine smooth muscle possesses β_2-receptors. These are activated selectively by both ritodrine and terbutaline.[9]

DOSING

Although long-term oral β_2-agonist therapy is ineffective in the prevention of preterm labor and delivery before 37 weeks' gestation, the primary indications for these medications are treatment of uterine hypertonus and acute preterm labor. Doses of terbutaline 0.25 mg intravenously or subcutaneously may be repeated and titrated to a maternal heart rate 20% or 30% above baseline, but terbutaline therapy should be used with caution in patients with cardiopulmonary disease.[13] In 2011, the US Food and Drug Administration (FDA) placed a Black Box Warning on terbulatine's label stating that the medication should not be used for prolonged tocolysis (48-72 hours) because of the risk of serious maternal cardiac toxicity and death.[13] Although ritodrine is the only medication approved by the FDA for tocolysis, it is no longer available in the United States.[9]

ADVERSE EFFECTS

The most common side effects of these drugs are related to maternal and fetal β_1 stimulation of the heart and β_2 effects on the pulmonary and endocrine systems. β-Mimetic agents induce transient hyperglycemia and hypokalemia. Although severe hyperglycemia is rare and typically resolves after discontinuation of β-agonist therapy, the increased blood glucose can result in hypokalemia and should be monitored closely in these patients. In some patients, the side effects of these agents may be serious and include tachycardia, myocardial ischemia, dysrhythmias, and pulmonary edema. Twin gestation, infection, and magnesium administration are risk factors for the development of pulmonary edema. β_2 Stimulation can also cause hypotension and cerebral ischemia.[14]

Calcium Channel Blockers

INDICATIONS

Data show that CCBs are superior to β-agonists in reducing preterm labor and improving neonatal outcomes.[15] They are considered first-line tocolytic agents. Nifedipine is the most commonly used CCB due to its affinity for smooth muscle over cardiac muscle.

MECHANISM OF ACTION

CCBs block calcium entry into the cell and release of calcium from the sarcoplasmic reticulum. This results in inhibition of the actin-myosin complex and produces relaxation of uterine smooth muscle.[9]

DOSING

Nifedipine is administered orally or sublingually, 10 to 20 mg every 4 to 6 hours.[15]

ADVERSE EFFECTS

Side effects are usually minimal but can include flushing, headache, and hypotension.[9] The combination of CCBs and general anesthesia can produce hypotension and cardiac conduction abnormalities.[16] However, severe hypotension resulting in reduced uteroplacental perfusion is rare, and adverse fetal effects have not been reported. Pulmonary edema can also occur and is more likely with concurrent administration of β-agonists and/or magnesium.[17] Also, because both oxytocin and PG agonists work via calcium channels, they may be of limited use when treating hemorrhage due to uterine atony[9] in patients recently treated with calcium channel blockers. In such cases, large-bore intravenous access, uterotonics, and blood products should be readily available.

Prostaglandin Synthetase Inhibitors (Nonsteroidal Anti-inflammatory Drugs)

INDICATIONS

These medications are most effective at prolonging pregnancy by 2 to 7 days in the setting of preterm labor.[4] Indomethacin, sulindac, and ketorolac can be used, but their use is limited to 72 hours before 32 weeks' gestation due to severe fetal side effects (eg, premature closing of the ductus arteriosus [after 32 weeks], oligohydramnios [with nimesulide], and necrotizing enterocolitis).[18] Selective cyclooxygenase-2 (COX-2) inhibitors (rofecoxib and nimesulide) may cause fewer adverse effects than their nonselective counterparts. However, these drugs are no longer considered first-line therapy in the treatment of preterm labor.[4]

MECHANISM OF ACTION

PG synthetase inhibitors irreversibly inhibit COX-1 and COX-2. This prevents the production of PGE_2 and $PGF_2\alpha$ from arachidonic acid; both are smooth muscle stimulants.[9]

DOSING

Indomethacin is the most commonly used drug in this class and is administered orally. A 50-mg loading dose is followed by 25 mg every 4 to 6 hours for 48 to 72 hours.[9]

ADVERSE EFFECTS

Although maternal side effects are generally minimal, platelet dysfunction and bleeding, reduced renal perfusion, renal insufficiency, increased systemic vascular resistance, triggering of aspirin-induced asthma, nausea, and heartburn can all occur.

Nitroglycerin

INDICATIONS

Nitroglycerin (NTG) provides rapid, short-acting uterine relaxation. Although NTG can produce profound uterine relaxation, it is mainly used for procedures such as external cephalic version, manual removal of placenta, uterine inversion, head entrapment, extraction of a second twin, and reversal of tetanic uterine contraction.[19] It has not been shown to be an effective treatment for preterm labor.[20]

MECHANISM OF ACTION

NTG increases cyclic GMP concentrations by guanylate cyclase activation and subsequent inhibition of calcium influx and smooth muscle contraction.

DOSING

NTG is administered intravenously, sublingually, or as a sublingual aerosol. When given intravenously, doses typically start at 50 µg. However, incremental doses up to 1850 μg have been reported without side effects. The dose is primarily dependent on the hemodynamic stability of the patient, with redosing dependent on hemodynamic stability.

ADVERSE EFFECTS

Transient hypotension can occur due to the effects of NTG on smooth muscle. However, due to the extremely short half-life of NTG, treatment with intravenous fluids and vasopressors are infrequently required. Maternal headache may also occur, but no adverse effects have been documented in the fetus.

Oxytocin Antagonists

INDICATIONS

Atosiban is a competitive inhibitor of oxytocin receptors and is used to treat preterm labor. Although originally thought to be superior to other tocolytics, a 2005 Cochrane database review found atosiban to be only as effective as β-agonists or placebo.[21] It is considered a second-line therapy behind CCBs because of its low side-effect profile.

MECHANISM OF ACTION

Atosiban reversibly binds and inhibits decidual and myometrial oxytocin receptors.[9]

DOSING

Atosiban is administered as an intravenous infusion at 300 μg/min.[9]

ADVERSE EFFECTS

Although atosiban binds very selectively to oxytocin receptors and the myometrium remains sensitive to oxytocin after atosiban administration, it has minimal maternal side effects. It does not cross the placenta and has no effect on the fetus.

Uterotonic Medications

Uterotonics increase contraction and tone of the uterus and are most commonly used to treat uterine atony (Table 5-3). Uterine atony is the most common cause of postpartum hemorrhage[22] and a leading cause of maternal mortality in the postpartum period. Judicious and timely use of these medications is often necessary.[23] Other uses include cervical ripening, induction of labor, or termination of pregnancy. Three classes of uterotonics are currently used: oxytocin, ergot alkaloids, and PGs.

Oxytocin

INDICATIONS

Oxytocin is a nonapeptide that is produced by the hypothalamus and stored in the posterior pituitary. Pitocin, the synthetic preparation of this compound, is the first-line agent to induce postdelivery hemostasis and treat uterine atony. Pitocin has fewer antidiuretic hormone (ADH)–related side effects (eg, water intoxication)

Table 5-3. Uterotonics

Medication	Route of Administration	Dose	Side Effects
Oxytocin (Pitocin)	Infusion	20-80 μ/L	Hypotension with bolus or rapid infusion, nausea, emesis, water intoxication
Methylergonovine (Methergine)	Intramuscular	0.2 mg IM q2-4h, up to 1 mg	Hypertension, vasoconstriction, nausea, emesis
15-Methyl prostaglandin $F_{2\alpha}$ (Hemabate)	Intramuscular, intrauterine	250 μg q15–90 min; repeat to total of 1 mg	Bronchospasm, systemic and pulmonary hypertension, nausea, emesis, diarrhea, flushing
Misoprostol (Cytotec)	Rectal, sublingual, oral	600-1000 mg; single dose	Tachycardia, fever

than oxytocin. It also used to induce contractions to initiate or augment labor and for contraction stress testing.

MECHANISM OF ACTION

Estrogen stimulates production of oxytocin receptors in the myometrium after 20 weeks of gestation. Oxytocin binds to these receptors and activates a G-protein pathway that increases calcium influx and PGs. The increase of both compounds then causes contraction of uterine smooth muscle.[24]

DOSING

To induce labor, an intravenous infusion of 1 to 2 mU/min is titrated up to 40 mU/min. Although the ED_{90} of oxytocin is 0.35 unit and the dose that eradicates 100% of the target pathogen is 0.5 unit, a dose of 20 to 80 units is diluted in 1 L of saline and given prophylactically over 15 to 30 minutes after every cesarean delivery.[9] Carbetocin, a long-acting synthetic derivative, has been found to be a very effective uterotonic but is not yet available in the United States.

ADVERSE EFFECTS

Oxytocin is structurally very similar to vasopressin and can have some ADH-related side effects such as water intoxication when given in high doses (ie, > 20 mU/min). Also, when there is a balance between catecholamine-inhibiting and oxytocin-stimulating contractions, a sudden reduction in catecholamines (such as related to rapid pain relief from neuraxial analgesia) can result in unopposed oxytocin effect and uterine tetany and nonreassuring fetal status. Uterine tetany should be treated by discontinuing the oxytocin infusion, if one is present, and administering NTG or terbutaline.

The vasodilatory effects of oxytocin can also produce significant hypotension and tachycardia, especially when administered as a bolus. In hemodynamically stable patients, bolus doses of up to 5 units over 5 minutes can be administered without adverse effects. However, larger doses should always be diluted. Even with these precautions, severe hypotension may develop in the setting of hypovolemia, ongoing blood loss, cardiopulmonary disease, and volatile anesthetic administration.[18]

Ergot Alkaloids

INDICATION

Methylergonovine, the synthetic derivative of ergonovine, is administered in cases of refractory uterine atony and postpartum hemorrhage. It causes less peripheral vasoconstriction than ergonovine and is considered a second-line agent for producing sustained uterine tone after oxytocin. When methylergonovine is coadministered with oxytocin, it improves uterine tone.

MECHANISM OF ACTION

Methylergonovine is a partial agonist of α-adrenergic, dopaminergic, and tryptaminergic receptors, but α-adrenergic receptors have the greatest role in promoting uterine contractility. Methylergonovine has greater selectivity for uterine receptors than for vascular receptors and thus is the ergot alkaloid of choice. It has a relatively long half-life and is not administered as a continuous infusion.[9]

DOSING

Methylergonovine, 0.2 mg intramuscularly, is typically administered when oxytocin is ineffective and prior to PG administration. It provides a uterotonic effect within 10 minutes and can be administered every 15 minutes, up to a dose of 1 mg. Duration of action is 3 to 6 hours. Intravenous administration is not recommended.

ADVERSE EFFECTS

Because of α-adrenergic stimulation, methylergonovine can cause severe peripheral vasoconstriction and hypertension, especially with intravenous administration. Hypertensive emergencies complicated by pulmonary edema, seizures, retinal and cerebral hemorrhage, and coronary artery vasospasm have been reported.[24] Methylergonovine also causes pulmonary artery constriction. Methylergonovine should not be given to patients with chronic hypertension, preeclampsia, coronary artery disease, pulmonary hypertension, or peripheral vascular disease. Blood pressure should be monitored in all patients who receive methylergonovine. Direct effects on the CNS emesis centers cause nausea and vomiting in 10% to 20% of patients.

Prostaglandins

INDICATION

PGE_1 analog, PGE_2, and $PGF_2\alpha$ are synthetic prostaglandins that produce dose-dependent increases in uterine tone. They are used for cervical ripening, to treat uterine atony, and to induce second trimester abortion. Hemabate is a $PGF_2\alpha$

derivative and uterotonic that is used in the management of uterine atony.[24] Cytotec is a rapid-onset PGE_1 analog and is used for the management of uterine atony,[25] particularly in women who experience atony that is refractory to parenteral oxytocic agents or in women with comorbidities.

MECHANISM OF ACTION

PGs are naturally occurring hormones that cause increased myometrial calcium concentrations and uterine contraction.[24]

DOSING

The use of PGE_1 analog (Cytotec) has replaced PGE_2 (Prostin) because of its favorable side-effect profile. It can be given rectally, sublingually, or orally for treatment of postpartum hemorrhage.[25] Hemabate is administered intramuscularly or intramyometrially in a 250-µg dose for postpartum hemorrhage. It can be repeated, up to a dose of 1 mg. It should not be administered intravenously.

ADVERSE EFFECTS

Hemabate can produce significant side effects. It is a potent systemic and pulmonary vasoconstrictor. All prostaglandins cause nausea, vomiting, diarrhea, and fever. These side effects should be treated with antiemetics and antidiarrheal agents. In addition, Hemabate causes increased systemic and pulmonary vascular resistance, mean arterial pressure and cardiac output.[24] Bronchoconstriction and hypoxemia due to ventilation-perfusion mismatch are also problematic. Therefore, this drug should not be used in patients with cardiac disease or pulmonary hypertension. It should be used with caution in patients with reactive airway disease. When deciding to use Hemabate in refractory uterine atony, the severity of the reactive airway disease should be weighed against the severity of the uterine atony.

PGE_1 has shown promise in the prevention and treatment of postpartum hemorrhage. In addition, it has no significant contraindications but may cause uterine hyperstimulation and uterine rupture in the setting of patients undergoing a trial of labor after cesarean delivery.

LOCAL ANESTHETICS

Local anesthetics are used commonly in obstetric anesthesiology to reduce the painful sensations of a normal vaginal delivery or to eliminate painful stimuli during surgical procedures or an assisted second stage delivery.

Structure

Local anesthetics are divided into two groups based on their structure. All local anesthetics have a lipophilic aromatic ring and hydrophilic compound linked to an intermediate hydrocarbon chain. The linkage of the hydrocarbon chain to the lipophilic portion is either an ester or amide bond.[26] Compounds with ester linkages between the aromatic ring and hydrocarbon chain are called amino-ester local anesthetics and include procaine, 2-chloroprocaine, tetracaine, and cocaine. Those with amide linkages are known as amino-amide local anesthetics and

Table 5-4. Commonly Used Local Anesthetics: Maximum Dose and Chemical Properties

		Maximum Dose (mg)			Relative Lipid Solubility	Relative Protein Binding
	Local Anesthetic	Plain	With Epi	pKa		
Esters	2–Chloroprocaine	800	1000	8.7	–	–
	Procaine	1000	NA	8.9	–	–
	Tetracaine	100 (topical)	NA	8.5	++	++
Amides	Lidocaine	300	500	7.8	++	++
	Ropivacaine	200	NA	8.1	+++	+++
	Bupivacaine	175	225	8.1	++++	+++
	Mepivacaine	300	400	7.6	++	++

Abbreviation: NA, not applicable.
Doses based on single epidural dose in a healthy 70-kg adult. Pregnancy, age, and comorbidities may influence dosing.

include lidocaine, bupivacaine, ropivacaine, and mepivacaine. There are important differences in metabolism and potential to produce allergic reactions between the two types of local anesthetics. The most commonly used local anesthetics, recommended single dosages, and physiochemical properties are listed in Table 5-4.

Mechanism of Action

Local anesthetics produce a temporary inhibition of nerve action potential formation by inhibiting sodium-gated ion channels in the nerve cell. The most commonly used local anesthetics are weak bases with a pKa (pH at which 50% of the molecules will be protonated) well above that of physiologic pH. Therefore, when a local anesthetic is injected, more than 50% of the local anesthetic will become protonated and will be unable to cross the cell membrane. It follows that local anesthetics with a pKa closer to physiologic pH, such as lidocaine, will have a faster onset; more molecules are available to inhibit the sodium channels inside the cell because only the uncharged form of local anesthetics is able to cross the lipid-rich cell membrane and bind to the sodium channel.[27] However, some local anesthetics with increased lipophilicity, such as 2-chloroprocaine, will have a fast onset despite a higher pKa. Once inside the cell, the local anesthetic molecule binds reversibly at a specific site on the inner pore of the sodium-gated ion channel, preventing the conformational change in the sodium channel necessary for passage of sodium ions and generation of the action potential.[27] This occurs more readily when the channel is in the inactivated closed state (ie, not the resting state). In this state, the local anesthetic stabilizes the sodium channel to prevent the permeability of sodium as well as to prevent changes to the rested-closed and activated-open states in response to nerve impulses. Nerves that fire more frequently (and rest less) have increased local anesthetic binding resulting in a phasic block. Dissociation from the channel depends on size, lipophilicity, and charge of the local anesthetic molecule.[28] Smaller molecules dissociate faster as do more lipophilic molecules, such as

2-chloroprocaine. However, extreme lipid solubility confers longer binding times (eg, bupivacaine) and is a major determinant of local anesthetic potency.

Pharmacokinetics

The pharmacokinetics of local anesthetics depend on the absorption, distribution, and clearance.[29] Local anesthetics are absorbed more rapidly in highly vascular spaces such as the epidural space and slower around peripheral nerves. Vasoconstrictors, such as epinephrine, slow absorption. In addition, when local anesthetics are highly bound, either to lipids or to protein (such as ropivacaine and bupivacaine), the rate of absorption is slowed and local anesthetic effect is increased. The volume of distribution is lower for highly protein bound drugs such as bupivacaine.

Metabolism

Following local anesthetic injection, peak plasma concentrations are determined by the rate of tissue redistribution and clearance of the local anesthetic. When local anesthetics have vasodilatory properties (eg, lidocaine, mepivacaine), there is greater systemic absorption and shorter duration of blockade. Metabolism of ester local anesthetics is by hydrolysis. Patients with atypical pseudocholinesterase are at risk for developing increased systemic concentrations of ester local anesthetics as well as prolonged blockade. Amide local anesthetics undergo metabolism by hepatic microsomal enzymes. However, lidocaine clearance is largely dependent on hepatic blood flow, whereas bupivacaine and ropivacaine clearance is more dependent on intrinsic hepatic enzymatic action.[29] Pulmonary extraction also occurs for some local anesthetics (eg, lidocaine, bupivacaine). Both first-pass pulmonary extraction and hepatic metabolism prevent accumulation of local anesthetics and reduce the risk of local anesthetic toxicity. However, in patients with liver disease or reduced hepatic blood flow, the rate of metabolism of amide local anesthetics can be decreased and the risk of systemic toxicity increased.

Types of Nerve Fibers and Sensitivity to Local Anesthetics

Nerve fibers are classified by their diameter, presence or absence of myelin, and their function (Table 5-5). As mentioned previously, a phasic block arises from the differential in nerve use/frequency of firing. A differential block between nerve types also depends on the diameter and myelination of the nerves. Myelinated axons have increased conduction velocity and are more sensitive to local anesthetics compared to unmyelinated nerves. Unmyelinated nerves require larger amounts of local anesthetic to achieve effective blockade because the sodium-gated channels of these nerves must be blocked along an entire sequential length of the nerve fiber. In contrast, the current is interrupted by nodes of Ranvier in myelinated nerves so that three consecutive nodes of Ranvier will prevent action potential propagation, thereby increasing their sensitivity to local anesthetics.[30] Large myelinated fibers are more sensitive to local anesthetics than smaller unmyelinated fibers. The susceptibility of various nerve fibers to local anesthetics is listed in Table 5-5.

Table 5-5. Peripheral Nerve Classification

Fiber Class	Subclass	Local Anesthetic Susceptibility	Function	Myelin	Diameter	Conduction Velocity
A	α	++	Motor	+	Largest	Fastest
	β	++	Proprioception, touch	+	↓	↓
	γ	++	Muscle tone	+	↓	↓
	δ	+++	Pain, touch, temperature	+	↓	↓
B		++++	Autonomic functions	+	↓	↓
C		+++	Autonomic functions, dull pain, temperature, touch	–	Smallest	Slowest

Additives

BICARBONATE

As mentioned previously, local anesthetics are weak bases with a pKa higher than physiologic pH. The addition of bicarbonate increases the pH of the local anesthetic, thereby, decreasing the amount of ionized local anesthetic, and speeds onset of action by facilitating more rapid transit across physiologic membranes.[28] The amount of bicarbonate needed is unique to each local anesthetic formulation in order to prevent flocculation.

EPINEPHRINE

When added to intrathecal preparations of local anesthetic, epinephrine increases lumbar and sacral block duration by producing vasoconstriction to limit systemic absorption.[31] Epinephrine also has a dose-sparing effect when added to epidural anesthesia. Epinephrine has two effects in this setting. One, it acts as an α_2-adrenergic agonist to produce analgesia. Two, it causes vasoconstriction, which reduces clearance of local anesthetic from the epidural space to reduce the risk of systemic toxicity.[32] This results in lower peak plasma concentrations of lidocaine and bupivacaine. Intrathecally, doses of 50 to 200 µg/mL and epidurally, doses of 1 to 5 µg/mL are commonly used.

PHENYLEPHRINE

The use of phenylephrine as a neuraxial anesthetic adjuvant has fallen out of favor due to its association with transient neurologic symptoms.[33]

Effects of Pregnancy on Local Anesthetic Requirements

The gravid uterus causes decreased venous return and distension of the epidural veins resulting in decreased intrathecal volume. In addition, the hormonal alterations of pregnancy, progesterone in particular, cause an increased susceptibility to the sodium channel blockade caused by local anesthetics. Cerebrospinal fluid in the pregnant patient also has a higher pH and lower $Paco_2$, increasing diffusion of nonionized local anesthetic across the nerve cell membrane.[34] Taken together, all of these factors cause a relatively higher spinal block at equivalent doses in the second and third trimesters of pregnancy.[35] The exact timing of return to nonpregnant dose-and-effect relationships is not known, but patients have nonpregnant local anesthetic requirements within 24 to 48 hours after delivery.[36]

Adverse Reactions to Local Anesthetics

Systemic toxicity often occurs after inadvertent intravascular injection or by absorption of local anesthetic from a regional or local injection site. The signs and symptoms of toxicity (Table 5-6) progress in a typical manner starting with drowsiness, perioral numbness and tinnitus.[37] These CNS symptoms progress to muscle twitching and generalized convulsions, coma, respiratory arrest and cardiovascular collapse. Cardiovascular effects arise both from the CNS and the direct dose-dependent inhibition of cardiac sodium-gated ion channels. The cardiac disturbances include QRS prolongation; PR prolongation; and dysrhythmias, including ventricular fibrillation. Local anesthetics differ in their cardiotoxic profiles. Lidocaine rarely causes ventricular dysrhythmias, whereas bupivacaine accumulates in cardiac tissues and has the most severe cardiac effects. The use of

Table 5-6. Signs and Symptoms of Local Anesthetic Systemic Toxicity (LAST)

		Signs and Symptoms
Central nervous system	Excitation	Agitation, confusion, muscle twitching, seizures
	Depression	Drowsiness, obtundation, coma, or apnea
	Nonspecific	Metallic taste, circumoral numbness, diplopia, tinnitus, dizziness
Cardiovascular system	Hyperdynamic (then...)	Hypertension, tachycardia, ventricular dysrhythmias
	Progressive hypotension	
	Rhythm disturbance	Conduction blockage, bradycardia, or asystole
	Ventricular dysrhythmias	Ventricular tachycardia, torsades de pointes, ventricular fibrillation

Consider LAST in any patient with altered mental status, neurologic symptoms, or cardiovascular instability after regional anesthesia. However, central nervous system signs may be subtle or absent. Cardiovascular signs are often the only manifestation of severe LAST. Toxic signs and symptoms may be delayed by 5 minutes or more and may be biphasic.
Data from Neal JM, Mulroy MF, Weinberg GL. American Society of Regional Anesthesia and Pain Medicine Checklist for Managing Local Anesthetic Systemic Toxicity: 2012 Version. *Reg Anesth Pain Med.* 2012;37:8-15.

incremental injection, frequent aspiration, test doses, and reduced local anesthetic concentration may account for the decreased incidence of local anesthetic toxicity in pregnancy. However, local anesthetic systemic toxicity has been recognized for decades as an important potential cause of maternal mortality.[38]

Treatment of Systemic Toxicity

Rapid treatment of convulsions and cardiotoxicity is needed to improve patient outcomes and survival.[39] Hypoxemia and acidosis exacerbate CNS and cardiac toxicity, so aggressive airway and respiratory management are necessary. Seizures should be treated with benzodiazepines with or without muscle relaxants to reduce acidosis due to convulsions and allow easier control of the airway. In addition to Advanced Cardiac Life Support, intralipid 20% is the treatment of choice for cardiotoxicity related to bupivacaine or ropivacaine intoxication. See Table 5-7 for checklist for treatment of local anesthetic systemic toxicity.[40]

Transient Neurologic Symptoms

It is well known that all local anesthetics can cause neurotoxicity with exposure at high concentrations for long periods of time. However, serious neurologic

Table 5-7. Checklist for Treatment of Local Anesthetic Systemic Toxicity (LAST)[a]

Call for help.

Initial management:
- Airway management: ventilate with 100% oxygen
- Seizure suppression: (1) benzodiazepines are preferred; (2) avoid propofol, especially in patients with cardiovascular instability
- Alert the nearest facility with cardiopulmonary bypass capability

Management of cardiac dysrhythmias:
- Basic and Advanced Cardiac Life Support (ACLS) may require prolonged effort. ACLS protocol may require adjustment of drug dosages (eg, epinephrine in small to moderate doses [individual dose <1 mg/kg]).
- Avoid vasopressin, calcium channel blockers, local anesthetics

If clinically unstable or symptoms progress, infuse 20% lipid emulsion (doses are for 70-kg patient)
- Bolus 1.5 mL/kg (lean body mass) over 1 minute (~100 mL)
- Then, continuous infusion at 0.25 mL/kg per minute (~18 mL/min; adjust by roller clamp; does not need to be exact)
- Repeat bolus once or twice for persistent cardiovascular collapse
- If hypotension persists, double infusion rate if persistent hypotension
- Continue infusion for at least 10 minutes after cardiovascular stability
- Upper limit for lipid emulsion ~10 mL/kg for 30 minutes

Post LAST events at www.lipidrescue.org and report use of lipid to www.lipidregistry.org

[a]Used with permission from Neal JM, et al. ASRA practice advisory on local anesthetic systemic toxicity. *Reg Anesth Pain Med.* 2010;35:152-161.

sequelae after regional anesthesia are rare and usually attributed to trauma during the procedure. Transient neurologic symptoms (TNS) consists of pain in the buttocks that radiates to the legs and resolves in a few days.[41] TNS is much more common with spinal anesthesia. Hyperbaric lidocaine in higher dosages is four times as likely to cause TNS than bupivacaine. This condition does not actually appear to be associated with any neurologic abnormalities and does not represent local anesthetic neurotoxicity. It occurs less often in pregnant patients than in nonpregnant patients.

Back Pain

Historically, 2-chloroprocaine has caused back pain. However, this appears to have been caused by the preservative ethylenediaminetetraacetic acid (EDTA), not the 2-chloroprocaine itself. Severe muscle spasms following injection of more than 25 mL of chloroprocaine are thought to be due to the localized hypocalcemia caused by leaching EDTA. After introduction of 2-chloroprocaine as a preservative-free solution in 1996, these reactions have largely disappeared.

Myotoxicity

Local anesthetics are myotoxic, and intramuscular injection can cause skeletal muscle damage.

Allergic Reactions

It is estimated that less than 1% of reported allergic reactions to local anesthetics are mediated by the immune system.[42] Systemic toxicity, epinephrine reactions, and vasovagal reactions probably account for most. However, amino ester hydrolysis produces para-aminobenzoic acid, a known allergen. Therefore, true allergic reactions to amino esters are more common. In addition, amino esters have shown allergic cross-sensitivity. Amino amides are not known to have any cross-sensitivity with the amino esters or with each other.

CASE STUDY

A 32-year-old G3, P0111 presents to labor and delivery triage at 32 2/7 weeks with painful contractions and a small amount of vaginal bleeding. She has a history of pregnancies complicated by preeclampsia and preterm labor, with one child born by cesarean section due to nonreassuring fetal well-being. She has had scant prenatal care with this pregnancy. Her past medical history is significant for mild intermittent asthma and obesity.

On presentation, her blood pressure is 165/105 mm Hg, heart rate 96 beats/min, respiratory rate 16 breaths/min, and oxygen saturation 97%. Once it is determined that she is actively contracting and dilated to 3 cm, she is admitted for antenatal steroids, tocolysis, and evaluation of increased blood pressure.

Questions

1. What medication would you use for tocolysis? How would you dose it? Can nonsteroidal anti-inflammatory drugs (NSAIDs) be used in this patient?

2. Is there any indication for the use of magnesium sulfate in this patient? How would you dose it? What type of monitoring and nursing assessments would you need to order while the patient is receiving magnesium?

3. What medications/interventions might be causing or contributing to the uterine atony?

4. What medication would you use first to treat the atony? How would you give it? What medication would you use next to treat the atony?

Answers

1. Nifedipine is the first-line tocolytic of choice. It is administered orally or sublingually every 4 to 6 hours in 10- to 20-mg doses. NSAIDs would be contraindicated in this patient as her pregnancy has progressed past 32 weeks.

2. Magnesium sulfate should be used in this patient as a neuroprotective agent for the fetus. It is dosed as a 4- to 6-g intravenous bolus over 20 minutes and then as a 1- to 2-g/h infusion. While it is being administered, the patient should have frequent assessment of her deep tendon reflexes, and her magnesium plasma levels should be checked regularly.

   The patient's contractions increase in frequency, and the fetus begins to have late decelerations. The obstetricians request that you provide anesthesia for an urgent cesarean section. You attempt a spinal anesthetic but are unable to place it due to the large size of the patient. The fetus now has a heart rate of 60 beats/min with maternal blood pressures in the 160/100 mm Hg range. You induce general endotracheal anesthesia. Once the airway is secured, the obstetricians perform an emergent cesarean section. The patient has severe uterine atony.

3. The administration of nifedipine and magnesium sulfate can both contribute to uterine atony as well as volatile anesthetics.

4. The first-line treatment for uterine atony is oxytocin. It is infused as 20 to 50 units diluted in a 1-L bag of saline. The next medications generally used to treat uterine atony are inadvisable in this patient because methylergonovine may increase blood pressures to a disastrous level and Hemabate may precipitate a bronchospastic crisis. Therefore, oral prostaglandin E_2 (misoprostol) may be the only other medicine that is safe to give in this situation.

REFERENCES

1. Martin JA, Hamilton BE, Ventura SJ, et al. Births: final data for 2009. National vital statistics reports. Centers for Disease Control and Prevention, National Center for Health Statistics, National Vital Statistics System. 2011;60:1-70.

2. Kashanian M, Akbarian AR, Soltanzadeh M. Atosiban and nifedipin for the treatment of preterm labor. *Int J Gynaecol Obstet.* 2005;91:10-14.

3. Anotayanonth S, Subhedar NV, Garner P, et al. Betamimetics for inhibiting preterm labour. *Cochrane Database Syst Rev.* 2004:CD004352.

4. King J, Flenady V, Cole S, et al. Cyclo-oxygenase (COX) inhibitors for treating preterm labour. *Cochrane Database Syst Rev.* 2005:CD001992.

5. Crowther CA, Hiller JE, Doyle LW. Magnesium sulphate for preventing preterm birth in threatened preterm labour. *Cochrane Database Syst Rev.* 2002:CD001060.

6. Mercer BM, Merlino AA; Society for Maternal-Fetal Medicine. Magnesium sulfate for preterm labor and preterm birth. *Obstet Gynecol.* 2009;114:650-668.

7. American College of Obstetricians and Gynecologists Committee on Obstetric Practice. Committee Opinion No. 455: Magnesium sulfate before anticipated preterm birth for neuroprotection. *Obstet Gynecol.* 2010;115:669-671.

8. Iseri LT, French JH. Magnesium: nature's physiologic calcium blocker. *Am Heart J.* 1984;108:188-193.

9. Hyagriv NS IJ, Romero R. Preterm birth. In: Gabbe SG NJ, Simpson JL, Landon MB, Glan HL, Jauniaux ER, Driscoll DA, eds. *Obstetrics: Normal and Problem Pregnancies.* 6th ed. Philadelphia, PA: WB Saunders; 2012:627-658.

10. Standley CA, Batia L, Yueh G. Magnesium sulfate effectively reduces blood pressure in an animal model of preeclampsia. *J Matern Fetal Neonatal Med.* 2006;19:171-176.

11. Danladi KY, Sotunmbi PT, Eyelade OR. The effects of magnesium sulphate-pretreatment on suxamethonium-induced complications during induction of general endotracheal anaesthesia. *Afr J Med Med Sci.* 2007;36:43-47.

12. Hino H, Kaneko I, Miyazawa A, et al. Prolonged neuromuscular blockade with vecuronium in patient with triple pregnancy treated with magnesium sulfate. *Masui.* 1997;46:266-270.

13. MedWatch Safety Alerts for Human Medical Products. http://www.fda.gov/Safety/MedWatch/SafetyInformation/SafetyAlertsforHumanMedicalProducts/default.htm. Accessed July 8, 2014.

14. Benedetti TJ. Life-threatening complications of betamimetic therapy for preterm labor inhibition. *Clin Perinatol.* 1986;13:843-852.

15. King JF, Flenady VJ, Papatsonis DN, et al. Calcium channel blockers for inhibiting preterm labour. *Cochrane Database Syst Rev.* 2003:CD002255.

16. Hysing ES, Chelly JE, Jacobson L, et al. Hemodynamic interactions when combining verapamil, acute changes in extracellular ionized calcium concentration and enflurane, halothane or isoflurane in chronically instrumented dogs. *Acta Anaesth Scand.* 1992;36:806-811.

17. Abbas OM, Nassar AH, Kanj NA, et al. Acute pulmonary edema during tocolytic therapy with nifedipine. *Am J Obstet Gynecol.* 2006;195:e3-e4.

18. Vermillion ST, Newman RB. Recent indomethacin tocolysis is not associated with neonatal complications in preterm infants. *Am J Obstet Gynecol.* 1999;181:1083-1086.

19. Morgan PJ, Kung R, Tarshis J. Nitroglycerin as a uterine relaxant: a systematic review. *J Obstet Gynaecol Can.* 2002;24:403-409.

20. El-Sayed YY, Riley ET, Holbrook RH Jr, et al. Randomized comparison of intravenous nitroglycerin and magnesium sulfate for treatment of preterm labor. *Obstet Gynecol.* 1999;93:79-83.

21. Papatsonis D, Flenady V, Cole S, et al. Oxytocin receptor antagonists for inhibiting preterm labour. *Cochrane Database Syst Rev.* 2005:CD004452.

22. American College of Obstetricians and Gynecologists. Practice Bulletin: Clinical Management Guidelines for Obstetrician-Gynecologists, Number 76, October 2006: postpartum hemorrhage. *Obstet Gynecol.* 2006;108:1039-1047.

23. Clark SL, Hankins GD. Preventing maternal death: 10 clinical diamonds. *Obstet Gynecol.* 2012;119:360-364.

24. Francois KE, Foley MR. Antepartum and postpartum hemorrhage. In: Gabbe SG, Niebyl JR, Simpson JL, et al, eds. *Obstetrics: Normal and Problem Pregnancies.* 6th ed. Philadelphia, PA: WB Saunders; 2012:415-444.

25. O'Brien P, El-Refaey H, Gordon A, et al. Rectally administered misoprostol for the treatment of postpartum hemorrhage unresponsive to oxytocin and ergometrine: a descriptive study. *Obstet Gynecol.* 1998;92:212-214.

26. Catterall W. Local anesthetics. In: Brunton L, ed. *Goodman and Gilman's The Pharmacological Basis of Therapeutics*. 11th ed. New York, NY: McGraw Hill; 2007.

27. Butterworth JFT, Strichartz GR. Molecular mechanisms of local anesthesia: a review. *Anesthesiology*. 1990;72:711-734.

28. Courtney KR. Size-dependent kinetics associated with drug block of sodium current. *Biophys J*. 1984;45:42-44.

29. Tucker GT. Pharmacokinetics of local anaesthetics. *Br J Anaesth*. 1986;58:717-731.

30. Franz DN, Perry RS. Mechanisms for differential block among single myelinated and non-myelinated axons by procaine. *J Physiol*. 1974;236:193-210.

31. Chiu AA, Liu S, Carpenter RL, et al. The effects of epinephrine on lidocaine spinal anesthesia: a cross-over study. *Anesth Analg*. 1995;80:735-739.

32. Polley LS, Columb MO, Naughton NN, et al. Effect of epidural epinephrine on the minimum local analgesic concentration of epidural bupivacaine in labor. *Anesthesiology*. 2002;96:1123-1128.

33. Sakura S, Sumi M, Sakaguchi Y, et al. The addition of phenylephrine contributes to the development of transient neurologic symptoms after spinal anesthesia with 0.5% tetracaine. *Anesthesiology*. 1997;87:771-778.

34. Hirabayashi Y, Shimizu R, Saitoh K, et al. Acid-base state of cerebrospinal fluid during pregnancy and its effect on spread of spinal anaesthesia. *Br J Anaesth*. 1996;77:352-555.

35. Hirabayashi Y, Shimizu R, Saitoh K, et al. Spread of subarachnoid hyperbaric amethocaine in pregnant women. *Br J Anaesth*. 1995;74:384-386.

36. Abouleish EI. Postpartum tubal ligation requires more bupivacaine for spinal anesthesia than does cesarean section. *Anesth Analg*. 1986;65:897-900.

37. Mather LE, Copeland SE, Ladd LA. Acute toxicity of local anesthetics: underlying pharmacokinetic and pharmacodynamic concepts. *Reg Anesth Pain Med*. 2005;30:553-566.

38. Bern S, Weinberg G. Local anesthetic toxicity and lipid resuscitation in pregnancy. *Curr Opin Anaesthiol*. 2011;24:262-267.

39. Weinberg GL. Lipid emulsion infusion: resuscitation for local anesthetic and other drug overdose. *Anesthesiology*. 2012;117:180-187.

40. Neal JM, Mulroy MF, Weinberg GL. American Society of Regional Anesthesia and Pain Medicine checklist for managing local anesthetic systemic toxicity: 2012. *Reg Anesth Pain Med*. 2012;37:16-18.

41. Faccenda KA, Finucane BT. Complications of regional anaesthesia Incidence and prevention. *Drug Saf*. 2001;24:413-442.

42. Finucane BT. Allergies to local anesthetics—the real truth. *Can J Anaesth*. 2003;50:869-874.

Neuraxial Labor Analgesia and Effect on Labor

6

Jeanette Bauchat and Cynthia A. Wong

The ideal labor analgesia should provide satisfactory maternal pain relief but not interfere with labor progression or outcome while minimizing adverse side effects to the mother and fetus. Although no single analgesia technique is ideal for all parturients, neuraxial analgesia (epidural, spinal, or combined spinal-epidural) is arguably the analgesic technique closest to the ideal for most women.

PAIN OF LABOR

Pain in the first stage of labor is caused primarily by cervical dilation transmitted via visceral afferent fibers to the T10 to L1 spinal cord segments. As labor progresses and the fetus descends in the birth canal, pain is also caused by vaginal and perineal distension transmitted via somatic afferent fibers traveling in the pudendal nerve to the S2 to S4 spinal cord segments. The pain of cervical dilation tends to be visceral and diffuse in nature. The sacral pain is somatic and localized.

ADVANTAGES AND DISADVANTAGES OF NEURAXIAL LABOR ANALGESIA

Advantages and disadvantages of neuraxial analgesia are listed in Table 6-1. Neuraxial analgesia is the most effective form of pain relief in labor.[1] However, administration of neuraxial analgesia requires the continued presence of a trained anesthesia provider. Although neuraxial labor analgesia is effective and safe in the majority of young healthy women, some women experience complications. Dense neuraxial analgesia may adversely affect the mode of vaginal delivery.

Alternate options for nonpharmacologic pain relief, particularly in early labor, include sterile water injections, water therapy, continuous labor support, touch and massage, and maternal movement and positioning.[2,3] Systemic opioids are the most common form of pharmacologic alternative to neuraxial labor analgesia, but analgesia is incomplete and maternal and fetal respiratory depression limit the dose.

INDICATIONS AND CONTRAINDICATIONS OF NEURAXIAL LABOR ANALGESIA

Indications for Neuraxial Labor Analgesia

Neuraxial labor analgesia is an elective procedure in the majority of young, healthy parturients. If there is no contraindication, neuraxial analgesia should be provided upon request. Both the American College of Obstetricians and Gynecologists and the American Society of Anesthesiologists have endorsed the following statement: "There is no other circumstance where it is considered acceptable for an individual to experience untreated severe pain, amenable to safe intervention, while under a physician's care. In the absence of a medical contraindication, maternal request is a sufficient medical indication for pain relief during labor."[4]

Table 6-1. Advantages and Disadvantages of Neuraxial Labor Analgesia

Maternal	
Advantages	Disadvantages
More effective than parenteral analgesia	Procedure requires anesthesia provider
Improves uteroplacental blood flow	Procedure with risk of complications
Blunts maternal sympathetic response to pain	Medications with side effects
	+/− Increase the rate of instrumental delivery
Rapid conversion from labor analgesia to surgical anesthesia for cesarean delivery	+/− Affects duration of labor
Fetal	
Advantages	Disadvantages
Lower exposure to medication than intravenous techniques	Possibility of maternal hypotension
Less exposure to maternal catecholamines	Possibility of uterine tachysystole (tetanic contraction)

Table 6-2. Absolute Contraindications to Epidural or Spinal Analgesia

- Patient refusal
- Increased intracranial pressure from a mass lesion
- Infection at the site of neuraxial placement
- Frank coagulopathy
- Uncorrected maternal hypovolemia
- Inadequate training/experience of the provider with the technique

Neuraxial labor analgesia may be medically indicated in some parturients. Epidural analgesia can be initiated early in labor to avoid the risks of general anesthesia for an emergency cesarean delivery in the setting of anticipated difficult airway, fetal intolerance to labor, or evolving coagulopathy (eg, HELLP [hemolysis, elevated liver enzymes, low platelet count] syndrome). Neuraxial analgesia may also contribute to the safe management of labor and delivery in patients with comorbid conditions, including preeclampsia with severe features (eg, blood pressure control, evolving airway edema), cardiac disease (eg, reduced catecholamines, afterload reduction), and autonomic hyperreflexia.

Contraindications to Neuraxial Labor Analgesia

Absolute contraindications to neuraxial analgesia are listed in Table 6-2. Relative contraindications to neuraxial techniques may include maternal systemic infection, anticoagulation, and some neurologic conditions. With prior administration of appropriate antibiotics to treat maternal systemic infection, transmission of the infection to the spinal or epidural space is unlikely, but neuraxial analgesia could worsen hemodynamic stability in patients with evolving sepsis. Pharmacologic anticoagulation increases the risk of spinal-epidural hematoma. It is important to refer to The American Society of Regional Anesthesia and Pain Medicine guidelines for the safe initiation and termination of neuraxial techniques in previously or currently anticoagulated patients.[5] Neuraxial anesthesia is likely safe in most patients with underlying neurologic conditions, but a thorough preprocedure neurologic examination and a comprehensive discussion with these patients regarding potential risks associated with neuraxial techniques is imperative.

Benefits of neuraxial analgesia administration must be weighed against the risks for any individual patient, and the anesthesiologist must be able to discuss these with the parturient and her obstetric providers and make appropriate recommendations.

PREPARATION FOR INITIATION OF NEURAXIAL LABOR ANALGESIA

The American Society of Anesthesiologists has published "Practice Guidelines for Obstetric Anesthesia" to guide anesthesiologists in the appropriate management of neuraxial labor analgesia and other aspects of anesthetic management of

Table 6-3. Preparation for Neuraxial Labor Analgesia

- Communicate with obstetric provider
- Review the patient's obstetric history
- Perform a focused preanesthetic evaluation
  ○ Maternal obstetric, anesthetic and health history
  ○ Focused physical examination (vital signs, airway, heart, lungs, back)
- Review or order relevant laboratory values and imaging studies
  ○ Consider need for blood typing and screening or cross-matching
- Formulate anesthetic plan
- Obtain informed consent
- Perform equipment check (routine and emergency resuscitation equipment)
- Check adequacy of and/or obtain intravenous access
- Apply maternal (blood pressure and pulse oximetry) and fetal heart rate monitors
- Perform a team "time-out" with the nurse and patient

parturients.[6] A checklist for the preparation for neuraxial labor analgesia is outlined in Table 6-3.

Communication with the parturient's obstetrician or midwife is important to ensure that he or she is aware the parturient is requesting neuraxial analgesia and allows exchange of information regarding the parturient's obstetric and medical history. A preanesthetic evaluation and focused physical examination is essential, allowing one to anticipate problems that may arise during labor or cesarean delivery, identify contraindications to neuraxial analgesia, and anticipate changes in the parturient's medical conditions. Blood typing and screening or cross-matching should be considered in women at high risk of postpartum hemorrhage. An anesthetic plan should be based on the anesthetic consultation and written informed consent should be obtained. Women generally want full disclosure, and despite pain and prior use of opioid analgesia are able to give informed consent.[7]

Resuscitation equipment and medications should be available to manage complications of neuraxial techniques, including hypotension, local anesthetic systemic toxicity, total spinal anesthesia, emergency cesarean delivery, massive postpartum hemorrhage, and respiratory depression (Table 6-4).

Adequacy of intravenous access should be assessed before performing a neuraxial technique. In the setting of spinal anesthesia for cesarean delivery, administering a crystalloid fluid bolus prior to initiation of anesthesia (preload) has no benefit compared to administering the bolus at the time of initiation of anesthesia (coload). Although the authors routinely administer a 500-mL crystalloid fluid coload to healthy parturients for initiation of low-dose neuraxial labor analgesia, evidence to support this practice is lacking. Phenylephrine is now considered the vasopressor of choice to treat hypotension in the setting of spinal anesthesia for cesarean delivery because it results in less neonatal acidosis than ephedrine. Influence of vasopressor choice on neonatal outcome in the setting of hypotension induced by neuraxial labor analgesia has not been studied; however, given the frequency of this side effect following neuraxial techniques in labor, a vasopressor(s) should be readily available.

Table 6-4. Resuscitation Drugs and Equipment

- Drugs
  - Sedative-hypnotic agents (propofol, ketamine, midazolam)
  - Succinylcholine
  - Vasopressors (ephedrine, phenylephrine, epinephrine)
  - Atropine
  - Calcium chloride
  - Sodium bicarbonate
  - Naloxone
- Equipment
  - Oxygen source
  - Suction source with tubing and suction catheter
  - Self-inflating bag for positive pressure ventilation
  - Face masks
  - Oral airways
  - Laryngoscope and assortment of blades
  - Endotracheal tubes and stylets
  - Eschmann stylet (bougie)
  - Qualitative carbon dioxide detector

Maternal blood pressure is measured every 2 to 2.5 minutes during and immediately after the neuraxial procedure for 15 to 20 minutes, and every 30 minutes during maintenance of epidural analgesia. Fetal heart rate should be continuously monitored by a trained professional during (if possible) and following the procedure. Fetal heart rate decelerations may occur secondary to maternal hypotension or uterine tachysystole (see below).

Communication should be ongoing among the anesthesiologists, midwives/obstetricians and nurses throughout labor to ensure accurate and timely exchange of information.

NEURAXIAL LABOR ANALGESIC TECHNIQUES

Continuous lumbar epidural analgesia, the primary technique for labor analgesia, has been used for many years. Anesthetic solution injected into the lumber epidural space spreads cephalad and caudad, providing sensory blockade to afferent pain fibers for both cervical dilation (T10-L1 dermatomes) and vaginal and perineal dilation (S2-S4 dermatomes). Analgesia is initiated with bolus injection of medication through the epidural needle, catheter or both, and maintained with continuous or intermittent administration of medication. An epidural catheter allows rapid conversion from labor analgesia to surgical anesthesia in the event a cesarean delivery is required. Disadvantages of epidural analgesia include a slower onset of analgesia and need for larger doses of medication to initiate analgesia (increasing risk of maternal systemic toxicity and fetal exposure) compared to combined spinal-epidural analgesia.

Combined spinal-epidural analgesia (CSE) is a popular technique because of the faster onset of analgesia, particularly in the sacral area, compared to traditional epidural analgesia.[8] Rapid onset of sacral analgesia is necessary in women in the late active phase of the first stage of labor, women in the second stage of labor, and in women whose labors are progressing rapidly. A needle-through-needle technique using a 25-gauge or smaller pencil-point spinal needle is used to initiate analgesia; an epidural catheter is sited for maintenance of analgesia. Additional advantages of combined spinal-epidural analgesia compared to traditional epidural analgesia include the ability to achieve rapid analgesia using a lipid-soluble opioid-only intrathecal injection, particularly in early labor. This results in less maternal hypotension and motor blockade, maintaining the ability to ambulate. The CSE technique requires a dural puncture, although the risk of postdural puncture headache has not been shown to be greater than a traditional epidural technique. The incidence of pruritus is higher with an intrathecal compared to epidural opioid injection.[8]

Continuous spinal analgesia is typically only used in the setting of unintentional dural puncture with an epidural needle, because only epidural catheters are available in the United States. Because of the large-bore needle required to place the catheter, this technique is associated with a high rate of postdural puncture headache. Continuous spinal analgesia can be used for labor analgesia and converted to an anesthetic for cesarean delivery. The potential for overdose and high-spinal anesthesia or total spinal anesthesia if a spinal catheter is mistaken for an epidural catheter is a real safety concern; all anesthesia providers must be aware of the presence of a spinal catheter on the labor and delivery unit and the catheter and medication pump must be clearly marked as a spinal catheter.

Caudal epidural analgesia is used infrequently because it is technically more difficult to place a caudal than a lumber catheter. Large volumes are required to achieve analgesia to the low thoracic level, thus increasing the risk of maternal local anesthetic systemic toxicity and fetal exposure to medication. This technique may be an option in women with lumbar spine instrumentation.

Single-shot spinal analgesia provides immediate pain relief with a low dose of medication but has a limited duration of action. Therefore, it use is usually limited to imminent vaginal deliveries or in settings in which an epidural catheter cannot be inserted.

INITIATION OF NEURAXIAL LABOR ANALGESIA

An example of the sequence of events for initiating neuraxial labor analgesia is outlined in Table 6-5. The parturient is positioned in either the sitting or lateral position. Sitting is particularly advantageous in obese parturients due to the ease in which midline can be identified. The lateral position may have the advantages of a lower risk of maternal hypotension, allowing easier access to fetal monitoring and improving maternal comfort. The use of preprocedure ultrasonography may help identify midline and interspinous spaces, but whether it improves labor analgesia outcomes is currently not known. Following the neuraxial procedure, the mother should be placed in a lateral position to avoid aortocaval compression and maximize maternal cerebral perfusion if hypotension occurs.

Epidural test doses are given at initiation of epidural analgesia in an attempt to reduce the likelihood that large doses of epidural medication are administered

Table 6-5. Initiation of Epidural Labor Analgesia

- Complete "Preparation for Neuraxial Labor Analgesia" checklist (Table 6-3)
- Position patient (lateral or sitting position)
- Initiate maternal blood pressure and pulse oximetry as well as fetal heart rate monitoring
- Intravenous bolus administration of a balanced salt solution (eg, 500 mL of lactated Ringer's solution)
- Utilizing sterile technique, locate the epidural space, administer an intrathecal dose if a combined spinal-epidural is the choice technique, and site epidural catheter in the epidural space
- Administer an epidural test dose
- If no spinal dose was administered, initiate epidural analgesia with 5-15 mL of epidural local anesthetic-opioid solution in 5-mL increments
- Monitor maternal blood pressure every 2-3 minutes for 15-20 minutes or until the parturient is hemodynamically stable
- Assess pain score and extent of sensory (both cephalad and caudad) and motor block
- Initiate epidural maintenance analgesia

through a malpositioned catheter (intravascular or intrathecal). Some practitioners argue that an epidural test dose may not be necessary if low-dose local anesthetic solutions are injected incrementally through the epidural catheter after negative aspiration; the authors believe that the test dose adds safety, particularly in the event of an emergency cesarean delivery when a rapid injection of a high-concentration local anesthetic solution is required. Aspiration of blood or cerebrospinal fluid is a more reliable sign of intrathecal or intravascular catheter placement with a multiorifice compared to a single-orifice catheter. Common test dose regimens are listed in Table 6-6.

DRUG CHOICES FOR INITIATION OF EPIDURAL AND SPINAL LABOR ANALGESIA

The most common method of achieving effective neuraxial analgesia while minimizing side effects uses low-dose local anesthetic solution in combination with a lipid-soluble opioid. The addition of lipid-soluble opioids to a local anesthetic solution for initiation of epidural or spinal labor analgesia decreases latency, prolongs duration of analgesia, improves the quality of analgesia, and decreases the total local anesthetic requirement.[9] The overall opioid requirement is also reduced when used in combination with epidural or intrathecal local anesthetic, effectively reducing side effects of nausea, vomiting, pruritus, and respiratory depression. The typical drugs and dosages used to initiate epidural or spinal labor analgesia are listed in Table 6-7.

In general, a higher epidural loading dose is required for initiation of analgesia in active versus latent labor. There is a dose-sparing effect achieved by administering a high-volume/low-concentration local anesthetic solution compared to a low-volume/high-concentration solution.[10] The intrathecal dose, as part of a CSE technique for initiation of labor analgesia, provides rapid onset of pain relief with lower doses of drug than traditional epidural analgesia. The spinal injection may provide complete analgesia with opioid alone in early labor. Local anesthetics are injected intrathecally in combination with opioids for active labor because as sole

Table 6-6. Epidural Test Dose Regimens

Test Dose Components	Positive Intravascular Test Dose	Positive Intrathecal Test Dose
Lidocaine 1.5% with epinephrine 1:200,000, 3 mL	Increase HR > 20 bpm within 60 s	Motor blockade in 3-5 min[a]
Bupivacaine 0.25% with epinephrine 1:200,000,3 mL	Increase HR > 20 bpm within 60 s	Motor blockade in 3-5 min[a]
Lidocaine 100 mg Bupivacaine 25 mg Chloroprocaine 90 mg	Tinnitus, perioral numbness, "dizziness"	
Fentanyl 100 µg	"Dizziness" or sedation	
Air 1 mL	Mill wheel murmur on Doppler placed over right heart	
Lidocaine 40-60 mg Bupivacaine 7.5 mg	Not applicable	Motor blockade in 3-5 min[a]

Abbreviation: HR, heart rate.
[a]Weakness in hip flexion. The test dose is less sensitive in pregnant women, patients on β-blockers and anesthetized patients.
Modified from Yilmaz M, Wong CA. Technique of neuraxial anesthesia. In: Wong CA, ed. *Spinal and Epidural Anesthesia.* New York, NY: McGraw-Hill; 2007:27-73.

agents, local anesthetics do not provide adequate analgesia unless used in high doses, thus causing the undesirable effect of lower extremity motor blockade.

Local Anesthetics

Bupivacaine, an amide local anesthetic, is commonly used to initiate and maintain labor analgesia. Because it is highly protein-bound in the maternal circulation,

Table 6-7. Drugs for Initiation of Epidural and Spinal Labor Analgesia

Drug	Epidural Analgesia[a]	Spinal Analgesia
Local Anesthetics[b]		
Bupivacaine	0.0625%-0.125%	1.25-2.5 mg
Ropivacaine	0.08%-0.2%	2.0-3.5 mg
Levobupivacaine	0.0625%-0.125%	2.0-3.5 mg
Opioids[b]		
Fentanyl	50-100 µg	15-25 µg
Sufentanil	5-10 µg	1.5-5 µg
Morphine[c]	N/A	0.125-0.25 mg

Abbreviation: N/A, not applicable.
[a]Volume required for initiation of epidural labor analgesia is 5 to 20 mL of local anesthetic, with higher volumes used with lower concentration of local anesthetic.
[b]Local anesthetic and opioid doses are reduced when drugs are combined or following a local anesthetic test dose.
[c]Not commonly used for initiation of labor analgesia due to long latency.

uteroplacental transfer of drug is limited. Bupivacaine is most commonly combined with fentanyl or sufentanil for initiation of labor analgesia. Typical onset of epidural analgesia is 8 to 10 minutes, with peak effect at 20 minutes and duration of 90 minutes, depending on the total dose and stage of labor. The typical formulation of plain bupivacaine is hypobaric with respect to cerebrospinal fluid and provides more effective analgesia than hyperbaric bupivacaine when administered in low doses in the intrathecal space.

Ropivacaine, an amide local anesthetic formulated as a single levorotary enantiomer, is similar to bupivacaine in structure and pharmacodynamics. In studies comparing ropivacaine to bupivacaine, ropivacaine was initially believed to cause less motor blockade and less cardiotoxicity than bupivacaine. However, when adjusted for potency (ropivacaine is less potent than bupivacaine), ropivacaine does not have any advantage over bupivacaine for labor epidural analgesia.[11] Ropivacaine is not approved for use as an intrathecal injection in the United States.

Levobupivacaine is the purified levorotary enantiomer of racemic bupivacaine and is therefore less cardiotoxic than bupivacaine. The risk of local anesthetic systemic toxicity (LAST) is rare using low-concentration solutions; thus, there do not appear to be any clinical advantages to using it compare to bupivacaine for labor analgesia. It is not available in the United States.

Lidocaine, an amide local anesthetic, is typically not used for initiation or maintenance of labor analgesia because of the short duration of action and higher umbilical vein to maternal vein drug concentration ratio than bupivacaine.

2-Chloroprocaine is an ester local anesthetic with limited utility for labor analgesia due to its short duration of action. Epidural administration of 2-chloroprocaine has a rapid onset (5-10 minutes) of analgesia that lasts 40 minutes with a low risk of systemic toxicity, making it a useful medication for instrumental vaginal or emergency cesarean delivery.

Opioids

Fentanyl and sufentanil, lipid-soluble opioids, are most commonly used for initiation of labor analgesia. High lipid solubility facilitates penetration through the dura (epidural injection) and entry into the spinal cord (intrathecal or epidural injection), resulting in faster onset of analgesia, shorter duration of action, and higher systemic absorption than with water-soluble opioids. Fentanyl and sufentanil both provide complete pain relief in early labor when used as sole agents for intrathecal injection. The duration of analgesia with intrathecal fentanyl alone varies from 80 to 120 minutes and has an analgesic plateau at 25 μg and worsening side effects (eg, pruritus) with increasing doses.[12] Sufentanil has greater lipid solubility than fentanyl, resulting in greater spinal cord penetration and potentially faster and better analgesia. Its higher lipid solubility results in higher volumes of distribution and lower maternal plasma concentrations with resultant lower fetal umbilical vein and plasma levels when given as an epidural injection compared to fentanyl. The actual clinical differences between the two drugs are small. Intrathecal sufentanil has a longer duration of action than fentanyl but similar side-effect profile.[13] Given that epidural maintenance analgesia is routinely initiated soon after the spinal dose, the longer duration of action of sufentanil may not be clinically relevant. In the United States, sufentanil is used less often than fentanyl because historically, it was more expensive than fentanyl. In addition, it is formulated commercially in a high concentration (50 μg/mL); thus is must be diluted before use, making it less practical and more prone to drug error.

Morphine, a water-soluble opioid, is impractical for routine use in labor analgesia due to its long latency and prolonged effects after delivery. Low doses of intrathecal morphine (0.1-0.25 mg), when combined with bupivacaine and lipid-soluble opioid for initiation of analgesia, make an acceptable alternative for active labor when epidural maintenance medications or resources are not available. Higher doses of intrathecal morphine (0.5-2 mg) are not effective for the second stage of labor and have unacceptably high incidence of side effects, including somnolence, nausea and vomiting, pruritus, and respiratory depression.

Diamorphine (heroin) is available in the United Kingdom and is used in combination with low-dose local anesthetics for labor analgesia, but no studies have compared it directly to fentanyl or sufentanil.

Meperidine is an opioid with local anesthetic properties, but there is no evidence that it is superior to low-dose local anesthetic with lipid-soluble opioid. Intrathecal meperidine (10 mg) can be used as a sole agent for spinal labor analgesia, but it is associated with more nausea and vomiting and is best reserved for patients who have a contraindication to local anesthetic-opioid labor analgesia.

Alfentanil is a lipid-soluble opioid whose analgesic properties have not been directly compared with fentanyl and sufentanil for labor analgesia, but it would presumably be inferior given its lower lipid solubility. Hydromorphone is not well studied for labor analgesia, but its latency and duration of action of lies between fentanyl and morphine. Butorphanol has strong κ-receptor activity, and studies utilizing this drug in labor demonstrated side effects such as transient sinusoidal fetal heart rate pattern and maternal somnolence or dysphoria.

Adjuvants to Local Anesthetics and Opioids for Labor Analgesia

Other medications have been used for their synergistic effects with local anesthetics and opioids to prolong duration of action, improve analgesia and reduce required anesthetic doses with the intent of reducing side effects (Table 6-8). Although these drugs may be used as alternatives or adjuvants, they should not be used routinely due to their high incidence of side effects and little to no advantage compared to local anesthetic-opioid analgesia alone.

Clonidine, an α_2-adrenergic receptor binder, inhibits neurotransmitter release in the dorsal horn of the spinal cord. Clonidine, when administered in the epidural or intrathecal space, improves quality and duration of labor analgesia. Although it provides adequate analgesia with no motor blockade, the high incidence of maternal hypotension, sedation and fetal heart rate abnormalities limits its use. The US Food and Drug Administration specifically warns against its use in obstetric patients because of the risk of hypotension.

Epinephrine acts as an analgesic adjuvant by binding directly to α-adrenergic receptors (inhibiting neurotransmitter release in the spinal cord) and causing

Table 6-8. Adjuvants to Neuraxial Labor Analgesia

	Epidural Analgesia		Spinal Analgesia
Adjuvant Drug	**Initiation Bolus Dose**	**Maintenance Infusion Dose**[a]	**Initiation Bolus Dose**
Epinephrine	25-75 µg[b]	25-50 µg/h[b]	2.25-200 µg
Clonidine	75-100 µg	19-37 µg/h	15-30 µg

[a]Usually coadministered with a low-concentration local anesthetic infusion (eg, bupivacaine < 0.08%), 10 to 20 mL/h.
[b]Usually administered in a 1:800,000 to 1:200,000 solution (1.25-5 µg/mL) with a local anesthetic and/or opioid.

vasoconstriction (preventing systemic absorption of drugs in the neuraxial space). It prolongs the effects of local anesthetic-opioid analgesia, allowing a decrease in concentration of local anesthetic; however, it increases the incidence of motor blockade and does not improve the quality of analgesia.

MAINTENANCE OF LABOR ANALGESIA

Analgesia must be maintained for at least several hours following initiation of neuraxial analgesia in most parturients. Maintenance of analgesia is accomplished by administering medication through an epidural catheter for the duration of labor. A long-acting, low-dose amide local anesthetic combined with a lipid-soluble opioid is the most common medication solution used for maintenance of labor analgesia.

Patients should be monitored by the anesthesia provider during maintenance of epidural analgesia. Assessment and documentation of the quality of analgesia, sensory and motor blockade, and maternal hemodynamics should be made intermittently throughout labor.

Drugs for Maintenance of Epidural Analgesia

Typical drugs and drug concentrations for maintenance of epidural analgesia are listed in Table 6-9. Bupivacaine and ropivacaine have both been used for maintenance analgesia with no clear advantage of one over the other.[11] Although the risk of breakthrough pain (thus requiring more interventions to treat inadequate analgesia) is higher using low-concentration compared to high-concentration local anesthetic solutions, high-concentration solutions are associated with more hypotension and motor blockade. Some studies have found that the incidence of instrumental vaginal delivery is lower using low-dose compared to high-dose local anesthetic solutions for maintenance of epidural analgesia.[14] Lidocaine and 2-chloroprocaine are not used for maintenance solutions because of their short duration of action. Epinephrine is sometimes added to the local anesthetic–opioid solution allowing further decrease in concentration of local anesthetic; however, there appears to be no clinical benefit because epinephrine potentiates both the sensory and motor blockade.

Table 6-9. Anesthetic Solutions for Epidural Maintenance Infusions Utilizing Continuous Infusion or Patient-Controlled Epidural Analgesia (PCEA)[a]

Drug[b]	Concentration
Local anesthetics	
Bupivacaine	0.05-0.125%
Ropivacaine	0.08-0.2%
Opioids	
Fentanyl	1.5-3 µg/mL
Sufentanil	0.2-0.33 µg/mL

[a]Continous infusions are typically 8 to 12 mL/h. Typical PCEA settings are background infusion: 2 to 12 mL, demand boluses: 4 to 10 mL, lockout interval: 10 to 30 minutes.
[b]Local anesthetic is most often combined with opioid.

Maintenance Techniques

Historically, manual intermittent boluses of medication were administered by the anesthesia provider for maintenance of epidural analgesia. Although this mode of administration was effective, it was not ideal given the inevitable regression of analgesia, which triggered requests for additional medication and depended on the ready availability of the nursing staff and anesthesia provider to avoid "windows" of pain. Continuous infusions, delivered via a mechanical pump, were found to have a safety profile similar to intermittent manual boluses with more constant analgesia, greater maternal satisfaction, and less need for anesthesia provider intervention. However, infusions compared to boluses of the same local anesthetic concentration results in use of greater volume of local anesthetic solution and greater degree of motor block.[15]

In modern practice, intermittent boluses with or without a background infusion are given using a patient-controlled epidural analgesia (PCEA) technique for maintenance of epidural analgesia. The most effective method of administering epidural medication with PCEA appears to be high-volume, low-concentration local anesthetic with lipid-soluble opioid. Optimal PCEA settings probably depend on the drug concentrations and may be patient-dependent. Although data are inconsistent, a background infusion likely results in more constant analgesia and reduces anesthesia provider interventions compared with no continuous infusion, and it may allow the patient to get more rest.[16] An hourly background infusion rate of one-third to one-half the total hourly anesthetic dose has been suggested.[16] Higher volume patient-administered boluses (> 5 mL) appear to be more effective than smaller boluses. Higher bolus volumes are used with longer time intervals and the PCEA pumps should be programmed with maximum limits to prevent overdose. Pumps capable of administering automated (programmed) intermittent boluses have been recently introduced and may facilitate bolus administration while allowing the patient to rest.

PCEA pumps should be distinct from the intravenous pumps to minimize accidental adjustments of epidural medication or administration of incorrect medications into the epidural catheter by other hospital providers. Hospital policy should clearly state who can administer or adjust epidural infusion pumps, but only trained anesthesia providers should order adjustment of epidural infusion rates, volume or medication content. Ideally, pharmacists should prepare epidural solutions to ensure sterility.

Maintenance of Spinal Analgesia

Continuous spinal analgesia for maintenance of labor analgesia is indicated in cases of unintentional dural puncture during the initial attempted placement of an epidural catheter. It is also used more rarely for specific indications (eg, morbid obesity, abnormal spine pathology).

The same medications and drug concentrations used for maintenance of epidural analgesia are used for spinal analgesia but at lower infusion rates, typically 2 mL/h. The infusion pump can be set with PCEA bolus administration (1-3 mL) to minimize disconnections of the catheter-infusion tubing and risk of infection or iatrogenic overdose. Our practice is not to give the PCEA button to the patient but rather administer these PCEA boluses via the anesthesia provider, thus encouraging frequent evaluation of the patient with a spinal catheter to assess pain, blood pressure, and sensory and motor blockade.

ANALGESIA AND ANESTHESIA FOR OPERATIVE VAGINAL DELIVERY

In the second stage of labor, pain is caused by vaginal and perineal distension via somatic nerve fibers in the S2 to S4 dermatomes. These are large nerves that may need more local anesthetic to provide adequate sacral analgesia. Some patients require higher concentration and volumes of local anesthetic than can be self-administered via the PCEA for second stage labor analgesia. Unfortunately, this additional injection of medication prior to delivery may cause motor blockade, high sensory block, and minimal sensation of perineal pressure to assist with maternal explosive efforts.

Supplemental analgesia is frequently necessary for women undergoing an assisted vaginal delivery, episiotomy, or repair of episiotomy or complex vaginal laceration. Table 6-10 describes techniques to provide analgesia/anesthesia for these circumstances.

MANAGEMENT OF BREAKTHROUGH PAIN

Despite complete relief of labor pain with the initiation of neuraxial anesthesia, breakthrough pain may occur during maintenance of epidural analgesia. It is important to have a conversation about the possibility of breakthrough pain during the preanesthetic evaluation and consenting process; otherwise, patients may become highly dissatisfied if the expectation is that epidural analgesia will provide complete relief of pain for the duration of labor. Table 6-11 lists suggested procedures for evaluating and treating breakthrough pain during labor.

Table 6-10. Anesthesia for Vaginal Delivery

Epidural anesthesia
- 2% or 3% 2-chloroprocaine or 2% lidocaine: 5-10 mL
Spinal anesthesia
- Hyperbaric bupivacaine 6-8 mg or hyperbaric lidocaine 25-50 mg[a]
Combined spinal-epidural anesthesia
- Intrathecal bupivacaine 2.5-5 mg + fentanyl 15-25 μg
- Administer additional drugs through epidural catheter if inadequate analgesia or cesarean delivery is necessary

---

[a]Administer a higher dose of bupivacaine if likelihood of instrumental delivery failure is high, resulting in a high likelihood of cesarean delivery, or perform combined spinal-epidural anesthesia anesthesia.

When evaluating a patient for breakthrough pain, it is important to evaluate not only epidural catheter function, but also review the obstetric history, progress of labor and current position of the fetus. If a woman undergoing a trial of labor after cesarean delivery complains of breakthrough pain, uterine rupture must be considered and this concern communicated with the obstetrician. Women with more advanced labor generally require higher drug doses to maintain analgesia. Patients should be asked to rate and describe the location and character of the pain. Solution injected into the lumbar epidural space preferentially distributes in the cephalad, not caudad direction. This distribution may result in so-called "sacral sparring." Thus, sensory blockade should be evaluated in both low thoracic and sacral dermatomes. Some parturients have breakthrough pain despite apparently

Table 6-11. Assessment and Management of Inadequate Neuraxial Analgesia

---

- Review and assess progress of labor
  - Rule out other causes of breakthrough pain (eg, bladder distension, uterine rupture)
- Evaluate the anesthetic
  - Is the catheter in the epidural space (ie, is sensory blockade present)?
  - If not, replace epidural catheter
- Catheter is in the epidural space, but there is inadequate sensory blockade (does not extend from T10 to S4):
  - Inject 10-20 mL of dilute local anesthetic solution with or without opioid
  - If this maneuver is successful, alter the maintenance technique (eg, increase infusion rate or concentration of local anesthetic)
  - If this maneuver fails, replace epidural catheter
- Catheter is in the epidural space, but the sensory blockade is asymmetric:
  - Place the patient on her side with the less blocked side in the dependent position
  - Inject 10-20 mL of dilute local anesthetic solution with or without opioid
  - If this maneuver fails, replace epidural catheter
- Catheter is in the epidural space, the sensory block is T10-S4, but the patient has pain
  - Inject a more concentrated solution of local anesthetic with or without an opioid
  - Alter the maintenance technique (eg, increase concentration of local anesthetic solution)

adequate sensory blockade due to increased pain from cephalopelvic disproportion or abnormal position of the fetus (eg, occiput posterior). These patients require a denser block (ie, higher concentration of local anesthetic).

ADVERSE SIDE EFFECTS OF NEURAXIAL LABOR ANALGESIA

Hypotension

The sympathectomy induced by neuraxial blockade may cause hypotension due to peripheral vasodilation and increased venous capacitance. The incidence of hypotension (usually defined as a 20%-30% decrease in baseline systolic blood pressure) after initiation of neuraxial labor analgesia is approximately 10%.[8] Because uteroplacental perfusion is not autoregulated and is directly related to maternal blood pressure, a decrease in maternal blood pressure results in decreased uteroplacental perfusion. Uncorrected maternal hypotension, particularly in maternal-fetal dyads with preexisting uteroplacental insufficiency (eg, preeclampsia), may result in fetal acidosis and hypoxia. Thus, maternal blood pressure should be monitored frequently (every 2-3 minutes) after the initiation of neuraxial analgesia and treated if low. Traditionally, small intravenous bolus doses of ephedrine (5-10 mg) have been used to treat maternal hypotension. Given that phenylephrine is arguably the vasopressor of choice to treat hypotension associated with spinal anesthesia for cesarean delivery, many practitioners now use small bolus doses of phenylephrine (50-100 µg) to treat hypotension during labor.

Other techniques to mitigate hypotension include avoidance of aortocaval compression. A rapid intravenous fluid bolus administered immediately prior or during the initiation of neuraxial analgesia is insufficient to prevent hypotension, but it may mitigate the severity of hypotension, especially if the parturient is dehydrated.

Uterine Tachysystole and Fetal Bradycardia

Fetal bradycardia has been observed after the initiation of both CSE and epidural labor analgesia, usually in the first 20 to 40 minutes. The etiology is unclear, but it has been proposed that the bradycardia is associated with an increase in uterine tone, resulting in decreased uteroplacental perfusion (the uterus is perfused during uterine diastole) and subsequent fetal hypoxemia.[17] The initiation of neuraxial analgesia results in an abrupt decrease in circulating maternal epinephrine levels. Epinephrine, via its β_2-adrenergic agonist effects, is a uterine tocolytic. Therefore, a decrease in epinephrine levels may cause uterine tachysystole and a subsequent decrease in uteroplacental perfusion. Data are inconsistent, but some studies suggest that the incidence of fetal bradycardia may be higher after spinal opioid compared to epidural opioids or epidural or spinal local anesthetic initiation of analgesia.[18] However, no study comparing the two techniques has identified a difference in the risk of emergency cesarean delivery. The fetal bradycardia usually resolves with conservative measures of in utero resuscitation, including relief of aortocaval compression, intravenous fluid bolus, supplemental maternal oxygen administration, discontinuing exogenous oxytocin, treatment of any maternal hypotension, and fetal scalp stimulation. Persistent tachysystole can be treated with subcutaneous terbutaline (0.25 mg) or intravenous (50-100 µg) or sublingual nitroglycerin (400-800 µg).

Pruritus

Pruritus is the most common side effect of neuraxial opioids; the incidence and severity are dose-dependent and are higher following spinal compared to epidural injection. The mechanism is unclear but appears to be mediated through µ-opioid receptors. The mechanism is not related to histamine release, and antihistamines are ineffective for treatment. The pruritus is usually most severe in the initial minutes following initiation of neuraxial analgesia. Most women do not require treatment. The symptoms are typically self-limiting, and the severity markedly diminishes after the first hour. Severe pruritus is successfully treated with a µ-opioid antagonist (eg, intravenous naloxone 40 µg) or an agonist-antagonist (eg, intravenous nalbuphine 2.5 mg).

Fever

Epidural analgesia has been associated with maternal fever in a subset of women.[19] The reported incidence ranges from 1% to 46%. The etiology is not clear but does not seem to be related to infection. However, markers of inflammation are higher in women with fever than those without it. The significance of epidural-associated maternal fever is not known but of concern. Maternal inflammation and fever have been associated with detrimental effects to the fetal brain. Additionally, chorioamnionitis is a clinical diagnosis that results in treatment to both the mother and the neonate, and epidural-associated fever may complicate the diagnosis of chorioamnionitis.

Shivering

Shivering is common during labor and may occur more frequently after epidural analgesia. Several factors, including hormonal changes, likely influence thermoregulatory responses during labor. The mechanism(s) are unclear, but some shivering has been shown to be nonthermoregulatory.[20]

Nausea and Vomiting

Nausea and vomiting are frequent during labor. Possible etiologies include pregnancy, pain, direct opioid effects on the chemoreceptor trigger zone in the area postrema and the vestibular apparatus, or opioid-induced delayed gastric emptying. The incidence of nausea and vomiting is significantly lower in women who receive neuraxial compared to systemic opioid analgesia.[21] For unclear reasons, the incidence is also lower in women who receive neuraxial opioids for labor, compared to the neuraxial administration of the same drugs for postoperative analgesia. Hypotension should be ruled out as a cause for neuraxial analgesia–associated nausea and vomiting.

Urinary Retention

The bladder and urethral sphincters receive sympathetic innervation from the low thoracic and high lumbar sympathetic fibers as well as parasympathetic innervation from sacral fibers. Neuraxial local anesthetic blockade interferes with bladder detrusor muscle function and internal and external sphincter function. Neuraxial opioids cause suppression of detrusor muscle contractility and decreased urge sensation by inhibition of sacral parasympathetic outflow. It is unclear to what extent neuraxial analgesia contributes to urinary retention during labor; parturients without neuraxial analgesia also frequently require bladder catheterization. Observational studies suggest that women with neuraxial analgesia have a higher rate of intrapartum and postpartum urinary retention than women who receive non-neuraxial or no analgesia; however, it is unclear whether the relationship is causal.[22] Parturients with neuraxial analgesia should be regularly assessed for urinary retention, especially if they complain of breakthrough pain. Some women are able to void when told their bladder is full; however, some may require catheterization to empty the bladder.

Delayed Gastric Emptying

Labor may result in delayed gastric emptying, and this delay is exacerbated by opioid administration, no matter the route. Delayed gastric emptying may contribute to nausea and vomiting, and it may increase the risk of pulmonary aspiration during the induction of general anesthesia.

COMPLICATIONS OF NEURAXIAL LABOR ANALGESIA

Unintentional Dural Puncture

A meta-analysis of studies of epidural procedures in obstetric patients estimated the incidence of unintentional dural puncture with an epidural needle at 1.5% (95% confidence interval [CI] 1.5-1.5).[23] Dural puncture may be detected at the time the epidural needle is advanced or after the "epidural" catheter is threaded unintentionally into the subarachnoid space. The anesthesia provider may elect to provide continuous spinal analgesia or may elect to resite the epidural catheter, usually at a different interspace. The incidence of postdural puncture headache after unintentional dural puncture with an epidural needle in the obstetric patient is slightly greater than 50%.[23]

Respiratory Depression

Respiratory depression may occur as a result of opioid administration by any route and is dose-dependent. Respiratory depression after the neuraxial administration of a lipid-soluble opioid occurs within 2 hours of injection. The risk appears greater if parenteral opioids are administered prior to neuraxial administration. The American Society of Anesthesiologists Practice Guidelines for the Prevention, Detection, and Management of Respiratory Depression Associated with Neuraxial Opioid Administration state that continual (ie, repeated regularly and frequently in steady rapid succession) monitoring should be performed for the first 20 minutes and that monitoring should continue at least once per hour for a minimum of 2 hours after neuraxial administration of a lipid-soluble opioid.[24] Monitoring should be performed at least once an hour for a continuous infusion.

Local Anesthetic Systemic Toxicity

Unintentional intravascular injection of local anesthetic, causing LAST, is a catastrophic complication of epidural anesthesia. The incidence is rare during epidural labor analgesia because of the use of low-dose local anesthetic solutions. Precautions against an unintentional intravascular injection are listed in Table 6-12. Recent reports suggest intravenous lipid emulsion therapy may improve rescue rates after LAST. The American Society of Regional Anesthesia and Pain Medicine updated 2012 Practice Advisory on Local Anesthetic Systemic Toxicity lists the level of evidence for lipid emulsion therapy as a category B (data derived from nonrandomized or laboratory studies, supported by multiple case reports or case series) and recommend considering its use at the first signs of LAST, immediately following airway management and initiation of cardiovascular resuscitation (1.5 mL/kg 20% lipid emulsion bolus, followed by 0.25 mL/kg per minute infusion for at least 10 minutes after circulatory stability is achieved).[25]

High or Total Spinal Anesthesia

High or total spinal anesthesia may result from the unrecognized and unintentional injection of high doses of local anesthetic into the subarachnoid space through a needle or catheter thought to be in the epidural space. A catheter that was originally sited in the epidural space may migrate to the subarachnoid space. Alternatively, a high cephalad blockade may result from an overdose of local anesthetic in the epidural or subdural space. The presence of a hole in the dura, made by recognized or unrecognized dural puncture with an epidural needle, increases the risk of a high block after epidural bolus injection of local anesthetic.

Symptoms of high spinal anesthesia include agitation, profound hypotension, dyspnea, inability to phonate, and loss of consciousness. Loss of consciousness is usually a result of brainstem hypoperfusion, not brain anesthesia. Symptoms usually appear within minutes after unintentional intrathecal injection but may take longer after an epidural or unintentional subdural injection (10-25 minutes). During

Table 6-12. Recommendations for Prevention of Local Anesthetic Toxicity

- Aspirate the needle or catheter before each injection.
- Consider use of an intravascular marker (eg, epinephrine or fentanyl) if injecting potentially toxic doses of local anesthetic (ie, use a test dose).
- Inject incremental doses (eg, 3-5 mL aliquots), pausing 15-30 seconds between each injection.
- Design systems to prevent accidental intravenous administration via an in situ peripheral or central intravenous catheter (eg, store epidural solutions in a different place than intravenous solutions).

continuous infusion analgesia, a gradual increase in the cephalad level of anesthesia, and an increase in the density of neuroblockade, may indicate intrathecal infusion of local anesthetic. Therefore, after any neuraxial local anesthetic injection, the anesthesia provider must observe the parturient for signs of high spinal anesthesia. Treatment includes management of the airway, ventilation, and oxygenation, and support of circulation. The patient may be paralyzed but not unconscious; therefore, sedative-hypnotics should be administered after the patient is stabilized.

Back Pain

More than 50% of women complain of back pain during and after pregnancy. Although several observation studies have linked epidural analgesia to postpartum back pain, randomized controlled trials comparing epidural to systemic opioid analgesia have not found an increased rate of back pain in women who receive epidural labor analgesia.[26] Short-term back tenderness may result from local tissue trauma at the site of skin puncture but usually resolves in several days.

ADVERSE EFFECTS OF NEURAXIAL LABOR ANALGESIA ON THE PROGRESS OF LABOR

Effects of Neuraxial Labor Analgesia on the Mode of Delivery

Observational studies suggest an association between neuraxial labor analgesia and increased risk of operative delivery. However, both randomized controlled trials and impact studies have consistently concluded that neuraxial analgesia does not cause an increased risk of cesarean delivery. Impact studies are before/after studies in which the outcome is measured (usually retrospectively) before the introduction of treatment (in this case, the availability of neuraxial labor analgesia), and after the introduction of treatment. Numerous impact studies have found that the introduction of a labor analgesia service, leading to a marked increase in the rate of neuraxial analgesia over a relatively short period of time, is not associated with an increased cesarean delivery rate.[27] For example, epidural analgesia was introduced into a large US military hospital in 1993.[28] The rate of epidural analgesia increased from 0% to more than 85%; the adjusted relative risk of cesarean delivery between the 1-year period immediate before the introduction of epidural analgesia, and the 1-year period after the introduction year was 0.8 (95% CI, 0.6-1.2).

Randomized controlled trials of the effect of neuraxial labor analgesia on the cesarean delivery rate are difficult to conduct. Optimally, a study of the effect of labor analgesia would randomize women to analgesia or no analgesia. However, because randomizing women to no analgesia is unethical, almost all randomized controlled trials have compared neuraxial analgesia to a control group who received systemic opioid analgesia. An additional limitation is that these studies cannot be blinded because the quality of analgesia is markedly different between the two techniques. Hence, neither obstetricians (who make the decision to proceed to intrapartum cesarean delivery) nor parturients are blinded to the treatment allocation group. In a 2011 meta-analysis of 27 randomized controlled trials that included

8417 parturients, the relative risk of cesarean delivery for epidural analgesia versus systemic opioid was 1.10 (95% CI 0.97-1.25) with minimal heterogeneity among studies.[1]

Controversy has existed regarding the timing of initiation of neuraxial analgesia. Observational studies suggest that early labor initiation of neuraxial analgesia (latent phase) is associated with in increased rate of cesarean delivery compared to initiation later in labor (active phase). However, randomized controlled trials comparing early labor (< 4 cm cervical dilation) to later initiation (women in the late group received systemic opioid analgesia until cervical dilation ≥ 4 cm) have consistently found that early initiation does not increase the risk of cesarean delivery.[21,29] Thus, the practice of encouraging women to wait until active labor to request neuraxial analgesia should be abandoned, and women should receive analgesia at any time in labor it is requested.

The findings in observational trials of an association between neuraxial analgesia and cesarean delivery are likely explained by selection bias. Studies have shown that women who have more painful labor have a higher cesarean delivery rate (likely because dysfunctional labor, larger fetuses, or malpositioned fetuses cause more pain and are risk factors for cesarean delivery), and women with more pain request neuraxial analgesia at a higher rate.[30]

The data regarding the effect of neuraxial labor analgesia on the risk of instrumental vaginal delivery are less consistent. A meta-analysis of seven impact studies (N = 28,443) found no difference in the instrumental vaginal delivery rate before and after the introduction of neuraxial labor analgesia (percent change 0.75%; 95% CI −1.2%-2.8%).[27] In contrast, a meta-analysis of randomized controlled trials of neuraxial versus systemic opioid analgesia, in which instrumental vaginal delivery was reported as a secondary outcome, found the risk of instrumental delivery was greater in women randomized to receive neuraxial analgesia (relative risk 1.42; 95% CI 1.28-1.57; risk difference 5%; number needed to treat 20).[1]

The risk of instrumental vaginal delivery may be influenced by the density of neuraxial analgesia. For example, a large, multicenter trial randomized women to one of three groups: epidural analgesia with 0.25% bupivacaine, epidural analgesia with 0.1% bupivacaine with fentanyl, or CSE analgesia maintained with 0.1% bupivacaine with fentanyl.[14] The risk of instrumental vaginal delivery was higher in the epidural 0.25% bupivacaine group compared to the two lower dose groups. Other studies have found similar results. Thus, taken together, studies suggest that neuraxial analgesia may increase the risk of instrumental vaginal delivery, but this risk can be minimized by using low-dose local anesthetic solutions and maintenance techniques that minimize total local anesthetic dose (eg, bolus versus continuous infusion techniques).

Effects of Neuraxial Labor Analgesia on the Duration of Labor

Randomized controlled trials of neuraxial labor compared to systemic opioid analgesia have assessed the duration of labor as secondary outcomes. A meta-analysis of 12 studies found no difference in the duration of the first stage of labor between groups.[1] However, the 95% CI was wide (−13 to 50 minutes) and the hetero-geneity among trials was significant. In contrast, the meta-analysis (13 trials) found the duration of the second stage of labor was significantly longer in women randomized to receive neuraxial analgesia (mean difference 14 minutes; 95% CI 7-21). Again, heterogeneity was significant. However, although the second stage was longer in the neuraxial group, there was no evidence that fetal outcomes were adversely affected.

CASE STUDY

A 30-year-old G3, P0 at 41.5 weeks' gestation is undergoing induction of labor due to "postdates." Her only significant medical history is a deep vein thrombosis discovered 5 years ago after a long road trip, which prompted a workup and subse-quent finding of factor V Leiden. During her pregnancy she was given prophylactic enoxaparin until 37 weeks' gestation, at which time she was switched to unfrac-tionated heparin 5000 U subcutaneous injection (twice a day). The patient's cervix is currently dilated to 2 cm, and she is complaining of 10/10 pain. The patient is requesting neuraxial analgesia, and the obstetrician has approved this request.

Questions

1. Which of the following blood tests is the *most* appropriate before initiating neuraxial analgesia:
   A. Hemoglobin/hematocrit
   B. Activated partial thromboplastin time (aPTT)
   C. Antibody screen (type and screen)
   D. Platelet count

2. Which of the following neuraxial procedures/drug combinations is *most* appro-priate for initiating analgesia in this patient?
   A. Combined spinal-epidural: plain bupivacaine 2.5 mg + fentanyl 15 μg
   B. Combined spinal-epidural: hyperbaric bupivacaine 2.5 mg + fentanyl 15 μg
   C. Epidural: fentanyl 50 μg
   D. Epidural: 10 mL of 0.25% bupivacaine + fentanyl 100 μg

3. Maintenance analgesia consisted of a patient-controlled epidural analgesia (PCEA) with a 8-mL/h background infusion of 0.0625% bupivacaine + fentanyl 2 μg/mL and patient-controlled epidural boluses of 8 mL every 10 minutes. Ten hours later, the nurse calls to report the patient is experiencing 7/10 sacral pain. The cervical examination is 9 cm, and the patient has a S4 – T9 bilateral sensory block. Which of the following approaches best describes the *most* appropriate next step?
   A. Administer 10 mL of the PCEA solution
   B. Sit the patient upright and administer epidural fentanyl 100 μg
   C. Administer 0.125% bupivacaine 10 mL
   D. Withhold additional analgesia because the patient is preparing to "push"

4. Which of the following drugs is *most* appropriate to administer for the treatment of the breakthrough pain?

    A. 10 mL ropivacaine 0.2%

    B. 15 mL lidocaine 2%

    C. 15 mL bupivacaine 0.25%

    D. Clonidine 100 µg

5. A cesarean delivery is deemed necessary for arrest of dilation at 6 cm cervical dilation following 26 hours of labor. Which of the following factors *most* likely contributed to an increased risk of cesarean delivery in this patient?

    A. Initiation of neuraxial analgesia at 2-cm cervical dilation

    B. Use of increased concentration of local anesthetic for breakthrough pain

    C. Induction of labor

    D. Use of neuraxial opioids

6. Following administration of 20 mL of lidocaine 2% + 1:200,000 epinephrine + bicarbonate in the operating room, the patient suddenly becomes unresponsive. Which of the following tasks is the *most* appropriate next step?

    A. Deliver the infant

    B. Ventilate the patient

    C. Administer lipid emulsion

    D. Check the blood glucose

Answers

1. **D.** Although the American Society of Anesthesiologists (ASA) Guidelines for Obstetric Anesthesia do not endorse routine request for platelet counts in healthy, laboring women requesting neuraxial analgesia, this patient has been taking subcutaneous heparin, which places her at risk of thrombocytopenia from heparin-induced thrombocytopenia. The American Society of Regional Anesthesia and Pain Medicine guidelines for neuraxial anesthesia and anticoagulation do not consider prophylactic subcutaneous heparin a contraindication to neuraxial placement, and an activated prothrombin time does not need to be obtained. The ASA Guidelines do not recommend routine assessment of antibody status in the intrapartum period; this is a routine antenatal assessment.

2. **A.** Hyperbaric bupivacaine does not provide adequate analgesia in early labor because it does not provide sensory blockade to the thoracic levels. Epidural fentanyl 50 µg is inadequate for labor analgesia. Higher doses are usually not used, because systemic absorption causes an unacceptably high incidence of adverse effects and analgesia may still not be complete. Ten milliliters of 0.25% bupivacaine (25 mg) is a large dose of bupivacaine for early labor and will result in a high incidence of hypotension and undesirable degree of motor block.

3. **C.** If the extent of thoracic and sacral sensory blockade is satisfactory (S4-T10), then the patient is likely having breakthrough pain due to an abnormal labor (ie, cephalopelvic disproportion or occiput posterior position of the fetal head), which typically requires higher doses of local anesthetic to achieve adequate labor analgesia. It is important to evaluate the progress of labor with the obstetrician or midwife to confirm abnormal labor progression or sacral sparing if the patient is advanced in labor. Position change alone will not correct or improve a unilateral epidural sensory block or sacral sparing. In advanced labor, the patient may experience inadequate analgesia in the sacral area due to larger nerve roots, increased distance from the epidural catheter placement site and more severe pain. Sacral pain from vaginal and perineal distention is somatic pain, and therefore an opioid alone, without a local anesthetic, may not treat the pain. A redose is appropriate in advanced labor, because adequate expulsive force can be achieved without sacral sensation. Ten milliliters of 0.125% bupivacaine is unlikely to result in dense motor blockade.

4. **A.** Lidocaine 2% is the concentration used for epidural anesthesia for cesarean delivery and will result in dense analgesia with motor blockade. Fifteen milliliters of 0.25% bupivacaine will also result in dense analgesia and is likely an overdose for this patient. The clonidine dose is too high and may result in hypotension and sedation.

5. **C.** There are well-conducted randomized controlled studies demonstrating no increased risk of cesarean delivery due to neuraxial anesthetic techniques or timing of administration of neuraxial techniques. There are no studies evaluating the effects of intravenous opioids or neuraxial opioids on labor progression. Nulliparous women who are induced are at greater risk of cesarean delivery than those who present in spontaneous labor.

6. **B.** The first task in treating an unresponsive patient is to ventilate the patient and then obtain control of the airway. The patient may have had total spinal anesthesia from migration of the epidural catheter into the intrathecal space; local anesthetic toxicity from migration of the epidural catheter into an epidural vein; or even a medical condition such as supine hypotension syndrome, massive pulmonary embolism, or amniotic fluid embolism. The cause is secondary until this patient's airway is secured.

REFERENCES

1. Anim-Somuah M, Smyth RM, Jones L. Epidural versus non-epidural or no analgesia in labour. *Cochrane Database Syst Rev.* 2011;12:CD000331.
2. Simkin P, Bolding A. Update on nonpharmacologic approaches to relieve labor pain and prevent suffering. *J Midwifery Womens Health.* 2004;49(6):489-504.
3. Smith CA, Collins CT, Cyna AM, Crowther CA. Complementary and alternative therapies for pain management in labour. *Cochrane Database Syst Rev.* 2006(4):CD003521.
4. American College of Obstetricians and Gynecologists. Analgesia and cesarean delivery rates. Committee Opinion No. 339: *Obstet Gynecol.* 2006;107(6):1487-1488.
5. Horlocker TT, Wedel DJ, Rowlingson JC, et al. Regional anesthesia in the patient receiving antithrombotic or thrombolytic therapy: American Society of Regional Anesthesia and Pain Medicine Evidence-Based Guidelines, 3rd ed. *Reg Anesth Pain Med.* 2010;35(1):64-101.

6. Practice guidelines for obstetric anesthesia: an updated report by the American Society of Anesthesiologists Task Force on Obstetric Anesthesia. *Anesthesiology.* 2007;106(4):843-863.

7. Bethune L, Harper N, Lucas DN, et al. Complications of obstetric regional analgesia: how much information is enough? *Int J Obstet Anesth.* 2004;13(1):30-34.

8. Simmons SW, Cyna AM, Dennis AT, Hughes D. Combined spinal-epidural versus epidural analgesia in labour. *Cochrane Database Syst Rev.* 2007(3):CD003401.

9. Van de Velde M. Neuraxial opioids for labour analgesia: analgesic efficiency and effect on labour. *Curr Opin Anaesthesiol.* 2002;15(3):299-303.

10. Lyons GR, Kocarev MG, Wilson RC, Columb MO. A comparison of minimum local anesthetic volumes and doses of epidural bupivacaine (0.125% w/v and 0.25% w/v) for analgesia in labor. *Anesth Analg.* 2007;104(2):412-415.

11. Beilin Y, Halpern S. Focused review: ropivacaine versus bupivacaine for epidural labor analgesia. *Anesth Analg.* 2010;111(2):482-487.

12. Palmer CM, Cork RC, Hays R, Van Maren G, Alves D. The dose-response relation of intrathecal fentanyl for labor analgesia. *Anesthesiology.* 1998;88(2):355-361.

13. Herman NL, Calicott R, Van Decar TK, Conlin G, Tilton J. Determination of the dose-response relationship for intrathecal sufentanil in laboring patients. *Anesth Analg.* 1997;84(6):1256-1261.

14. Comparative Obstetric Mobile Epidural Trial Study Group UK. Effect of low-dose mobile versus traditional epidural techniques on mode of delivery: a randomised controlled trial. *Lancet.* 2001;358(9275):19-23.

15. Bogod DG, Rosen M, Rees GA. Extradural infusion of 0.125% bupivacaine at 10 mL/hr to women during labor. *Br J Anaesth.* 1987;59(3):325-330.

16. Halpern SH, Carvalho B. Patient-controlled epidural analgesia for labor. *Anesth Analg.* 2009;108(3): 921-928.

17. Clarke VT, Smiley RM, Finster M. Uterine hyperactivity after intrathecal injection of fentanyl for analgesia during labor: a cause of fetal bradycardia? *Anesthesiology.* 1994;81(4):1083.

18. Abrao KC, Francisco RP, Miyadahira S, Cicarelli DD, Zugaib M. Elevation of uterine basal tone and fetal heart rate abnormalities after labor analgesia: a randomized controlled trial. *Obstet Gynecol.* 2009;113(1):41-47.

19. Segal S. Labor epidural analgesia and maternal fever. *Anesth Analg.* 2010;111(6):1467-1475.

20. Panzer O, Ghazanfari N, Sessler DI, et al. Shivering and shivering-like tremor during labor with and without epidural analgesia. *Anesthesiology.* 1999;90(6):1609-1616.

21. Wong CA, Scavone BM, Peaceman AM, et al. The risk of cesarean delivery with neuraxial analgesia given early versus late in labor. *N Engl J Med.* 2005;352(7):655-665.

22. Weiniger CF, Wand S, Nadjari M, et al. Post-void residual volume in labor: a prospective study comparing parturients with and without epidural analgesia. *Acta Anaesthesiol Scand.* 2006;50(10):1297-1303.

23. Choi PT, Galinski SE, Takeuchi L, et al. PDPH is a common complication of neuraxial blockade in parturients: a meta-analysis of obstetrical studies. *Can J Anaesth.* 2003;50(5):460-469.

24. Horlocker TT, Burton AW, Connis RT, et al. Practice guidelines for the prevention, detection, and management of respiratory depression associated with neuraxial opioid administration. *Anesthesiology.* 2009;110(2):218-230.

25. Neal JM, Mulroy MF, Weinberg GL, et al. American Society of Regional Anesthesia and Pain Medicine checklist for managing local anesthetic systemic toxicity: 2012 version. *Reg Anesth Pain Med* 2012; 37 (1): 16-8.

26. Loughnan BA, Carli F, Romney M, Dore CJ, Gordon H. Epidural analgesia and backache: a randomized controlled comparison with intramuscular meperidine for analgesia during labour. *Br J Anaesth.* 2002;89(3):466-472.

27. Segal S, Su M, Gilbert P. The effect of a rapid change in availability of epidural analgesia on the cesarean delivery rate: a meta-analysis. *Am J Obstet Gynecol.* 2000;183(4):974-978.

28. Zhang J, Yancey MK, Klebanoff MA, Schwarz J, Schweitzer D. Does epidural analgesia prolong labor and increase risk of cesarean delivery? A natural experiment. *Am J Obstet Gynecol.* 2001;185(1):128-134.

29. Wassen MM, Zuijlen J, Roumen FJ, et al. Early versus late epidural analgesia and risk of instrumental delivery in nulliparous women: a systematic review. *BJOG.* 2011;118(6):655-661.

30. Hess PE, Pratt SD, Soni AK, Sarna MC, Oriol NE. An association between severe labor pain and cesarean delivery. *Anesth Analg.* 2000;90(4):881-886.

Ultrasound in Obstetric Anesthesia

7

Kamal Kumar and Timothy P. Turkstra

INTRODUCTION

Ultrasound has emerged as a valuable tool in anesthesia practice, "unblinding" many of what were once "blind" procedures. Because ultrasound is a radiation-free imaging tool, it has gained popularity for patient management in many areas of medicine. In anesthesia practice, it has become important for line placement[1] and provides some distinct advantages in placement of regional anesthesia.[2] The educational benefits of ultrasound imaging for teaching regional anesthesia have also been elucidated.[3,4]

In obstetric anesthesia, central neuraxial blockade analgesia is the most common anesthetic technique. The availability of ultrasound has naturally extended interest in this modality from peripheral nerve blocks to facilitating spinal/epidural techniques in obstetrics. Successful use of spinal ultrasound to aid in the placement of epidural and spinal injection in obstetric anesthesia was first reported in 1984.[5] Recently, as ultrasound machines with higher quality images have become more affordable and more commonly available, their popularity has increased further.

Several studies conducted to assess the effectiveness of spinal ultrasound for epidural anesthesia have shown that an ultrasound-guided neuraxial approach can reduce the number of attempts and the procedure time while at the same time increasing the block success rate.[6-8] These studies have provided a foundation for National Institute of Clinical Excellence (NICE) guidelines related to ultrasound imaging to facilitate instrumentation of the epidural space.[9] The benefits of routine ultrasound imaging for intrathecal anesthetic placement are less clear.

ULTRASOUND TECHNOLOGY

Ultrasound imaging is based on high-frequency sound waves that are transmitted and received by a transducer (1-20 MHz). The transducer detects both the intensity of the echo and the time required to travel back to the source, which enables the calculation of the distance of the reflecting interface. Different layers of tissue produce a separate reflection of the ultrasound signal. At each interface, some of the wave is reflected back and detected by the transducer. The proportion of reflected to transmitted wave depends on acoustic impedance of tissues forming the interface. Bone reflects the majority of the energy, so few structures beyond bone can be visualized. Ultrasound examination of spine is challenging because the area of interest is deep and shielded by a complex, articulated cage of bones. For these reasons, images of the spinal structures are best observed with a low-frequency, curved ultrasound probe (2-5 MHz). Although higher frequency allows higher image resolution, the low frequency ultrasound beam provides deeper penetration, at the expense of image resolution.

Two acoustic windows are effective for lumbar spine sonographic assessment: one seen on the transverse approach and one seen on the longitudinal paramedian approach. The information from these two scanning planes complements each other.

IMPLICATIONS OF ULTRASOUND IN OBSTETRIC ANESTHESIA

Educational Implications

Ultrasound can be an important teaching tool in anesthesia. Sonographic visualization of anatomical structures can help improve understanding of spatial relationships and increase confidence in trainees, potentially reducing complications. In obstetric anesthesia, the learning curve for labor epidural placement has improved significantly with the advent of ultrasound imaging for teaching epidural anesthesia.[3] Preprocedure ultrasound examination has reduced the number of attempts and failures[10] for placing epidural catheters by anesthesiology trainees. It can be used as a preoperative assessment tool for predicting the feasibility/difficulty of neuraxial blockade.[11,12] It appears that resident learning can be improved with the addition of ultrasound imaging.

Clinical Implications

- Neuraxial blockade
- Acute and chronic pain control
- Vascular access
- Cardiac evaluation

NEURAXIAL BLOCK

Ultrasonic assessment of the lumbar spine in assisting neuraxial anesthesia placement has become increasingly used in obstetric anesthesia. The efficacy and safety of ultrasound-guided neuraxial blocks in obstetrics have been evaluated by several studies.[3,5-9] The conventional method used to perform neuraxial blocks is based on using palpation to identify bony landmarks. Pregnancy-associated weight gain and presacral edema can obscure anatomic landmarks and render palpation more complex and challenging. This can lead to an increase in the likelihood of block failure or complications, which can also be augmented with obesity, spine abnormalities, and prior back surgery. Ultrasound prepuncture scanning can provide information on the sonoanatomy of the lumbar spine. Studies have shown that the success rate of ultrasound-guided epidural insertions at first attempt was 30% to 60% greater when compared with the conventional epidural palpation technique.[13] For intrathecal anesthetic placement, the benefits are less clear.

Advantages of Neuraxial Ultrasound

- More accurate location of midline
- Accurate determination of interspace level
- Suggestion of optimal needle puncture point and the angle of the puncture
- Estimation of depth of the epidural space
- Valuable teaching tool
- Increased in efficacy and decreased in duration of procedure
- May decrease the number of attempts and hence trauma
- Potential reduction in the number of unintentional dural punctures and other complications
- Useful in identifying atypical anatomy, including that associated with obesity, scoliosis, and previous spinal instrumentation

Ultrasound Examination of the Lumbar Spine

A systematic approach to ultrasound imaging of the spine has been described and builds on a detailed knowledge of lumbar spine anatomy. In 2008, The National Institute for Health and Clinical Excellence (NICE) issued guidelines for the use of lumber ultrasound imaging.[9] Commonly used approaches to access the acoustical windows of lumbar spines are longitudinal paramedian and the transverse approaches. The pattern of images is described as the "saw sign" in the longitudinal paramedian approach (Figure 7-1) and "flying bat" in the transverse approach (Figure 7-2). In the "saw sign," the teeth of the "saw" represent the articular processes and the spaces between the teeth represent the interspinous spaces, which consist of the ligamentum flavum/posterior longitudinal ligament and the vertebral body.[14] Due to wider acoustic window in longitudinal approach, the ultrasonic images obtained in this plane are superior in quality compared with those obtained in the transverse plane, but the information obtained from each of these views complement each other.

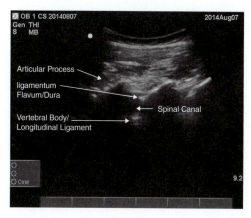

Figure 7-1. "Saw sign" in longitudinal paramedian approach.

Sonoanatomical Landmarks Seen in the Longitudinal Paramedian Approach

- Sacrum
- Lamina
- Ligamentum flavum and dorsal dura mater
- Spinal canal
- Vertebral body/longitudinal ligament

Sonoanatomical Landmarks Seen in the Transverse Approach

- Transverse process
- Articular process
- Spinous process

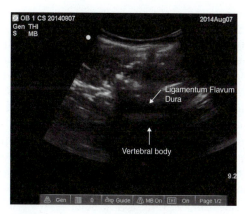

Figure 7-2. "Flying bat sign" in transverse approach.

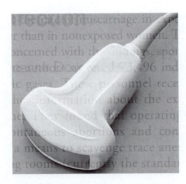

Figure 7-3. Low-frequency curved transducer.

- Ligamentum flavum
- Spinal canal
- Vertebral body/longitudinal ligament

Stepwise Approach for Neuraxial Ultrasound

SELECT AN APPROPRIATE TRANSDUCER TO OBTAIN THE BEST IMAGE

A low-frequency (2-5 MHz) curved transducer is required for spine ultrasound (Figure 7-3). Depth settings of 9 to 14 cm should be used to view all of the relevant structures. The angle of the transducer should be perpendicular to the structures of interest because the ultrasound waves returned to the transducer to the maximum extent at this angle. This helps to obtain the optimum quality image.

ENSURE THAT THE PATIENT IS IN THE PROPER POSITION

The patient should be placed in the flexed forward position and curled inward. This may be accomplished in either the lateral decubitus or sitting position.

START BY SCANNING FIRST IN THE LONGITUDINAL PLANE

This is the preferred plane for counting the interspace levels. The probe is initially placed over the sacral area, 2 to 3 cm to the left of the midline and slightly angled to the center of the spinal canal. At this point, the sacrum is visualized as a continuous bright line (Figure 7-4A). The probe is then slowly moved cephalad until a hyperechoic sawlike image is seen (Figure 7-5). The exact level of each interspace (L5-S1 to L1-L2) can then be marked at this point (Figure 7-4B).

Once the interspaces are marked and the level to be scanned is identified, the transverse scanning can be performed by positioning the probe horizontally and perpendicular to the long axis of the spine at the marked levels. With this approach, the midline of the spine corresponding to the spinous process is identified as a small hyperechoic signal immediately underneath the skin (Figure 7-6B).

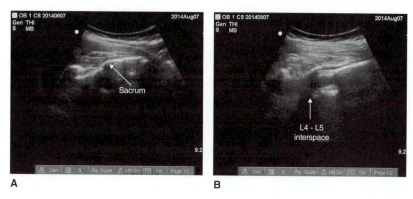

A   B

Figure 7-4. Longitudinal scan showing Sacrum.

The probe is then moved slightly cephalad or caudad to capture a view of the best acoustic window of an interspace. Once the clear image of the interspace is obtained, the image is frozen and the transducer is kept still, and the skin is marked at the center of both the upper and the lateral aspects of the transducer. The transducer is then removed, and lines are drawn to connect these marks. The needle insertion point is determined by the intersection of these two lines.

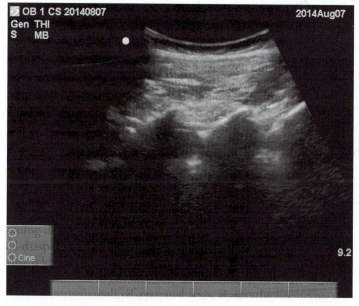

Figure 7-5. Longitudinal paramedian spine view.

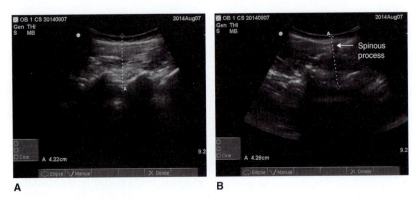

Figure 7-6. Distance to the ligamentum flavum.

The distance to the ligamentum flavum can also be measured using the ultrasound image at this time (Figure 7-6).

ACUTE PAIN MANAGEMENT

Acute pain management after cesarean section remains challenging. A significant component of postcesarean pain is incisional pain from the anterior abdominal wall which is supplied by the anterior rami of T7-L1. These nerves, after exiting the spinal column, proceed through the lateral abdominal wall within the transversus abdominal fascial plane and then terminate in the anterior abdominal wall. With a transversus abdominal plane (TAP) block, these nerves can be blocked with a bilateral injection to supplement other postoperative pain modalities, such as intraspinal opioids. Ultrasound guidance for TAP block has increased the efficacy and success of this block.[15,16] Studies have shown that a multimodal postoperative analgesic approach along with ultrasound TAP block provides superior pain relief in terms of decreased pain scores and postoperative opioid consumption, which can also reduce undesirable side effects of systemic narcotics.[10,17] See Figure 7-7 for the further use of ultrasound and a TAP block.

VASCULAR ACCESS

The use of ultrasound for central venous cannulation has become a standard of care in anesthesia practice.[1] The NICE guidelines[1] recommend the use of ultrasound as a standard practice in central venous access.

Benefits of Ultrasound Guidance Vascular Access

- Detection of anatomic variations and exact vessel location.
- Avoidance of central veins with preexisting thrombosis.
- An excellent teaching tool to improve the understanding of the procedure.

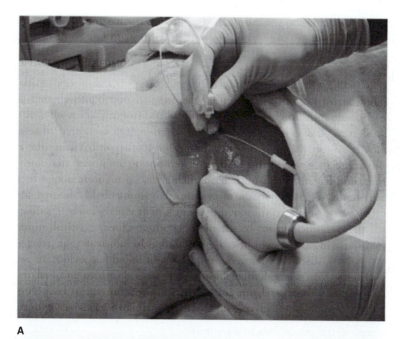

A

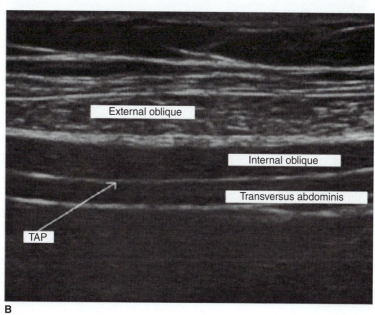

B

Figure 7-7. Transversus abdominal plane TAP plane.

- Increased the success rate and reduced complications such as accidental arterial puncture, failed placement, malposition of the catheter tip, hematoma, pneumothorax, and hemothorax.

- Ultrasound has been proven very useful in "difficult to cannulate" conditions such as patients who are morbidly obese, hypovolemic, or coagulopathic or in those patients who cannot tolerate recumbent position and also when landmark-based cannulation has failed.

- The use of ultrasound is also becoming popular for peripheral venous cannulation and also for arterial cannulation to monitor invasive blood pressure.

PERIOPERATIVE CARDIAC EVALUATION AND MONITORING

Although a detailed discussion about transthoracic echocardiography (TTE) is beyond the scope of this chapter, it is a safe, portable, and noninvasive modality for determining cardiovascular function. The anterior and left displacement of the heart, combined with an elevated diaphragm, are unique characteristics in a pregnant woman, which facilitate TTE examination, and partial left lateral tilt assist with parasternal and apical views. TTE may be used for obstetric applications in routine locations such as the birthing suite, emergency department, operating theater, and in the postanesthetic care unit.

ROLE IN OBSTETRIC ANESTHESIA[15,18,19]

- The rapid obstetric screening echocardiography scan can be used to rapidly assess the critically ill pregnant women.
- Assist in diagnosis of intraoperative and postoperative hypotension despite adequate fluid resuscitation.
- Peripartum cardiac disease is a leading cause of maternal mortality. The use of TTE and early diagnosis of peripartum cardiomyopathy, tamponade, or pulmonary embolism may help to formulate a management plan.
- Implementation of TTE in routine practice of obstetrics may assist quality assurance.
- TTE probe can be used to assess fetal heart rate.
- It may be an opportunity to increase our knowledge base surrounding parturients and improve obstetric care.

CONCLUSION

The use of ultrasound has been shown to be beneficial in clinical practice and is becoming increasingly popular. Obstetric anesthesiologists and trainees should be encouraged to utilize this technology in routine practice.

ACKNOWLEDGMENT

A special thanks to Dr. Kevin Armstrong and Dr. Rakesh Vijayshanker for their help for images.

REFERENCES

1. Guidance for the use of ultrasound locating devices for placing central venous catheters. 2002. National Institute for Clinical Excellence (NICE). Sep 1, 2002.
2. Neal JM, Brull R, Chan VW, et al. The ASRA evidence-based medicine assessment of ultrasound-guided regional anesthesia and pain medicine: *Reg Anesth Pain Med*. 2010;35(2 suppl 1):S1-S9.
3. Orebaugh SL, Williams BA, Kentor ML. Ultrasound guidance with nerve stimulation reduces the time necessary for resident peripheral nerve blockade. *Reg Anesth Pain Med*. 2007;32(5):448-454.
4. Vallejo MC, Phelps AL, Singh S, Orebaugh SL, Sah N. Ultrasound decreases the failed labor epidural rate in resident trainees. *Int J Obstet Anesth*. 2010;19(4):373-378.
5. Currie JM. Measurement of the depth to the extradural space using ultrasound. *Br J Anaesth*. 1984;56(4):345-347.
6. Grau T, Leipold RW, Conradi R, Martin E, Motsch J. Ultrasound imaging facilitates localization of the epidural space during combined spinal-epidural anesthesia. *Reg Anaesth*. 2001;26:64-67.
7. Grau T, Leipold RW, Conradi R, Martin E, Motsch J. Ultrasonography and peridural anesthesia. Technical possibilities and limitations of ultrasonic examination of the epidural space. *Anaesthesist*. 2001;50(2):94-101.
8. Grau T, Bartusseck E, Conradi R, Martin E, Motsch J. Ultrasound imaging improves learning curves in obstetric epidural anesthesia: a preliminary study. *Can J Anaesth*. 2003;50:1047-1050.
9. IPG 249 Ultrasound-guided catheterisation of the epidural space. 2008. National Institute of Clinical Excellence (NICE). Jan 1, 2008.
10. Mishriky BM, George RB, Habib AS. Transversus abdominis plane block for analgesia after Cesarean delivery: a systematic review and meta-analysis. *Can J Anaesth*. 2012;59(8):766-778.
11. Chin KJ, Chan V. Ultrasonography as a preoperative assessment tool: predicting the feasibility of central neuraxial blockade. *Anesth Analg*. 2010;110(1):252-253.
12. Weed JT, Taenzer AH, Finkel KJ, Sites BD. Evaluation of pre-procedure ultrasound examination as a screening tool for difficult spinal anesthesia. *Anaesthesia*. 2011;66:925-930.
13. Balki M. Locating the epidural space in obstetric patients-ultrasound a useful tool: continuing professional development. *Can J Anaesth*. 2010;57(12):1111-1126.
14. Carvalho J. Ultrasound-facilitated epidurals and spinals in obstetrics. *Anesthesiol Clin*. 2008;26:145-158.
15. Belavy D, Cowlishaw PJ, Howes M, Phillips F. Ultrasound-guided transversus abdominis plane block for analgesia after caesarean delivery. *Br J Anaesth*. 2009;103:726-730.
16. Baaj J, Alsatli R, Majaj H, Babay Z, Thallaj A. Efficacy of ultrasound guided transversus abdominis plane (TAP) block for post cesarean section delivery analgesia—a double-blind, placebo-controlled, randomized study. *Middle East J Anaesthesiol*. 2010;20:821-826.
17. Siddiqui MR, Sajid MS, Uncles DR, Cheek L, Baig MK. A meta-analysis on the clinical effectiveness of transversus abdominis plane block. *J Clin Anesth*. 2011;23(1):7-14.
18. Dennis AT. Transthoracic echocardiography in obstetric anesthesia and obstetric critical illness. *Int J Obstet Anesth*. 2011;20(2):160-168.
19. Dennis A, Stenson A. The use of transthoracic echocardiography in postpartum hypotension. *Anesth Analg*. 2012;115(5):1033.

Non-neuraxial Labor Analgesia

Ingrid Browne and Mairead Deighan

8

Labor is different for every woman, and the methods chosen for pain relief will depend on the obstetric/medical condition, the techniques locally available, and the preference of the patient. Neuraxial analgesia is the most effective method. However, there are many mothers who wish to avoid intervention or in whom the technique is contraindicated or impossible to perform. Contraindications for regional labor analgesia may include coagulopathy, local infection, allergy to local anesthetics, and uncorrected hypovolemia. Difficulties in placing epidurals can arise from anatomical deformities, postsurgical spine corrections, and obesity. For this group of parturients, alternative methods may be required and often will involve alternatives to neuraxial analgesia such as nonpharmacologic and pharmacologic techniques.

NONPHARMACOLOGIC LABOR ANALGESIA

Childbirth Education

Antenatal childbirth education is a critical first step for a labor analgesia plan. This dates back to the 1930s, when Grantley Dick-Read in England suggested that childbirth did not require medical intervention if the mother was adequately prepared. In the 1950s, Dr Lamaze, a French obstetrician, developed psychoprophylaxis. This technique involves education regarding the physiologic process of labor and delivery with trained relaxation response to contractions. The technique also uses patterned breathing with two goals: increasing maternal oxygenation and interfering with pain signal transmission to the cerebral cortex from the uterus. Although antenatal education will undoubtedly alleviate some of the fear and anxiety associated with labor, it is unrealistic to suggest that it will lead to painless childbirth for the majority of mothers.

Doulas

Coming from the Greek word for "servant or slave," a *doula* is a woman trained to attend to the emotional and physical needs of the parturient. Research has suggested that continuous support and encouragement from doulas throughout labor reduces the need for epidural, analgesic interventions, and the rate of operative deliveries.[1]

Transcutaneous Electrical Nerve Stimulation

Transcutaneous electrical nerve stimulation (TENS) is a noninvasive method using surface electrodes placed over the T10-L1 dermatomes and is most effective in early labor. A second set of electrodes can be placed over the S2-S4 dermatomes for second stage pain relief. Conventional TENS utilizes low-intensity, high-frequency biphasic pulsed currents in a repetitive manner with pulse durations of 50 to 250 ms and pulse frequencies of 1 to 200/s. The efficacy of TENS relates to the gate control theory of pain. The electrical current is postulated to reduce pain via nociceptive inhibition at a presynaptic level in the dorsal horn of the spinal cord, thus limiting central transmission of pain impulses. The electrical cutaneous stimulation preferentially activates low-threshold myelinated nerve fibers. This afferent activity inhibits propagation of nociception in small unmyelinated C fibers by blocking transmission to the target cells located within laminae 2 and 3 of the substantia gelatinosa of the dorsal horn.[2] Another proposed theory is that TENS enhances the release of endorphins and enkephalins, which are naturally occurring neuropeptides.[2] Currently, there is no evidence that TENS is superior to placebo; however, it is minimally invasive, allows mobilization during use, and is widely available.[3]

Hydrotherapy

Immersion in warm water to where the abdomen is covered is thought to benefit the mother by facilitating muscular relaxation. There is some evidence that it can reduce women's perceptions of pain and the demand for regional analgesia in the first stage of labor.[4] It is not associated with adverse outcomes on duration of labor, operative delivery, or neonatal outcome.[5] Continuous fetal monitoring cannot be carried out in the birthing pool, so it is not suitable for mothers carrying an at-risk fetus. Similarly, for mothers requiring any kind of continuous monitoring, intravenous infusions, or pharmacologic analgesia, the birthing pool is inadvisable.

Hypnosis, Acupuncture, Aromatherapy, and Reflexology

Hypnosis can be described as an altered state of consciousness with reduced awareness of external stimuli and an increased response to verbal or nonverbal communications. Highly motivated mothers can learn self-hypnosis to dampen the perception of pain and the physiologic responses to pain. Currently, available evidence suggests that it does lead to increased maternal satisfaction and reduces the need for pharmacologic pain relief, including epidurals, in labor.[6]

Acupuncture involves the insertion of fine needles into the body to a depth of 2.5 to 3 cm at specified areas. There are about 400 acupuncture points and

20 meridians connecting these points. Each of the 20 meridians corresponds to an organ. The acupuncture points used in labor are on the hands, feet, and ears. Acupuncture is thought to stimulate the body to produce endorphins and thereby reduce pain. There are few studies concerning its use in obstetric practice, but it does appear to reduce pain and analgesic requirements in labor.[7]

Aromatherapy utilizes the healing power of plants, and reflexology involves manipulating and pressing parts of the feet. There is no strong evidence that either of these is effective in the management of labor pain. However, some mothers gain emotional support and satisfaction from the aforementioned alternative therapies and, because they are harmless, there is little reason to discourage their use.

PHARMACOLOGIC LABOR ANALGESIA

Inhalational Agents

Since Sir James Young Simpson began using chloroform ether for labor pain relief in 1847, volatile agents and anesthetic gases have been used in childbirth. In the United Kingdom and Europe, a mixture of 50% nitrous oxide and 50% oxygen (Entonox) is used extensively. Nitrous oxide has a low blood-gas partition coefficient and accordingly, a rapid onset and offset of action. It is self-administered through a mouthpiece incorporating a two-stage reducing and on-demand valve. Should the mother become drowsy, the delivery system will be released before unconsciousness occurs. Entonox needs to be inhaled for at least 45 seconds to achieve maximum analgesic effect, so deep inhalation must start as soon as the contraction is first felt. It may cause disorientation, drowsiness, and nausea in some mothers. However, it does relieve labor pain to some degree, and it is easy to use, inexpensive, has minimal accumulation with intermittent use, and is safe for mother and fetus.

Sevoflurane has a physical profile similar to nitrous oxide. As well as having a rapid uptake and washout rate, it is nonirritant. Some research has suggested that in subanesthetic concentrations (0.8%), sevoflurane provides better pain relief than Entonox in the first stage of labor.[8] Sevoflurane may also be associated with less nausea and vomiting. Despite this, it has not been widely utilized because of the potential risk of somnolence and technical difficulties related to an effective scavenging system.

Systemic Opioids

MEPERIDINE

Meperidine is a synthetic phenylpiperidine derivative designed originally as an anticholinergic agent, but subsequently it was found to have analgesic properties. Since its introduction as an analgesic in 1940, it has become one of the most common opioids used in early labor. It has been given intramuscularly in doses of 50 to 150 mg. Its analgesic effects are experienced after 10 to 15 minutes and last for up to 3 hours. It provides only very modest analgesia, but because it is inexpensive and easy to administer, its use is widespread.[9] Meperidine, in common with other opioids, causes sedation, delayed gastric emptying, nausea and vomiting, and dose-dependent respiratory depression.

Meperidine crosses the placenta, with the maximum fetal plasma concentration occurring 2 to 3 hours after maternal intramuscular administration. It can cause decreased variability on the cardiotocograph and greater fetal acidosis during labor than occurs with epidurals. Neonatal effects are compounded by the metabolite normeperidine, which has mild activity. This accumulates in the fetus due to delayed clearance and causes sedation and respiratory depression. Infants of mothers given meperidine have also been found to have impaired neurobehavioral scores.[10] Meperidine also raises the seizure threshold, and patients tend to be sleepier, less attentive, and less successful at establishing breast feeding.[11]

OTHER PARENTERAL OPIOIDS

Morphine has a longer duration of action than other opioids and is therefore used more cautiously in labor. With similar side effects to meperidine, it rapidly crosses the placenta and can cause sedation and neonatal depression.

Diamorphine, a synthetic form of heroin, is more potent than meperidine and can be administered intramuscularly in doses of 5 to 7.5 mg. It is popular as a labor analgesic in some parts of the United Kingdom; however, is not widely available in other countries.

Fentanyl is also a phenylpiperidine derivative with a rapid onset of action. It exhibits a longer context-sensitive half-life than both morphine and meperidine with repeated doses, leading to potential drug accumulation in both the fetus and the mother.

OPIOID AGONIST-ANTAGONIST DERIVATIVES

Buprenorphine is a partial μ and δ agonist and a κ antagonist. It is 20 to 30 times more potent than morphine but its common side effects include nausea and sedation.

Butorphanol is a κ agonist and a partial μ agonist and antagonist. It is five times more potent than morphine. It causes less nausea and vomiting but produces excessive sedation. Unlike meperidine, its metabolites are inactive. Butorphanol can be associated with a drug-induced form of sinusoidal fetal heart rate pattern, which can be alarming, because this fetal heart rate pattern usually signifies fetal hypoxia/anemia if not associated with butorphanol administration.

Nalbuphine is a partial δ and κ agonist and a μ antagonist. It is less potent than morphine. Although it appears to cause less nausea and vomiting, it does result in a greater degree of sedation and dizziness.

The unfavorable side-effect profile of these drugs has limited their usage in obstetric pain relief.

Intravenous Patient-Controlled Analgesia

Intravenous patient-controlled analgesia (IV PCA) is more effective than parenteral analgesia but requires adequate equipment and staffing. Parenteral opioids can be titrated to result in moderate analgesia, enabling the mother to have a degree of control.

Remifentanil, an ultrashort-acting opioid, has unique characteristics, making it an "ideal" drug for labor IV PCA. It is a pure μ agonist with an ester linkage that

Table 8-1. Suggested Regimens for Intravenous Patient-Controlled Analgesia

Drug	Bolus Dose	Lockout Time
Remifentanil	30-50 μg	2 minutes
Meperidine	10-15 mg	10 minutes
Fentanyl	l10-25 μg	5 minutes

results in rapid metabolism by nonspecific plasma and tissue esterases. Its duration of action is thus determined by metabolism and not distribution, and because of an abundance of esterases, the duration of administration does not affect the duration of action. The drug has a rapid onset with peak effect at 60 to 90 seconds and also exhibits rapid clearance (2800 mL/min). Remifentanil also appears to be safe for the fetus. Research suggests that remifentanil crosses the placenta but is swiftly metabolized and/or redistributed.[9] Remifentanil has maternal side effects; in common with all opioids, sedation and respiratory depression are the two most concerning. Maternal oxygen saturation, heart rate, respiratory rate, blood pressure, and sedation level should be monitored continuously. With the drug's short duration of action, however, any problems should be quickly and easily reversed. It is generally administered using a bolus dose of 30 to 50 μg and a lockout time of 2 minutes.

Fentanyl and meperidine have also been used for IV PCA for labor. Dosage regimens are presented in Table 8-1. Studies suggest that remifentanil provides better pain relief and higher maternal satisfaction than both meperidine and fentanyl, with no difference in fetal outcome.[11,12] Remifentanil's effect does appear to decrease after 2 hours,[13] and so it may be more effective in parous women who are likely to have shorter labors.

Non-neuraxial Blocks (Performed by Obstetricians)

A paracervical block is a bilateral injection of low-dose bupivacaine around the paracervical (Frankenhauser's) ganglia that can provide up to 2 hours of uterine and cervical anesthesia during the first stage of labor. However, there may be reduced uterine blood flow or increased uterine tone, which may result in fetal asphyxia.

A pudendal block is a bilateral blockade of this nerve (S2, S3, S4) that can produce vaginal, vulvar, and perineal anesthesia for the second stage of labor. It is safe and gives effective analgesia for spontaneous vaginal and low-forceps delivery. The pudendal nerve may be blocked via the transvaginal or transperineal route. However, success bilaterally can be as low as 50%. Maternal or fetal complications of pudendal nerve block are unusual but may include fetal trauma or direct injection of local anesthetic into the fetus.

The distribution of the sensory pathways for labor pain and the targets of the analgesic effects of different techniques of regional anesthesia are shown in Figure 8-1.[14]

In summary, there are many analgesic options for laboring mothers who cannot avail themselves of neuraxial analgesic techniques or those who would like an alternative option.

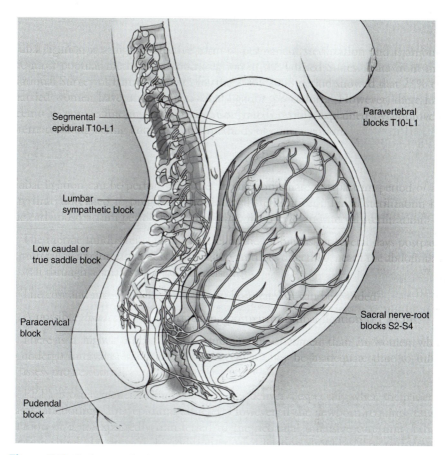

Figure 8-1. Pathways of Labor Pain. Labor pain has a visceral component and a somatic component. Uterine contractions may result in myometrial ischemia, causing the release of potassium, bradykinin, histamine, and serotonin. In addition, stretching and distention of the lower segments of the uterus and the cervix stimulate mechanoreceptors. These noxious impulses follow sensory-nerve fibers that accompany sympathetic nerve endings, traveling through the paracervical region and the pelvic and hypogastric plexus to enter the lumbar sympathetic chain. Through the white rami communicantes of the T10, T11, T12, and L1 spinal nerves, they enter the dorsal horn of the spinal cord. These pathways could be mapped successfully by a demonstration that blockade at different levels along this path (sacral nerve-root blocks S2 through S4, pudendal block, paracervical block, low caudal or true saddle block, lumbar sympathetic block, segmental epidural blocks T10 through L1, and paravertebral blocks T10 through L1) can alleviate the visceral component of labor pain. (Reproduced from: Elzschig HK, Lieberman ES, Camann WR. Medical progress: regional anesthesia and analgesia for labor and delivery. NEJM. 2003;348(4):319-332.)

CASE STUDY

You are asked to see a patient in the Anesthetic Antenatal Preassessment Clinic. She is a 33-year-old woman at 36 weeks' gestation in her first pregnancy. She has a history of severe congenital scoliosis, partially corrected at 12 years of age with Harrington rods. She would like to discuss analgesic options for labor.

Questions

1. What do you advise the patient initially?

2. What nonregional options are available to her for analgesia?

3. The patient asks about IV PCA with remifentanil but she is concerned that it may affect the infant. What do you tell her to allay her fears?

Answers

1. A patient with previous spinal corrective surgery may have obliterated or distorted epidural space anatomy due to surgical scarring in the area. Cephalopelvic disproportion is increased in scoliotic women, and they are at increased risk for assisted or operative delivery. Placement of epidural catheter may be difficult due to scarring. It is important to explain potential difficulties with regional techniques from the outset of the consultation so that the patient does not have unrealistic expectations for labor analgesia.

   Firstly, epidural analgesia, if successfully placed, may provide patchy analgesia and not be 100% reliable should an operative delivery be deemed necessary. Combined spinal epidural or single shot spinal using intrathecal opioid or local anesthetic combination have been used with good effect but there may not be adequate spread of the local anesthetic due to distorted spinal anatomy. Continuous spinal anesthesia may successfully allow titration of analgesia or anesthesia as required. Nonregional techniques as discussed below should also be offered as adjunctive therapy. If an operative delivery is required, general anesthesia should also be discussed, especially with an emergency caesarean section.

2. Adequate antenatal preparation by attending birthing classes is important. Initial noninvasive methods such as TENS may be beneficial in early labor. Acupuncture or acupressure, if available, may offer relief. Considering learned coping strategies such as Lamaze techniques, hypnobirthing, would be an adjunct to other nonregional methods. At the time of delivery, a pudendal block or infiltration of the perineum with local anesthetic by the obstetrician is often sufficient for analgesia for assisted deliveries using forceps or ventouse methods.

   Parenteral opioids may be given in early labor but may cause fetal depression and maternal respiratory depression.

3. Remifentanil is an ultra-short-acting opioid that has been shown to be a more effective analgesic than meperidine (pethidine *demerol*). It is a suitable medication that can be effective delivered using a PCA device. It does cross the placenta, but due to its rapid metabolism by the body, it is not associated with long-lasting

neonatal and maternal sedation or somnolence or neonatal respiratory depression. When administered with adequate monitoring for both mother and fetus/neonate, it offers a safe, although somewhat less effective alternative to epidural analgesia. It has not been demonstrated to cause any more maternal hypoxia or desaturations than with use of pethidine.

REFERENCES

1. McGrath SK, Kennell JH. A randomized controlled trial of continuous labor support for middle-class couples: effect on caesarean delivery rates. *Birth.* 2008;35(2):92-97.

2. Jones I, Johnson M. Transcutaneous electrical nerve stimulation. *Contin Educ Anaesth Crit Care Pain.* 2009;9:130-135.

3. Dowswell T, Bedwell C, Lavender T, Neilson JP. Transcutaneous electrical nerve stimulation (TENS) for pain relief in labor. *Cochrane Database Syst Rev.* 2009;(2):CD007214.

4. Aird IA, Luckas MJ, Buckett WM, Bousfield P. Effects of intra-partum hydrotherapy on labour related parameters. *Aust N Z J Obstet Gynaecol.* 1997;37:137-142.

5. Cluett ER, Nikodem VC, McCandlish RE, Burns EE. Immersion in water in pregnancy, labor and birth. *Cochrane Database Syst Rev.* 2004;(2):CD000111.

6. Smith CA, Collins CT, Cyna AM, Crowther CA. Complementary and alternative therapies for pain management in labor. *Cochrane Database Syst Rev.* 2006;(4):CD003521.

7. Hantoushzadeh S, Alhusseini N, Lebaschi AH. The effects of acupuncture during labor on nulliparous women: a randomized controlled trial. *Aust N Z J Obstet Gynaecol.* 2007;47(1):26-30.

8. Yeo ST, Holdcroft A, Yentis SM, Stewart A, Bassett P. Analgesia with sevoflurane during labor: ii. Sevoflurane compared with Entonox for labour analgesia. *Br J Anaesth.* 2007;98(1):110-115.

9. Bricker L, Lavender T. Parenteral opioids for labor pain relief: a systematic review. *Am J Obstet Gynaecol.* 2002;186(5 suppl Nature):S94-S109.

10. Wittels B, Scott DT, Sinatra RS. Exogenous opioids in human breast milk and acute neonatal neurobehaviour: a preliminary study. *Anaesthesiology.* 1990;73(5):864-869.

11. Reynolds F. Labour analgesia and the baby: good news is no news. *Int J Obstet Anesth.* 2011;20(1):38-50.

12. Kan RE, Hughes SC, Rosen MA, et al. Intravenous remifentanil. Placental transfer, maternal and neonatal effects. *Anaesthesiology.* 1998;88:1467-1474.

13. Volikas I, Male D. A comparison of pethidine and remifentanil patient-controlled analgesia in labour. *Int J Obstet Anesth.* 2001;10(2):86-90.

14. Cammann W, et al. Regional anesthesia and analgesia for labor and delivery. *NEJM.* 2003;348(4):320; Figure 1.

Anesthesia for Cesarean Section and Postoperative Analgesia

9

Paloma Toledo

INTRODUCTION

The increase in the cesarean delivery rate in the United States has reached near epidemic proportions. As of 2010, approximately 30% of all births in the United States occurred via cesarean delivery, and projections estimate a continued increase over time. Therefore, attention to the anesthetic management of these patients will continue to be of increasing importance.

The typical sequence of events for providing anesthesia for cesarean delivery is as follows:

1. Preoperative assessment and consent

2. Aspiration prophylaxis

3. Placement of monitors

4. Administration of antibiotics

5. Patient positioning

6. Administration of surgical anesthesia

7. Fluid coloading

8. Management of hypotension

9. Administration of uterotonics

10. Postoperative analgesia planning

Each of the components will be discussed in the following sections.

PREOPERATIVE ASSESSMENT AND CONSENT

Assessment

Prior to initiation of anesthesia, a thorough preoperative assessment should be completed. In addition to regular components of the history in obstetric patients, specific attention should also be given to relevant obstetric issues such as medical conditions that may complicate surgery (ie, obesity, hypertensive disorders of pregnancy, gestational diabetes) and number of previous cesarean deliveries.[1]

Physical examination should include an examination of the back if neuraxial anesthesia is planned.[1] An airway examination should be timed close to surgery because evidence has shown that there may be changes in the Mallampati classification of the airway with pregnancy/labor.[2]

Routine laboratory tests may not be necessary for all women prior to cesarean delivery. However, there is controversy among practicing anesthesiologists regarding whether a routine platelet count should be obtained prior to regional anesthesia. Certainly, in high-risk patients, such as parturients with severe preeclampsia, gestational thrombocytopenia, or history of coagulation disorders, a platelet count and/or coagulation studies may be necessary. A sample of the patient's blood should be sent to the blood bank for all cesarean deliveries. The decision to type and screen or type and cross-match blood should be made based on the likelihood of requiring a blood transfusion.

Consent

During the consent process, the patient should be informed of the risks and benefits of the anesthetic planned for the procedure. Although there are many potential risks with neuraxial and general anesthesia, generally the most common risks should be discussed. For neuraxial anesthesia, these should include infection, bleeding, risk of postdural puncture headache, hypotension, and patchy/failed block requiring a repeat puncture or conversion to general anesthesia.

ASPIRATION PROPHYLAXIS

The estimated incidence of pulmonary aspiration in women undergoing cesarean delivery is 1 in 661 and appears to be decreasing. The decline is likely to be multifactorial, is related to the increased use of neuraxial anesthesia and decreased use of

Table 9-1. Commonly Used Aspiration Prophylaxis Medications

Agent	Onset Time	Duration	Mechanism of Action	Common Dose
Nonparticulate antacid 0.3 M sodium citrate	Immediate action	60 min	Increases gastric pH	30 mL
H_2-receptor antagonists Ranitidine Famotidine	15-30 min	2 h	Increases gastric pH and reduces volume of secretions	50 mg IV 20 mg IV
Dopamine antagonist Metoclopramide	1-3 min	1-2 h	Increases gastric motility; antiemetic effect	10 mg IV

general anesthesia, adherence to fasting guidelines in obstetric practice, and routine use of antacid prophylaxis.

The American Society of Anesthesiologists (ASA) recommends withholding clear liquids for 2 hours prior to elective cesarean delivery and withholding solids for 6 to 8 hours, depending on the fat content of the meal and the presence of comorbidities such as diabetes.[1] For women who are in labor, it is controversial whether they should be allowed to eat light meals during labor. A Cochrane review evaluating oral intake in labor found no difference in labor or neonatal outcomes when low-risk patients were allowed liquid/solid intake[3] and concluded that low-risk patients should be allowed to eat and drink. The difficulty with these studies is that aspiration is a relatively rare event, and the meta-analyses did not have sufficient statistical power to assess maternal aspiration as a primary outcome. Although active labor combined with or without neuraxial analgesia does slow gastric emptying, particularly especially with prior administration of opioids, most institutions do allow laboring women to drink clear liquids in labor but do not allow ingestion of solid food because of the perceived increased aspiration risk.

Prior to cesarean delivery, pharmacologic aspiration prophylaxis should be given. Three classes of drugs are routinely used: nonparticulate antacids, H_2-receptor antagonists, and dopamine antagonists. Of the three, in an emergency, the most important to administer is the nonparticulate antacid as it has the fastest onset and decreases gastric acidity. Table 9-1 summarizes the onset, mechanism of action, and common doses of these agents.

PLACEMENT OF MONITORS

As with all surgical procedures, ASA standard monitors are required. Whether or not the electrocardiogram (ECG) leads need to be on the patient during placement of neuraxial anesthesia is controversial. Temperature assessment is only required during cesarean deliveries under general anesthesia. The American College of Obstetrics and Gynecology states that fetal heart rate should be documented prior to surgery in all but the direst emergencies.

Invasive hemodynamic monitoring is not required for routine cesarean deliveries in healthy parturients, but should be considered on a case-by-case basis for high-risk deliveries or patients with cardiopulmonary disease.

ADMINISTRATION OF ANTIBIOTICS

The use of prophylactic antibiotics for cesarean delivery reduces maternal infectious morbidity. However, the timing of the antibiotic administration has been controversial. It was previously thought that administration of antibiotics prior to umbilical cord clamping would interfere with neonatal sepsis evaluation should it be necessary, as well as lead to antibiotic resistance in the newborn. However, several randomized controlled trials have demonstrated that there is a decrease in endometritis and/or wound infection when antibiotics are administered prior to skin incision, as opposed to at umbilical cord clamping, with no increased adverse effects on the mother or fetus. Indeed, wound infection rates when antibiotics are held until cord clamp are equivalent to not having given antibiotics at all. Given this evidence, the American College of Obstetrics and Gynecology recently issued a Committee Opinion in which they recommend *that antibiotic prophylaxis be administered within 60 minutes of the start of a cesarean delivery*.[4] Exceptions to this include patients who have already received appropriate antibiotics (such as those being treated for chorioamnionitis) or those patients who are undergoing emergency cesarean deliveries. In the latter situation, antibiotics should be administered as soon as they are available. Considering that placement of regional anesthesia may be difficult in some parturients, we suggest that antibiotics be administered after induction of regional anesthesia during skin preparation; in this way, the interval between antibiotic administration and surgical incision will always be within 60 minutes.

PATIENT POSITIONING

Prior to delivery of the infant, the patient should be placed in left uterine displacement. A minimum of 15-degree leftward tilt prevents aortocaval compression syndrome, which results from the gravid uterus resting on the aorta and vena cava. This in turn leads to reduced venous return to the heart. After delivery of the infant, the left tilt may be removed.

ADMINISTRATION OF SURGICAL ANESTHESIA

The type of anesthesia selected for cesarean delivery needs to be tailored to the individual woman's situation. The anesthetic plan is usually determined by the urgency of the cesarean delivery and maternal/fetal condition. There are three types of anesthesia for cesarean delivery: (1) general anesthesia; (2) neuraxial anesthesia, which includes (a) spinal anesthesia, (b) epidural anesthesia, (c) combined spinal-epidural anesthesia, and (d) continuous spinal anesthesia; and (3) Infiltration of local anesthesia, which is rarely used. The flow chart in Figure 9-1 describes an approach to deciding on an initial anesthetic plan for a cesarean delivery.

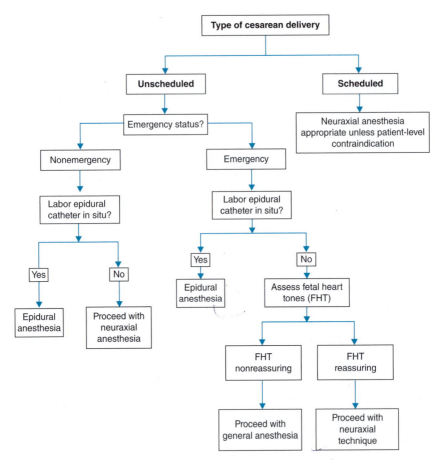

Figure 9-1. Proposed algorithm to guide anesthetic decision-making.

General Anesthesia

General anesthesia may be required in dire emergency situations where there is immediate threat to the mother or infant, when there is insufficient time to initiate neuraxial anesthesia, or in women who have contraindications to neuraxial anesthesia. Other reasons for the use of general anesthesia include hypovolemia (due to maternal hemorrhage) and infection. Due to the physiologic changes of pregnancy, all patients undergoing general anesthesia are considered to be at risk for aspiration; therefore, in addition to aspiration prophylaxis, rapid sequence intubation with cricoid pressure should be performed. The advantage of general anesthesia is that it allows the shortest "decision-to-incision" interval when compared to a de novo neuraxial technique. The trade-offs are a lower initial 1-minute Apgar score and an increased likelihood of uterine atony and bleeding related to the effects of halogenated agents.[5]

The following is a common approach to general anesthesia.[6] Induction should occur after denitrogenation, skin decontamination, and confirmation that the surgical team is prepared to proceed with surgery in order to shorten the induction-to-delivery interval and reduce the potential for neonatal depression. After induction and intubation, the surgical team should be told to commence, and the patient should be ventilated with 100% oxygen and up to 1 minimum alveolar concentration (MAC) of a potent inhalational agent. Following delivery of the infant, the FiO_2 may be decreased to 30% and 70% nitrous oxide added, while maintaining a one-half MAC of inhalational agent. At this point, benzodiazepines and opioids may be administered. The stomach should be decompressed with an orogastric tube, and the temperature should be monitored. For most surgeries, it is not necessary to administer additional muscle relaxant beyond the intubating dose. Because the risk of hemorrhage is increased with general anesthesia,[7] it may be prudent to increase the dose of oxytocin administered after delivery. Patients should be extubated awake and monitored in a postanesthesia recovery unit. It is critical that postanesthesia care units have systems and resources in place identical to those of main operating rooms. Indeed, recent evidence suggests that anesthesia-related deaths due to airway obstruction or hypoventilation occurred during emergence and recovery, not during the conduct of general anesthesia.[8]

Neuraxial Anesthesia

The overwhelming majority of cesarean deliveries are performed using neuraxial anesthesia, with the most common anesthetic being a single-shot spinal. Table 9-2 describes the advantages, disadvantages, common scenarios, and common dosing strategies for each neuraxial anesthetic regimen.

With all neuraxial techniques, a T4-T6 dermatomal level should be established prior to commencement of the surgery; otherwise the patient may experience breakthrough pain and require supplemental opioids or conversion to general anesthesia. The assessment of sensory level should be to touch/pinprick because the discrepancy between cold and touch may exceed two dermatomes.[9]

Common dosing regimens for spinal anesthesia include a local anesthetic agent with a short-acting opioid. The addition of an opioid allows for a reduction in local anesthetic dose, thus decreasing the incidence of hypotension and other local anesthetic-related side effects. For women without clinical contraindications, morphine is often added for extended postoperative analgesia. For patients in whom the duration of surgery is anticipated to exceed the usual duration of the spinal, anesthetic epinephrine may be added to the spinal to enhance anesthesia, or alternatively, an epidural or combined spinal-epidural technique may be chosen.

In some instances, epidural anesthesia may be chosen for cesarean delivery. However, the most likely scenario for epidural use is that there is a well-functioning epidural catheter at the time the decision to deliver via cesarean delivery is made in a laboring woman, and the block reinforced accordingly. The patient may not require as much epidural local anesthetic as a patient who is receiving de novo epidural anesthesia.

Table 9-2. Neuraxial Anesthesia Options

Anesthesia	Advantage	Disadvantage	Common Clinical Scenarios	Common Regimens
Spinal anesthesia	Rapid onset Simple, reliable technique	Limited duration of anesthesia	Primary/repeat cesarean delivery	**Local anesthetic:** Bupivacaine 9-12 mg Lidocaine 60-70 mg **Opioid:** Fentanyl 15 µg Sufentanil 10 µg **± Long-acting opioid:** (Morphine 100-150 µg) **± Epinephrine:** 100-200 µg
Epidural anesthesia	Titratable Catheter may be used for prolonged postoperative analgesia	Slower in onset than spinal anesthesia Complex technique	Anticipated duration of surgery longer than duration of spinal Concern for difficult intubation Epidural catheter in situ in laboring patient Patient in whom dural puncture is contraindicated	**Local anesthetic:** Lidocaine 2% 15-20 mL with sodium bicarbonate and epinephrine 75-100 µg (if using a 1:200,000) Chloroprocaine 3% 15-20 mL **After delivery of infant:** Epidural morphine 3.0-3.5 mg
Combined spinal-epidural anesthesia	Rapid onset with spinal component Titratable with epidural catheter May be used for postoperative analgesia	Cost Delayed recognition of dysfunctional epidural catheter Complexity of technique	Anticipated duration of surgery longer than duration of spinal	Spinal dose as for spinal anesthesia Test dose epidural catheter and after two-dermatome regression. Redose epidural (~5 mL) at regular intervals
Continuous spinal anesthesia	Rapid, reliable onset May be used for postoperative analgesia	Increased risk of postdural puncture headache Complexity of technique Potential for unintended injection of nonapproved substances resulting in neurotoxicity	Inadvertent dural puncture during epidural placement Morbidly obese parturients	Spinal dose as for spinal anesthesia If intrathecal catheter in situ for labor, incrementally dose spinal catheter to avoid high spinal

EPIDURAL ANESTHESIA IN WOMEN WITH IN-DWELLING LABOR EPIDURAL CATHETERS

Urgency will dictate which local anesthetic is used. For emergency cesarean deliveries (those in which there is an immediate threat to the life of mother or fetus), 3% chloroprocaine would be the most expeditious choice.[10] In less emergent settings, such as where nonreassuring status is less threatening or responds to therapy, or where the parturient requires delivery but there is no fetal compromise (arrest of dilation or arrest of descent), a slower onset local anesthetic such as 2% lidocaine may be chosen. The advantage of lidocaine over chloroprocaine may be that that chloroprocaine interferes with the efficacy of subsequently administered epidural morphine.[11] The mechanism of this interaction is not completely understood but may be related to a metabolite-induced receptor effect or to a window effect where the chloroprocaine effect has vanished but the morphine effect is slower. When feasible, induction of the anesthetic should commence in the patient's room with blood pressure monitoring, as this has been demonstrated to increase the likelihood of success.

INFILTRATION OF LOCAL ANESTHESIA

In situations where an anesthesiologist is not readily available, a cesarean delivery may be performed under local anesthesia. Complete description of this technique is beyond the scope of this chapter. However, briefly, 0.5% lidocaine is used to sequentially anesthetize the skin, subcutaneous tissues, fascia, and peritoneum. This technique requires that the obstetrician make a vertical abdominal incision and not exteriorize the uterus.

FLUID COLOADING: PREVENTION OF HYPOTENSION WITH REGIONAL ANESTHESIA

Hypotension is the most common complication of spinal anesthesia during cesarean delivery.[12] Side effects of hypotension include nausea/vomiting, loss of consciousness, maternal cardiac arrest, and decreased uteroplacental perfusion resulting in neonatal acidosis.

For many years, a fluid preload of 500 mL to 1 L of crystalloid was advocated to prevent maternal hypotension; however, current evidence suggests that crystalloid preloads alone are ineffective in preventing hypotension. In contrast to preload, crystalloid coloading has been shown to reduce both hypotension and vasopressor requirements.[13] The use of colloids has been investigated as a preload and coload. It seems that colloids are more effective than crystalloids when given as a preload[14] and possibly more effective than crystalloids when administered as a coload.[15] Although these initial results are promising, the cost, as well as the increased risk of side effects with colloids (pruritus, coagulation abnormalities, and severe allergic reactions), may limit their use in routine obstetric practice. Therefore, considering the evidence at this time, *a crystalloid coload through a free-flowing wide-bore intravenous catheter is recommended for prevention of hypotension.* Other strategies for management of hypotension are discussed in the following section.

MANAGEMENT OF HYPOTENSION

Phenylephrine and ephedrine are the two most commonly used vasopressors for treatment of hypotension during cesarean delivery. Ephedrine had been the first-line vasopressor for many years because it was thought to cause less reduction in uterine blood flow in animal studies. However, in the past decade, *phenylephrine has become the preferred vasopressor* in preventing/treating hypotension because recent studies have shown that the small doses used in obstetric anesthesia do not reduce utero-placental perfusion. As important is the fact that ephedrine use may be associated with neonatal acidosis related to placental transfer of the drug and a resultant imbalance between fetal oxygen demand and supply, often manifested by fetal tachycardia.[16]

Due to down-regulation of adrenergic receptors during normal pregnancy, higher doses of vasopressors may be required for treatment of hypotension in pregnant women without preeclampsia compared to nonpregnant women. A recent up-down sequential allocation study found the 90% effective dose (ED_{90}) of phenylephrine in spinal anesthesia-induced hypotension to be 150 µg.[17] A suggested starting dose for ephedrine would be 5 to 10 mg.

Much attention has been focused recently on the method of delivery for phenylephrine and whether there is benefit to an infusion of drug versus mini-boluses. Many of the early studies evaluating phenylephrine infusions used a high-dose phenylephrine infusion (100 µg/min) technique. A more recent study compared physician-delivered boluses to four fixed-rate phenylephrine infusions (25, 50, 75, and 100 µg/min) after initiation of spinal anesthesia. The authors did not find any benefit to the infusions compared to physician-delivered boluses with respect to the number of times physicians needed to intervene for hypertension or hypotension.[18] Furthermore, there were no differences in blood pressure control, intraoperative nausea, or need for antiemetics among the five groups. However, with escalating doses of phenylephrine, there was the potential for more reactive hypertension. In conclusion, current evidence does not support the use of a fixed-rate phenylephrine infusion; however, if an infusion is to be used, clinicians should start with lower doses (25-50 µg/min), because these doses are associated with less reactive hypertension.

ADMINISTRATION OF UTEROTONICS

Oxytocin is considered the first-line agent for hastening involution of the uterus and prevention of postpartum hemorrhage following cesarean delivery. However, the optimal dose and route of delivery are not well established. Sometimes, oxytocin is administered as a bolus intravenous injection, with common doses ranging from 2 to 5 international units (IU). Bolus administration of oxytocin has been associated with many undesirable cardiovascular side effects, such as hypotension, tachycardia, and ECG changes that may be suggestive of myocardial ischemia.[19] Recent evidence suggests that adequate uterine tone can be achieved with bolus doses as low as 0.5 to 0.03 IU and with fewer side effects.[20] Many institutions have therefore transitioned to the use of oxytocin infusions following umbilical cord

Table 9-3. Additional Uterotonic Medications

Name	Mechanism of Action	Side Effects	Contraindications	Common Dose
Ergot alkaloids (Methergine)	Direct activation of uterine smooth muscle	Coronary vasoconstriction, hypertension, bradycardia	Severe hypertension (preeclampsia)	200 µg IM q30min
Prostaglandin 15-methyl $F_{2\alpha}$ (Hemabate)	Activate uterine smooth muscle	Bronchoconstriction, hypertension, nausea/vomiting	Asthma	250 µg IM q15min

clamping at cesarean delivery. The ED_{90} for oxytocin delivered as an infusion has been estimated to be 0.4 IU/min.[21] Current evidence does not suggest a benefit to administering a bolus of oxytocin prior to initiation of an oxytocin infusion.[22] Higher doses of oxytocin may be necessary after prolonged labor with oxytocin induction/augmentation, because animal evidence suggests that there is receptor desensitization with increasing doses of oxytocin.[23]

Postpartum hemorrhage is one of the leading causes of maternal mortality worldwide. Mortality from hemorrhage is due, in part, to an underappreciation of the amount of blood lost[24] and a subsequent delay in initiating treatment for the hemorrhage. In the setting of postpartum hemorrhage due to atony, additional uterotonic agents may be necessary. In addition to oxytocin, the two most commonly used classes of agents are ergot alkaloids and prostaglandin 15-methyl-$F_{2\alpha}$. Their mechanism of action, side effects, contraindications, and common doses are listed in Table 9-3.

POSTOPERATIVE ANALGESIA PLANNING

There are two components to postoperative pain-somatic (incisional) and visceral (uterine) pain. Options for postoperative analgesia are described below.

Neuraxial Opioids

Neuraxial morphine is the most efficacious technique to achieve prolonged postoperative analgesia of both visceral and somatic pain. Spinally administered morphine acts primarily at the mu receptors in the spinal cord, whereas epidurally administered morphine acts through spinal and supraspinal opioid receptors.[25] The duration of action of neuraxially administered morphine is between 12 and 24 hours. An extended-release epidural morphine has been developed; however, the potential for delayed respiratory depression extends beyond that of conventional morphine, thus the need for increased respiratory monitoring (48 hours). Also, there is potential for lysis of the lipid capsules containing morphine if local anesthetic is administered, thus causing an uncontrolled release of morphine.[26] Patients who receive neuraxial opioids should receive scheduled parenteral nonsteroidal anti-inflammatory agents (NSAIDs) postoperatively for treatment of visceral pain.

Parenteral Analgesia

In patients who do not receive neuraxial morphine, intravenous narcotics and NSAIDs should be administered. Opioids are often delivered via intravenous patient-controlled analgesia until the patient is able to tolerate oral medications.

Transversus Abdominis Plane Blockade

The transversus abdominis plane (TAP) block is an adjuvant analgesic technique that has become popular in the past 10 years. It has gained acceptance with the use of ultrasound guidance to improve accuracy of the block to prevent visceral damage, intraperitoneal injection, and liver laceration. Briefly, local anesthetic is deposited in the fascial plane between the transversus abdominis and the internal oblique using ultrasound guidance. Several nerves lie in the TAP: lower thoracic nerves (T7-T11), subcostal nerve, and the two branches of first lumbar nerve (the iliohypogastric and ilioinguinal nerves).

Early studies with the TAP block in cesarean delivery patients found a reduction in morphine consumption and prolonged first request to analgesia as compared to women not receiving the block[27]; however, patients in these studies did not receive neuraxial morphine. There has been only one randomized controlled trial that evaluated the efficacy of TAP block in women who had received intrathecal morphine, and found no benefit to TAP block beyond the analgesia provided by neuraxial morphine.[28] Another recently published study randomized patients undergoing elective cesarean deliveries to one of four groups, either intrathecal morphine with a 2-mg/kg bilateral bupivacaine TAP block or sham TAP, or intrathecal saline with a bupivacaine TAP block or sham TAP. Patients in the intrathecal morphine group had the best analgesia with movement at 6 hours postpartum, and the lowest morphine consumption in the first 12 hours. These studies confirm that intrathecal morphine is the most efficacious technique for providing postoperative analgesia due to its ability to provide somatic as well as visceral analgesia. Thus, TAP block should be reserved for three patient populations: (1) those patients who undergo general anesthesia for cesarean delivery, (2) those who did not receive neuraxial morphine, and (3) those patients who have breakthrough incisional pain despite having received neuraxial morphine.

COMPLICATIONS OF ANESTHESIA

Aspiration

As mentioned in the antacid prophylaxis section, aspiration may be a complication of general anesthesia or whenever at-risk pregnant women are unable to protect their airway from whatever cause. Although the incidence is decreasing, aspiration prophylaxis should be taken in all parturients undergoing cesarean delivery, even if under regional anesthesia, because of the potential risk of intraoperative conversion to general anesthesia.

Awareness

The incidence of awareness following general anesthesia in the obstetric patient population is low, with current estimates of 0.1% to 0.2%.[29]

Difficult Intubation

Due to the physiologic changes of pregnancy (increased capillary engorgement with resultant decreased internal tracheal diameter), there is the potential for increased difficulty with intubation in pregnant patients. Obstetric anesthesia providers should know the American Society of Anesthesiologists Difficult Airway Algorithm. General anesthesia should not be undertaken without a full assessment of the airway. If difficulty is anticipated, consideration should be given to alternative anesthetic techniques. There should be the full range of airway devices on the obstetric unit both for intubation and rescue as necessary.

High Spinal

A high spinal may occur following spinal anesthesia. However, more frequently it is an unintended complication of epidural anesthesia (epidural medications inadvertently injected intrathecally or subdurally) or when a spinal anesthetic is placed subsequent to failed de novo epidural anesthesia for cesarean delivery or after epidural analgesia for labor. If a patient experiences a high spinal, it is important to oxygenate by assisting with ventilation or even intubate, maintain left uterine displacement, and treat hypotension until the level recedes.

Local Anesthetic Systemic Toxicity

The possibility of local anesthetic systemic toxicity (LAST) exists in obstetric anesthesia with the initiation of epidural anesthesia or with TAP blockade. Providers should be aware of the signs and symptoms of LAST and treatment algorithms. The American Society of Regional Anesthesia published a practice advisory on LAST in 2010, which can be found on their website (www.asra.com). In the case of long-acting amide local anesthetic cardiotoxicity, consideration should be given to the administration of lipid emulsion as an adjunct to Advanced Cardiac Life Support to facilitate resuscitation. If a maternal cardiac arrest occurs, a hysterotomy should be promptly performed if there is no return of cardiac activity within 5 minutes, because closed chest cardiac massage may be ineffective with aortocaval compression.

Neonatal Depression

Infants delivered under general anesthesia have a higher incidence of fetal acidemia and lower 1-minute Apgar scores than those delivered under neuraxial anesthesia.[5] With prolonged uterine incision-to-delivery intervals (> 3 minutes), there is a higher incidence of acidosis and neonatal depression.[30]

REFERENCES

1. Practice guidelines for obstetric anesthesia. An updated report by the American Society of Anesthesiologists Task Force on Obstetric Anesthesia. *Anesthesiology.* 2007;106:843-863.

2. Boutonnet M, Faitot V, Katz A, Salomon L, Keita H. Mallampati class changes during pregnancy, labour, and after delivery: can these be predicted? *Br J Anaesth.* 2010;104:67-70.

3. Singata M, Tranmer J, Gyte GM. Restricting oral fluid and food intake during labour. *Cochrane Database Syst Rev.* 2010:CD003930.

4. American College of Obstetricians and Gynecologists (ACOG). Antimicrobial prophylaxis for cesarean delivery: timing of administration. ACOG Committee Opinion No. 465. *Obstet Gynecol.* 2010;116:791-792.

5. Tonni G, Ferrari B, De Felice C, Ventura A. Fetal acid-base and neonatal status after general and neuraxial anesthesia for elective cesarean section. *Int J Gynaecol Obstet.* 2007;97:143-146.

6. Scavone BM, Toledo P, Higgins N, Wojciechowski K, McCarthy RJ. A randomized controlled trial of the impact of simulation-based training on resident performance during a simulated obstetric anesthesia emergency. *Simul Healthc.* 2010;5:320-324.

7. Chang CC, Wang IT, Chen YH, Lin HC. Anesthetic management as a risk factor for postpartum hemorrhage after cesarean deliveries. *Am J Obstet Gynecol.* 2011;205:462.e461-e467.

8. Mhyre JM, Riesner MN, Polley LS, Naughton NN. A series of anesthesia-related maternal deaths in Michigan, 1985-2003. *Anesthesiology.* 2007;106:1096-1104.

9. Russell IF. A comparison of cold, pinprick and touch for assessing the level of spinal block at caesarean section. *Int J Obstet Anesth.* 2004;13:146-152.

10. Gaiser RR, Cheek TG, Gutsche BB. Epidural lidocaine versus 2-chloroprocaine for fetal distress requiring urgent cesarean section. *Int J Obstet Anesth.* 1994;3:208-210.

11. Toledo P, McCarthy RJ, Ebarvia MJ, Huser CJ, Wong CA. The interaction between epidural 2-chloroprocaine and morphine: a randomized controlled trial of the effect of drug administration timing on the efficacy of morphine analgesia. *Anesth Analg.* 2009;109:168-173.

12. Cyna AM, Andrew M, Emmett RS, Middleton P, Simmons SW. Techniques for preventing hypotension during spinal anaesthesia for caesarean section. *Cochrane Database Syst Rev.* 2006:CD002251.

13. Dyer RA, Farina Z, Joubert IA, et al. Crystalloid preload versus rapid crystalloid administration after induction of spinal anaesthesia (coload) for elective caesarean section. *Anaesth Intensive Care.* 2004;32:351-357.

14. Riley ET, Cohen SE, Rubenstein AJ, Flanagan B. Prevention of hypotension after spinal anesthesia for cesarean section: six percent hetastarch versus lactated Ringer's solution. *Anesth Analg.* 1995;81:838-842.

15. McDonald S, Fernando R, Ashpole K, Columb M. Maternal cardiac output changes after crystalloid or colloid coload following spinal anesthesia for elective cesarean delivery: a randomized controlled trial. *Anesth Analg.* 2011;113:803-810.

16. Ngan Kee WD, Khaw KS. Vasopressors in obstetrics: what should we be using? *Curr Opin Anaesthesiol.* 2006;19:238-243.

17. George RB, McKeen D, Columb MO, Habib AS. Up-down determination of the 90% effective dose of phenylephrine for the treatment of spinal anesthesia-induced hypotension in parturients undergoing cesarean delivery. *Anesth Analg.* 2010;110:154-158.

18. Allen TK, George RB, White WD, Muir HA, Habib AS. A double-blind, placebo-controlled trial of four fixed rate infusion regimens of phenylephrine for hemodynamic support during spinal anesthesia for cesarean delivery. *Anesth Analg.* 2010;111:1221-1229.

19. Thomas JS, Koh SH, Cooper GM. Haemodynamic effects of oxytocin given as i.v. bolus or infusion on women undergoing Caesarean section. *Br J Anaesth.* 2007;98:116-119.

20. Butwick AJ, Coleman L, Cohen SE, Riley ET, Carvalho B. Minimum effective bolus dose of oxytocin during elective Caesarean delivery. *Br J Anaesth.* 2010;104:338-343.

21. George RB, McKeen D, Chaplin AC, McLeod L. Up-down determination of the ED(90) of oxytocin infusions for the prevention of postpartum uterine atony in parturients undergoing Cesarean delivery. *Can J Anaesth.* 2010;57:578-582.

22. King KJ, Douglas MJ, Unger W, Wong A, King RA. Five unit bolus oxytocin at cesarean delivery in women at risk of atony: a randomized, double-blind, controlled trial. *Anesth Analg.* 2010;111:1460-1466.

23. Magalhaes JK, Carvalho JC, Parkes RK, Kingdom J, Li Y, Balki M. Oxytocin pretreatment decreases oxytocin-induced myometrial contractions in pregnant rats in a concentration-dependent but not time-dependent manner. *Reprod Sci.* 2009;16:501-508.

24. Toledo P, McCarthy RJ, Hewlett BJ, Fitzgerald PC, Wong CA. The accuracy of blood loss estimation after simulated vaginal delivery. *Anesth Analg.* 2007;105:1736-1740, table of contents.

25. Gadsden J, Hart S, Santos AC. Post-cesarean delivery analgesia. *Anesth Analg.* 2005;101:S62-S69.

26. Atkinson Ralls L, Drover DR, Clavijo CF, Carvalho B. Prior epidural lidocaine alters the pharmaco-kinetics and drug effects of extended-release epidural morphine (DepoDur®) after cesarean delivery. *Anesth Analg.* 2011;113:251-258.

27. McDonnell JG, Curley G, Carney J, et al. The analgesic efficacy of transversus abdominis plane block after cesarean delivery: a randomized controlled trial. *Anesth Analg.* 2008;106:186-191.

28. Costello JF, Moore AR, Wieczorek PM, Macarthur AJ, Balki M, Carvalho JC. The transversus abdominis plane block, when used as part of a multimodal regimen inclusive of intrathecal morphine, does not improve analgesia after cesarean delivery. *Reg Anesth Pain Med.* 2009;34:586-589.

29. Robins K, Lyons G. Intraoperative awareness during general anesthesia for cesarean delivery. *Anesth Analg.* 2009;109:886-890.

30. Datta S, Ostheimer GW, Weiss JB, Brown WU Jr, Alper MH. Neonatal effect of prolonged anesthetic induction for cesarean section. *Obstet Gynecol.* 1981;58:331-335.

Anesthesia for Preterm Labor, Multiple Gestations, and Abnormal Presentations

10

Daria M. Moaveni and J. Sudharma Ranasinghe

TOPICS

PRETERM LABOR

Introduction

Prematurity is a serious cause of adverse perinatal outcome. It is a contributing factor in 75% of neonatal deaths and may result in neonatal neurologic injury.[1] Preterm labor is defined as the onset of labor prior to 37 weeks' gestation. Anesthetic management includes analgesia for labor and vaginal delivery, as well as anesthesia for cesarean delivery if indicated. Furthermore, the anesthesiologist may become involved in managing the effects of tocolytic agents.

Risk Factors for Preterm Labor

Genetic, hormonal, psychosocial, and environmental factors are believed to be associated with preterm labor. Risk factors, identified in fewer than 50% of cases, include, but are not limited to nonwhite race, low socioeconomic status, history of preterm delivery, multiple gestation, preterm premature rupture of membranes, abnormal uterine anatomy, abnormal cervical anatomy, genital or systemic infection, trauma, abdominal surgery, fetal genetic abnormalities, fetal death, and tobacco/substance use.[2]

Pathophysiology of Preterm Labor

Initiation of labor is complex and multifactorial, and it includes genetic as well as hormonal factors. The characteristics of both term and preterm labor include cervical dilation and effacement, increased uterine contractility, and activation of the amniochorionic membrane. In term gestation, these changes are routine conclusions to pregnancy. However, in preterm labor, these changes are initiated through pathologic mechanisms.[3] During normal pregnancy, activation of the fetal hypothalamic-pituitary-adrenal axis contributes to labor initiation. Secretion of adrenocorticotropic hormone (ACTH) increases in response to release of corticotropin-releasing hormone from the hypothalamus. ACTH, in turn stimulates the adrenal glands to secrete cortisol.[4] This leads to an inflammatory response resulting in increased myometrial prostaglandin, which in turn produces an increase in intracellular calcium, with subsequent initiation of uterine contractions.[2] Thus, any stimulus that can initiate the inflammatory cascade of mediators can lead to uterine contractions, even prior to term of pregnancy.

Diagnosis

Preterm labor occurs at 20 to 37 weeks' gestation. Uterine contraction frequency should be at least 4 or more in a 20-minute period, or 8 or more in a 60-minute period. There must be either ongoing cervical changes, cervical dilation of at least 2 cm, or effacement of at least 80%.[2] False labor is characterized by irregular contractions that do not increase in frequency, duration, or strength. Also, there is no change in cervical dilation or effacement with false labor.[3]

Tocolytics versus Delivery

Not all patients with preterm labor progress to preterm delivery. Preterm delivery is associated with the potential for increased neonatal morbidity and mortality; therefore, prevention of delivery, or at least prolongation of pregnancy, is desirable. Tocolytic medications inhibit uterine contractions and should be considered for parturients at 20 to 34 weeks' gestation with reassuring fetal status and absence of infection[2] who are in preterm labor. Contraindications to tocolysis include fetal death, fetal anomalies incompatible with life, nonreassuring fetal status, chorioamnionitis or fever of unknown origin, severe hemorrhage, severe chronic hypertension or pregnancy complicated by preeclampsia[3] or other maternal contraindication.

TOCOLYTICS

Tocolytics can decrease the frequency, strength, and duration of contractions. They do not generally stop preterm labor but may be effective in prolonging the time to delivery by 2 to 7 days. This allows time for antenatal steroid administration to promote fetal lung maturity, or for transfer to a tertiary care facility with an appropriate capacity for handling preterm births.[1] Four classes of medications are used to decrease uterine contractions during preterm labor: β-adrenergic agonists, calcium channel blockers, cyclooxygenase inhibitors (nonsteroidal anti-inflammatory drugs), and magnesium. The preferred agent of choice depends on the presence of maternal comorbidities and the ability to tolerate the side effects. A summary of available agents are listed in Table 10-1.[1,2,4,5]

Table 10-1. Tocolytic Agents Used in Preterm Labor

Type of Agent	Dosage	Mechanism of Action	Side Effects (Maternal)	Side Effects (Fetal-Neonatal)	Contraindications	Interactions with Anesthesia
β$_2$ Agonist (terbutaline)	0.25 mg SQ q20min	Decreases myometrial contractions	Tachycardia, dysrhythmia, hypotension, myocardial infarction, hyperglycemia, pulmonary edema, nausea/vomiting, hyperinsulinemia	Hypoinsulinemia, hypoglycemia, intravascular hemorrhage, hyperbilirubinemia	Dysrhythmia, uncontrolled diabetes, uncontrolled thyroid disease	Need to monitor blood pressure, heart rate, and rhythm closely
Calcium channel blockers (nifedipine)	20-30 mg SL/PO, then 10-20 mg PO q4-6h	Decreases calcium uptake into cells and decreases calcium release from sarcoplasmic reticulum, thus decreasing myometrial contractions	Hypotension, flushing, headache, nausea, vomiting, pulmonary edema, dyspnea	Nonreassuring fetal status due to maternal hypotension	Cardiac disease, renal disease, hepatic disease, hypotension, magnesium	Increased risk of hypotension and reflex tachycardia
Cyclooxygenase inhibitors (indomethacin)	50-100 mg PO or PR, then 25-50 mg q4h	Inhibiting prostaglandin production thereby reduces intracellular calcium, thus decreasing myometrial contractions	Heartburn, nausea	Closure of ductus arteriosus, pulmonary hypertension, oligohydramnios, hyperbilirubinemia	Thrombocytopenia, coagulation disorders, renal disease, gastritis, nonsteroidal anti-inflammatory drug sensitivities	Neuraxial blockade can be performed safely[5]
Magnesium (magnesium sulfate)	4-6 g IV loading dose, then 1-2 g/h IV infusion	Competitor of calcium at the receptor, decreasing calcium uptake into the myometrium	Muscle weakness, diplopia, flushing, lethargy, headache, pulmonary edema, cardiac arrest	Hypotonia, respiratory depression, lethargy	Maternal neuromuscular disorders	Hypotension due to neuraxial blockade may be accentuated. May prolong action of nondepolarizing muscle relaxant

SUMMARY: TOCOLYTIC AGENTS

Studies have failed to demonstrate any specific tocolytic agent that is being more efficacious than another in prolonging preterm labor.[6,7] Thus, medications are chosen based on individual considerations such as maternal comorbidities, gestational age, and the potential for side effects. Magnesium and nifedipine have been reported to be the preferred first-line tocolytics in the United States.[8] Nifedipine has the advantage of being an effective tocolytic with minimal side effects.[6,9] Terbutaline is often avoided due to its effects on the maternal and fetal cardiovascular systems. Cyclooxygenase inhibitors have fallen out of favor due to the potential risk of ductus arteriosus closure and fetal pulmonary hypertension.

Antenatal Steroids

The purpose of antenatal steroid administration is to decrease the risk of respiratory distress syndrome (RDS) in the neonate. Fetal surfactant is composed of phospholipids that decrease the surface tension of alveolar walls and thus prevent collapse. Secretion of surfactant begins at about 24 weeks' gestation and is completed by 34 weeks' gestation. Therefore, mothers at gestational ages between 24 and 34 weeks who are at risk of preterm delivery within 7 days, should be considered for steroid therapy. Use of antenatal steroids before preterm delivery decreases the incidence of RDS, intraventricular hemorrhage, and neonatal death.[10] Two regimens are recommended in pregnant women between 24 and 34 weeks' gestation who are at risk for preterm delivery within 7 days: (1) two doses of betamethasone 12 mg intramuscularly at an interval of 24 hours or (2) four doses of dexamethasone 6 mg intramuscularly at an interval of 12 hours.[10]

Analgesia for Preterm Labor and Vaginal Delivery

Prematurity does not preclude maternal analgesia. Regional analgesia remains the most effective route of analgesia and may be beneficial in providing perineal relaxation and a controlled delivery of the fetal head. Furthermore, an early regional technique is recommended because delivery of the preterm fetus may occur at less than 10-cm cervical dilation.[2] Also, the preterm fetus is at higher risk for developing hypoxia and acidosis, and a well-functioning regional analgesic can easily be converted quickly to an anesthetic should an emergency cesarean delivery may be warranted (thus avoiding the need for general anesthesia). Combined spinal-epidural (CSE) analgesia is also an efficient modality that provides rapid onset of analgesia during labor and effective anesthesia for cesarean delivery via the epidural component. Use of intrathecal opioids has been reported to be associated with fetal bradycardia in *healthy* neonates; this is related to sudden decrease in catecholamines and subsequent increased uterine contraction due to hyperactivity of α-adrenergic agonists or greater responsiveness to endogenous or exogenously administered oxytocin.[11] The preterm fetus may not have the well-defined characteristics and responses in heart rate of a term fetus. For that reason, it is important that there be good communication among the members of the delivery team. Often, as a norm, a preterm fetus may have heart rates greater than 160 beats/min and decreased variability.[2]

Anesthesia for Cesarean Delivery for the Parturient in Preterm Labor

Cesarean delivery for the parturient in preterm labor is indicated for nonreassuring fetal status, history of previous cesarean delivery (not allowed to labor), and for breech presentation. It is important to obtain a comprehensive preanesthetic evaluation, paying particular attention to tocolytic side effects. For emergent and "stat" situations related to fetal heart rate abnormalities, it is important to reevaluate fetal heart rate once in the operating room because often the fetal heart rate may have improved and consideration may be given to regional as compared to general anesthesia if time allows.

REGIONAL ANESTHESIA

Neuraxial anesthesia is the preferred anesthetic technique for cesarean delivery, avoiding the airway risks associated with general anesthesia. Regional anesthesia also reduces the potential for transient fetal effects of central nervous system–depressing anesthetic agents. A single-shot or CSE anesthesia provides rapid onset of dense sensory blockade. If the fetus is breech and there has been significant cervical dilation, the lateral rather than sitting position may be preferred for initiation of neuraxial blockade to avoid umbilical cord prolapse. Neonatal resuscitation may be required; thus, a neonatologist should be present for delivery.

GENERAL ANESTHESIA

General anesthesia is usually reserved if there is rapid dilation in a preterm breech with head entrapment; if there is dire nonreassuring fetal status where any delay may adversely affect outcome; or where there may be maternal contraindication to neuraxial blockade, usually related to the side effects of tocolytics. Rapid sequence induction is performed with standard induction agents (thiopental, propofol, ketamine, or etomidate) and muscle relaxant (succinylcholine at 1-1.5 mg/kg). If the patient has been given magnesium, avoid nondepolarizing neuromuscular blockers, or administer a small dose, because the effects will be prolonged. The use of a neuromuscular monitor to measure the depth of blockade and guide drug administration should be routine. There has been concern regarding the potential for neurocognitive effects in the newborn related to in utero exposure to anesthetic agents. All the anesthetic agents have been implicated, with the exception of local anesthetics as used in regional obstetric anesthesia. Thus, wherever possible, we believe that the use of regional is preferred to general anesthesia for both maternal and fetal considerations. However, it is also our belief that fetal hypoxia and acidosis are far worse for the developing fetal brain and in dire situations, if a preexisting regional anesthetic is not in place, general anesthesia may be required simply because it can be induced quickly.[12]

MULTIPLE GESTATION

Multiple gestation refers to a pregnancy with twins or higher order multiples (eg, triplets, quadruplets).

Incidence

In the United States, the twin birth rate rose 70% between 1980 and 2004. Since then the twin birth rate has been stable.[13] In 2005, twin births represented 3% of all births and triplets and higher order multiples accounted for 0.2% of all births. In 2008, the twin birth rate in the United States was 32.6 per 1000 births and the rates of higher order multiple births (triplets, quadruplets, quintuplets, sextuplets and septuplets) was 147.6 per 100,000 births.[13] The increase in incidence of multiparity may be related to growth in assisted reproductive therapies (in vitro fertilization, ovulation-inducing drugs, and artificial insemination) and pregnancy in older women.

Twin Pregnancy

There are two types of twin pregnancies: dizygotic (66%) (more common) and monozygotic (approximately 30%). In the case of dizygotic twins, two separate ova are fertilized. Dizygotic twins have separate amnions, chorions, and placentae. Monozygotic twins develop from a single fertilized ovum, which splits into two distinct individuals after conception. Twinning (splitting) cannot occur beyond 15 days after fertilization. An early splitting (ie, within 3 days after fertilization) produces separate chorions and amnions. The twins have separate placentas but can also have a single fused one. Approximately 30% of monozygotic twins are dichorionic diamniotic. Splitting between 4 and 8 days after fertilization results in monozygotic monochorionic diamniotic placentation (Figure 10-1). Approximately 70% of monozygotic twins are monochorionic diamniotic. If splitting occurs 8 to 13 days after fertilization, monochorionic monoamniotic placentation occurs. Only 1% of (monozygotic) twins have this form of placentation. If splitting occurs between 13 and 15 days after fertilization, the fertilized ovum splits only partially, resulting in conjoined twins with a monochorionic monoamniotic placenta.

Is It Important to Distinguish Monochorionic From Dichorionic Twins?

Yes, this is because monochorionic twin pregnancies have a much higher rate of complications than dichorionic twin pregnancies. The placentae of nearly all monochorionic twin (monochorionic monoamniotic or monochorionic diamniotic) have vascular communications. Most of these anastomoses are of little fetal consequence because distribution of blood supply is well balanced. However, deeper vascular anastomoses can result in net transfusion of blood from one twin (the donor) to the other twin (the recipient), leading to twin-twin transfusion syndrome (TTTS). The donor twin is usually smaller, suffers from anemia, hypovolemia, and produces less urine. Because urine is the main component of amniotic fluid, the amniotic fluid surrounding the donor will decrease. Severe oligohydramnios can result in the "stuck twin phenomena" (ie, the twins appear "stuck" up against the wall of the uterus in a fixed position).[14] The recipient twin may also develop complications; he or she receives an excess of blood from the donor twin and may develop polyhydramnios, polycythemia, and cardiac failure. In contrast to the donor twin, polyhydramnios develops in the sac because of increased fetal urine output.

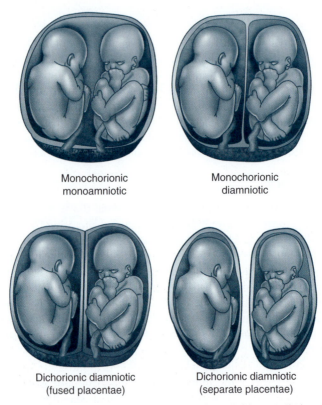

Monochorionic
monoamniotic

Monochorionic
diamniotic

Dichorionic diamniotic
(fused placentae)

Dichorionic diamniotic
(separate placentae)

Figure 10-1. Placentation in twin pregnancies. From Cleary-Goldman J, Chitkara U, Berkowitz R. Multiple gestations. In: Gabbe SG, Niebyl JR, Simpson JL, eds. *Obstetrics: Normal and Problem Pregnancies.* 5th ed. New York, NY: Churchill Livingstone; 2007:736.

TTTS complicates about 15% of *monochorionic* twin pregnancies, usually between 18 and 26 weeks' gestation.[14] Complications include significant neurologic injury to the fetus and even fetal death. Current therapeutic options for TTTS include drainage of excessive fluid (amniocentesis), surgical separation of connecting vessels in the placenta by means of laser (selective laser photocoagulation of communicating vessels [SLPCV]), amniotic septostomy (creating connection between amniotic membrane), and selective feticide. The goal of amniocentesis is to decrease the likelihood of preterm labor by reducing the amniotic fluid volume in the sac of the recipient twin. In contrast, septostomy equilibrates pressures between the two amniotic cavities.[15]

Is It Possible to Distinguish Between Monochorionic and Dichorionic Twins?

The distinction between monochorionic and dichorionic twins can be made on ultrasound scan with 100% accuracy early in pregnancy (ie, before the 14th week of pregnancy). Later on in pregnancy, it becomes far more difficult and will depend on the interpretation of membrane thickness.[15]

Risks of a Multiple Gestation

FETAL COMPLICATIONS

Multifetal pregnancies are high-risk pregnancies. Twins are five times and triplets nearly 15 times more likely than singletons to die within a month of birth.[16] The major issues that affect neonatal outcome with multiple fetal pregnancies include preterm delivery, low birth weight, and intrauterine growth retardation. The mean gestational age at delivery is approximately 35 weeks for twins, 32 weeks for triplets and 30 weeks for quadruplets.[14] The risk of severe intrauterine growth retardation and fetal death are increased significantly when the twins share a common placenta (monochorionic). TTTS syndrome occurs in monochorionic/monoamniotic or monochorionic/diamniotic twins.

Cerebral palsy is estimated to occur four times more often in twin infants and 17 times more often in triplets than in singleton infants. It is possible that the increased risk of cerebral damage is due to the higher incidence of premature birth and low birth weight in twin sets compared with singleton pregnancies.[17]

Congenital anomalies are also more common in twins than a single fetus. The defects commonly involve the CNS, cardiovascular system and gastrointestinal system. Monozygotic twins have an increased prevalence of deformity secondary to twinning, vascular anastomosis, and intrauterine crowding.[18]

Vanishing twin syndrome may also occur. As many as one-half of all twin pregnancies result in the delivery of only a single fetus; the second twin "vanishes." Acute exsanguination of the surviving twin into the relaxed circulation of the deceased twin can result in intrauterine CNS ischemia.[15]

Delivery room management of multiple gestation requires adequate personnel skilled in neonatal resuscitation. Multifetal pregnancies have a significantly higher rate of malpresentation and cesarean delivery; malpresentation increases the risk of umbilical cord prolapse.

MATERNAL COMPLICATIONS

The potential for maternal morbidity and mortality increases in proportion to the number of fetuses. There is increased incidence of premature rupture of membranes/preterm labor, preeclampsia/eclampsia, gestational diabetes mellitus, placental abruption, disseminated intravascular coagulation, pulmonary embolism, operative delivery, and postpartum hemorrhage associated with multiple pregnancy.

In women with multiple gestations, maternal weight increases at a greater rate after 30 weeks' gestation.[19] Because of exaggeration of physiologic changes of pregnancy associated with multiple pregnancy, these mothers are at higher risk for difficult intubation, pulmonary aspiration of gastric contents, and supine hypotension syndrome compared to singleton pregnancy.

For instance, there is a 20% greater increase in cardiac output, an additional 500-mL increase of blood volume, and a more frequent occurrence of anemia compared to women with a singleton fetus.[2] Greater oxygen consumption and decreased functional residual capacity increase the risk of maternal hypoxemia during apnea. Therefore, adequate denitrogenation is essential prior to induction of general anesthesia.

When preterm labor occurs, the mother may receive tocolytic therapy, such as β-adrenergic agonists and magnesium therapy. Those who fail tocolytic therapy may require administration of anesthesia for delivery. The side effects of tocolytic agents are more pronounced in these mothers and may include increased risk of pulmonary edema, postpartum hemorrhage, and altered response to anesthetic agents.

Typically, the method of delivery depends on the gestational age and presentation of twin A (first twin) along with the clinical conditions of the mother and baby. Most obstetricians allow a trial of labor if both twins maintain a vertex presentation. The American College of Obstetricians and Gynecologists (ACOG) currently recommends cesarean delivery when one twin is noncephalic.[20] Following vaginal delivery of the first twin, the method of delivery of the second twin depends on presentation of the fetus, fetal heart rate, and maternal hemorrhage. Intrauterine manipulation of fetus for vaginal delivery or cesarean delivery may be needed for safe delivery. Cesarean delivery is the usual method of delivery for higher-order multiple births (eg, triplets, quadruplets).

Anesthetic Management

SURGERY FOR TWIN-TWIN TRANSFUSION SYNDROME

Local anesthetic infiltration of the abdominal wall is usually sufficient to allow percutaneous procedures such as amniocentesis and SLPCV. Supplemental maternal analgesia and anxiolysis can be achieved by maternal administration of midazolam, opioids, or low-dose propofol infusion. This also may provide some fetal analgesia and immobility via placental transfer. Continuous infusion of remifentanil also has been used to improve fetal immobility and maternal sedation.[21]

LABOR AND DELIVERY

Regional analgesia results in the most effective labor analgesia and offers several advantages during a trial of labor of twin gestation. It prevents early pushing and facilitates a controlled, atraumatic delivery of the after coming head. Because there is a greater risk of cesarean delivery in twin pregnancy, any questionable epidural catheters should be replaced promptly during labor.

Managing a delivery in a patient with multiple gestation should occur in the operating room with preparation for emergency cesarean delivery (double set-up). Effective neuraxial anesthesia facilitates internal podalic version, breech extraction of the second twin, or emergency extension of anesthesia for cesarean delivery, if necessary. Prevention of hypotension and avoidance of aortocaval compression are important. In some cases, uterine relaxation may be required to facilitate internal version and breech extraction. Sublingual (400-800 μg) or intravenous (50-250 μg) nitroglycerin may provide adequate uterine relaxation in most cases. If this is inadequate and/or emergency cesarean delivery is warranted, rapid sequence induction of general anesthesia with endotracheal intubation and potent inhalational agent may be needed.

ABNORMAL PRESENTATION

Introduction

Fetal presentation is defined by the fetal body part that descends first during the second stage of labor and can be palpated via vaginal examination. The bony anatomy of the maternal pelvis must be traversed for successful vaginal delivery. Normally, the fetal head presents first, allowing for a series of six cardinal fetal movements of vaginal delivery. Abnormal presentation may cause more severe labor pain, arrest of descent, fetal heart rate abnormalities, and these may lead to urgent, emergent, or "stat" cesarean deliveries. Knowledge of the various types of abnormal presentations and their obstetric management allows for proper analgesic and anesthetic care of the parturient.

Definitions

An understanding of the definitions of abnormal presentation is required for anesthetic planning.[19,22,23]

PRESENTATION

Fetal body part that overlies the pelvic inlet—
   Cephalic: head
      Vertex: head flexed; chin in contact with trunk
      Face: head hyperextended; occiput in contact with upper back
      Brow: head midway between flexion and hyperextension
   Breech: buttocks and/or lower extremities
      Complete: hip and knee flexed
      Frank: hip flexed and knee extended
      Incomplete: complete breech with deflexion of a hip and/or knee
      Footling: feet (one or both) below the breech
   Shoulder: shoulder
   Compound: fetal extremity presents *with* the main presenting fetal part; may be associated with prolapsed cord

FETAL LIE

Alignment of the fetal spine relative to the maternal spine—
   Longitudinal: fetal spine is parallel to maternal spine
   Transverse: fetal spine is perpendicular to maternal spine
   Oblique: fetal spine is neither parallel nor perpendicular to maternal spine

POSITION

Location of a specific fetal bone relative to the *maternal pelvis*. Fetal bones used to describe position are—
   Occiput: defines the cephalic-vertex presentation
   Mentum: defines the cephalic-face presentation
   Sacrum: defines the breech presentation
   Acromion: defines the shoulder presentation

ATTITUDE

Relationship of fetal head to fetal trunk—
  Flexed: head is flexed down toward trunk
  Military: head is in neutral position
  Hyperextended: head is extended away from trunk

ENGAGEMENT

Widest diameter fetal presenting part passing through pelvic inlet

STATION

Location of fetal presenting part relative to ischial spines. This describes the descent of the fetus through the pelvis and vagina. Ischial spines are at 0 station and the range is −5 to +5. Negative stations are cephalad to the ischial spines, whereas positive stations are caudad to the ischial spines.

Breech Presentation

Breech presentation is the most common nonvertex fetal presentation. It occurs in 3% to 4% of full-term pregnancies[22] and may be diagnosed by physical examination or ultrasound. It is relatively common during early gestation, but by 34 weeks, most fetuses are in the vertex position. Risk factors for breech presentation include abnormalities of the uterus, pelvis, or fetus, as well as obstetric conditions. A list of risk factors is presented in Table 10-2.[19,24]

FETAL AND MATERNAL MORBIDITY AND MORTALITY

Both the fetus and the mother may have increased morbidity associated with breech presentation, both during vaginal and cesarean delivery. Fetal complications associated with breech vaginal delivery are primarily related to congenital anomalies and birth trauma, including fracture of long bones, brachial plexus injury, arrest of delivery of head, fetal asphyxia, seizures, hypotonia, and fetal death.[22] Most worrisome is the increased risk of umbilical cord prolapse (Table 10-3). Because a large body part such as the head or buttocks does not cover the dilated cervix, umbilical cord prolapse is more common with incomplete and complete breech presentations. Umbilical cord prolapse is an obstetrical emergency and requires emergent or "stat" cesarean delivery.

Table 10-2. Risk Factors for Breech Presentation

Uterus: fibroids, septate uterus
Pelvis: pelvic tumor
Fetus: multiple fetuses, macrosomia, prematurity, hydrocephalus, myotonic dystrophy, joint contractures
Placenta: cornual-fundal placenta, placenta previa
Obstetric conditions: multiparity, previous breech, polyhydramnios, oligohydramnios

Table 10-3. Type of Breech Presentation and Risk of Umbilical Cord Prolapse[a]

Type of Breech	Percentage of All Breech	Risk of Umbilical Cord Prolapse (%)
Frank	48-73	0.5
Incomplete	12-38	15-18
Complete	5-12	4-6

[a]Modified from Koffel B. Abnormal presentation and multiple gestation. In: Chestnut DH, Polley LS, Tsen LC, et al. *Chestnut's Obstetric Anesthesia Principles and Practice.* 4th ed. Philadelphia, PA: Mosby Elsevier; 2009:780-781.

Maternal complications during vaginal delivery include chorioamnionitis, perineal trauma, and postpartum hemorrhage. Complications related to unplanned emergency cesarean deliveries include maternal infection, hemorrhage, and hysterectomy.[25]

OBSTETRIC MANAGEMENT

The preferred method of delivery of breech presentation in the United States is cesarean delivery. The 2006 ACOG Committee Opinion on Mode of Term Singleton Breech Delivery states that because most obstetricians are no longer experienced in vaginal breech delivery, cesarean delivery is preferred. A planned vaginal breech delivery is acceptable only if the obstetrician is experienced in this procedure and hospital guidelines are followed.[26] These recommendations are based on the large randomized controlled Term Breech Trial, which concluded that neonatal morbidity and mortality were significantly reduced with planned cesarean delivery compared to planned vaginal breech delivery for single frank or complete breech presentations at 37 weeks' gestation or longer.[22] However, external cephalic version may convert a breech to vertex and result in a vaginal delivery.

EXTERNAL CEPHALIC VERSION

External cephalic version (ECV) is a maneuver done by an obstetrician that changes the fetal presentation from breech to vertex. The purpose of ECV is to allow for cephalic-vertex presentation and vaginal delivery, thus avoiding cesarean delivery. Although the fetus may return to the breech position, ECV performed at about 36 to 39 weeks' gestation increases the probability of the fetus remaining in the cephalic position.[24] ACOG recommends obstetricians to offer and perform ECV when appropriate.[26] The average success rate of ECV is approximately 60%. Risks of the procedure include fetal heart rate abnormalities, rupture of membranes, vaginal bleeding, fetomaternal hemorrhage, and placental abruption.[27]

Anesthetic Management ECV should be performed in a setting where an emergency cesarean delivery can be performed promptly and safely. Both neuraxial (spinal, epidural, and CSE) and intravenous analgesic (fentanyl) have been used successfully. Although success rates are reported to be similar with the two techniques, maternal pain scores were lower and satisfaction scores higher with neuraxial analgesia as compared to intravenous opioids.[28] Apart from satisfactory analgesia, the neuraxial technique also provides adequate relaxation of abdominal muscles, which helps increase the success of ECV. Placement of an epidural catheter (in epidural or CSE technique) helps provide successful labor analgesia in case of induction of labor after successful ECV. The catheter could also be used if needed for emergency cesarean delivery. Both analgesic doses (spinal bupivacaine 2.5 mg plus fentanyl 20 μg, epidural 0.25% bupivacaine) and anesthetic doses (spinal bupivacaine 7.5 mg, epidural 2% lidocaine plus fentanyl 100 μg to obtain a T6 sensory level) have been used in successful version.[27,29] Although the results of studies are conflicting, generally speaking, when compared to *analgesia* for ECV, *anesthesia* for ECV may significantly improve success.[27] This difference may be due to improved abdominal relaxation with anesthetic as compared to analgesic doses of local anesthetic. Risks of regional analgesia and anesthesia for ECV include those associated with neuraxial blockade such as hypotension, postdural puncture headache, and so on.

Vaginal Breech Delivery

Vaginal breech delivery is rarely performed in the United States today. As stated previously, the Term Breech Trial published in 2000 showed a significantly increased rate of neonatal morbidity and mortality with vaginal breech delivery compared to cesarean delivery[22] attributable to vanishing experience. However, obstetricians skilled in vaginal breech delivery may still perform this procedure under specific hospital guidelines.

Analgesia for Labor and Vaginal Breech Delivery The anesthetic management of vaginal breech labor and delivery includes analgesia for labor pain, inhibition of uncontrolled pushing during the first stage of labor, relaxation of the pelvic floor during second stage of labor, and preparedness for emergency cesarean delivery.[19] Regional analgesia can accomplish all of these goals.

During the first stage of labor, pushing may cause the fetal lower extremities and abdomen to enter the partially dilated cervix. The head is significantly larger and will remain in the uterine cavity, thus causing fetal head entrapment. In the second stage of labor, a successful vaginal delivery requires adequate maternal pushing for delivery to the level of the umbilicus. Finally, during extraction of the fetus, profound perineum relaxation is needed. Delivery may be spontaneous or assisted with forceps.[24]

Continuous neuraxial analgesia with dilute anesthetics (bupivacaine 0.0625%-0.125%) allows for effective labor pain relief, adequate pushing in second stage of labor, and adequate perineal muscle relaxation if forceps are used for delivery.[30,31] The epidural catheter can be used to administer 3% 2-chloroprocaine or 2% lidocaine if denser anesthesia is required for mechanical extraction.[19] Importantly, the catheter can also be used to administer anesthesia for emergency cesarean delivery at any time during the course of labor. Straight epidural catheter or spinal catheter placement may be favored over combined spinal-epidural, such that catheter function can be verified immediately after placement.

Nitroglycerin (1-2 sprays [400 μg/spray or 50-500 μg intravenously]) may be used to produce uterine relaxation if needed.[19]

In the event of emergency cesarean delivery, 3% 2-chloroprocaine may be used to establish surgical anesthesia using the epidural catheter.[19] Patients without catheters may be given a single-shot spinal or combined spinal-epidural for emergent cesarean delivery. This must be performed in the lateral position, because umbilical cord prolapse may occur in the sitting position. Where there is no time or no preexisting epidural in place, general anesthesia may be necessary for emergency cesarean delivery. Volatile anesthetics will produce uterine relaxation and facilitate abdominal breech delivery, but they must be reduced after delivery to decrease the risk of postpartum hemorrhage.

ANESTHESIA FOR CESAREAN DELIVERY FOR BREECH PRESENTATION

Elective Cesarean Delivery The majority of mothers with known breech presentation are scheduled for elective cesarean delivery at term. Neuraxial anesthesia (single-shot spinal, epidural, CSE, continuous spinal) is preferred to avoid risks related to general anesthesia. Standard anesthetic doses may be used for neuraxial anesthesia. However, even with cesarean delivery, there is a higher rate of birth trauma in breech deliveries compared to non-breech presentation.[24] Skin and uterine incisions may need to be more extensive for successful breech delivery. If regional anesthesia is contraindicated and general anesthesia is administered, uterine relaxation to augment breech delivery may be achieved with volatile anesthesia.

However, this must be reduced to amnesic levels after delivery to reduce the risk of postpartum hemorrhage from uterine atony. Neonates delivered breech via cesarean delivery more frequently require neonatal resuscitation than those delivered from the vertex presentation.[19]

Cesarean Delivery for Spontaneous Rupture of Membranes Parturients presenting in spontaneous labor with breech presentation may require either urgent or emergent cesarean deliveries, depending on fetal status. Umbilical cord prolapse may manifest as sudden fetal bradycardia with breech presentation. In the presence of reassuring fetal status, neuraxial anesthesia in the lateral position is preferred. General anesthesia is indicated for dire emergencies or where a regional block cannot be performed.

REFERENCES

1. American College of Obstetricians and Gynecologists (ACOG). ACOG Committee on Practice Bulletins—Obstetrics. Management of preterm labor. Practice Bulletin No. 43. May 2003. *Int J Gynaecol Obstet.* 2003;82(1):127-135.

2. Muir HA, Wong CA. Preterm labor and delivery. In: Chestnut DH, Polley LS, Tsen LC, et al. *Chestnut's Obstetric Anesthesia Principles and Practice.* 4th ed. Philadelphia, PA: Mosby Elsevier; 2009:749-777.

3. Iams JD, Romero R. Preterm birth. In: Gabbe SG, Niebyl JR, Simpson JL, et al. *Obstetrics: Normal and Problem Pregnancies.* 5th ed. Philadelphia, PA: Churchill Livingstone; 2007. Online version.

4. Hobel, CJ. Obstetric complications: preterm labor, PROM, IUGR, postterm pregnancy, and IUFD. In: Hacker NF, Moore JG, Gambone JC, et al. *Essentials of Obstetrics and Gynecology.* 4th ed. Philadelphia, PA: Elsevier Saunders; 2004:167-182.

5. Horlocker TT, Wedel DJ, Rowlingson JC, et al. Regional anesthesia in the patient receiving antithrombotic or thrombolytic therapy: American Society of Regional Anesthesia and Pain Medicine Evidence-Based Guidelines (3rd ed.). *Reg Anesth Pain Med.* 2010;35(1):64-101.

6. Blumenfeld YJ, Lyell DJ. Prematurity prevention: the role of acute tocolysis. *Curr Opin Obstet Gynecol.* 2009;21(2):136-141.

7. Han S, Crowther CA, Moore V. Magnesium maintenance therapy for preventing preterm birth after threatened preterm labour. *Cochrane Database Syst Rev*. 2010;(7):CD000940.

8. Fox NS, Gelber SE, Kalish RB, Chasen ST. Contemporary practice patterns and beliefs regarding tocolysis among U.S. maternal-fetal medicine specialists. *Obstet Gynecol*. 2008;112(1):42-47.

9. Nassar AH, Aoun J, Usta IM. Calcium channel blockers for the management of preterm birth: a review. *Am J Perinatol*. 2011;28(1):57-66. Epub 2010 July 16.

10. National Institutes of Health. Antenatal corticosteroids revisited: repeat courses—Consensus Development Conference Statement, August 17-18, 2000. *Obstet Gynecol*. 2001;98:144-150.

11. Mardirosoff C, Dumont L, Boulvain M, Tramèr MR. Fetal bradycardia due to intrathecal opioids for labour analgesia: a systematic review. *BJOG*. 2002;109(3):274-281.

12. Creeley CE, Olney JW. The young: neuroapoptosis induced by anesthetics and what to do about it. *Anesth Analg*. 2010;110:442-448.

13. Martin JA, Hamilton BE, Sutton PD, et al. Births: final data for 2007. *Natl Vital Stat Rep*. 2010:58:1-86.

14. Cunningham FG, Leveno KJ, Bloom SL, et al. *Williams Obstetrics*. 22nd ed. New York, NY: McGraw-Hill; 2005:911-948.

15. Quintero RA, Chmait RH. Operative fetoscopy in complicated monochorionic twins: current status and future direction. *Curr Opin Obstet Gynecol*. 2008;20:169-174.

16. Martin JA, Hamilton BE, Sutton PD, et al. Births: final data for 2005. *Natl Vital Stat Rep*. 2007:56:1-103.

17. Blickstein I. Cerebral palsy in multifoetal pregnancies. *Dev Med Child Neurol*. 2002;44:352-355.

18. American College of Obstetricians and Gynecologists (ACOG). Multiple gestation: complicated twin, triplet, and high order multifetal pregnancy. Practice Bulletin. No 56. Oct 2004.

19. Koffel B. Abnormal presentation and multiple gestation. In: Chestnut DH, Polley LS, Tsen LC, et al. *Chestnut's Obstetric Anesthesia Principles and Practice*. 4th ed. Philadelphia, PA: Mosby Elsevier; 2009:779-793.

20. Cleary-Goldman J, Chitkara U, Berkowitz R. Multiple gestations. In: Gabbe SgG, Niebyl JR, Simpson JL, eds. *Obstetrics: Normal and Problem Pregnancies*. 5th ed. New York, NY: Churchill Livingstone; 2007:733-770.

21. Van de Velde M, Van Schoubroeck D, Lewis LE, et al. Remifentanil for fetal immobilization and maternal sedation during fetoscopic surgery. A randomized double blind comparison with diazepam. *Anesth Analg*. 2005;101:251-258.

22. Hannah ME, Hannah WJ, Hewson SA, Hodnett ED, Saigal S, Willan AR. Planned caesarean section versus planned vaginal birth for breech presentation at term: a randomised multicentre trial. Term Breech Trial Collaborative Group. *Lancet*. 2000;356(9239):1375-1383.

23. Moore TR. Multifetal gestation and malpresentation. In: Hacker NF, Moore JG, Gambone JC, et al. *Essentials of Obstetrics and Gynecology*. 4th ed. Philadelphia, PA: Elsevier Saunders; 2004:183-196.

24. Lanni SM, Seeds JW. Malpresentations. In: Gabbe SG, Niebyl JR, Simpson JL, et al. *Obstetrics: Normal and Problem Pregnancies*. 5th ed. Philadelphia, PA: Churchill Livingstone; 2007. Online Version.

25. Binghaum P, Lilford R. Management of selected term breech presentation: assessment of the risks of selected vaginal delivery versus cesarean section for all cases. *Obstet Gynecol*. 1987;69:965-978.

26. American College of Obstetricians and Gynecologists (ACOG). ACOG Committee on Obstetric Practice. Mode of term singleton breech delivery. ACOG Committee Opinion No. 340. *Obstet Gynecol*. 2006;108(1):235-237.

27. Lavoie A, Guay J. Anesthetic dose neuraxial blockade increases the success rate of external fetal version: a meta-analysis. *Can J Anaesth*. 2010;57(5):408-414.

28. Sullivan JT, Grobman WA, Bauchat JR, et al. A randomized controlled trial of the effect of combined spinal-epidural analgesia on the success of external cephalic version for breech presentation. *Int J Obstet Anesth*. 2009;18(4):328-334.

29. Yoshida M, Matsuda H, Kawakami Y, et al. Effectiveness of epidural anesthesia for external cephalic versión. *J Perinatol*. 2010;30:580-583.

30. Benhamou D, Mercier FJ, Ben Ayed M, Auroy Y. Continuous epidural analgesia with bupivacaine 0.125% or bupivacaine 0.0625% plus sufentanil 0.25 mg·mL⁻¹: a study in singleton breech presentation. *Int J Obstet Anesth*. 2002;11(1):13-18.

31. Van Zundert A, Vaes L, Soetens M, et al. Are breech deliveries an indication for lumbar epidural analgesia? *Anesth Analg*. 1991;72(3):399-403.

Assessment of the Newborn and Neonatal Resuscitation

11

Deborah J. Stein and Thomas E. Bate

INTRODUCTION

Anesthesiologists are often involved in various aspects of care on a labor and delivery unit. However, the anesthesiologist's primary responsibility is to provide care to the mother, particularly during an anesthetic for cesarean or complicated vaginal delivery. Thus, on a labor and delivery unit, at least one person other than the members of surgical team should be qualified to provide neonatal resuscitation and be immediately available to assume responsibility for resuscitation of the depressed newborn.[1] Because the primary responsibility of the obstetrician and anesthesiologist is care of the mother, these individuals may not be able to shift care from the mother to the newborn. For the anesthesiologist, this may even be the case when the patient has a neuraxial anesthetic that is functioning adequately.[1] However, the anesthesiologist should offer assistance in situations including management of a difficult neonatal airway or during the absence of a designated qualified individual for resuscitation. The benefit to the child must be weighed against the risk to the mother in these special circumstances.[2] In the majority of situations, after assisted vaginal delivery or cesarean section, the mother is stable; therefore, if there is a need for neonatal resuscitation, the anesthesiologist should be available to help. In certain institutions, there may be an anesthesia care team caring for the mother (eg, an attending and a resident or fellow, or a nurse anesthetist). If the mother is stable, one member of this team may be free to help care for the neonate. It is important to keep in mind that soon after delivery the mother is undergoing tremendous physiologic changes and maternal status may change quickly. It still remains a judgment call for the anesthesiologist in charge to determine where his or her priorities lie—caring for either the mother or the newborn or caring for both.

149

History

Neonatal resuscitation has come a long way since the days of swinging the infant upside down and dilating the rectum with a raven's beak back in the 19th century.[3] Figure 11-1 is an illustration, reputedly of Dr. Bernhard Schultze himself, demonstrating the Schultze method of neonatal resuscitation.

There are approximately 4 million neonatal deaths per year worldwide, and 23% of these are the result of birth asphyxia.[4] In an attempt to improve outcome, the Neonatal Resuscitation Program (NRP) was developed by a joint American Academy of Pediatrics (AAP) and American Heart Association (AHA) committee, which produced its first textbook in 1987.[5] The NRP was initiated to ensure that at least one person trained in neonatal resuscitation be present in every hospital delivery, and it is designed to be uniform for all personnel who attend deliveries, including physicians and nurses. By the end of 2010, more than 2.9 million health care providers in the United States had been trained in the techniques of neonatal resuscitation.[5] It is strongly recommended that anyone who may be involved in

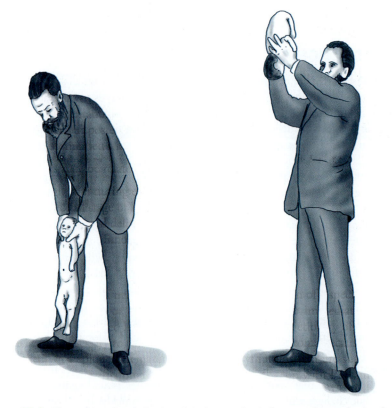

Figure 11-1. The outdated and obsolete Schultze method of neonatal resuscitation from the 19th century. From Schultze BS. *Der Scheintod Neugeborener.* Jena: Mauke's Verlag; 1871.

neonatal resuscitation should be trained and kept up-to-date with these neonatal resuscitation programs.

One of the most important factors demonstrated to provide better outcomes in neonatal resuscitation is communication among the caregivers. The other major criteria for success is that neonatal resuscitation is most effective when performed by a designated and coordinated team. Recent work in the field of neonatal resuscitation culminated in the guidelines mentioned above. Although these guidelines apply primarily to newborn infants undergoing transition from intra to extrauterine life, they may be applied within the first week to months after birth, should the clinician be called to a neonatal resuscitation.

Epidemiology

Delivery, although generally safe, may be complicated for some infants. Approximately, 10% of births will require some sort of assistance following delivery, and approximately 1% of these infants will require extensive resuscitation.[6] In the United States, there are approximately 5000 delivery rooms, with a total of 4,130,665 births registered in 2009.[7] According to these statistics, this will result in approximately 400,000 neonatal resuscitations a year, and thankfully the majority of these will result in a healthy newborn. Keep in mind that prolonged resuscitation in the newborn is a poor prognostic feature.

NEONATAL RESUSCITATION

Neonatal resuscitation should be planned in an organized fashion, with anticipation, preparation, evaluation, and management of the infant. Each item is described in detail below.

Anticipation: Identifying the At-Risk Mother and Fetus

Early knowledge of a complicated or high-risk pregnancy is important. In anticipating the need for resuscitation, it helps to monitor the progress of labor and fetal well-being. The need for resuscitation can be predicted in approximately 80% of cases.[2] Table 11-1 identifies some of the many antepartum and intrapartum risk factors to consider, which should put one on high alert for the need to resuscitate the neonate.[5] Another very useful method of assessing the fetus is fetal scalp blood sampling. Any time the procedure is carried out on the labor floor, the anesthesiologist should be informed beforehand and should be on standby for an urgent or emergent delivery. The fetal scalp sample values, both normal and abnormal, and their interpretations and resultant obstetric plans are outlined in Table 11-2.[8]

Preparation

As with most things in anesthesiology, problems that can be foreseen, anticipated, and prepared for in advance may be dealt with more successfully. In trauma, the "golden hour" is often described as being the crucial resuscitation steps taken in

Table 11-1. Risk Factors Suggesting a Greater Need for Neonatal Resuscitation

Antepartum Risk Factors	Intrapartum Risk Factors
• Maternal diabetes	• Emergency cesarean delivery
• Hypertensive disorder of pregnancy (including preeclampsia)	• Forceps or vacuum-assisted delivery
• Chronic hypertension	• Breech or other abnormal presentation
• Chronic maternal illness (eg, cardiovascular, thyroid, neurologic, pulmonary, renal)	• Preterm labor
	• Precipitous labor
• Anemia or isoimmunization	• Chorioamnionitis
• Previous fetal or neonatal death	• Prolonged rupture of membranes (> 18 hours before delivery)
• Bleeding in second or third trimester	• Prolonged labor (> 24 hours)
• Maternal infection (eg, GBS, HIV, CMV)	• Prolonged second stage of labor (> 2 hours)
• Polyhydramnios	• Fetal bradycardia
• Oligohydramnios	• Nonreassuring fetal heart rate pattern
• Premature rupture of membranes/preterm delivery	• Use of general anesthesia
	• Uterine tetany
• Post-term gestation	• Maternal administration of opioids within 4 hours of delivery
• Multiple gestation	
• Discrepancy between fetal size and dates (ie, last menstrual period)	• Meconium-stained amniotic fluid
	• Prolapsed cord
• Drug therapy (eg, lithium carbonate, magnesium, adrenergic-blocking drugs and adrenergic agonists)	• Placental abruption
	• Placenta previa
• Maternal substance abuse	• Significant intrapartum bleed (including trauma and hypovolemia)
• Fetal malformation or anomalies (including fetal hydrops)	• Macrosomia
• Diminished fetal activity	
• No prenatal care	
• Maternal age < 16 or > 35 years	

Data from Aucott SL, Zuckerman RL[2] and American Academy of Pediatrics and American Heart Association.[5]

the hour immediately after the initial trauma. In neonatal resuscitation, it may be considered that there is a "golden minute" immediately after the neonate is born. The initial two steps in the neonatal resuscitation algorithm take place over two 30-second intervals—the "golden minute." Despite prior assessment of risk during pregnancy and labor, there remains unpredictability about which newborns may require resuscitation; therefore, staff must be ready to resuscitate in all situations. A good resource to guide clinical practice in this regard is the 2010 update from the AHA and the AAP resuscitation guidelines,[6] some of which are discussed later in this chapter. It must be remembered that these guidelines are continually being challenged and updated, and some of the guidelines are already being reassessed.

In preparing for resuscitation of the newborn, one must become familiar with all the equipment that may be needed, and these should be checked on a regular

Table 11-2. Blood Gases/Fetal Blood Sampling

Normal
pH: 7.25-7.35 pCO_2: 40-50 mm Hg pO_2: 20-30 mm Hg Base excess: < 10 mmol/L
Nonreassuring Findings
pH: < 7.20 Base excess: ≤ 12 mmol/L
Metabolic Acidosis
pH: <7.25 pCO_2: 45-55 mm Hg pO_2: < 20 mm Hg Base excess: > 10 mmol/L
Respiratory Acidosis
pH: < 7.25 pCO_2: > 50 mm Hg pO_2: varies Base excess: < 10 mmol/L
Interpretation
Scalp pH ≥ 7.25 and fetal heart tracing (FHT) remains nonreassuring. Continue to observe labor. Repeat scalp sampling every 2-3 hours. Scalp pH ≥ 7.20 and FHT remains nonreassuring. Repeat scalp sample in 15-30 minutes. Scalp pH < 7.20. Repeat scalp sample immediately. If no change in pH, then immediate delivery.

Used with permission from Scott Moses, MD at Fpnotebook.com. Fetal scalp pH. http://www.fpnotebook.com/OB/Lab/FtalSclpPh.htm. Updated July 16, 2014.[8]

basis. It is essential to have equipment readily available and in good working condition. See Table 11-3 and Figure 11-2 for equipment that should be on hand.

Evaluation and Management

A prompt and accurate assessment of newborn should be performed immediately after birth. This will help to identify the infants who need immediate attention.

THE THREE TS

In assessment of the newborn, there are three questions that need to be answered immediately. These are the three Ts—tone, term, and tantrum. This translates as active or floppy, gestational age, and crying or breathing. If the answer is "yes" to all three questions—good tone, term gestation, and crying—no further intervention is required. If the answer is "no" to any questions, then resuscitation of some sort is required. The presence of meconium may also predispose the neonate to require some degree of resuscitation. Color in the neonate is difficult to assess

Table 11-3. Equipment

Suction Equipment

- Bulb syringe
- Mechanical suction and tubing
- Suction catheters: 5F or 6F, 8F, and 10F, 12F or 14F
- 8F feeding tube and 20-mL syringe
- Meconium aspiration device

Bag-and-Mask Equipment

- Neonatal resuscitation bag with a pressure-release valve or pressure manometer (the bag must be capable of delivering 90%-100% oxygen)
- Face masks: newborn and preterm sizes (masks with cushioned rim preferred)
- Oxygen source
- Compressed air source
- Oxygen blender to mix oxygen and compressed air with flow meter (flow rate up to 10 L/min) and tubing

Intubation Equipment

- Laryngoscope with straight blades: number 0, 00 (preterm) and number 1 (term)
- Extra bulbs and batteries for laryngoscope
- Tracheal tubes: 2.5, 3.0, 3.5, and 4.0 mm ID uncuffed
- Stylet (optional)
- Scissors
- Tape or securing device for tracheal tube
- Alcohol sponges
- CO_2 detector or capnograph
- Laryngeal mask airway

Medications

- Epinephrine 1:10,000 (0.1 mg/mL): 3-mL or 10-mL ampules
- Isotonic crystalloid (normal saline or Ringer's lactate) for volume expansion: 100 or 250 mL
- Sodium bicarbonate 4.2% (5 mEq/10 mL): 10-mL ampules
- Naloxone hydrochloride 0.4 mg/mL: 1-mL ampules (or 1.0 mg/mL, 2-mL ampules)
- Normal saline: 30 mL
- Dextrose 10%: 250 mL
- Feeding tube: 5F (optional)

Umbilical Vessel Catheterization Supplies

- Sterile gloves/hat/mask/gown
- Scalpel or scissors
- Povidone-iodine solution/prep solution
- Umbilical tape
- Umbilical catheters: 3.5F, 5F
- Three-way stopcock
- Syringes: 1-, 3-, 5-, 10-, 20-, and 50-mL
- Needles: 25-, 21-, and 18-gauge, or puncture device for needleless system

(continued)

Table 11-3. Equipment (Continued)

Miscellaneous
• Gloves and appropriate personal protection, gowns, masks, caps
• Radiant warmer or other heat source
• Firm, padded resuscitation surface
• Clock (timer optional)
• Warmed linens
• Stethoscope
• Tape: ½ or ¾ inch
• Cardiac monitor and electrodes and/or pulse oximeter with probe (optional for delivery room)
• Oropharyngeal airways
For Very Preterm Infants
• Size 00 laryngoscope blade (optional)
• Reclosable, food-grade plastic bag (1 gal size) or plastic wrap
• Chemically activated warming pad (optional)
• Transport incubator to maintain infant's temperature during move to the nursery
• Oxygen

Data from Aucott SL, Zuckerman RL[2] and American Academy of Pediatrics and American Heart Association.[5]

accurately and is a poor means of judging oxygenation.[9] It is no longer used as an initial form of assessment in NRP training.

The normal transition from intrauterine to extrauterine environment happens with three important changes after birth: replacement of fluid in the alveoli by air, dilation of pulmonary vessels by increased levels of oxygen, and rise in systemic pressure due to clamping of umbilical cord and resultant isolation of low-pressure placental circulation.[5]

This transition is facilitated by the initial cries and breathing of the infant. A respiratory rate of 30 to 60 breaths/min should be expected within 30 seconds of birth, and respirations should be regular by 90 seconds after delivery. A newborn that is not breathing may have either primary or secondary apnea. Animal work from the 1960s contributed to understanding of the pathophysiology of fetal asphyxia. When the fetus becomes hypoxic, it will attempt to breathe in utero. Further hypoxia leads to primary apnea. After 2 to 3 minutes, continuing hypoxia leads to primitive gasping reflex breaths. These are irregular and uncoordinated at a rate of 6 to 12 breaths/min; further hypoxia causes this gasping to cease and results in secondary (terminal) apnea, which may lead to bradycardia and hypotension.[10] The importance is that stimulation will be effective in restoration of breathing in primary apnea, but secondary apnea is a terminal event and positive pressure ventilation (PPV) needs to be initiated as quickly as possible. Figure 11-3 demonstrates the physiologic changes and the acid-base balance associated with the response of a mammalian fetus to total sustained asphyxia starting at time zero. It highlights the need to carry out assessment and resuscitation immediately and simultaneously.

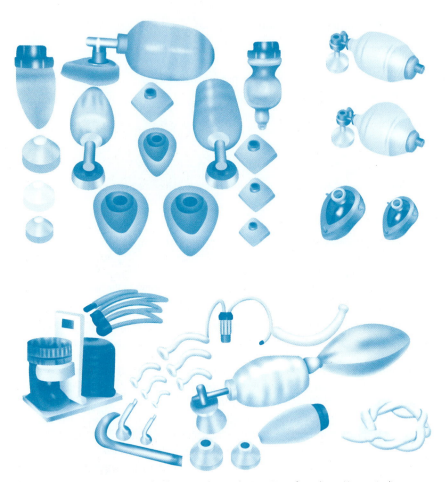

Figure 11-2. Various items for bag/mask ventilation. Data from http://www.indiamart. com/meditrininstruments/infant-careequipment.html.

The NRP concentrates on simple and sensitive methods of assessment and resuscitation for the newborn.

A stepwise progression is taught through the resuscitation flow diagram seen in Figure 11-4. Any deviations from these criteria can be promptly assessed and treated if abnormal. The pink boxes indicate assessments, and the various colored boxes show actions that may be required following these assessments. The subject of meconium aspiration, where treatment differs from the algorithm, is discussed later in the chapter. Initially, the discussion will focus on routine assessment of the neonate. Apgar score is not recommended as a means of determining the need for resuscitation in neonates. By definition, Apgar Scores are determined at 1 and 5 minutes. By 1 minute, the most important part of assessment and treatment should be well underway. However, Apgar scores are very useful for conveying

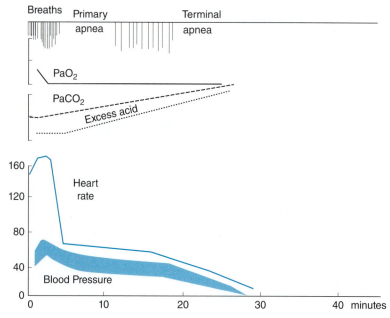

Figure 11-3. Diagrammatic representation of primary and secondary (terminal) apnea following the onset of acute total asphyxia at time 0. European Paediatric Life support. 3rd ed. 2011:102. Reproduced with the kind permission of the Resuscitation Council (UK).

information about responses to resuscitative efforts. A maximum score of 10 is obtained from five different categories shown in Table 11-4.

The assessment blocks should proceed with continuous assessment of resuscitation efforts. The steps in initial resuscitation are discussed below.

BLOCK A: AIRWAY

The initial steps in neonatal resuscitation are to dry and warm the newborn, position the head to open the airway and clear the airway as necessary (see Stimulation Technique/Meconium), and stimulate and maintain the patent airway. Stimulation involves rubbing the newborn while drying and gently tapping the feet. Aggressive stimulation (eg, slapping the back, shaking) and continued use of stimulation in an apneic infant should be avoided. Evaluate the neonate during and immediately following this first intervention. No more than 30 seconds should be taken for these steps; breathing and heart rate are simultaneously assessed. A stethoscope on the precordium is the best technique for determining the neonatal heart rate. Palpation at the base of the umbilical cord can be used in the first few minutes of life to measure the neonatal heart rate, but it is unreliable if the heart rate is less than 100 beats/min. If the newborn does not respond, the neonate may have secondary apnea and more aggressive intervention, such as mask ventilation and possibly intubation, is warranted.

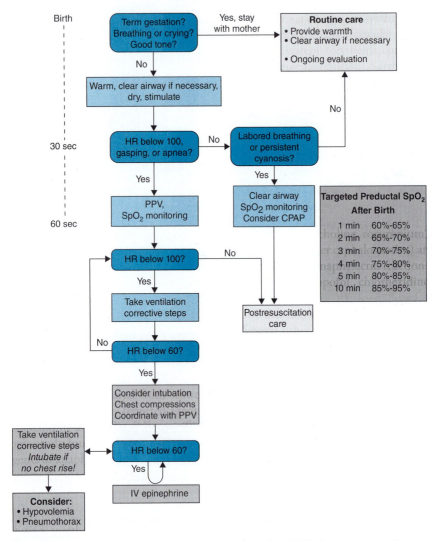

Figure 11-4. Neonatal Resuscitation Program algorithm. CPAP, continuous positive airway pressure; HR, heart rate; IV, intravenous; PPV, positive pressure ventilation. (Kattwinkel, et al. Special Report: Neonatal Resuscitation: 2010 American Heart Association Guidelines for Cardiopulmonary Resuscitation and Emergency Cardiovascular Care. *Pediatrics.* 2010;126(5):e1400-e1413; *Pediatrics.* 2011;128:176).

Supplemental Oxygen The immediate use of 100% oxygen during neonatal resuscitation is discouraged. Studies have demonstrated that when compared with 100% oxygen, resuscitation in asphyxiated infants initiated with air or air/oxygen blend resulted in improved survival and lower incidence of hypoxemia.[11,12] It is recommended that oxygen saturation should be maintained at preductal levels using

Table 11-4. Apgar Score

Parameter	0	1	2
Heart Rate (bpm)	Absent	< 100	> 100
Respiratory Effort	Absent	Irregular, slow, shallow, or gasping respirations	Robust, crying
Muscle Tone	Absent, limp	Some flexion of extremities	Active movement
Reflex Irritability (nasal catheter, oropharyngeal suctioning)	No response	Grimace	Active coughing and sneezing
Color	Cyanotic	Acrocyanotic (trunk pink, extremities blue)	Pink

From Chestnut MD. *Chestnut's Obstetric Anesthesia: Principles and Practice.* 4th ed. Philadelphia PA: Elsevier (Mosby); 2009.

air or blended oxygen mixture for both preterm and term neonates. The oxygen concentration could then be increased as needed to achieve the targeted oxygen saturation as shown in Figure 11-4.

BLOCK B: BREATHING

If the neonate is apneic, or the heart rate is below 100 beats/min, then Positive Pressure Ventilation should be started without delay. With the help of a self-inflating bag and properly fitting appropriate size masks (or endotracheal tube as indicated), assisted ventilation should be delivered at a rate of 40 to 60 per minute. If the heart rate fails to increase and/or inadequate chest excursions, denoting inadequacy of ventilation, persist, then prompt maneuvers such as repositioning of mask to attempt a better seal, reassessment of head position (with neck extension), and clearing of oropharyngeal secretions should be initiated. If there is respiratory distress, then continuous positive airway pressure (CPAP) can be considered by those familiar with the technique, although data supporting beneficial effects of CPAP on the outcome of neonates are still lacking.[6]

All personnel trained in NRP should be able to effectively provide PPV. If either PPV or CPAP is needed, a pulse oximeter is required to determine the need for supplemental oxygen. The pulse oximeter probe should be attached to the hand of the neonate first and only then plugged into the machine. The probe should be placed on the right side of the newborn so as to measure preductal saturation.[10]

Respiratory effort and heart rate should be reassessed after 30 seconds of effective ventilation. The primary goal of intervention, at this juncture, is to ensure adequate ventilation. In the majority of cases, after effective ventilation, the neonate's heart rate will increase to above 100 beats/min. As stated previously, in neonates, respiratory support is the key to successful resuscitation. If the neonatal heart rate continues to decrease despite adequate PPV and falls to less than 60 beats/min, then move to block C for continued resuscitation.

BLOCK C: CIRCULATION

Chest compressions should be started when the heart rate is below 60 beats/min, even with adequate ventilation, after 30 seconds, and should be performed with a ratio of 3:1 compressions to ventilations with 90 compressions and 30 breaths/min. A two-handed technique for chest compressions is recommended with both of the resuscitator's hands encircling the chest of the neonate as in Figure 11-5 During chest compressions, pressure should be applied at the lower third of the sternum to a depth of approximately one-third of anteroposterior depth of the chest at that point. The need for chest compressions goes hand-in-hand with intubation, which should be performed at this point, if it had not already been done. This ensures that assisted ventilation is being delivered optimally because chest compressions are likely to compete with effective ventilation.[6] Endotracheal intubation is also indicated during ineffective bag-and-mask ventilation, tracheal suctioning of less active meconium-stained newborn, or in special cases, such as in patients with congenital diaphragmatic hernia or in very low birth weight patients. Placement of the endotracheal tube should be confirmed by a carbon dioxide detector, although keep in mind that in cases of significantly decreased or absent pulmonary blood flow, it may fail to demonstrate the presence of CO_2 on exhalation. Other less ideal but commonly used methods to confirm endotracheal tube

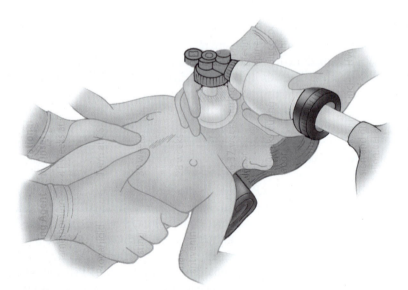

Figure 11-5. Two thumb-encircling hands chest compression in infant (two rescuers).
Frölich MA. Chapter 41. Obstetric Anesthesia. In: Butterworth JF, IV, Mackey DC, Wasnick JD. eds. Morgan & Mikhail's Clinical Anesthesiology, 5e. New York, NY: McGraw-Hill; 2013. http://accessmedicine.mhmedical.com/content.aspx?bookid=564&Sectionid=42800573. Accessed December 22, 2014

placement are auscultation of breath sounds, chest rise, and condensation in the endotracheal tube. In cases of difficult intubation, placement of laryngeal mask airway should be considered to achieve ventilation.[6]

At this point the neonate is reevaluated and reassessed and if the heart rate remains below 60 beats/min, then the resuscitative measures move onto block D.

BLOCK D: DRUGS

Epinephrine is administered at a dose of 0.01 to 0.03 mg/kg given intravenously. There are conflicting recommendations for administration of epinephrine via the endotracheal tube, and some clinicians may still choose to use this route if intravenous access cannot be obtained. Pulmonary absorption is slower and more unpredictable unpredictable than with intravenous administration, and doses of up to 0.1 mg/kg are likely to be needed. Intravenous access should be established through an umbilical vein catheterization. Intraosseous access can be used temporarily if initial umbilical vein catheterization attempts are unsuccessful.[4] The neonate must be reevaluated at every stage of the resuscitation. If the heart rate increases to above 60 beats/min, then chest compressions should be stopped. PPV should be continued until the heart rate has increased to above 100 beats/min.

ADJUVANTS

Other drugs and volume expansion are used in exceptional circumstances along with therapeutic hypothermia. These are discussed below.

Summary: Routine Resuscitation The resuscitation of a newborn is broken down into 30-second intervals while progressing through the flow diagram (Figure 11-4). It is essential to work as a team to accomplish each step of the resuscitation. If the need for neonatal resuscitation at a delivery is anticipated, the recruitment of additional skilled personnel should be undertaken prior to delivery. Prepare and check all the equipment that may be necessary prior to delivery of the neonate.

Stimulation Technique/Meconium At the time of delivery, brisk but gentle drying with a soft towel should be used to stimulate the infant to breathe. For premature infants who are placed in or under a polyethylene bag or sheet to prevent evaporative heat loss, drying beforehand is unnecessary and potentially counterproductive. Tactile stimulation for the premature neonate may be provided through the bag or sheet, if needed. In delivery of nonvigorous, meconium-exposed infants, intubation and suction of meconium from the trachea is indicated. Intubation should occur immediately after delivery, prior to the neonate's first breath and stimulation should be withheld until suction is completed. In this manner, it is possible to determine if the neonate has meconium below the vocal cords, which puts the newborn at risk for meconium aspiration syndrome. Slapping, shaking, spanking, or holding the newborn upside down, which may have been used in the past, are potentially dangerous actions and should not be used as methods of stimulation. During all handling of the neonate, care should be taken to ensure that the head and neck are supported in a neutral position, especially if muscle tone is low.[9]

Drug Administration Drugs are rarely indicated in newborn resuscitation because the majority of neonates requiring resuscitation will respond to supplemental oxygen and ventilation. If the neonate does not respond to ventilation and supplemental oxygen, then epinephrine may be used to boost heart rate and cardiac output to increase oxygen delivery. Narcotic antagonists and vasopressors, excluding epinephrine, may be useful drugs in a neonatal resuscitation, but they are not recommended in the delivery room. Intravenous glucose may be considered in certain circumstances, to avoid neonatal hypoglycemia.[3]

Volume expansion should be considered when blood loss is known or suspected and other resuscitative measures have been unsuccessful. An isotonic crystalloid solution or blood transfusion is recommended at 10 mL/kg.[6]

Induced Therapeutic Hypothermia It is recommended that infants born at greater than 36 weeks' gestation, with evolving moderate to severe hypoxic encephalopathy, be offered therapeutic hypothermia. Neonatal intensive care units should have protocols and strict parameters outlined for which neonates may be eligible for this treatment. Expert advice should be sought urgently regarding such protocols so the neonate may be transferred, if necessary, to an institution that can provide this service.

Resuscitation of Preterm Infants When a preterm delivery is anticipated, special preparation is required. Preterm infants may have immature lungs that are more susceptible to injury by PPV, and these neonates may be more difficult to ventilate. They have immature blood vessels in the brain, which makes them more susceptible to intraventricular hemorrhage. These neonates have thin skin and a large surface area, which can contribute to more rapid heat loss. To avoid excess heat loss, food-grade plastic bags can be used to wrap the infant in immediately after delivery. Premature infants are also at an increased risk of infection and more susceptible to hypovolemic shock related to their small blood volume when compared to term neonates.[6] However, rapid volume expansion with large amount of fluid may cause intraventricular hemorrhage in premature infants.[6]

Discontinuation Prognosis When resuscitative efforts have continued for more than 10 minutes in neonates, there is a very poor prognosis. If this is the situation, it is important to consider the presumed etiology of the need for resuscitation, the gestational age of the neonate at the time of delivery, and the parents' wishes when assessing the benefits of continuing resuscitative efforts.

FURTHER WORK

Historically, most of the guidelines for neonatal resuscitation have been based on personal and professional opinions. More and more randomized control trials are being conducted. The ultimate goal in neonatal resuscitation is to have interventions based on the best available scientific evidence. Despite the difficulty in conducting such trials in the delivery or operating rooms, clinicians need to strive to conduct further high-quality studies and audit outcomes and most importantly, continue to question themselves and reassess.

CASE STUDY

You are called into the delivery room just as an infant is being delivered. You are told that the pediatrician has been called but has not arrived. The patient is a multiparous woman at term whose membranes ruptured, and the fluid was noted to contain meconium. The parturient's labor has progressed rapidly and she has delivered precipitously.

Questions

1. What is your initial assessment of the infant?

2. What is your next step?

3. What is the key intervention that should be performed?

4. Should chest compressions be started?

5. What further options are available if the heart rate had continued to drop?

6. Where should this infant go? What are your plans for this infant?

Answers

1. In the initial assessment of the neonate, remember the three Ts—tone (floppy), term (gestational age), and tantrum (crying, breathing). The infant is covered in meconium and is making a poor, uncoordinated respiratory effort. You are handed the infant and note that it has poor tone.

2. This nonvigorous infant has a meconium aspiration risk. The neonatal heart rate should be assessed before stimulating the newborn. If the heart rate is more than 100 beats/min, the neonate should be intubated and the trachea suctioned for evidence of meconium. The infant's heart rate is 120 beats/min. Intubation of the trachea using a meconium aspirator recovers large amounts of meconium. The heart rate has now dropped to 80 beats/min on reevaluation.

3. At this juncture, because the neonatal heart rate has dropped below 100 beats/min, PPV is required. You apply a face mask but have difficulty inflating the lungs with a bag-and-mask, so you decide to intubate the infant's trachea. Following the tracheal intubation, the neonate's chest appears to rise well, breath sounds are heard equally bilaterally, and a CO_2 monitor confirms air exchange. You ventilate the neonate's lungs for 30 seconds, but despite these efforts, the neonate's heart rate drops further to 50 beats/min.

4. Yes. Chest compressions should be started because the neonatal heart rate is less than 60 beats/min. You have secured the airway; clinical examination suggests the intubation was successful; and a CO_2 exchanger is positive for expired CO_2, which confirms ventilation is optimal at present. A pulse oximeter should be attached if not done so already. Chest compressions are commenced and when the heart rate is reevaluated, it is 110 beats/min. Chest compressions should be stopped and the PPV continued until there is evidence of spontaneous

respiratory efforts. The need for continued intubation and supplemental oxygen should be reassessed.

5. Epinephrine intravenously would be the next step after securing umbilical vein catheterization of the neonate. At this point, volume expanders could be considered if there is suspicion of blood loss during delivery.

6. This has been an extensive neonatal resuscitation, and this infant should go to the neonatal intensive care unit for further stabilization, treatment, and monitoring.

REFERENCES

1. American Society of Anesthesiologists. Guidelines for Obstetric Anesthesia. Optimal Goals For Anesthesia Care in Obstetrics. 2010. www.asahq.org.

2. Aucott SW, Zuckerman RL. Neonatal assessment and resuscitation. In: Chestnut DH, Polley LS, Tsen LC, Wong CA, eds. *Chestnut's Obstetric Anesthesia: Principles and Practice*. 4th ed. Philadelphia, PA: Elsevier (Mosby); 2009:155-183.

3. O'Donnell CPF, Gibson AT, Davis PG. Review. Pinching, electrocution, ravens' beaks, and positive pressure ventilation: a brief history of neonatal resuscitation. *Arch Dis Child Fetal Neonatal Ed*. 2006; 91:F369-F373.

4. Black RE, Cousens S, Johnson HL, et al. Child Health Epidemiology Reference Group of WHO and UNICEF. Global, regional, and national causes of child mortality in 2008: a systematic analysis. *Lancet*. 2010;375(9730):1969-1987.

5. American Academy of Pediatrics and American Heart Association. *Textbook of Neonatal Resuscitation*. 6th ed. 2011.

6. Kattwinkel J, Perlman JM, Aziz K, et al. Neonatal resuscitation: 2010 American Heart Association Guidelines for cardiopulmonary resuscitation and emergency cardiovascular care. *Pediatrics*. 2010;126(5):e1400-e1413.

7. Martin JA, Hamilton BE, Ventura SJ, et al. Births: final data for 2009. *Division of Vital Statistics*. 2011;60(1).

8. FPnotebook. Fetal scalp pH. http://www.fpnotebook.com/OB/Lab/FtalSclpPh.htm. Updated July 16, 2014.

9. Australian Resuscitation Council (ARC), New Zealand Resuscitation Council (NZRC) Emergency Medicine Australasia Assessment of the Newborn Infant. ARC and NZRC Guideline 2010. 2011;23:426-427.

10. Mackway-Jones K, Molyneux E, Phillips B, Wieteska S. *Advanced Paediatric Life Support: The Practical Approach*. 4th ed. Malden, MA: Blackwell; 2005.

11. Davis PG, Tan A, O'Donnell PF, Schulze A. Resuscitation of newborn infants with 100% oxygen or air: a systemic review and meta-analysis. *Lancet*. 2004;364:1329-1333.

12. Rabi Y, Rabi D, Yee W. Room air resuscitation of the depressed newborn: a systemic review and meta-analysis. *Resuscitation*. 2007;72:353-363.

Anesthesia for Surgery During Pregnancy

12

Yaakov Beilin

INTRODUCTION

The incidence of surgery during pregnancy is between 0.3% and 2.0%.[1,2] There are approximately 4,000,000 deliveries per year in the United States; this translates to approximately 80,000 anesthetics per year administered to pregnant women for intercurrent surgical procedures. In actuality, this may be an underestimate due to surgery performed prior to clinical recognition of the pregnancy. Surgery may be required at any time during pregnancy, and appendectomy is the most frequently performed nonobstetric operation.[3]

Anesthesia for the pregnant woman is one of the rare situations where the anesthesiologist contends with two patients—the mother and the unborn fetus. Therefore, providing a safe anesthetic requires an understanding of the physiologic changes of pregnancy and the impact of anesthesia and surgery on the developing fetus.

PHYSIOLOGIC CHANGES OF PREGNANCY

The pregnant woman undergoes significant physiologic changes to allow adaptation for the developing fetus. These changes are discussed in Chapter 1 and summarized in Table 12-1.

FETAL CONSIDERATIONS

Drug Teratogenicity

A teratogen is a substance that produces an increase in the incidence of a defect that cannot be attributed to chance. To produce a defect, the teratogen must be

165

Table 12-1. Physiologic Changes of Pregnancy

Organ System	Nature of Change
Respiratory	
Minute ventilation	Increases by 50%
Tidal volume	Increases by 40%
Respiratory rate	Increases by 10%
Oxygen consumption	Increases by 20%
PaO_2	Increases by 10 mm Hg
Dead space	No change
Alveolar ventilation	Increases by 70%
$PaCO_2$	Decreases by 10 mm Hg
Arterial pH	No change
Serum HCO_3^-	Decreases by 4 mEq/L
Functional residual capacity	Decreases by 20%
Expiratory reserve volume	Decreases by 20%
Residual volume	Decreases by 20%
Vital capacity	No change
Cardiovascular	
Cardiac output	Increases by 30%-40%
Heart rate	Increases by 15%
Stroke volume	Increases by 30%
Total peripheral resistance	Decreases by 15%
Femoral venous pressure	Increases by 15%
Central venous pressure	No change
Systolic blood pressure	Decreases by 0%-15%
Diastolic blood pressure	Decreases by 10%-20%
Intravascular volume	Increases by 35%
Plasma volume	Increases by 45%
Red blood cell volume	Increases by 20%
Gastrointestinal	
Motility	Decreases
Stomach position	More cephalad and horizontal
Transaminases	Increases
Alkaline phosphatase	Increases
Pseudocholinesterase	Decreases by 20%
Hematologic	
Hemoglobin	Decreases
Coagulation factors	Increases
Platelet count	Decreases by 20%
Lymphocyte function	Decreases
Renal	
Renal blood flow	Increases
Glomerular filtration rate	Increases
Serum creatinine and blood urea nitrogen	Decreases
Creatinine clearance	Increases
Glucosuria	1-10 g/d
Proteinuria	300 mg/d
Nervous system	
Minimum alveolar concentration	Decreases by 40%
Endorphin levels	Increases

administered in a sufficient dose at a critical point in development. In humans, this critical point is during organogenesis, which extends from 15 to approximately 60 days gestational age. Each organ system has its own unique period of susceptibility depending on when it develops. For example, the heart differentiates between the third and sixth weeks and the palate between the six and eighth weeks. It is important to note that the central nervous system does not fully develop until after birth; therefore, the critical time for this system may extend beyond gestation.

Well-controlled randomized human studies are essentially impossible to perform because of either ethical considerations or the large number of patients required. A study designed to find a two fold increase in the incidence of a congenital defect with an incidence of 1:5000 (eg, anencephaly) would require more than 23,000 participants. Four approaches have been utilized to study the effects of anesthetic agents or anesthesia in the pregnant patient: (1) animal studies, (2) retrospective human studies, (3) studies of operating room personnel chronically exposed to trace concentrations of inhaled anesthetics, and (4) outcome studies of women who underwent surgery while pregnant.

Almost all anesthetic agents have been found teratogenic in some animal models. However, the results of animal studies are of limited value because of (1) species variations, (2) the doses of anesthetic agents used in animal studies were usually far greater than those used in humans, and (3) other factors such as hypercarbia, hypothermia, and hypoxemia (known teratogens) were neither measured or nor controlled. Species variation is particularly important. Thalidomide has no known teratogenic effects on rats and was approved by the US Food and Drug Administration (FDA) for use in humans. It is now known that thalidomide is teratogenic in humans.[4]

The FDA has established a risk classification system to help physicians weigh the risks and benefits when choosing therapeutic agents for the pregnant woman (Table 12-2).[5] To date, only five drugs are known to be teratogens, and none of

Table 12-2. United States Food and Drug Administration Category Ratings of Drugs During Pregnancy[a]

Category A: Controlled studies demonstrate no risk. Well-controlled studies in humans have not demonstrated risk to the fetus.

Category B: No evidence of risks in humans. Either animal studies have found a risk but human studies have not. Alternatively, animal studies are negative but adequate human studies have not been done.

Category C: Risk cannot be ruled out. Human studies have not been adequately performed and animal studies are positive or have not been conducted. Potential benefits may justify the risk.

Category D. Potential evidence of risk: Confirmed evidence of human risk. However, benefits may be acceptable despite the known risk (ie, no other medication is available to treat a life-threatening situation).

Category X: Contraindicated in pregnancy. Human or animal studies have shown fetal risk that clearly outweighs any possible benefit to the patient.

[a]Data from *Physicians' Desk Reference*. 69th ed. Montvale, NJ: PDR Network; 2015:211.

them are anesthetic agents. These drugs include thalidomide, isotrentinoin, coumarin, valproic acid, and folate antagonists.[6] Most anesthetic agents, including the intravenous induction agents, local anesthetics, opioids, and neuromuscular blocking drugs have been assigned a category B or C classification (Table 12-3). Indeed, only the benzodiazepines have been assigned as category D and none a

Table 12-3. United States Food and Drug Administration Category Ratings of Specific Anesthetic Agents

Anesthetic Agent	Classification
Induction agents	
Etomidate	C
Ketamine	C
Methohexital	B
Propofol	B
Thiopental	C
Inhaled agents	
Desflurane	B
Enflurane	B
Halothane	C
Isoflurane	C
Sevoflurane	B
Local anesthetics	
2-chloroprocaine	C
Bupivacaine	C
Lidocaine	B
Ropivacaine	B
Tetracaine	C
Opioids	
Alfentanil	C
Fentanyl	C
Sufentanil	C
Meperidine	B
Morphine	C
Neuromuscular blocking drugs	
Atracurium	C
Cisatracurium	B
Curare	C
Mivacurium	C
Pancuronium	C
Rocuronium	B
Succinylcholine	C
Vecuronium	C
Benzodiazepines	
Diazepam	D
Midazolam	D

category D. For the purposes of this chapter, discussion of individual anesthetic agents will be limited to those whose use is controversial—nitrous oxide and benzodiazepines.

NITROUS OXIDE

Nitrous oxide is a known teratogen in mammals and rapidly crosses the human placenta.[7] It had been presumed that the teratogenicity of nitrous oxide in animals is related to its oxidation of vitamin B_{12}, which then cannot function as a cofactor for the enzyme methionine synthetase. Methionine synthetase is needed for the formation of thymidine, a subunit of DNA. There is some evidence that the effects in animals of nitrous oxide are not related to possible effects on DNA synthesis. Pretreatment of rats exposed to nitrous oxide with folinic acid, which bypasses the methionine synthetase step in DNA synthesis, does not fully prevent congenital abnormalities,[8] and suppression of methionine synthetase occurs at low concentrations of nitrous oxide[9]—concentrations found safe in animal studies.[10] Despite these theoretical concerns, nitrous oxide has not been found to be associated with congenital abnormalities in humans.[1,2] The FDA has not given nitrous oxide a category classification because it is a medical gas and not directly regulated by the FDA.

BENZODIAZEPINES

Benzodiazepines exert their action through the inhibition of gamma-aminobutyric acid (GABA) receptors in the central nervous system. GABA has been shown to inhibit palate shelf reorientation, thus leading to cleft palate formation. Some investigators, in human retrospective studies, noted an association between diazepam ingestion in the first 6 weeks of pregnancy and cleft palate.[11] These findings have been questioned in prospective studies that did not demonstrate an association.[12] It is important to remember that in all these studies the assessment was in women chronically exposed to benzodiazepines and not in women with a one-time low dose exposure as typically occurs during surgery. The FDA has assigned benzodiazepines a category D designation and although controversial, this author prefers not to use benzodiazepines during nonobstetric surgery unless there is a compelling reason to do so.

Human Studies

There have been two approaches to assess the effects of anesthetic agents on pregnancy outcome: (1) large retrospective epidemiologic surveys of women chronically exposed to anesthetic gases and (2) retrospective database studies comparing women who underwent surgery while pregnant to those who did not.

EPIDEMIOLOGIC STUDIES

A number of epidemiologic studies were performed in the 1970s to determine the health hazards, including birth defects and spontaneous abortions, of chronic exposure to anesthetic gases.[13] All the studies produced similar results, and the most consistent finding was that the rate of miscarriage in exposed women is approximately 25% to 30% greater than in nonexposed women. The American Society of Anesthesiologists (ASA), concerned with the findings, sponsored a large study and found similar results.[14] The authors surveyed 73,496 individuals who may have been exposed to anesthetic gases. These personnel received questionnaires in the mail designed to gather information about the extent of their exposure and reproductive outcome. They found that operating room personnel had an increased risk of spontaneous abortions and congenital abnormalities. They recommended that a means to scavenge trace anesthetic gases should be mandatory in all operating rooms (currently the standard). However, all these studies were later criticized for their lack of a control group, low response rate to questionnaires, recall bias, and statistical inaccuracies.[15] An additional study with a different study design was unable to confirm these findings. Ericson and Kallen[16] used a Swedish birth registry and compared delivery outcome in nurses who worked in the operating room with those who worked on internal medicine wards. Because this is a registry study and not a survey study, it is not subject to the same issues that affect survey studies, especially the problem with recall bias. The researchers were not able to find a difference in miscarriage, perinatal deaths, or malformations among the groups.

OUTCOME STUDIES IN WOMEN WHO HAD SURGERY WHILE PREGNANT

There have also been a number of retrospective studies of pregnant women who have undergone surgery to seek an association between anesthesia and surgery and congenital defects, spontaneous abortions, or fetal demise, and the results were remarkably similar. The largest study to date was performed by Mazze and Kallen.[2] They linked the data from three Swedish health registries, the Medical Birth Registry, the Registry of Congenital malformations, and the Hospital Discharge registry for the 9-year period 1973-1981. They examined the data for four adverse outcomes: congenital defects, stillborn infants, infants born alive but who died within 7 days, and infants with birth weights less than 1500 g and less than 2500 g. They found 5405 women had undergone surgery during their pregnancy of a total of 720,000 pregnancies. In their data set, most procedures were performed during the first trimester (41.6%), and the incidence decreased during the second and third trimesters (34.8% and 23.5%, respectively). Many of the surgeries (54%) were performed with general anesthesia—almost all of them (more than 98%) with nitrous oxide. The researchers were not able to find an increase in congenital abnormalities or stillborn births among those who underwent surgery while pregnant during any trimester. However, the number of infants born with birth weights less than 1500 g and less than 2500 g, and the number of infants who died within 7 days of postnatal life was greater in those who underwent surgery while pregnant (Figure 12-1). This was true during all three trimesters. These risks could not be linked to either the specific anesthetic agents or the anesthetic technique. The increased risk to the fetus may be due to the condition that necessitated surgery in the first place, with the highest rate in gynecologic procedures.

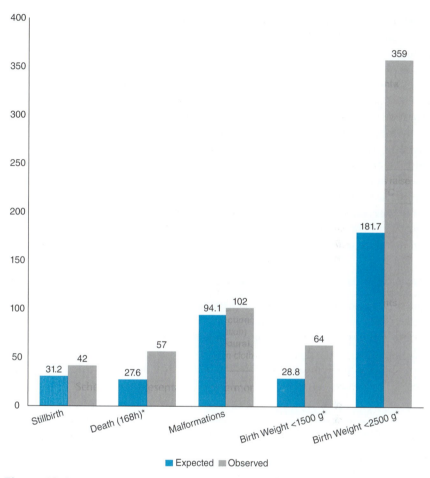

Figure 12-1. Total number of observed and expected outcomes among women having nonobstetric surgery during pregnancy. The incidence of infants of low or very low birth weight and infants who died within 168 hours were significantly increased. *P < .05. (Modified from Mazze RI, Källén B. Reproductive outcome after anesthesia and operation during pregnancy: a registry study of 5405 cases. *Am J Obstet Gynecol.* 1989;161:1178.)

Behavioral Teratology and Apoptosis in the Newborn Brain

It is well known that the halogenated agents, particularly halothane and enflurane, cause learning deficits in rodents.[17] Most anesthetic agents act by either blocking N-methyl-d-aspartate receptors or by enhancing GABA. Studies have demonstrated that when agents that act by either of these mechanisms (eg, ketamine, nitrous oxide, midazolam, barbiturates, and volatile agents) are administered to the rodent during the period of synaptogenesis, they induce widespread neuronal apoptosis in the developing brain.[18]

Although an association between anesthetic agents and neuronal apoptosis has been demonstrated in animal models, extrapolation from animal studies to humans is problematic at best. Whereas most organ systems have completed development by the end of the first trimester or earlier, the brain continues to develop until after delivery. The time of greatest concern is during synaptogenesis or rapid growth spurt, which lasts from the third trimester until 3 years of age. Randomized trials to confirm apoptosis in the human brain obviously cannot be performed, and evaluating the anesthetic effect on the brain is complicated. Recently, two separate authors assessed the effect of anesthesia and surgery on behavior later in life—one learning disabilities[19] and the other deviant behavior.[20] Both found an association between surgery and anesthesia and their outcome measures. The studies are far from conclusive because they were not randomized, but the studies certainly highlight the need for well-controlled studies. At this point, it is premature to make any changes in anesthesia practice based on the data to date, and the FDA at an advisory committee meeting came to the same conclusion.[21]

Avoidance of Intrauterine Fetal Asphyxia

The most important consideration for the fetus during nonobstetric surgery is the maintenance of a normal intrauterine physiologic milieu and avoidance of intrauterine fetal asphyxia. Fetal oxygenation is directly dependent on maternal arterial oxygen tension, oxygen carrying capacity, oxygen affinity, and uteroplacental perfusion. It is therefore critical to maintain a normal maternal PaO_2, $PaCO_2$, and uterine blood flow.

MATERNAL AND FETAL OXYGENATION

Mild to moderate maternal hypoxemia is generally well tolerated by the fetus because fetal hemoglobin has a high affinity for oxygen. However, severe hypoxia will lead to fetal death. General anesthesia is a particular risk for the pregnant woman because (1) management of the airway can be difficult and (2) the rate of hemoglobin oxygen desaturation is increased due to the decreased functional residual capacity and increased oxygen consumption. Care must also be taken with a neuraxial anesthetic because a high dermatomal level of anesthesia, a toxic local anesthetic reaction, or oversedation can also lead to a hypoxic event.

Elevated maternal oxygen tension commonly occurs during general anesthesia. However, because of placental shunting of blood, fetal PaO_2 never rises above 60 mm Hg even if maternal PaO_2 is 600 mm Hg. Therefore, maternal inspired oxygen concentration should not be limited.

MATERNAL CARBON DIOXIDE

Both maternal hypercapnia and hypocapnia can be detrimental to the fetus. Severe hypocapnia produced by excessive positive pressure ventilation may increase mean intrathoracic pressure, decrease venous return, and lead to decreased uterine blood flow. In addition, maternal alkalosis, as produced by hyperventilation, will decrease uterine blood flow by direct vasoconstriction and decrease oxygen delivery by shifting the maternal oxyhemoglobin dissociation curve to the left. Severe hypercapnia is detrimental because carbon dioxide readily crosses the placenta and is associated with fetal acidosis and myocardial depression.

UTEROPLACENTAL PERFUSION

Both drugs and anesthetic procedures affect uterine blood flow. Placental blood flow is directly proportional to the net perfusion pressure across the intervillous space and inversely proportional to the resistance. Perfusion pressure will be decreased by hypotension that may be due to the sympathectomy from local anesthetics administered as part of an epidural or spinal anesthetic, from aortocaval compression in the supine position, or from hemorrhage. Nonetheless, a moderate degree of hypotension, as is occasionally needed for neurosurgical procedures, has been safely used.[8] Medications that cause vasoconstriction (eg, α-adrenergic drugs or ketamine at doses greater than 2 mg/kg); hypocapnia as may occur with hyperventilation during general anesthesia; or increased catecholamines such as occurs during pain, apprehension, or light anesthesia will increase vascular resistance and decrease uteroplacental blood flow should therefore be avoided.

Phenylephrine used to be considered problematic because it is a vasoconstrictor and could lead to uterine vasoconstriction. Recent data from women undergoing cesarean delivery suggest that it may be the preferred vasopressor.[22] Whether these data can be extrapolated to the fetus not being delivered, as occurs during maternal nonobstetric surgery, is unclear, but this author uses phenylephrine in this scenario.

PREVENTION OF PREMATURE LABOR

Spontaneous abortions, premature labor and preterm delivery are the most significant risks to the fetus during maternal surgery.[1,2] It is unclear if this is due to the surgery, anesthetic, or underlying medical condition, but the greatest risk is during gynecologic or pelvic procedures when there is uterine manipulation. With respect to timing, the lowest risk occurs during the second trimester because the potential for teratogenicity is negligible and the risk of premature labor is low because uterine oxytocin receptors have not proliferated. The potent inhaled anesthetic agents decrease uterine tone and inhibit uterine contractions, so from this perspective they may be beneficial. Also, medications that increase uterine tone, such as ketamine at doses greater than 2 mg/kg, should theoretically be avoided. No study, however, has ever documented that any particular anesthetic agent or technique is associated with a greater or smaller incidence of abortion or preterm labor.

LAPAROSCOPIC SURGERY

Once considered an absolute contraindication during pregnancy, laparoscopic surgery is now routinely performed during pregnancy.[23] Reedy et al, in a survey study, compared five fetal outcome variables in pregnant women who had a laparotomy (n = 2181) versus those who had laparoscopy (n = 1522) between 4 and 20 weeks' gestation versus the general population who did not have surgery. They found that there was an increased risk of preterm delivery and low birth weight (less than 2500 g) in both surgical groups compared to the general population. But there was no difference in any of the other outcome variables between the two surgical groups.

Table 12-4. Guidelines for Laparoscopic Surgery During Pregnancy[a]

1. Indications for treatment of acute abdominal processes are the same in pregnant and non-pregnant patients.
2. Laparoscopy can be safely performed during any trimester of pregnancy.
3. Obstetric consultation can be obtained preoperatively and/or postoperatively based on the acuteness of the patient's disease and availability.
4. Pregnant patients should be placed with left uterine displacement to minimize compression of the vena cava and the aorta.
5. Fetal heart monitoring should occur preoperatively and postoperatively.
6. Initial access can be safely accomplished with an open or Hassan, Veress needle, or optical trocar.
7. Insufflation of 10-15 mm Hg can be safely used in the pregnant patient.
8. Intraoperative CO_2 monitoring by capnography should be used.
9. Intraoperative and postoperative pneumatic compression devices and early postoperative ambulation are recommended prophylaxis for deep venous thrombosis.
10. Tocolytic agents should not be used prophylactically but should be considered perioperatively when signs of preterm labor are present.

[a]Data from Guidelines Committee of the Society of American Gastrointestinal and Endoscopic Surgeons, Yumi H.[24]

Specific anesthetic considerations during laparoscopy include maintaining normocarbia, because carbon dioxide is commonly used to maintain a pneumoperitoneum. Adjusting maternal ventilation to maintain end tidal carbon dioxide between 30 and 35 mm Hg should avoid hypercarbia and fetal acidosis. The Society of American Gastrointestinal and Endoscopic Surgeons proposed guidelines for laparoscopic surgery during pregnancy. Surgical concerns include caution during placement of the trocars and maintaining low pneumoperitoneum pressures (less than 15 mm Hg) to maintain uterine perfusion[24] (Table 12-4).

Fetal Heart Rate Monitoring

Fetal heart rate (FHR) monitoring becomes feasible around 16 to 18 weeks with an external tocodynamometer. However, the indication for its use is less well defined, and it obviously cannot be used in abdominal procedures. One issue is how to act on the information? If the fetus is not viable and the FHR tracing is concerning, all that can be done is normalize the physiologic milieu. Is this sufficient reason to use the monitor when this would be done anyway? Katz et al[25] reported a case in which researchers were able to correct an abnormal FHR in a woman who was undergoing eye surgery by increasing the percentage of inspired oxygen given to the mother.

Another issue is who should interpret the tracing? Anesthetic agents may change the FHR baseline and decrease variability, and these changes need to be distinguished from fetal compromise. Furthermore, if a change is noted and the fetus is viable, will the obstetrician intervene with immediate delivery?

The American College of Obstetricians and Gynecologists issued a joint statement with the ASA on this issue.[26] General guidelines from the statement include:

1. A qualified individual should be readily available to interpret the FHR.
2. If the fetus is previable, it is generally sufficient to ascertain the FHR before and after the procedure, but that in "select circumstances, intraoperative monitoring may be considered to facilitate positioning or oxygenation interventions."
3. If the fetus is viable, then simultaneous FHR and contraction monitoring should be performed before and after the procedure and an obstetric provider should be available and willing to intervene for fetal indications.

The statement concludes by stating, "the decision to use fetal monitoring should be individualized" and "ultimately, each case warrants a team approach for optimal safety of the woman and fetus."[26]

GENERAL RECOMMENDATIONS FOR ANESTHETIC MANAGEMENT

Preoperative Management and Timing of Surgery

Whenever possible, anesthesia and surgery should be avoided during the first trimester. Although no anesthetic drug has been proven teratogenic in humans, it is prudent to minimize or eliminate fetal exposure if at all possible. Prior to initiating any anesthetic, an obstetrician should be consulted and FHR tones should be documented. Precautions against aspiration should be taken from as early as the 12th week, and a clear nonparticulate oral antacid, H_2-receptor blocker, and metoclopramide should be considered.

Apprehension should be allayed by reassurance from the anesthesiologist rather than with premedication, if possible. The patient should be informed that there is no known risk to the infant regarding congenital malformations but that there is an increased risk of abortion or premature labor depending on the site of surgery. This is a good opportunity to educate the patient as to the signs of premature labor (eg, back pain prior to term), which can occur up to 1 week after the procedure. The patient should be transported to the operating room with left uterine displacement to avoid aortocaval compression after 16 to 18 weeks' gestation.

Monitoring

In addition to the standard ASA intraoperative monitors, the FHR and uterine tone should be monitored, if at all possible. It is the best way to ensure maintenance of a normal fetal physiologic milieu. Monitoring and interpretation should be performed by an obstetrician or someone with expertise in FHR interpretation other than the anesthesiologist. Regardless of the decision to perform intraoperative FHR monitoring, the FHR and uterine contractions should be monitored before and after the surgery.

Anesthetic Technique

The type of anesthesia should be based on maternal indications, the site and nature of the surgery, and the anesthesiologist's experience. Because anesthetic drug effect may be enhanced during pregnancy, the dose of all anesthetic agents for regional or general anesthesia should be reduced. Although no study has found any difference in neonatal outcome in terms of congenital defects or preterm delivery, regional anesthesia may be preferable to general anesthesia to avoid the risk of pulmonary aspiration and decrease fetal drug exposure. Also, local anesthetics have not been found teratogenic, even in animal studies.

The most frequent risk of neuraxial anesthesia is hypotension, which may reduce uteroplacental perfusion. Prevention of hypotension is difficult because prehydration does not reliably reduce the incidence of hypotension. If hypotension occurs, ephedrine or phenylephrine can be used, but phenylephrine may be preferred.[22] More important is not which drug is chosen but that hypotension should be treated quickly.

General anesthesia should be preceded by careful evaluation of the airway, denitrogenation, and a rapid sequence induction with the application of cricoid pressure. Edema, weight gain, and increase in breast size may make tracheal intubation technically difficult. An array of laryngoscope blades and handles as well as other emergency airway management equipment should be available. Capillary engorgement of the mucosal lining of the upper airway accompanies pregnancy. This mandates extreme care during manipulation of the airway and the use of a smaller-than-normal tracheal tube. The use of a nasal airway and nasotracheal intubation should be avoided. A high inspired concentration of oxygen should be used (at least 50%) and arterial pCO_2 should be maintained at normal pregnancy levels (30-35 mm Hg).

Postoperative Care

FHR and uterine activity monitoring should continue postoperatively. Epidural or subarachnoid opioids are an excellent choice for pain management because they cause minimal sedation, and smaller doses can be utilized compared to the intramuscular or intravenous routes. Nonsteroidal anti-inflammatory drugs should be avoided because they may cause premature closure of the ductus arteriosus.[27]

Regardless of the technique, attention to detail and maintenance of a normal intrauterine physiologic milieu throughout the perioperative period, including the avoidance of hypotension, hypoxemia, hypercarbia, hypocarbia, hypothermia, and so on, is the key to a successful outcome.

CASE STUDY

A 24-year-old woman at 17 weeks' gestation presents to the emergency department complaining of abdominal pain, nausea, and vomiting. After physical examination, a presumptive diagnosis of appendicitis is made, and an emergency appendectomy is planned.

Questions

1. What are the anesthetic concerns when anesthetizing a pregnant woman?

2. What is a teratogen and which anesthetic agents are known teratogens?

3. What precautions should be taken to avoid intrauterine fetal asphyxia?

4. What general recommendations can be made when anesthetizing the pregnant woman for nonobstetric surgery?

Answers

1. Anesthetizing the pregnant woman is one of the only times an anesthesiologist must consider two patients simultaneously. The anesthetic concerns therefore relate to the mother in terms of the physiologic changes of pregnancy and to the fetus in terms of the possible teratogenic effects of anesthetic agents, avoidance of intrauterine fetal asphyxia, and prevention of premature labor.

2. A teratogen is a substance that produces an increase in the incidence of a particular defect that cannot be attributed to chance. None of the commonly used anesthetic agents are teratogens. The use of benzodiazepines is controversial because retrospective studies have found an association between benzodiazepines and cleft palate. They should only be used if the benefits outweigh the risks.

3. Intrauterine fetal asphyxia is avoided by maintaining normal maternal PaO_2, $PaCO_2$, and uterine blood flow. Uterine blood flow is primarily affected by changes in blood pressure. General anesthesia with tracheal intubation is a particularly vulnerable period because oxygen consumption is increased but oxygen reserve is decreased. Careful airway evaluation is necessary and specialized airway equipment should be available. During placement of neuraxial anesthesia, careful attention to blood pressure is required.

4. Whenever possible, anesthesia and surgery should be avoided during the first trimester. Prior to initiating any anesthetic, an obstetrician should be consulted and FHR tones should be documented. In addition to the routine intraoperative monitors, consideration should be given to monitoring the fetal heart tones during surgery. The type of anesthesia should be based on maternal indications, the site and nature of the surgery, and the anesthesiologist's experience. Unless otherwise contraindicated, local or regional anesthesia may be preferable to general anesthesia to avoid the risk of pulmonary aspiration and decrease fetal drug exposure. Regardless of the technique, maintenance of a normal intrauterine physiologic milieu throughout the perioperative period, including the avoidance of hypotension, hypoxemia, hypercarbia, hypocarbia, hypothermia, and so on, is the key to a successful outcome.

REFERENCES

1. Brodsky JB, Cohen EN, Brown BW, et al. Surgery during pregnancy and fetal outcome. *Am J Obstet Gynecol.* 1980;138:1165-1167.
2. Mazze RI, Kallen B. Reproductive outcome after anesthesia and operation during pregnancy: a registry study of 5405 cases. *Am J Obstet Gynecol.* 1989;161:1178-1185.
3. Kort B, Katz VL, Watson WJ. The effect of nonobstetric operation during pregnancy. *Surg Gynecol Obstet.* 1993;177:371-376.

4. Leck IM, Millar EL. Incidence of malformations since the introduction of thalidomide. *Br Med J.* 1962;2:16-20.

5. *Physicians' Desk Reference.* 64th ed. Montvale, NJ: PDR Network; 2009:215.

6. Nava-Ocampo AA, Koren G. Human teratogens and evidence-based teratogen risk counseling: the Motherisk approach. *Clin Obstet Gynecol.* 2007;50:123-131.

7. Marx GF, Joshi CW, Orkin LR. Placental transmission of nitrous oxide. *Anesthesiology.* 1970;32:429-432.

8. Keeling PA, Rocke DA, Nunn JF, et al. Folinic acid protection against nitrous oxide teratogenicity in the rat. *Br J Anaesth.* 1986;58:528-534.

9. Baden JM, Serra M, Mazze RI. Inhibition of rat fetal methionine synthetase by nitrous oxide. *Br J Anaesth.* 1987;59:1040-1043.

10. Mazze RI, Fujinaga M, Rice SA, et al. Reproductive and teratogenic effects of nitrous oxide, halothane, isoflurane and enflurane in Sprague-Dawley rats. *Anesthesiology.* 1986;64:339-344.

11. Safra MJ, Oakley GP Jr. Association between cleft lip with or without cleft palate and prenatal exposure to diazepam. *Lancet.* 1975;2:478-480.

12. Shiono PH, Mills JL. Oral clefts and diazepam use during pregnancy. *New Engl J Med.* 1984;311:919-920.

13. Cohen EN, Bellville JW, Brown BW Jr. Anesthesia, pregnancy, and miscarriage: a study of operating room nurses and anesthetists. *Anesthesiology.* 1971;35:343-347.

14. American Society of Anesthesiologists, Ad Hoc Committee. Occupational disease among operating room personnel: a national study. *Anesthesiology.* 1974;41:321-340.

15. Fink BR, Cullen BF. Anesthetic pollution: what is happening to us? *Anesthesiology.* 1976;45:79-83.

16. Ericson HA, Källén AJ. Hospitalization for miscarriage and delivery outcome among Swedish nurses working in operating rooms 1973-1978. *Anesth Analg.* 1985;64:981-988.

17. Chalon J, Tang CK, Ramanathan S, et al. Exposure to halothane and enflurane affects learning function of murine progeny. *Anesth Analg.* 1981;60:794-797.

18. Young C, Jevtovic-Todorovic V, Qin YQ, et al. Potential of ketamine and midazolam, individually or in combination, to induce apoptotic neurodegeneration in the infant mouse brain. *Br J Pharmacol.* 2005;146:189-197.

19. Wilder RT, Flick RP, Sprung J, et al. Early exposure to anesthesia and learning disabilities in a population-based birth cohort. *Anesthesiology.* 2009;110:796-804.

20. Kalkman CJ, Peelen L, Moons KG, et al. Behavior and development in children and age at the time of first anesthetic exposure. *Anesthesiology.* 2009;110:805-812.

21. Center for Drug Evaluation and Research, Food and Drug Administration, Department of Health and Human Services. Anesthetic and life support drugs. Advisory Committee Meeting, March 29, 2007. Available at www.fda.gov/ohrms/dockets/ac/07/transcripts/2007-4285t1.pdf.

22. Ngan Kee WD, Khaw KS, Ng FF. Prevention of hypotension during spinal anesthesia for cesarean delivery: an effective technique using combination phenylephrine infusion and crystalloid cohydration. *Anesthesiology.* 2005;103:744-750.

23. Reedy MB, Kallen B, Kuehl TJ: Laparoscopy during pregnancy: a study of five fetal outcome parameters with use of the Swedish Health Registry. *Am J Obstet Gynecol.* 1997;177:673-679.

24. Guidelines Committee of the Society of American Gastrointestinal and Endoscopic Surgeons, Yumi H. Guidelines for diagnosis, treatment, and use of laparoscopy for surgical problems during pregnancy: this statement was reviewed and approved by the Board of Governors of the Society of American Gastrointestinal and Endoscopic Surgeons (SAGES), September 2007. *Surg Endosc.* 2008;22:849-861.

25. Katz JD, Hook R, Barash PG. Fetal heart rate monitoring in pregnant patients undergoing surgery. *Am J Obstet Gynecol.* 1976;125:267-269.

26. American College of Obstetricians and Gynecologists (ACOG) Committee on Obstetric Practice. Nonobstetric surgery in pregnancy. ACOG Committee Opinion No. 284, 2003. *Obstet Gynecol.* 2003;102:431.

27. Heymann MA, Rudolph AM. Effects of acetylsalicylic acid on the ductus arteriosus and circulation in fetal lambs in utero. *Circ Res.* 1976;38:418-422.

Anesthesia for Obstetric Procedures not Involving Delivery

13

Mieke A. Soens and Lawrence C. Tsen

TOPICS

INTRODUCTION

Clinical obstetric anesthesia is most commonly associated with delivery of an infant; however, there are a number of other obstetric procedures and surgeries where the use of anesthesia can optimize maternal and fetal outcomes. Miscarriage or termination of pregnancy may occur in up to 30% of pregnancies, and when accompanied by retained fetal or placental tissues, removal is accomplished with a dilation and curettage (D&C) or dilation and evacuation (D&E); these typically occur within the first 12 weeks following conception. Between 1% and 2% of pregnancies are associated with an incompetent cervix; a minority of these cases will require cervical cerclage, which is typically placed during the second trimester. Percutaneous umbilical blood sampling (PUBS) is most commonly performed in the second or third trimester for fetal indications, and late in the third trimester, external cephalic version may be attempted to turn a breech fetus into the cephalic position. Tubal ligations are most frequently performed within the first 48 hours' postpartum, with a second peak occurrence at 6 to 8 weeks' postpartum, when most of the pregnancy-related changes have resolved. Knowledge of the anatomic and physiologic alterations with different stages of pregnancy, as well as the relevant innervation (Figure 13-1), can optimize the planning and conduct of anesthesia; such knowledge will improve the ability of these procedures to be conducted safely and successfully, and augment the patients' experience, comfort, and satisfaction.

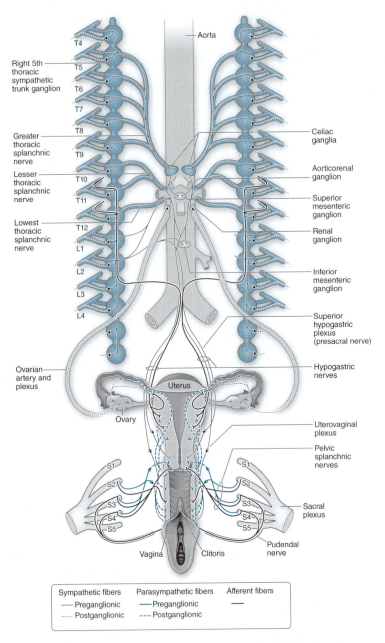

Figure 13-1. Innervation (and relevant obstetric procedure) of the female reproductive organs. The fallopian tubes (tubal ligation) are innervated by T11–L1 via the hypogastric nerves. The uterus (cerclage, dilation and curettage or dilation and evacuation, and external cephalic version) is innervated by T10–L1 and S2–S4 by the uterovaginal and sacral plexus. The umbilical cord (percutaneous umbilical blood sampling) has been observed to be devoid of innervation. Relevant sensory blockade by local, regional, or neuraxial anesthesia techniques may need to include additional sensory levels to account for the placement of surgical instrumentation and the possibility for referred pain.

POSTPARTUM TUBAL LIGATION

Tubal ligation is a highly effective form of permanent sterilization and is among the most popular methods of contraception in the United States. Data from the National Survey of Family Growth for the 2006-2008 period showed that 21% of married women have undergone a tubal ligation procedure.[1] However, there has been a recent decline in tubal sterilization rate, possibly explained by improved alternative long-acting and reversible methods of contraception.

Timing

Tubal ligation can be performed either in the immediate postpartum period or at any time unrelated to pregnancy (ie, interval sterilization). Tubal sterilization in the early postpartum period has several *advantages* over an interval sterilization:

- The uterine fundus remains at the level of the umbilicus for several days postpartum, allowing for easy access to the fallopian tubes directly beneath the abdominal wall through a small subumbilical incision.

- The cost and inconvenience of a second hospital visit can be avoided.

A possible *disadvantage* of performing postpartum tubal ligation (PPTL) is:

- There is a higher probability of regret in these women than in women who undergo interval sterilization,[2,3] because there may be inadequate time to fully assess the newborn.

PPTL is often requested immediately after delivery, especially when the patient has a functioning labor epidural catheter. However, if the newborn requires resuscitation or is unexpectedly transferred to the neonatal intensive care unit, tubal ligation should be delayed. In addition, a tubal ligation should not be performed at a time when it might compromise other aspects of patient care.[3,4]

Preoperative Evaluation

All patients require a thorough preoperative assessment prior to the procedure. For immediate PPTL, the patient's hemodynamic status and uterine tone should be evaluated carefully because blood loss is often underestimated during delivery.[5] Patients should have fasted for 6 to 8 hours, depending on the type of food ingested, and aspiration prophylaxis should be considered.[4] Gastric emptying of solids is delayed during labor and in the postpartum period; in contrast, gastric emptying of clear liquids is not delayed in the peripartum period unless opioids are administered during labor.[6-9]

Anesthetic Management

Neuraxial anesthesia is preferred to general anesthesia for most tubal ligations.[4] Choice of neuraxial technique will depend on the existence of a functional epidural catheter and the interval from delivery to tubal ligation.

EPIDURAL ANESTHESIA

The presence of a functioning labor epidural catheter allows for the provision of an anesthetic for immediate PPTL. A sensory level of at least T5-T6 is needed to block visceral pain during exposure and manipulation of the fallopian tubes. Most commonly, 2% lidocaine with epinephrine with fentanyl 100 μg is used; 3% 2-chloroprocaine, a local anesthetic of shorter duration, may be used as well (Table 13-1). Some epidural catheters that have provided adequate analgesia during labor may fail to provide adequate anesthesia for PPTL, particularly if the interval since delivery is longer.[4] One observational study demonstrated a significant decline in epidural catheter "reactivation" success when the postdelivery interval was greater than 24 hours,[10] and another study observed highest success rates when the interval was less than 4 hours.[11] As a consequence, if the procedure will most likely be delayed beyond 24 hours, an elective spinal anesthetic technique may be a better option. The functioning of the epidural catheter should be carefully evaluated prior to reactivation; in cases of unilateral or incomplete block or inadequate pain relief during labor analgesia, any plan to use the existing epidural catheter should be abandoned.

Failure of epidural catheter reactivation may result in complications, including high or total spinal anesthesia if a spinal technique is performed shortly after epidural administration of large volumes (> 10 mL) of local anesthetics. PPTL is an elective procedure; therefore, in situations where the epidural anesthesia produced is suboptimal, it may be better to allow any block to recede before attempting spinal anesthesia.

Table 13-1. Local Anesthetic Agents

Local Anesthetic	Dose	Duration[a]	Comments
3% Chloroprocaine	S: E: 450-600 mg (15-20 mL)	Short (30-45 min)	Preservative-free form available for spinal use Can be used for paracervical block
2% Lidocaine	S: 45-60 mg (2.5-3 mL) E: 300-400 mg (15-20 mL)	Medium (45 min-1.5 h)	Can be used for paracervical block Epinephrine often added to prolong block
1.5% Mepivacaine	S: 45-60 mg (3-4 mL) E: 225-300 mg (15-20 mL)	Medium (45 min-1.5 h)	Can be used for paracervical block
0.75% Bupivacaine	S: 10-15 mg E: Not used	Long (1.5-3 h)	

Abbreviations: E, epidural; S, spinal.
[a]Duration is given as a range, due to the influence of administration location (eg, spinal space, epidural space or mucosal/subcutaneous tissues), baricity of the solution (whether dextrose is added), patient characteristics (eg, height, weight), and the presence of other additives (eg, epinephrine or opioids).

SPINAL ANESTHESIA

In patients who do not have a functioning epidural catheter, spinal anesthesia can be performed. Some anesthesiologists prefer spinal anesthesia, regardless of whether an epidural catheter is in place. Spinal anestheisa for postpartum tubal ligation has been shown to be associated with a reduction in overal operating room time and charges compared with attempted reactivation of an epidural catheter placed during labor.[12] This should be weighed against the small but increased probability of headache after dural puncture.

Some studies suggest that patients undergoing PPTL require more spinal bupivacaine compared to patients undergoing cesarean delivery, to achieve the same level and duration of anesthesia.[13-14] Pregnancy is associated with an enhanced spread and sensitivity to local anesthetics. This alteration in sensitivity has been attributed to decreased cerebrospinal fluid (CSF) volume secondary to vertebral venous plexus engorgement and increased intra-abdominal pressure,[15,16] as well as enhanced neural susceptibility to local anesthetics, which may be related to high progesterone levels.[17,18] Dose requirements return to nonpregnant levels within 24 to 48 hours' postpartum,[13] which may be related to an increase in CSF volume following relief of vena caval compression or due to the rapid decrease in progesterone levels following delivery. Nevertheless, given the short nature of the procedure, low doses of local anesthetics have been reported to be adequate for postpartum sterilization. A dose-finding study for hyperbaric bupivacaine found that 7.5 mg provided adequate anesthesia for PPTL, lasting approximately 60 minutes. The time of onset to peak sensory level in this study was approximately 20 minutes. Although larger doses can be associated with prolonged motor block and recovery times,[19] a dose of 12 mg of hyperbaric bupivacaine has been shown to be effective and safe in providing surgical anesthesia for PPTL.[14] To avoid general anesthesia in case of a failed single-shot spinal, a dose greater than 10 mg of hyperbaric bupivacaine has been suggested for routine use.[14]

GENERAL ANESTHESIA

General anesthesia is frequently avoided, particularly when the tubal ligation is performed in the immediate postpartum period, when the effects of pregnancy are still present with regard to slowing of gastric emptying[6-9] and decreased lower esophageal sphincter tone. Should general anesthesia be selected, particularly during the immediate postpartum period, such procedures should be used as an opportunity to apply "obstetric" airway management techniques, including a rapid sequence induction, use of a videolaryngoscopy intubation device, and greater attention during extubation and recovery.[20]

Similar to local anesthetics, volatile agents may have decreased minimum alveolar concentration (MAC) values during pregnancy, which also has been attributed to increased progesterone concentration. MAC values usually return to normal 12 to 24 hours after delivery.[21] Uterine atony may occur in the immediate postpartum period, and as a consequence, volatile agents should be maintained at levels that will not reduce the uterine response to oxytocin (0.5 MAC).[22]

Many patients undergoing surgery in the postpartum period are breastfeeding. Because most anesthetics are cleared rapidly, the quantity excreted is insignificant with minimal to no neonatal clinical effects.

CERVICAL CERCLAGE

Cervical cerclage, a surgical procedure to keep the cervical os closed during pregnancy with a purse-string type of stitch, is used for treatment of cervical incompetence. This is a condition characterized by painless cervical dilation with or without herniation and rupture of fetal membranes. These patients typically have a history of recurrent second trimester pregnancy loss. Cervical incompetence can be caused by congenital, anatomical, hormonal, or elastin/collagen abnormalities; alternatively, it is associated with a history of cervical trauma or surgery.

The absolute benefit of cervical cerclage to prevent preterm birth has been questioned; however, most patients with a diagnosis of cervical incompetence undergo cervical cerclage placement.[23] An individual patient data meta-analysis found a nonsignificant trend toward reduction of pregnancy loss or neonatal death in patients with singleton pregnancies, whereas for the small number of multiple gestation pregnancies that were evaluated, a worsened outcome was observed.[24]

Obstetric Considerations

Cervical cerclage can be performed using either a transvaginal or transabdominal approach. The transabdominal approach is typically reserved for those patients in whom a transvaginal cerclage has failed or if no substantial cervical tissue is present.[25] The most commonly performed transvaginal cerclage procedures are the McDonald cerclage and the modified Shirodkar cerclage. In both procedures, a circumferential suture is placed around the cervix at or near the level of the internal cervical os. With the McDonald cerclage, the cervical mucosa is left intact. With the Shirodkar cerclage, in contrast, the mucosa is incised anteriorly and posteriorly, and the ligature is placed submucosally.

COMPLICATIONS

Immediate complications include bleeding, rupture of fetal membranes (especially in case of bulging membranes), and preterm labor. Delayed complications include infection, cervical scarring, and stenosis.

CONTRAINDICATIONS

A cerclage should not be performed in patients with preterm labor, vaginal bleeding, fetal anomalies, fetal death, rupture of membranes, and chorioamnionitis.

Anesthetic Options

Anesthetic options include neuraxial anesthesia and general anesthesia.

Regional Anesthesia

SPINAL ANESTHESIA

Spinal anesthesia is an excellent choice, because it results in rapid, predictable onset of sacral anesthesia, which is desirable for this procedure. Left uterine displacement should be performed if the pregnancy is greater than 18 to 20 weeks' gestation. A sensory level from T10 through the sacral dermatomes is required to cover both the cervix (T10-L1) and vagina and perineum (S2-S4). Hyperbaric 1.5% mepivacaine (45-60 mg), 1.5% lidocaine (45-60 mg), or 0.75% bupivacaine (7.5-10 mg) can be used for this procedure. Because placement of a cervical cerclage is a very short procedure (generally less than 30-45 minutes) frequently performed in an ambulatory setting, short-acting local anesthetics are preferable. A dose of 0.75% bupivacaine as low as 5.25 mg (0.7 mL) with addition of 20 µg of fentanyl (total injectate volume of 3 mL with addition of 0.9% saline) was reported to be successful in cervical cerclage.[26]

The use of preservative-free 3% 2-chloroprocaine is an option, despite several reports in the early 1980s of neurologic deficits associated with possible intrathecal injection of epidural chloroprocaine. These neurotoxic effects were most likely due to presence of the preservative sodium bisulfite and the high doses of chloroprocaine used. Spinal anesthesia with chloroprocaine has been associated with faster block resolution and earlier hospital discharge when compared to bupivacaine[27] or lidocaine.[28] Of interest, chloroprocaine has an increased density compared to CSF and is therefore hyperbaric without the addition of dextrose. These qualities make preservative-free chloroprocaine (45-60 mg) an acceptable alternative for spinal anesthesia for cervical cerclage.

Epidural Anesthesia Lumbar epidural anesthesia can also be performed. However, occasional sacral nerve sparing can make it a less ideal anesthetic compared to spinal anesthesia.

GENERAL ANESTHESIA

Endotracheal intubation is preferable when the gestational age is greater than 18 to 20 weeks. At earlier gestational ages, a laryngeal mask airway may be acceptable. Total intravenous anesthesia using fentanyl and propofol with spontaneous breathing via mask in patients with gestational age of 14 to 16 weeks was reported to be a safe alternative to general anesthesia via endotracheal intubation for cervical cerclage.[29]

Some anesthesiologists advocate the use of general anesthesia for emergency cerclage procedures in the presence of bulging of the fetal membranes, because volatile agents relax uterine smooth muscle and decrease intrauterine pressure. However, general anesthesia, particularly in response to presence or removal of an airway conduit, may result in coughing, nausea, and emesis, which can increase intrauterine pressure. Although this may be minimized with neuraxial anesthesia, studies comparing obstetric outcomes after administration of neuraxial versus general anesthesia have found no differences in maternal or fetal outcomes.[30]

Cerclage Removal

A cerclage will typically be removed at 37 to 38 weeks' gestation, unless rupture of fetal membranes or the onset of labor occurs. If labor proceeds with the cerclage in place, uterine rupture can occur. Labor frequently commences either spontaneously or with pharmacologic induction within a few hours or days after cerclage removal. Anesthesia is usually necessary for removal of a Shirodkar cerclage but not a McDonald cerclage. If anesthesia is required and the patient is expected to remain in the hospital for labor, a combined spinal epidural (CSE) technique with a short-acting local anesthetic is an attractive option. The spinal component provides adequate anesthesia for cerclage removal, with the epidural catheter being used later for labor analgesia. If the procedure is performed as an outpatient, a short-duration spinal anesthetic can be performed.

DILATION AND CURETTAGE OR EVACUATION

Indications

Both D&C and D&E procedures are quite similar in that both involve opening the uterine cervix and instrumenting the uterine lining. A D&E also involves vacuum suction. The procedures are most commonly performed for spontaneous or elective abortions or when retained tissues of conception are still present. Most spontaneous abortions manifest clinically between 8 and 14 weeks' gestation and result in complete expulsion of products of conception without any intervention. A *term* abortion refers to a pregnancy loss or termination before 20 weeks' gestation or when the fetal weight is less than 500 g. A *missed* abortion may result in a fetal death that goes unrecognized for several weeks and can be complicated by disseminated intravascular coagulation.

A D&E procedure can also be indicated in a patient with postpartum hemorrhage due to retained products of conception.

Obstetric Procedure

The procedures are performed with the patient in the lithotomy position. After speculum insertion, the cervix is cleansed with povidone-iodine or the equivalent. The obstetrician may choose to perform a paracervical block. However, if another form of anesthesia is used simultaneously, the short duration of the block may be of limited value. The D&E procedure begins with the cervix being dilated gradually, with metal or hygroscopic dilators, followed by mechanical destruction and evacuation of the fetal parts. After complete removal of the fetus, a large-bore vacuum curette is used to remove the placenta and remaining tissue.

Anesthetic Options

Anesthetic options for the D&E procedure include a paracervical block and sedation, spinal, epidural, or general anesthesia. When deciding as to which anesthetic would be most appropriate, the anesthesiologist should consider whether the patient is hemodynamically stable, has lost a significant amount of blood, has a full stomach, or is septic.

For patients with first or second trimester pregnancy loss and who have been "nothing by mouth" for 6 to 8 hours, a paracervical block with intravenous sedation will most often suffice. Routine monitors should be applied, including capnography. Airway equipment and suction should be available and checked before the procedure. We often use midazolam 2 mg, fentanyl 100 μg, and propofol titrated to the desired amount of sedation or anesthesia. Alternatively, neuraxial anesthesia can be used, provided that the patient is hemodynamically stable and has not suffered significant blood loss. A sensory level from T10 through the sacral dermatomes is required. This can be obtained with spinal 1.5% mepivacaine 45 to 60 mg with dextrose or preservative-free 3% 2-chloroprocaine 45 to 60 mg. However, it is important to keep in mind that both spontaneous and elective abortions are emotionally difficult, and the patient will often prefer general anesthesia. In patients who have suffered significant blood loss, general anesthesia with endotracheal intubation is preferred to secure their airway prior to potentially aggressive fluid replacement (with extravasation into the peripheral and airway tissues) and to minimize the chance of gastric contents entering the lungs. Ketamine or etomidate are good induction agents, because they preserve or minimally affect cardiac output, respectively. Supplementation or provision of total intravenous anesthesia can minimize the dose-dependent uterine relaxation produced by volatile anesthetic agents.

EXTERNAL CEPHALIC VERSION

Breech presentation occurs in 3% to 4% of pregnancies at term.[31] Breech delivery is associated with significantly increased neonatal morbidity and mortality, even when accomplished by cesarean delivery. The American College of Obstetricians and Gynecologists therefore recommend that external cephalic version be offered to all women near term with a fetus in breech presentation.[31]

Obstetric Considerations

With external cephalic version, the obstetrician applies manual, external pressure on the abdomen to change the fetus' position from a breech to a cephalic presentation, with the goal of ultimately achieving a vaginal delivery. Although external cephalic version (ECV) at 34 to 35 weeks' gestation may have higher initial success rates, most obstetricians will wait until 37 to 38 weeks' gestation to decrease the risk of the fetus spontaneously returning to breech presentation or needing to be immediately delivered prematurely.[32] Also, compared to ECV at 37 or 38 weeks, earlier ECV was not shown to reduce the rate of cesarean delivery.[32] The success rate for external cephalic version is estimated to be approximately 60%, although there is a wide variation in this estimate.[31] Several factors have been proposed to increase the success rate of external cephalic version, including tocolytic agents and regional anesthesia.[31]

RISKS AND COMPLICATIONS

Because external cephalic version can be complicated by transient fetal bradycardia, continuous fetal heart rate monitoring should be utilized. Other rare complications include vaginal bleeding or placental abruption.

Anesthetic Considerations

A systematic review and meta-analysis of studies on external cephalic version, found a significant improvement in the success rate with regional anesthesia. The number needed to treat was 5, meaning that for every 5 patients receiving regional anesthesia, 1 additional version will be successful.[32] Regional anesthesia is thought to increase the success rate for external cephalic version by relaxing the maternal abdominal wall and improving maternal tolerance to the procedure.

Anesthetic doses of local anesthetics (spinal bupivacaine 7.5 mg or epidural 2% lidocaine to obtain a T6 sensory level) have been associated with higher success rates when compared to analgesic doses of local anesthetics (spinal bupivacaine 2.5 mg or epidural 2% lidocaine 45 mg).[33] Catheter-based anesthesia techniques, such as a CSE or continuous epidural technique, may be the optimal anesthetic option, because they provide the ability to provide labor analgesia during labor after successful ECV or cesarean anesthesia for emergency delivery, should the need arise.

PERCUTANEOUS UMBILICAL BLOOD SAMPLING

PUBS is a procedure in which a blood sample is collected from the fetus. This sample can be used for diagnosis and treatment of severe anemia or hydrops, as well as for genetic analysis or for diagnosis of certain infections.

Obstetric Procedure

The procedure is performed under ultrasound guidance. After disinfection of the maternal abdomen with povidone-iodine or equivalent, local anesthetic is injected at the insertion site. Subsequently, a 22-gauge spinal needle is used to access the umbilical vein and blood is withdrawn. In case of fetal anemia, a neuromuscular blocking agent can be administered to the fetus followed by a blood transfusion. The procedure usually takes less than 10 minutes.

Anesthetic Considerations

Most often this procedure is performed under local anesthesia administered at the insertion site by the obstetrician. Some discomfort and cramping is usually experienced when the needle passes through the uterus to access the umbilical vein, for which fentanyl 50 to 100 μg could be administered.

REFERENCES

1. Mosher WD, Jones J. Use of contraception in the United States: 1982-2008. National Center for Health Statistics. *Vital Health Stat.* 2010;23(29):1-44.
2. Kariminia A, Saunders DM, Chamberlain M. Risk factors for strong regret and subsequent IVF request after having tubal ligation. *Aust N Z J Obstet Gynaecol.* 2002;42:5:526-529.

3. Hills SD, Marchbanks PA, Tylor LR, Peterson HB. Poststerilization regret: findings from the United States Collaborative Review of Sterilization. *Obstet Gynecol.* 1999;93(6):889-895.

4. Bucklin B. Postpartum tubal ligation: timing and other anesthetic considerations. *Clin Obstet Gynecol.* 2003;46:657-666.

5. Practice Guidelines for Obstetric Anesthesia. An updated report by the American Society of Anesthesiologists Task Force on Obstetric Anesthesia. *Anesthesiology.* 2007;106:843-863.

6. Toledo P, McCarthy RJ, Hewlett BJ, et al. The accuracy of blood loss estimation after simulated vaginal delivery. *Anesth Analg.* 2007;105:1736-1740.

7. Wong CA, Loffredi M, Ganchiff JN, et al. Gastric emptying of water in term pregnancy. *Anesthesiology.* 2002;96:1395-1400.

8. Jayaram A, Bowen MP, Deshpande S, Carp HM. Ultrasound examination of the stomach contents of women in the postpartum period. *Anesth Analg.* 1997;84:522-526.

9. Scrutton MJ, Metcalfe GA, Lowy C, et al. Eating in labour: a randomized controlled trial assessing the risks and benefits. *Anaesthesia.* 1999;54:329-334.

10. Carp H, Jayaram A, Stoll M. Ultrasound examination of the stomach contents in parturients. *Anesth Analg.* 1992;74:683-687.

11. Goodman EJ, Dumas SD. The rate of successful reactivation of labor epidural catheters for postpartum tubal ligation surgery. *Reg Anesth Pain Med.* 1998;23:258-261.

12. Vincent RD, Reid RW. Epidural anesthesia for postpartum tubal ligation using epidural catheters placed during labor. *J Clin Anaesth.* 1993;5:289-291.

13. Viscomi CM, Rathmell JP. Labor epidural catheter reactivation or spinal anesthesia for delayed postpartum tubal ligation: a cost comparison. *J Clin Anaesth.* 1995;7:380-383.

14. Abouleish EI. Postpartum tubal ligation requires more bupivacaine for spinal anesthesia than does cesarean section. *Anesth Analg.* 1986;65:897-900.

15. Teoh WH, Ithnin F, Sia ATH. Comparison of an equal-dose spinal anesthetic for cesarean section and for post partum tubal ligation. *Int J Obstet Anesth.* 2008;17:228-232.

16. Hirabayashi Y, Shimizu R, Fukuda H, Saitoh K, Igarashi T. Soft tissue anatomy within the vertebral canal in pregnant women. *Br J Anaesth.* 1996;77:153-156.

17. Hogan QH, Prost R, Kulier A, Taylor ML, Liu S, Mark L. Magnetic resonance imaging of cerebrospinal volume and the influence of body habitus and abdominal pressure. *Anesthesiology.* 1996;84:1341-1349.

18. Popitz-Bergez FA, Leeson S, Thalhammer JG, Strichartz GR. Intraneural lidocaine uptake compared with analgesic differences between pregnant and nonpregnant rats. *Reg Anesth.* 1997;22:363-371.

19. Datta S, Hurley RJ, Naulty JS, et al. Plasma and cerebrospinal fluid progesterone concentrations in pregnant and nonpregnant women. *Anesth Analg.* 1986;65:950-954.

20. Huffnagle SL, Norris MC, Huffnagle HJ, Leighton BL, Arkoosh VA. Intrathecal hyperbaric bupivacaine dose response in postpartum tubal ligation patients. *Reg Anesth Pain Med.* 2002;27:284-288.

21. Tsen LC, Kodali BS. Can general anesthesia for cesarean delivery be completely avoided? An anesthetic perspective. *Expert Rev Obstet Gynecol.* 2010;5:517-524.

22. Zhou HH, Norman P, DeLima LGR, Mehta M, Bass D. The minimum alveolar concentration of isoflurane in patients undergoing bilateral tubal ligation in the postpartum period. *Anesthesiology.* 1995;82:1364-1368.

23. Yildiz K, Dogru K, Dalgic H, et al. Inhibitory effects of desflurane and sevoflurane on oxytocin-induced contractions of isolated pregnant human myometrium. *Acta Anaesthesiol Scand.* 2005;49:1355-1359.

24. Smith V, Devane D, Begley CM, Clarke M, Higgins S. A systematic review and quality assessment of systematic reviews of randomized trials of interventions for preventing and treating preterm birth. *Eur J Obstet Gynecol Reprod Biol.* 2009;142:3-11.

25. Jorgensen AL, Alfirevic Z, Smith CT, Williamson PR. Cervical stitch (cerclage) for preventing pregnancy loss: individual patient data meta-analysis. *BJOG.* 2007;114:1460-1476.

26. Beilin Y, Zahn J, Abramovitz S. et al. Subarachnoid small-dose bupivacaine versus lidocaine for cervical cerclaje. *Anesth Analg.* 2003;97:56-61.

27. Zaveri V, Aghajafari F, Amankwah K, Hannah M. Abdominal versus vaginal cerclage after a failed transvaginal cerclage: a systematic review. *Am J Obstet Gynecol.* 2002;187:868-872.

28. Lacasse MA, Roy JD, Forget J, et al. Comparison of bupivacaine and 2-chloroprocaine for spinal anesthesia for outpatient surgery: a double-blind randomized trial. *Can J Anaesth.* 2011;58:384-391.

29. Prasanna, Sarma K, Adhikari RK, et al. A comparative study of conventional general anesthesia with total intravenous anesthesia (TIVA) in cervical cerclage—prospective randomized study. *J Anaesth Clin Pharmacol.* 20110;26(1):27-30

30. Yoon HJ, Hong JY, Kim SH. The effect of anesthetic method for prophylactic cerclage on plasma oxytocin: a randomized trial. Int. J. Obstet. Anesth. 2008;17:26-30.

31. American College of Obstetricians and Gynecologists (ACOG). External cephalic version. ACOG Practice Bulletin No. 13. Washington, DC: American College of Obstetricians and Gynecologists; 2000.

32. Hutton EK, Hannah ME, Ross SJ, et al. The early external cephalic version (ECV) 2 trial: an international multicenter randomized controlled trial of timing of ECV for breech pregnancies. *BJOG.* 2011;118:564-577.

33. Cluver C, Hofmeyr GJ, Sinclair M. Interventions for helping to turn breech babies to head first presentation when using external cephalic version. *Cochrane Database Syst Rev.* 2012 Jan 18;1:CD000184.

Section 3

Anesthetic Complications

Anesthetic Complications due to Airway Management/Aspiration

14

Kamilla Greenidge and Scott Segal

INTRODUCTION

The term *difficult airway* most commonly refers to difficulty in placing an endotracheal tube through the vocal cords with the use of direct laryngoscopy. However, it can also refer to difficulty in providing adequate mask ventilation.[1] Despite advances in airway management and rescue, the incidence of airway difficulty encountered in the pregnant population resulting in inability to intubate is still estimated by some to be 1 in 300, a value eight times higher than that seen in the general population.[2-4] In the past, aspiration was considered a major cause of maternal morbidity and mortality.[5] It follows that complications of airway management and failed or difficult intubation after induction of general anesthesia in near term pregnant women may be significant contributors to anesthesia-related maternal complications, and avoidance of difficult airway scenarios be of paramount concern to the obstetric anesthesiologist. Indeed, failure to intubate was the leading cause of anesthesia related maternal mortality from 1979 to 1990.[6] Historically, this has led anesthesiologists to reduce the use of general anesthesia and thus the rate of airway catastrophe at the time of induction of general anesthesia for cesarean delivery. More recently, however, because of improved difficult airway protocols and rescue equipment, including the use of the laryngeal mask airway, increased use of regional anesthesia, and overall increased awareness, the

192

maternal death rate from airway complications, particularly at induction of general anesthesia, appears to be decreasing.[7,8] The following discussion focuses on airway and gastrointestinal changes in pregnancy, managing the difficult airway, and aspiration.

UPPER AIRWAY AND RESPIRATORY MECHANICS

Pregnancy, labor, delivery, and the puerperium induce significant changes in upper airway anatomy and respiratory mechanics (Table 14-1). Higher levels of estrogen and an increase in maternal blood volume contribute to capillary engorgement, mucosal edema, and tissue friability in the parturient's airway. This airway edema can be significantly worsened by preeclampsia, respiratory tract infection, expulsive efforts during the second stage of labor, and excessive fluid administration. Mallampati score increases during gestation and more so during labor.[9] Because of these airway changes, it is generally recommended to use smaller sized endotracheal tubes for general anesthesia in pregnant women.[4] Direct laryngoscopy should be performed carefully so as to minimize trauma and subsequent bleeding. Nasal endotracheal intubation should be used cautiously and with careful attention to vasoconstriction of the nasal mucosa.[10]

Respiratory physiologic changes during pregnancy relevant to airway management include an increase in minute ventilation, an increase in oxygen consumption, and a decrease in functional residual capacity (FRC) to 80% of the nonpregnant value by term gestation. The decreased FRC brings the lung closer to closing capacity, which further predisposes parturients to atelectasis. For these reasons, pregnant women near term become hypoxemic more rapidly than do non-pregnant women during episodes of apnea. For example, during rapid sequence induction of general anesthesia, the PaO_2 of parturients decreases at more than twice the rate of that in nonpregnant women (139 versus 58 mm Hg/min).[11]

As is the case before any anesthetic, it is critical to perform a thorough airway assessment in obstetric patients. Assessment of Mallampati classification, atlanto-occipital extension, thyromental distance, and mandibular protrusion are four useful examinations for predicting difficulty with laryngoscopy. However, because no single test is sufficient to identify a patient with a difficult airway, anesthesia

Table 14-1. Risk Factors for Airway Complications During Pregnancy[a]

Airway edema
Decreased FRC
Increased oxygen consumption
Weight gain
Enlarged breasts
Full dentition
Decreased lower esophageal sphincter tone
Decreased gastric emptying during labor

[a]Adapted from Chestnut DH, Polley LS, Tsen LC, Wong CA, eds. *Obstetric Anesthesia.* 4th ed. Philadelphia, PA: Mosby-Elsevier; 2009:651.

providers should perform a complete airway evaluation in obstetric patients, as outlined in the American Society of Anesthesiologists (ASA) Practice Guidelines.[1] Regardless of when the airway was first examined, labor and pushing may all affect the Mallampati score, and it should be rechecked when closer to anesthetic intervention.

NEURAXIAL ANALGESIA AND ANESTHESIA AS PROPHYLAXIS

The widespread acceptance of neuraxial analgesic techniques for obstetric patients has improved maternal and fetal outcome by reducing the need for general anesthesia and airway manipulation.[8] Neuraxial techniques provide a mechanism by which anesthesia for cesarean delivery can be delivered in a safe and predictable manner, even in urgent situations. Advances in the delivery of neuraxial anesthesia that have made it safer include (1) administration of an epidural test dose, (2) use of a dilute solution of local anesthetic for epidural analgesia, (3) administration of the therapeutic dose of local anesthetic in incremental boluses through an epidural catheter, (4) maintenance of adequate left uterine displacement to prevent aortocaval compression, and (5) prompt and aggressive treatment of hypotension.[8]

There is also a greater acceptance of early or prophylactic placement of an epidural catheter in high-risk parturients. A *prophylactic* epidural catheter is one that is placed and tested with a small dose of local anesthetic; analgesia is not established until active labor occurs, the patient requests analgesia, and/or an operative delivery is required. Such a catheter provides a readily available conduit for providing neuraxial analgesia or anesthesia, especially if rapid onset (eg, emergency operative delivery) is desirable, thus avoiding airway manipulation. An early epidural catheter is placed in a controlled setting and allows time for catheter manipulation and replacement, if necessary, before further pathophysiologic changes (eg, decrease in platelet count, worsening airway edema) occur.[12]

Given that a failed neuraxial anesthetic may require conversion to general anesthesia, it is generally recommended that some form of pharmacologic prophylaxis should be administered to alter gastric pH in all parturients requiring surgical intervention, whether or not they receive general or neuraxial anesthesia.[12] The anatomic and physiologic changes of pregnancy (eg, reduced lower esophageal sphincter tone, delayed gastric emptying) increase the risk of aspiration in labor (although likely not prior to the onset of labor).[13] Failed or difficult intubation is also associated with aspiration (see Pulmonary Aspiration in Obstetrics, below).

In light of the increased utilization of neuraxial anesthesia, one might expect the frequency of failed endotracheal intubations to have decreased. Yet, despite the dramatic increase in use of neuraxial techniques, Rahman and Jenkins demonstrated that over an 11-year period while the number of cesarean deliveries doubled, the frequency of failed endotracheal intubation remained constant.[3] This study, and others, suggests that the majority of cases of failed tracheal intubation occurred during emergencies, outside normal working hours, and involved anesthesia trainees. Unfortunately, modern day trainees are not well experienced in obstetric general anesthesia. Hawthorn et al suggested that trainees' exposure to general anesthesia in obstetrics has decreased simply because there are more trainees.[6] However, it is also clear that trainee exposure has been reduced as a result of there being fewer general anesthetics in obstetrics due to the overwhelming preference for regional techniques.[14] These data suggest there may be room for improvement in obstetric anesthesiology training programs, perhaps in the area of anesthesia simulation.[15]

The etiology of airway-related mortality appears to be shifting. In a review of anesthesia-related mortality in Michigan, Mhyre and colleagues reviewed 850 maternal deaths and were unable to find a single case of failed intubation during elective cesarean delivery. They demonstrated that anesthesia-related deaths from airway obstruction or hypoventilation took place during emergence, extubation, or recovery—not during the induction of general anesthesia—as previously observed. Also of note in this landmark study, system errors contributed to the majority of maternal deaths—specifically, lapses in standard postoperative monitoring and inadequate supervision by an anesthesiologist.[8] The ASA guideline for postoperative care[16] suggests that pulse oximetry is associated with early detection of hypoxemia and recommends periodic assessment of airway patency, respiratory rate, and oxygen saturation measured by pulse oximetry during emergence and recovery. The data from this study suggest also that the rate of failed intubation is now overstated and that the presence of an emergency itself is a significant risk factor for failed intubation.[8]

The most recent Confidential Enquiries into Maternal Deaths[17] (2006-2008) reported that of the seven maternal deaths in the United Kingdom during this period as a result of direct anesthetic causes, two were the result of failure to ventilate the lungs, one was an aspiration of gastric contents on emergence from general anesthesia, and one was the result of postoperative "opiate toxicity." The first case of "failure to ventilate" involved an unrecognized esophageal intubation through an intubating laryngeal mask airway after it was utilized for rescue during induction of general anesthesia. The second failure to ventilate case occurred in a patient with a known difficult airway that suffered dislodgement of her preexisting tracheostomy appliance postoperatively in the intensive care unit. This most recent survey suggests that vigilance around airway management should be extended to the entire perioperative period, not only during induction of general anesthesia and extubation.

Several authors have warned that a higher incidence of failed intubation in obstetric patients should be expected in the future.[3,6,15] One reason for this concern is that there is a significant increase in the use of neuraxial analgesic and there are limited opportunities to teach and practice the skills necessary for obstetric airway management. Another reason is the changing demographics of the obstetric population. The prevalence of obesity is rising at an alarming rate in both developed and developing countries worldwide. Obesity itself is an independent risk factor associated with airway management problems during pregnancy.[17] In addition, anesthesiologists today provide care for older parturients having more comorbidities, in part as a result of delayed childbearing and the use of assisted reproductive technologies. These comorbid conditions may exacerbate the effects of hypoxemia, hypercarbia, and acidosis during a delayed or failed intubation.[15,17] Clearly, more work needs to be done, and many experts believe that the obstetric anesthesia community has a responsibility to become more aggressive in encouraging research and in developing clinical protocols that specifically address airway issues in the obstetric population.

THE UNANTICIPATED DIFFICULT AIRWAY

Even with the best attempts to adequately assess an airway preoperatively, it is possible that unanticipated difficulty with airway management can still occur. This may be due to an unrecognized anatomic variation, airway edema from preeclampsia, airway changes during labor, failure of bedside airway examination techniques, or some other unforeseen cause. Adequate equipment suitable for a variety of airway techniques should be available in all obstetric anesthetizing locations (Table 14-2). Initial management consists of repositioning the patient to achieve the proper sniffing position. Use of a different laryngoscope blade, video-assisted laryngoscope, a gum elastic bougie (Eschmann stylet), and/or a smaller diameter endotracheal tube should also be considered. In experienced hands, the authors suggest that subsequent laryngoscopy attempts should be performed only by the most experienced operator available, be limited to no more than two or three attempts, and that the second or third attempt should be performed only in those cases in which a portion of the laryngeal anatomy is visible (grade III or better). If a grade IV laryngoscopic view is identified with the initial laryngoscopy, the anesthesia provider should immediately focus on ensuring adequate oxygenation and ventilation of the mother (Figure 14-1).[18]

Oxygenation and ventilation take priority over intubation when the hemoglobin saturation decreases below 90%, cyanosis develops, or after two intubation attempts fail. Each attempt entails one insertion of the relevant airway equipment by a single provider, and should be completed in 1 minute. A review of the ASA obstetric closed claims data suggests that repeated attempts at intubation may result in progressive difficulty in ventilation that ultimately leads to complete airway obstruction.[18]

Table 14-2. Suggested Airway Equipment to Maintain for the Induction of Obstetric Anesthesia

Face mask and oral airways
Gauze and a tongue blade
Two working laryngoscope handles
Macintosh blades sizes 3 and 4
6.5 styletted endotracheal tube with an empty 10-mL syringe connected to the pilot balloon
Backup endotracheal tubes in a range of sizes
Gum elastic bougie
Primary extraglottic airway appropriate for a 70- to 100-kg person
Suction adequate to remove secretions

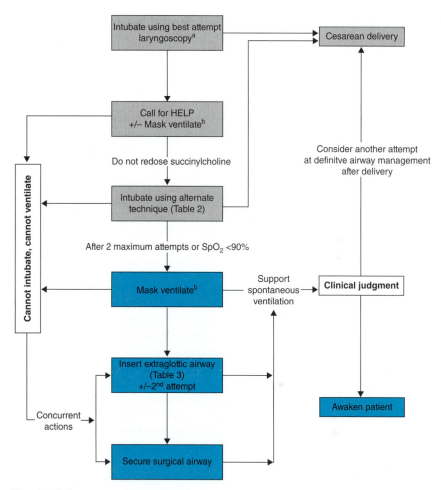

Figure 14-1. Suggested algorithm for ensuring adequate oxygenation and ventilation.
[a]Adjust cricoid pressure; backward, upward, rightward pressure (BURP); bougie; minor position adjustments. [b]Oral airway, jaw thrust, adjust cricoid pressure, two-handed technique. Used with permission from Mhyre JM, Healy D.[18]

EXTUBATION OF A KNOWN DIFFICULT AIRWAY

When caring for the patient with a difficult airway, consideration should always be given to the possibility of airway compromise after extubation. This is of particular importance in patients who have a disease process that may increase the risk of development of airway edema, those who have had a prolonged surgery, those who received a large amount of fluid or blood products, those who are obese, or those who have a history of obstructive sleep apnea.[19] This is illustrated by an increasing number of anesthesia-related deaths that largely involved postoperative airway obstruction and hypoventilation.[17] Therefore, patients, particularly those with the aforementioned risk factors, should be monitored appropriately postoperatively with continuous pulse oximetry, dedicated nursing care, and possibly capnography or other measure of ventilation.

Studies attempting to stratify risk factors that can reliably predict difficulty with extubation have been inconclusive. Many providers rely on the leak test to assess readiness for extubation of patients with the potential for airway edema and subsequent obstruction. The goal is to assess whether airway caliber is adequate for ventilation. The test is performed by deflating the endotracheal tube cuff and occluding the proximal end of the tube. The patient should be evaluated for the ability to spontaneously breathe around the tube or changes in tidal volume with the cuff deflated. Inability to do so suggests a higher likelihood of airway occlusion on extubation, but it is important to note that a negative leak test does not necessarily indicate that the patient would fail extubation. Indeed, some have questioned the validity of the test in predicting the need for reintubation.[20,21] Preferably, extubation should be performed in a controlled setting and after a full assessment of patient's strength, level of consciousness, and ability to follow commands.

PULMONARY ASPIRATION IN OBSTETRICS

Aspiration of gastric contents into the lung is one of the most feared complications of anesthesia, particularly in obstetrics. Indeed, the first reported complication of anesthesia was likely an aspiration event.[22] The modern view of aspiration in obstetrics was developed by Mendelson,[23] an anesthesiologist and scientist who reported in 1946 a series of patients and animal experiments describing the pathophysiology of the acid aspiration syndrome. His work led to the widespread use of prophylactic antacid use, nothing-by-mouth policies during labor, and greater use of regional anesthesia administered by well-trained anesthesiologists.

Historically, women undergoing a cesarean delivery were said to have at least a three fold higher risk of aspiration than do those patients in the general population undergoing anesthesia. However, more recent data suggest that emergency surgery and obesity, both becoming more common, contribute significantly to the risk of aspiration rather than pregnancy per se.[24] In fact, data from the Confidential Enquiries into Maternal Deaths indicate that death from pulmonary aspiration in obstetrics has declined and is now exceedingly rare—less than 1 in 3.2 million deliveries.[17] In a recent large audit of approximately 12,800 obstetric general anesthetics (out of 720,000 deliveries) in the United Kingdom, there were five cases of aspiration, four of which were in the setting of a failed intubation.[25] The estimated overall incidence of 1 per 2560, or about 4 per 10,000, approximates the risk of aspiration in nonpregnant individuals. Conversely, one large observational study found one aspiration event in more than 1000 uses of general anesthetics for cesarean delivery, implying a higher incidence. Notably, there were eight witnessed episodes of regurgitation, with five occurring at extubation. This emphasizes the need for vigilance during emergence as well as induction of anesthesia.[2]

The decline in aspiration events is probably multifactorial. First, there is greater use of neuraxial anesthesia and conversely fewer general anesthetics. When general anesthesia is needed in a laboring patient, a rapid sequence induction is routinely used.

Second, there is frequent use of antacids, histamine (H_2)-receptor antagonists, and/ or proton pump inhibitors to reduce gastric volume and raise gastric pH. Third, there is greater awareness of aspiration risks and better training of anesthesia providers. Fourth, the establishment and enforcement of nothing-by-mouth policies have also likely contributed to this decline. All of these maneuvers are controversial, and some have questioned their contribution to reduced aspiration events, with the exception of the widespread and growing use of regional techniques.[13,26,27]

Pathophysiology

Pregnancy itself does not significantly alter basal gastric acid secretion or the rate of gastric emptying. However, the rate of gastric emptying is decreased during advanced labor; this is presumably due in part to the pain and stress associated with labor, because these are also known to delay gastric emptying. Furthermore, the administration of systemic opioids delay gastric emptying in both pregnant and nonpregnant patients.[28] It is well established that boluses of epidural fentanyl 50 to 100 μg delay gastric emptying in laboring women. Continuous epidural infusion of low-dose local anesthetic with fentanyl, however, does not appear to delay gastric emptying until the total dose of fentanyl exceeds 100 μg.[28]

The inhalation of gastric contents that are particulate or acidic in nature can lead to acute lung injury, and this is referred to as aspiration pneumonitis. It generally occurs either during induction of general anesthesia or during emergence when the airway is unsecured. However, it can occur at any time in a patient with a depressed level of consciousness due to anesthesia, sedation, seizures, or drug overdose. Largely, the morbidity and mortality related to aspiration depends on the volume of the aspirate; the pH of the aspirate; and whether it is solid, particulate, or liquid. Aspirates with a pH less than 2.5 or containing particulate material can lead to severe lung injury. Aspiration of small volumes of neutral liquid results in a very low rate of morbidity and mortality, whereas aspiration of large volumes of neutral liquid results in a higher mortality rate, presumably as a result of the disruption of surfactant by a large volume of liquid.[29]

The pathophysiology of the aspiration syndrome was first characterized in the 1940s by Mendelson. It is an inflammatory process, not generally infectious, that induces acute pulmonary injury. The inflammatory response is most pronounced after aspiration of acidic aspirates and material containing small particulate matter.[30] The aspirate induces a chemical burn, often leading to bronchospasm, which results in alveolar exudates composed of edema, albumin, fibrin, cellular debris, and red blood cells. Ultimately, there is an increase in intra-alveolar water and protein with a loss of lung volume, leading to a reduction in lung compliance with intrapulmonary shunting of blood. This results in hypoxemia and an increase in pulmonary vascular resistance. After the initial injury, there is an intense inflammatory response with the release of cytokines, interleukins, and tumor necrosis factor. The pathophysiologic process that ensues is similar to acute lung injury or acute respiratory distress syndrome. Most patients will have an abnormal chest x-ray, but this may take several hours before becoming apparent.

Prophylaxis and Management

Prophylaxis of acid aspiration remains a matter of some controversy. Given the very low incidence of the complication, it is difficult to perform studies with sufficient statistical power. Nonetheless, most authors advocate the oral administration of a clear nonparticulate antacid as the most common method of pharmacologic aspiration prophylaxis in obstetric patients. Sodium citrate (0.3 M) 30 mL should be administered within 30 minutes of induction of anesthesia to ensure optimal neutralization of stomach acid. Use of other agents such as H_2 blockers and proton pump inhibitors is less common, and the advantages of these agents over nonparticulate antacids are unclear. It is true that the combination of these parenteral agents with oral antacids more reliably increases gastric pH.[26] Rapid sequence induction of anesthesia, with omission of mask ventilation and use of cricoid pressure, is widely recommended as the standard of care, but these interventions, too, are the subject of controversy, at least in fasted, elective cases.[13,27,31] Indeed, there are series totaling nearly 5000 cesarean deliveries performed with use of a laryngeal mask airway without evidence of aspiration.[32-34] An additional controversy surrounds nothing-by-mouth policies for laboring patients. Traditionally, once in active labor or after activation of epidural analgesia, pregnant patients were made strictly "nothing by mouth" or allowed only ice chips. More recently, however, the ingestion of modest amounts of clear liquids during labor, and up to 2 hours before scheduled cesarean delivery, has been advocated by both anesthesiologists[12] and the American College of Obstetricians and Gynecologists (ACOG).[35] The ASA recommends that more restrictive policies be considered for high-risk parturients (eg, diabetes, difficult airway, morbid obesity). Consumption of solid food in labor has been advocated by natural childbirth proponents and others, but two randomized, controlled trials failed to show any benefits with respect to progress of labor or neonatal outcome.[36,37] Gastric volumes were higher among patients who ate and emesis volumes greater in those who ate and vomited,[36] although vomiting itself was not increased.[37] Both ACOG and ASA suggest that solid food should not be consumed in labor.

Management of an aspiration event in the pregnant population is similar to that in the nonpregnant population and is largely supportive. The trachea should be thoroughly suctioned. Bronchoalveolar lavage is not recommended because it is possible to further spread particulate matter deeper in to the lung. Bronchoscopy may be used where indicated to remove large particles of food. Bronchospasm is likely to accompany an aspiration event and should be treated as indicated. Prophylactic antibiotic therapy is not recommended unless the patient's clinical course suggests an infection is present. Corticosteroids are not recommended.

SUMMARY

Historically, failed intubation during the induction of general anesthesia was a significant cause of anesthesia related maternal death. In fact, in 1991 through 1997, problems associated with airway management, sometimes complicated by aspiration, were the most significant cause of anesthesia-related maternal death.

This led to major changes in anesthetic practice, including increased use of regional anesthesia in obstetrics and adherence to difficult airway algorithms. Today, the vast majority of cesarean deliveries are performed under neuraxial anesthesia. This shift from general to regional anesthesia has dramatically diminished the need for airway manipulation in obstetrics. Nonetheless, anesthesia providers must still contend with airway management particularly in emergency obstetric surgery, which significantly predisposes to difficult intubation and/or an aspiration event. Anesthesiologists should thus remain vigilant throughout the peripartum period to avoid these potentially fatal complications.

REFERENCES

1. Apfelbaum JL, Hagberg CA, Caplan RA, et al. Practice guidelines for management of the difficult airway: an updated report by the American Society of Anesthesiologists Task Force on Management of the Difficult Airway. *Anesthesiology.* 2013;118(2):251-270.
2. McDonnell NJ, Paech MJ, Clavisi OM, Scott KL. Difficult and failed intubation in obstetric anaesthesia: an observational study of airway management and complications associated with general anaesthesia for caesarean section. *Int J Obstet Anesth.* 2008;17(4):292-297.
3. Rahman K, Jenkins JG. Failed tracheal intubation in obstetrics: no more frequent but still managed badly. *Anaesthesia.* Feb 2005;60(2):168-171.
4. Munnur U, de Boisblanc B, Suresh MS. Airway problems in pregnancy. *Crit Care Med.* 2005;33 (10 suppl):S259-S268.
5. Merrill RB, Hingson RA. Study of incidence of maternal mortality from aspiration of vomitus during anesthesia occurring in major obstetric hospitals in United States. *Curr Res Anesth Analg.* 1951;30(3):121-135.
6. Hawthorne L, Wilson R, Lyons G, Dresner M. Failed intubation revisited: 17-yr experience in a teaching maternity unit. *Br J Anaesth.* 1996;76(5):680-684.
7. Cooper GM, McClure JH. Anaesthesia chapter from Saving Mothers' Lives; reviewing maternal deaths to make pregnancy safer. *Br J Anaesth.* 2008;100(1):17-22.
8. Mhyre JM, Riesner MN, Polley LS, Naughton NN. A series of anesthesia-related maternal deaths in Michigan, 1985-2003. *Anesthesiology.* 2007;106(6):1096-1104.
9. Kodali BS, Chandrasekhar S, Bulich LN, Topulos GP, Datta S. Airway changes during labor and delivery. *Anesthesiology.* 2008;108(3):357-362.
10. Arendt KW, Khan K, Curry TB, Tsen LC. Topical vasoconstrictor use for nasal intubation during pregnancy complicated by cardiomyopathy and preeclampsia. *Int J Obstet Anesth.* 2011;20(3):246-249.
11. Archer GW, Jr, Marx GF. Arterial oxygen tension during apnoea in parturient women. *Br J Anaesth.* 1974;46(5):358-360.
12. Practice guidelines for obstetric anesthesia: an updated report by the American Society of Anesthesiologists Task Force on Obstetric Anesthesia. *Anesthesiology.* 2007;106(4):843-863.
13. de Souza DG, Doar LH, Mehta SH, Tiouririne M. Aspiration prophylaxis and rapid sequence induction for elective cesarean delivery: time to reassess old dogma? *Anesth Analg.* 2010;110(5):1503-1505.
14. Palanisamy A, Mitani AA, Tsen LC. General anesthesia for cesarean delivery at a tertiary care hospital from 2000 to 2005: a retrospective analysis and 10-year update. *Int J Obstet Anesth.* 2011;20(1):10-16.
15. Arendt KW, Segal S. Present and emerging strategies for reducing anesthesia-related maternal morbidity and mortality. *Curr Opin Anaesthesiol.* 2009;22(3):330-335.
16. Apfelbaum JL, Silverstein JH, Chung FF, et al. Practice guidelines for postanesthetic care: an updated report by the American Society of Anesthesiologists Task Force on Postanesthetic Care. *Anesthesiology.* 2013;118(2):291-307.
17. Cantwell R, Clutton-Brock T, Cooper G, et al. Saving mothers' lives: reviewing maternal deaths to make motherhood safer: 2006-2008. The eighth report of the confidential enquiries into maternal deaths in the United Kingdom. *BJOG.* 2011;118 (suppl 1):1-203.
18. Mhyre JM, Healy D. The unanticipated difficult intubation in obstetrics. *Anesth Analg.* 2011;112(3): 648-652.

19. Rout CC. Anaesthesia and analgesia for the critically ill parturient. *Best Pract Res Clin Obstet Gynaecol.* 2001;15(4):507-522.

20. Shin SH, Heath K, Reed S, Collins J, Weireter LJ, Britt LD. The cuff leak test is not predictive of successful extubation. *Am Surg.* 2008;74(12):1182-1185.

21. Zhou T, Zhang HP, Chen WW, et al. Cuff-leak test for predicting postextubation airway complications: a systematic review. *J Evid Based Med.* 2011;4(4):242-254.

22. Simpson JY. Remarks on the alleged case of death from the action of chloroform. *Lancet.* 1848;1:175.

23. Mendelson CL. The aspiration of stomach contents into the lungs during obstetric anesthesia. *Am J Obstet Gynecol.* 1946;52:191-205.

24. Kluger MT, Short TG. Aspiration during anaesthesia: a review of 133 cases from the Australian Anaesthetic Incident Monitoring Study (AIMS). *Anaesthesia.* 1999;54(1):19-26.

25. Quinn AC, Milne D, Columb M, Gorton H, Knight M. Failed tracheal intubation in obstetric anaesthesia: 2 yr national case-control study in the UK. *Br J Anaesth.* 2013;110(1):74-80.

26. Paranjothy S, Griffiths JD, Broughton HK, Gyte GM, Brown HC, Thomas J. Interventions at caesarean section for reducing the risk of aspiration pneumonitis. *Int J Obstet Anesth.* 2011;20(2):142-148.

27. Holmes N, Martin D, Begley AM. Cricoid pressure: a review of the literature. *J Perioper Pract.* 2011;21(7):234-238.

28. Zimmermann DL, Breen TW, Fick G. Adding fentanyl 0.0002% to epidural bupivacaine 0.125% does not delay gastric emptying in laboring parturients. *Anesth Analg.* 1996;82(3):612-616.

29. James CF, Modell JH, Gibbs CP, Kuck EJ, Ruiz BC. Pulmonary aspiration—effects of volume and pH in the rat. *Anesth Analg.* 1984;63(7):665-668.

30. Knight PR, Rutter T, Tait AR, Coleman E, Johnson K. Pathogenesis of gastric particulate lung injury: a comparison and interaction with acidic pneumonitis. *Anesth Analg.* 1993;77(4):754-760.

31. El-Orbany M, Connolly LA. Rapid sequence induction and intubation: current controversy. *Anesth Analg.* 2010;110(5):1318-1325.

32. Yao WY, Li SY, Sng BL, Lim Y, Sia AT. The LMA Supreme in 700 parturients undergoing Cesarean delivery: an observational study. *Can J Anaesth.* 2012;59(7):648-654.

33. Han TH, Brimacombe J, Lee EJ, Yang HS. The laryngeal mask airway is effective (and probably safe) in selected healthy parturients for elective Cesarean section: a prospective study of 1067 cases. *Can J Anaesth.* 2001;48(11):1117-1121.

34. Halaseh BK, Sukkar ZF, Hassan LH, Sia AT, Bushnaq WA, Adarbeh H. The use of ProSeal laryngeal mask airway in caesarean section—experience in 3000 cases. *Anaesth Intensive Care.* 2010;38(6): 1023-1028.

35. Amercian College of Obstetricians and Gynecology (ACOG). ACOG Committee Opinion No. 441: Oral intake during labor. *Obste Gynecol.* 2009;114(3):714.

36. Scrutton MJ, Metcalfe GA, Lowy C, Seed PT, O'Sullivan G. Eating in labour. A randomised controlled trial assessing the risks and benefits. *Anaesthesia.* Apr 1999;54(4):329-334.

37. O'Sullivan G, Liu B, Hart D, Seed P, Shennan A. Effect of food intake during labour on obstetric outcome: randomised controlled trial. *BMJ.* 2009;338:b784.

Postdural Puncture Headache

15

Jonathan Epstein and Jacquiline Geier

Postdural puncture headache (PDPH) continues to be one of the most common complications of neuraxial anesthesia used in obstetrics. It is critical that the obstetric anesthesiologist be able to recognize the difference between PDPH, the incidence of which may approach 40%, and other causes of postpartum headache.[1] PDPH is also the third most common cause of litigation stemming from neuraxial anesthesia.[2] In fact, claims related to maternal death and newborn death/brain damage have steadily decreased since 1990, but PDPH settlements have seen a steady increase.[3] Retrospective analysis indicates that the most frequently cited reason for a patient's deciding to pursue legal action was a lack of full disclosure regarding potential for PDPH and/or lack of follow-up by the anesthesiologist.[2] Although the headache itself is the usual official complaint, it seems that poor communication and an absence of empathy is what actually drives the majority of these legal actions. Accordingly, patients should be counseled about the risks of PDPH prior to every neuraxial anesthetic. If a Tuohy needle accidentally punctures the dura, it is imperative that, after the patient is comfortable, the potential risk of headache be once again explained. At that time, the patient should be advised of specific treatment options and reassured that adequate follow-up will be available.

WHAT CAUSES A POSTDURAL HEADACHE?

The symptoms of PDPH are thought to be due to leakage of cerebrospinal fluid (CSF) through a dural defect produced by the dural puncture. If the rate of CSF leakage exceeds the rate of production of CSF (approximately 550-700 mL/d, with 120-150 mL present in the subarachnoid space at any given time), then on assuming an upright position, the downward traction on the pain-sensitive intracranial veins, meninges, and cranial nerves results in headache. Other contributing factors to patient discomfort may be related to a compensatory vasodilation to account for loss of intracranial CSF volume as the body attempts to achieve homeostasis by maintaining a constant intracranial volume.[4]

HOW OFTEN DOES A POSTDURAL HEADACHE OCCUR AND WHO GETS IT?

It is important to remember that PDPH may arise either from an intentional dural puncture for a spinal anesthetic or an unintended dural puncture from the placement of an epidural needle. The overall incidence of unintentional dural puncture during attempted epidural placement lies somewhere in the range of 0.5% to 2.0%, depending on the experience of the clinician and characteristics of the patient.[5] Whether the patient actually develops a headache is dependent on a number of variables. The landmark study by Vandam et al. identified three independent risk factors for developing a headache after unintended dural puncture in the general population. Female, younger, and pregnant patients were more likely than male, older, and nonpregnant patients to develop headache after dural puncture with identical needles.[6]

The needle gauge is the other major determinant for developing a headache. As one might expect, the larger bore the needle, the more CSF leakage, which, in turn, leads to a more significant headache. See Table 15-1 and Figure 15-1 for more information.[7]

The other characteristic of the needle that can affect headache rate is whether it is a cutting or a pencil point needle. The lower incidence of headache after a dural puncture with a pencil point needle is the result of "spreading" the dural fibers, rather than cutting them as with a conventional Quincke-type needle. This

Table 15-1. Effect of Gauge and Type of Needle on Incidence of PDPH[a]

Gauge/Type of Spinal	Incidence of Postdural
18-gauge Tuohy	70-80
22-gauge Quincke	20-40
25-gauge Quincke	10-15
22-gauge pencil point	1-2
25-gauge pencil point	<1

[a]Data from Cesarini M, Torrielli F, Lahaye F, et al.[7]

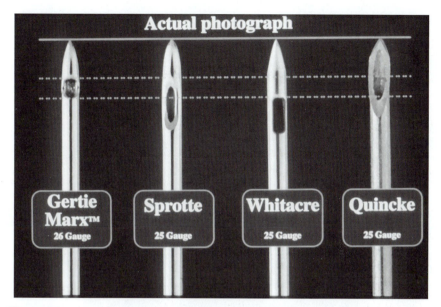

Figure 15-1. From Left to Right: Three examples of pencil-point needles (Gertie Marx, Sprotte, and Whitacre) and a cutting needle (Quincke).

theoretically allows the dura to heal faster than with a similar-bore cutting needle. See Figure 15-2.

For many years, conventional wisdom suggested that morbid obesity was protective against PDPH. Initially, this hypothesis was based on the fact that fewer obese women received epidural blood patches. This, however, could be interpreted in one of two ways. One, it could be that fewer obese patients were having severe headache symptoms or, two, conversely, that providers were more hesitant about performing a blood patch on obese women who had already been "wet-tapped." Further confounding the evidence is the fact that morbidly obese women have a higher cesarean delivery rate than nonobese women and as a result are given neuraxial morphine for postoperative pain relief, which in and of itself may alter the natural progression of the headache. More recent literature seems to support the notion that PDPH is rarer in the obese population but likely related to increased intra-abdominal pressure that is transmitted to the epidural space, thereby reducing CSF leakage and baseline CSF volume as compared to women with normal body habitus.[8]

SYMPTOMS AND COMPLICATIONS OF POSTDURAL PUNCTURE HEADACHE

The natural history of PDPH is self-limiting. Between 70% and 80% of cases of PDPH generally resolve within 7 days or less, and between 88% and 95% of the headaches resolve within 6 weeks. In a small minority of cases, the symptoms may persist for weeks or even months.[6]

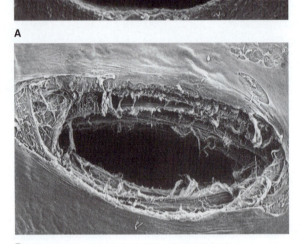

A

B

Figure 15-2. (A) Scanning electron micrograph of a dural puncture hole made by a 25-gauge Quincke (cutting) needle. (B) Scanning electron micrograph of a dural puncture hole made by a 25-gauge Whitacre (pencil point) needle. Used with permission from Covino BG, Scott DB, Lambert DH. Handbook of Spinal Anaesthesia and Analgesia. WB Saunders, Philadelphia (1994).

Symptoms of PDPH typically include a positional headache in the frontal or occipital regions. Other presentations may include diplopia, tinnitus and/or changes in hearing, dizziness, and nuchal myalgia. Most of these symptoms can be explained by loss of CSF volume or compensatory measures to account for its loss. For example, as a result of CSF loss, diplopia is a direct result of traction on the sixth cranial nerve, and hearing loss is thought to be secondary to alterations of hair cell position in the inner ear.

Beyond difficulties in performing activities of daily living, PDPH can be a precursor to serious medical problems. Subdural hematoma may occur due to traction and pulling on the bridging subdural veins caused by intracranial hypotension as a result of CSF leakage. The actual incidence of subdural hematoma following dural puncture is unknown, but if it occurs, it has been successfully treated with either surgical decompression or epidural blood patch. Because subdural hematoma is more likely to be diagnosed following neurologic changes, or worsening of the headache, many practitioners are more likely to provide aggressive management (ie, an epidural blood patch), in the presence of more severe symptoms.[9]

The hearing loss and diplopia that can be part of the initial presentation of PDPH can rarely outlast the headache itself. They occasionally persist for months with case reports of changes in hearing persisting indefinitely.[10]

TREATMENT

The options for treating PDPH can be divided into two categories: conservative and aggressive.

Conservative Management

Conservative management involves maintaining a supine position, hydration, caffeine, nonsteroidal anti-inflammatory drugs, and the butalbital-acetaminophen-caffeine combination (Fioricet). Lying flat simply alleviates severity of symptoms but does not decrease the incidence of headache. It is important to remember that the theory behind hydrating patients is that patients with relative hypovolemia will produce less CSF. However, once a patient is euvolemic, additional hydration only exacerbates the symptoms of the headache by forcing patients to frequently walk to the bathroom. If a patient is taking oral fluids ab libitum, additional intravenous supplementation is not indicated. Other conservative strategies for ameliorating PDPH focus on countering the vasodilation that occurs as the body attempts to preserve brain homeostasis in the face of decreased intracranial volume due to CSF leakage. Caffeine is a cerebral vasoconstrictor, but normal oral intake does not appear to reduce long-term severity of headache or obviate the need for an epidural blood patch, although there may be some transient benefit.[11] However, as a central nervous stimulant, there have been reports of seizures after high doses of intravenous administration of caffeine, particularly if blood is withdrawn for injection in a blood patch.

Other cerebral vasoconstrictors that have been used with varying success include theophylline and sumatriptan. According to meta-analysis, theophylline demonstrated a lower "mean sum of pain" when visual analog scores (VAS) were tabulated, but sumatriptan was not found to differ from placebo scores. Gabapentin, however, resulted in lower VAS at 1, 2, 3, and 4 days of administration. The reason is unclear but may be related to its structural similarity to gamma-aminobutyric acid, or its action at calcium channels. The Cochrane review was careful to caution that its meta-analysis was based on few trials that were, for the most part, poorly powered.[12]

Fioricet is often used as a first-line therapeutic agent. As previously stated, it consists of acetaminophen for pain relief as well as butalbital and caffeine for their vasoconstrictor effect.

Aggressive Management

More invasive measures postpuncture may include converting the anesthetic to a continuous spinal, which may reduce the incidence of headache. If a headache does occur, an epidural blood patch (EBP) may be performed.

INTRATHECAL CATHETER

In 2003, Ayad et al. published a study involving three groups of women after unintended dural puncture: the first group simply had the epidural placed at a different level.[13] In addition, there were two additional groups, one where an intrathecal catheter was placed through the puncture site and removed after vaginal delivery, and the other where the intrathecal catheter was not removed until 24 hours after delivery. The group that had the epidural catheter replaced at a different site had a PDPH rate of 91%, the group that had the intrathecal catheter in place for labor had a lower PDPH rate of 51.4%, and the group that had the catheter left in place for 24 hours had the lowest PDPH rate—of only 6.2%.[13] The authors speculated that the reduction in headache with the intrathecal catheters was related to a mechanical obstruction to the outflow of CSF, and in the case of the delayed catheter removal, it has been proposed that an inflammatory reaction accelerates the healing process around the dural defect. However, others have contested that point, noting that all medical plastics used in humans undergo testing to ensure their inert nature. To date, no well-powered, large, prospective study has confirmed these findings, and there remains concern over the potential for misuse of an intrathecal catheter on the floor. Indeed, in a letter to the editor, Rosenblatt et al. questioned the safety of running an intrathecal anesthetic on a busy labor floor manned by both attending and trainees. The authors of the letter pointed out that an epidural dose administered through an intrathecal catheter could easily result in the death of the parturient and her fetus, whereas, the major downside of replacing the epidural would most likely be a self-limited headache that in the vast majority of cases is amenable to treatment.[14]

Most recently, in a 2013 meta-analysis was performed on nine studies of intrathecal catheters placed after inadvertent dural puncture. Heesen et al. were able to identify a significant decrease in the number of patients requiring epidural blood patch after intrathecal catheter had been placed.[15] The effect size of the Ayad study was not seen in the meta-analysis. When all studies, including Ayad's, were reviewed, the actual incidence of PDPH was not statistically significant. Nevertheless, placing the intrathecal catheter may be a valuable intervention to decrease the severity of the PDPH.

EPIDURAL BLOOD PATCH

EBP has been most successful in treating PDPH for more than 40 years. The mechanism of action is not completely understood. Because there is often almost immediate relief after an EBP, there must be a mechanism involving additional factors than just CSF volume restoration. It is hypothesized that the initial relief can be attributed to increased lumbar CSF pressures that are transmitted cranially,[16] thus restoring intracranial pressures and reversing reflex cerebral vasodilation. The longer acting relief then may come as a result of the "patching" of the dural puncture by clot and subsequent repletion of the CSF volume. The initial estimates of EBP suggested that the success rate was as high as 90%. More recent and larger studies have placed the overall success rate at closer to 61% to 75%.[17] Commonly, the initial success of the procedure may be as high as 90%, but over the next 24 hours the overall success regresses back to that 60% to 75%. If a second EBP is

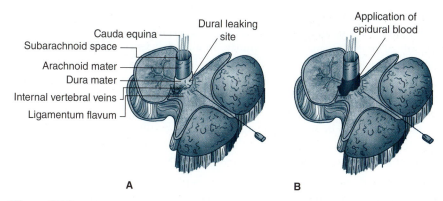

Figure 15-3. Schematic cross-section of the vertebral column, showing the cauda equina and surrounding membranes with the dural leakage site before (A) and after (B) application of an epidural blood patch. (From Oedit R, van Kooten F, Bakker SLM, Dippel DWJ.[18])

performed, this too carries a success rate of 60% to 75%, making the overall success rate of two EBPs approximately 90%. (See Figure 15-3.)[18]

A full and detailed consent should be obtained, including a discussion regarding the risk of repuncturing dura and the other associated risks of performing an epidural, namely, bleeding, infection, and neurologic damage. As with any regional technique, contraindications include patient refusal, coagulopathy, infection at injection site, systemic infection, and increased intracranial pressure.

Once the epidural space is identified, 15 to 20 mL of blood is obtained aseptically and injected into the epidural space. The blood must be injected slowly and should be stopped if increased pressure or pain is elicited in the back, down the legs, or in the head/neck. The optimal dose of the EBP has yet to be established. Generally, 12 to 20 mL should be sufficient, with the larger volume appearing to be more efficacious if tolerated.[19] Studies using technetium-labeled red blood cells have demonstrated more cephalad than caudad spread of blood and that a 12- to 15-mL injection usually spreads between five and nine spinal segments. The success rate of the EBP is improved if the patient lies supine immediately after injection for at least 1 and possibly 2 hours.[20] from observational studies, it has been suggested that a blood patch may not be as effective if performed within the first 24 hours of dural puncture—for several reasons.[21] One is that a larger hole may cause an earlier onset headache and may, theoretically, be more difficult to treat based on its size. Other theories revolve around ability to form a clot within the first 24 hours. For instance, local anesthetic and CSF may have anticoagulant properties and may prevent the blood from clotting over the dural defect. Alternatively, it is certainly possible that a longer time interval from puncture to EBP may add healing on its own and may account for the improved results observed with a delayed EBP.

While the EBP is the current gold standard for treatment, it is not without its own unique risks. The risks can essentially be divided into two groups, infectious and neurologic. Although a high fever or sepsis would be a contraindication to EBP, it is unclear whether a low-grade fever treated by antibiotics would be a contraindication.

However, there are reports of meningitis following EBP and, as blood is an exceptional culture medium, the utmost care must be taken to perform the procedure in a sterile manner. In patients with human immunodeficiency virus (HIV), the risk of seeding the central nervous system (CNS) with HIV is less of a concern due to the fact that the virus first appears in the CNS during primary infection and thus is already present in the CNS. Other concerns involve the hematogenous spread of metastatic disease in cancer victims. As with all therapies, the potential benefits of the EBP should be weighed against the risks of seeding the CNS with tumor. In one case report, fibrin glue rather than the patients' own blood was successfully used for an EBP in a nonobstetric patient with leukemia.[22]

Neurologic Complications Neurologic complications of the EBP can be categorized into lumbosacral, intracranial, and inflammatory-mediated processes. The possible lumbosacral complications of EBP include transient low back pain, radicular back pain, cauda equina syndrome, and lumbovertebral syndrome (back pain with lower extremity neurologic impairment). Diaz et al, in a case series, described an association between compressive symptoms and epidural blood patch with injected volume greater than 35 mL as opposed to noncompressive symptoms (radicular irritation), which were associated with a mean volume of 17 mL.[23] Abouleish et al conducted a longitudinal study in 118 patients having an EBP and found the most common neurologic symptom to be low back pain with 16% of patients with this symptom experiencing persistent back pain of 27 day mean duration.[24] Intracranial complications are rare and include the potential for subdural hematoma, cranial nerve palsies, and seizures. Diaz et al suggested that delaying treatment in patients having cranial nerve manifestations (ie, diplopia, hearing changes) could result in a protracted course. They described two patients having received a blood patch within 4 days of the onset of cranial nerve symptoms, which resolved within 6 weeks, whereas three patients who were treated late (9-11 days after onset of cranial nerve symptoms) experienced a persistent palsy of 3 to 4 months' duration.[23] It is also important to rule out primary intracranial pathology as well as late-onset eclampsia when patients experience seizures. Inflammatory processes that may mimic PDPH include acute meningeal irritation and arachnoiditis. Arachnoiditis is thought to be caused by free radical damage to nerve roots by degraded hemoglobin and can be diagnosed by history as well as findings of nerve root clumping and adhesions on magnetic resonance imaging (MRI). As with any new-onset neurologic deficit, those associated with an EBP necessitate prompt investigation and management.

HEADACHES UNRELATED TO DURAL PUNCTURE: PNEUMOCEPHALUS, POSTERIOR REVERSIBLE ENCEPHALOPATHY SYNDROME, CORTICAL VEIN THROMBOSIS, AND DURAL SINUS THROMBOSIS

Pneumocephalus presents as sudden onset of severe headache with or without neck pain, back pain, and mental status changes. It is usually caused by the unintended injection of air subarachnoid when used to identify the epidural space. On computed tomography (CT) scan, intracranial air can be visualized. The symptoms can be positional and typically resolve within the first week. Patients should receive oxygen supplementation because it may shorten the duration of the headache.[25] Nitrous oxide should be avoided in patients with pneumocephalus due to the potential for bubble expansion.

Posterior reversible encephalopathy syndrome (PRES) is a curious name for a disease entity that need not be posterior or reversible. Symptomatology includes headache, seizures, altered mental status, visual changes, and focal neurologic deficits. It occurs in varied populations. Patients who are at risk may have preeclampsia, uremia, hemolytic-uremic syndrome, or exposure to immunosuppressant drugs. Twenty-five percent of PRES cases occur in pregnant patients. Radiologic features usually include symmetric areas of cerebral edema involving the white matter surrounding the posterior circulation; this is thought to be due to changes in blood-brain barrier integrity similar to hypertensive encephalopathy. Thus, aggressive treatment of hypertension and seizure prophylaxis is necessary to reverse the process and prevent irreversible cytotoxic edema.[26]

Related to the hypercoagulability of pregnancy, parturients are also at increased risk for cortical vein thrombosis (CVT). This disease process may also be difficult to distinguish from PDPH as it too may have a postural component. CVT has an incidence of 10 to 20 per 100,000 deliveries in developed countries but may be more frequent in developing countries.[27] Symptoms include focal neurologic signs, seizures, and coma and cerebral infarction may occur if diagnosis is delayed. The diagnosis may be made by MRI. Treatment is largely symptomatic and aimed at anticoagulation and seizure prevention.[28] More aggressive treatment with thrombolysis is currently being investigated.

Even more infrequent than CVT may be dural sinus thrombosis. Symptoms may include headache, abnormal vision, and any of the symptoms of stroke and seizures. The diagnosis is usually made by CT scan or MRI using radiocontrast, thus allowing visualization of obstruction of the venous sinuses by the thrombus. A high degree of suspicion must be present to make this very rare diagnosis. Treatment should involve anticoagulation.

CONCLUSION

PDPH is one of the most common complications of neuraxial anesthesia. Given the high incidence of peripartum headaches in general, it is imperative that when consulted, obstetric anesthesiologists consider all of the myriad possible etiologies. Although there are some innocuous sources of peripartum headache, postdural puncture headache is a complication that should not be taken lightly. Most of these headaches will spontaneously resolve, or be mitigated either by conservative, or aggressive management, but there is the potential for significant morbidity. Accordingly, patients should always be apprised of their options at every stage of the headache and its resolution.

REFERENCES

1. Goldszmidt E, Kern R, Chaput A, Macarthur A. The incidence and etiology of postpartum headaches: a prospective cohort study. *Can J Anaesth*. 2005;52:971-977.
2. Chadwick HS, Posner KL, Caplan RA, Ward RJ, Cheney FW. A comparison of obstetric and nonobstetric anesthesia malpractice claims. *Anesthesiology*. 1991;74:242-249.

3. Davies JM, Posner KL, Lee LA, Cheney FW, Domino KB. Liability associated with obstetric anesthesia: a closed claims analysis. *Anesthesiology*. 2009;110(1):131-139.

4. Grant R, Condon B, Patterson J, et al. Changes in cranial CSF volume during hypercapnia and hypocapnea. *J Neurol Neurosurg Psychiatry*. 1989;52:218-222.

5. Choi PT, Galinski SE, Takeuchi L, et al. PDPH is a common complication of neuraxial blockade in parturients: a meta-analysis of obstetrical studies. *Can J Anaesth*. 2003;50:460-469.

6. Vandam LD, Dripps RD. Long term follow up of patients who received 10,098 spinal anesthetics. *JAMA*. 1956;161:586-590.

7. Cesarini M, Torrielli F, Lahaye F, et al. Sprotte needle for intrathecal anaesthesia for Caesarean section: incidence of postdural puncture headache. *Anaesthesia*. 1990;45:656-658.

8. Ray A, Hildreth A, Esen UI. Morbid obesity and intra-partum care. *J Obset Gynecol*. 2008;28:301-304.

9. Zeidan A, Farhat O, Maaliki H, Baraka A. Does postdural puncture headache left untreated lead to subdural hematoma? Case report and review of the literature. *Int J Obst Anesth*. 2006;15:50-58.

10. Nishio I, Williams BA, Williams JP. Diplopia: a complication of dural puncture. *Anesthesiology*. 2004;100:158-164.

11. Camann WR, Murray RS, Mushlin PS, Lambert DH. Effects of oral caffeine on postdural puncture headache: a double-blind, placebo controlled trial. *Anesth Analg*. 1990;70:181-184.

12. Basurto Ona X, Martínez García L, Solà I, Bonfill Cosp X. Drug therapy for treating post-dural puncture headache. *Cochrane Database Syst Rev*. 2011;8:CD007887.

13. Ayad S, Demian Y, Narouze SN, Tetzlaff JE: Subarachnoid catheter placement after wet tap for analgesia in labor: influence on the risk of headache in obstetric patients. *Reg Anesth Pain Med*. 2003;28:512-515.

14. Rosenblatt MA, Bernstein HH, Beilin Y. Are subarachnoid catheters really safe? *Reg Anesth Pain Med*. 2004;29:298.

15. Heesen M, Klohr S, Rossain R, Walters M, Straub S, van de Velde M. Insertion os an intrathecal catheter following accidental dural puncture: a meta-analysis. *Int J Obstet Anesth*. 2013;22:26-30.

16. Coombs DW, Hooper D: Subarachnoid pressure with epidural blood patch. *Reg Anesth*. 1979;4:3-6.

17. Taivainen T, Pitkanen M, Tuominen M, Rosenberg PH. Efficacy of epidural blood patch for postdural puncture headache. *Acta Anaesthesiol Scand*. 1993;37:702-705.

18. Oedit, R, van Kooten F, Bakker SLM, Dippel DWJ. Efficacy of the epidural blood patch for the treatment of post lumbar puncture headache BLOPP: a randomised, observer-blind, controlled clinical trial [ISRCTN 71598245]. *BMC Neurology*. 2005,5:12.

19. Szeinfeld M, Ihmeidan IH, Moser MM, et al. Epidural blood patch: evaluation of the volume and spread of blood injected into the epidural space. *Anesthesiology*. 1986;64:820-822.

20. Martin R, Jourdain S, et al. Duration of decubitus position after epidural blood patch. *Can J Anaesth*. 1994;41:23-25.

21. Safa-Tisseront V, Thormann F, Malassine P, et al. Effectiveness of epidural blood patch in the management of post-dural puncture headache. *Anesthesiology*. 2001;95:334-339.

22. Decramer I, Fuzier V, Franchitto N, Samii K. Is use of epidural fibrin glue patch in patients with metastatic cancer appropriate? *Eur J Anaesthesiol*. 2005;22:724-725.

23. Diaz JH, Weed JT. Correlation of adverse neurological outcomes with increasing volumes and delayed administration of autologous epidural blood patches for postdural puncture headaches. *Pain Pract*. 2005;5:216-222.

24. Abouleish E, Vega S, Blendinger I, Tio TO. Long-term follow-up of epidural blood patch. *Anesth Analg*. 1975;54:459-463.

25. Smarkusky L, DeCarvalho H, Bermudez A, Gonzalez-Quintero VH. Acute onset headache complicating labor epidural caused by intrapartum pneumocephalus. *Obstet Gynecol*. 2006;108:795-798.

26. Pande AR, Ando K, Ishikura R, et al. Clinicoradiological factors influencing the reversibility of posterior reversible encephalopathy syndrome: a multicenter study. *Radiat Med*. 2006;24:659-668.

27. Lockhart EM, Baysinger CL. Intracranial venous thrombosis in the parturient. *Anesthesiology*. 2007;107:652-658.

28. Bousser MG. Cerebral venous thrombosis: diagnosis and management. *J Neurol*. 2000;247:252-258.

Peripheral Nerve Injury Associated With Labor

16

Barbara Orlando and Jonathan Epstein

The majority of complications involving peripheral nerves are unrelated to the anesthetic technique and more likely due to obstetric circumstances. A survey of 6057 women who delivered in Chicago[1] reported an incidence of lower extremity nerve injuries of approximately 1% (24 lateral femoral cutaneous nerve, 22 femoral nerve, 3 peroneal nerve, 3 lumbosacral plexus, 2 sciatic nerve, 3 obturator nerve, and 5 radicular injuries).[1] Significant risk factors for peripheral nerve injury (PNI) were nulliparity and a prolonged second stage of labor, but not neuraxial anesthesia. The findings of this survey corroborate those of the Leeds study,[2] stating that "that postpartum neurologic dysfunction is more frequent if specifically sought, and support the clinical impression that significant neurological deficits occur irrespective of the use of regional anaesthesia."

EPIDEMIOLOGY

The detection of PNI may be spuriously increasing as a result of the routine follow-up performed by the anesthesia team in the immediate postpartum period to detect complications linked to the practice of neuraxial anesthesia (eg, postdural puncture headache, epidural hematoma, nerve root damage). On the other hand, with the changes in obstetric practices regarding intolerance for protracted labor and difficult forceps delivery, the prevalence of these complications will likely decrease. The new obstetric guidelines show a preference for cesarean delivery as opposed to prolonged labor and forceps assistance in these situations.

Neurologic complaints due to factors associated with labor and delivery are seen in 1.6 to 4.8/10,000 of parturients, and those attributed to the possible deficits related to regional anesthetic techniques are found in 0 to 1.2/10,000 of parturients.[3]

MECHANISMS OF PERIPHERAL NERVE INJURY

Acute nerve injury may occur as a consequence of transection, traction, compression of a nerve, or vascular injury.[4]

- Compression or traction on a nerve can result in compromised perineural blood flow and lead to ischemia. This may cause focal demyelination and conduction block. However, symptoms are usually transient, because the focal demyelization is a reversible phenomenon.
- In more serious injuries, the axons of the nerve can be damaged. In this case, the damage can be permanent, or if temporary, the symptoms will disappear slowly.
- Neuraxial anesthesia can mask the early symptoms of PNI. Residual numbness or weakness can be attributed falsely to residual local anesthetic effect. Thus, a high index of suspicion for PNI must be maintained in the face of unintended extended sensory or motor block.

RISK FACTORS FOR PERIPHERAL NERVE INJURY

Risk factors may be maternal or fetal.[5,6]

- Maternal obesity
- Abnormal presentation
- Persistent occiput posterior position
- Fetal macrosomia/fetus large for gestational age

  Risk factors may be related to the labor.[5,6]

- Breakthrough pain during epidural labor analgesia
- Prolonged second stage of labor
- Difficult instrumental delivery
- Prolonged use of the lithotomy position

SYMPTOMS

PNIs typically result in a neurologic deficit in the distribution of a specific peripheral nerve. Neurologic or neurosurgical consultation and immediate imaging studies should be obtained if there is any question about the etiology of prolonged anesthesia; it is necessary to rule out an epidural/spinal hematoma because PNI can be confused with epidural hematoma. However, symptoms that are suggestive of PNI versus epidural hematoma include absence of back pain with PNI, unilateral block, and regression (rather than progression) of the symptoms. When the roots are touched at the level of the spinal cord, secondary to neuraxial anesthesia, the distribution of the symptoms will be more extended. As for PNI, depending on the nerve damaged, the symptoms and circumstances of the injury will be different (Figure 16-1).[7,8]

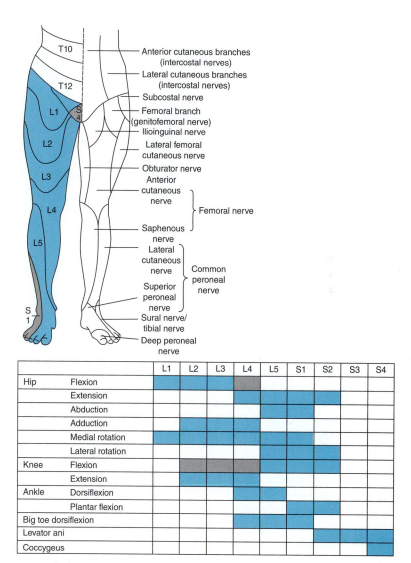

		L1	L2	L3	L4	L5	S1	S2	S3	S4
Hip	Flexion	■	■	■	■					
	Extension				■	■	■	■		
	Abduction				■	■	■			
	Adduction		■	■	■					
	Medial rotation	■	■				■			
	Lateral rotation				■	■	■	■		
Knee	Flexion		■	■	■	■	■	■		
	Extension		■	■	■					
Ankle	Dorsiflexion				■	■				
	Plantar flexion						■	■		
Big toe dorsiflexion					■	■	■			
Levator ani								■	■	■
Coccygeus								■	■	■

Figure 16-1. Sensory innervation of the lower extremity. Precise identification of the location of the deficit will aid in assessing improvement and suggest possible etiologies for the deficit.

TYPES OF PERIPHERAL NERVE INJURY

Lumbosacral Trunk: L4 and L5 Roots

ANATOMY

The lumbosacral trunk (LST) follows very closely the ala of the sacrum near the sacroiliac joint. The psoas muscle offers protection of the LST except at its terminal portion near the pelvic edge, where the S1 nerve root meets with the LST to form the

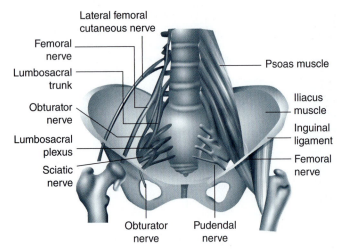

Figure 16-2. Dermatomal distribution of activities commonly impaired by peripheral nerve injuries.

sciatic nerve (Figure 16-2).[9] In that area, the LST becomes susceptible to compression of the fetal head (usually the forehead), as the head descends through the pelvis.

RISK FACTORS

This complication is more likely with cephalopelvic disproportion, prolonged labor with difficult/instrumental vaginal delivery, fetal macrosomia, and malpresentation (occiput posterior or brow presentation). In addition, it may occur with certain pelvic features such as platypelloid pelvis, shallow anterior sacral ala, and flattened sacral promontory.

SYMPTOMS

Symptoms include foot drop and varying degrees of lower extremity weakness, sensation changes, pain, and diminished reflexes in L4-L5 territory.

Sciatic Nerve Injury

ANATOMY

The sciatic nerve (SN) is formed by the ventral rami of L4-S3. The SN exits the pelvis via the greater sciatic foramen, inferior to the piriformis muscle, and then travels posterior to the buttock and thigh where it splits into the tibial nerve and the common peroneal nerve.

The SN primarily supplies the muscles of the lower leg, including the calf, ankle, and the back of the knee. It also supplies sensation to the sole and lateral aspect of the foot, the lateral aspect of the lower leg, and the back of the thigh.

RISK FACTORS

Risk factors for injury to the SN include a high lithotomy position with prolonged hip hyperflexion and excessive external rotation, as can be seen during a difficult vaginal delivery. Additionally, the fetal head at the pelvic edge can also compress the SN as the fetus descends into the pelvis. SN compression during cesarean delivery has also been described. The likely etiology would be a result of prolonged compression of the nerve against the operating room table in a supine patient with slight left lateral decubitus position.

SYMPTOMS

Injury to the SN will cause motor loss of the muscles of the posterior thigh, leg, and foot (see Common Peroneal Nerve Injury). Also, it will lead to sensory loss over the distribution described above.

Common Peroneal Nerve Injury

ANATOMY

The common peroneal nerve (CPN) is one of two branches of the SN. It separates from the posterior tibial branch of the SN above the popliteal fossa, then passes over the lateral head of fibula and descends down the lateral calf, splitting into a superficial and deep branch. It is very vulnerable to injury as it travels superficially around the neck of the fibula (Figure 16-3). The deep and superficial peroneal branches provide sensation to the anterior and lateral parts of the legs and to the dorsum of the foot. They also innervate muscles in the legs responsible for eversion and dorsiflexion of the foot as well as extension of the toes.

RISK FACTORS

Risk factors for injury to the CPN include prolonged squatting during childbirth, hyperflexion of the knees during delivery, and direct compression of the nerve over the fibular head by the patient holding her legs with fingers placed over the anterior tibia and palms over the fibular head. Likewise, certain types of stirrups that may be used for pushing during the second stage of labor may also cause compression of the CPN but is more common during gynecologic surgery in lithotomy position.

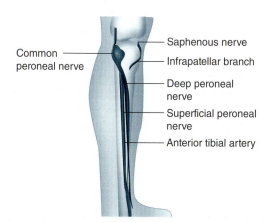

Common peroneal nerve

Saphenous nerve

Infrapatellar branch

Deep peroneal nerve

Superficial peroneal nerve

Anterior tibial artery

Figure 16-3. The lumbosacral plexus in the pelvis.

Symptoms

The main manifestation of CPN injury is a foot drop on the affected site associated with paresthesia on the dorsum of the foot and anterolateral aspect of the leg.

Femoral Nerve Injury

Anatomy

The femoral nerve (FN) is a branch of the lumbar plexus that enters the thigh just under the inguinal ligament and lateral to the femoral vein and artery (mnemonic *NAV*, for *n*erve, *a*rtery, *v*ein, from lateral to medial). The FN ends as the saphenous nerve, the largest cutaneous branch of the FN and only sensory branch innervating the medial aspect of the leg and foot. The SN innervates the remainder of the leg.

Risk Factors

Risk factors for injury to the FN include prolonged pushing in extreme flexion. In contrast to other PNIs, cephalopelvic disproportion is not implicated in this nerve injury because the femoral nerve does not traverse the true pelvis.

Symptoms

The FN provides sensation to the anterior side of thigh, and medial aspect of the leg and foot up to the big toe. The main presentation of FN injury is a motor deficit including weakness of hip flexion and knee extension. It is common for the patient to tell you that she has "trouble standing up from the sitting position."

Lateral Femoral Cutaneous Nerve Injury

Anatomy

The lateral femoral cutaneous nerve (LFCN) is a branch of the FN and exits the pelvis under the inguinal ligament and becomes medial and inferior to the anterior superior iliac spine.

Risk Factors

Risk factors for LFCN injury include prolonged pushing with hip flexion because the nerve is compressed under the inguinal ligament. The clinician should recommend frequent leg repositioning during labor, as well as avoiding prolonged hip flexion and shortening pushing time. Ideally, the fetus should descend passively before starting to push. A wide Pfannenstiel incision during cesarean section may transect the LFCN and it may also be compressed by self-retaining retractors.

Symptoms

The LFCN has no motor component and when injured is responsible for meralgia paresthesia syndrome, which typically presents with burning, pain, and/or numbness of the anterolateral thigh.

Obturator Nerve Injury

ANATOMY

The obturator nerve (ON) arises from the ventral divisions of the second, third, and fourth lumbar nerves (L2, L3, and L4). It descends through the fibers of the psoas major muscle and emerges from the medial border near the edge of the pelvis. The nerve then passes behind the common iliac arteries to the upper part of the obturator foramen, where it enters the thigh and passes through the obturator canal. It then divides into an anterior and a posterior branch. The ON is responsible for the sensory innervation of the skin of the medial aspect of the thigh and for the motor innervation of the adductor muscles of the lower extremity.

RISK FACTORS

The ON can be compressed by the fetal head as it descends into the pelvis. It can also be injured during forceps delivery or during prolonged lithotomy position (because of the angulation of the nerve as it leaves the obturator foramen). A pudendal nerve block with a resultant hematoma can also damage the ON by entrapment.

SYMPTOMS

Symptoms of ON injury include medial thigh or groin pain, weakness with leg adduction, and sensory loss in the medial thigh of the affected side.

Upper Extremities Nerve Injury

These injuries are seen mostly during cesarean delivery under general anesthesia (which is less and less frequent due to advances in regional anesthesia). They are due to the inappropriate positioning of the arms on the arm boards and include injury of the brachial plexus (hyperabduction) or ulnar nerve injury (compression on the armboard at the level of the elbow). Radial nerve injury can occur with compression of the nerve at the level of the humerus (spiral groove) when the parturient rests her arms against the birthing bar during vaginal delivery.

SUMMARY

Most PNIs during obstetric care are due to maternal factors, such as morbid obesity, or two obstetric factors—prolonged labor and malposition of the fetal head. Indeed, the most likely cause of PNIs is the mother's assuming unphysiologic positions that can result in stretch or compression of lower extremity nerves as they exit the pelvis.

REFERENCES

1. Wong CA, Scavone BM, Dugan S, et al. Incidence of postpartum lumbosacral spine and lower extremity nerve injuries. *Obstet Gynecol*. 2003;101:279-288.
2. Dar AQ, Robinson AP, Lyons G. Postpartum neurological symptoms following regional blockade: a prospective study with case controls. *Int J Obstet Anesth*. 2002;11:85-90.
3. Zakowski MI. Postoperative complications associated with regional anesthesia in the parturient. In: Norris M, ed. *Obstetric Anesthesia*. 2nd ed. Philadelphia, PA: Lippincott Williams & Wilkins; 1999.

4. McDonald A. Obstetrical nerve injury. *Perinatal Outreach Program of Southwestern Ontario.* Spring 2008;31:1-4.

5. Bamgbade OA, Rutter TW, Nafiu OO, Dorje P. Postoperative complications in obese and nonobese patients. *World J Surg.* 2007;31:556-560.

6. Chestnut DH, Wong CA, Tsen LC, eds. *Chestnut's Obstetric Anesthesia: Principles and Practice.* 4th ed. Philadelphia, PA: Mosby/Elsevier; 2009.

7. Redick LF. Maternal perinatal nerve palsies. *Postgrad Obstet Gynecol.* 1992;12:1-6.

8. Russell R. Assessment of motor blockade during epidural analgesia in labour. *Int J Obstet Anesth.* 1992;4:230-234.

9. Cole JT. Maternal obstetric paralysis. *Am J Obstet Gynecol.* 1946;52:374.

Anaphylaxis During Pregnancy

17

Kal Chaudhuri

INTRODUCTION

The word *anaphylaxis* (ana: backward; phylaxis: guard, or "against protection") was coined by Paul Portier and Charles Richet, two scientists who unexpectedly induced acute anaphylaxis in their experimental dogs during an attempt to produce vaccines for prophylaxis against a toxin (actinotoxin) from a sea anemone, *Actinia sulcata*.[1] Anaphylaxis is a severe, life-threatening, systemic event caused by immediate hypersensitivity reaction. Although it is relatively infrequent during pregnancy, the potentially fatal effects on the mother and the unborn baby warrant prompt recognition and immediate management. Severe anaphylaxis, in general, affects 1 to 3 per 10,000 population,[2] but the incidence during anesthesia is reported to range from as high as 1 in 4000 to 1 in 25,000.[3] The prevalence of anaphylaxis in pregnant patients is approximately 3 per 100,000 deliveries.[4]

PATHOPHYSIOLOGY

Anaphylaxis is a systemic form of immediate hypersensitivity reaction caused by immunoglobulin E (IgE)–mediated release of mediators from mast cells and basophils. Exposure to allergen in a susceptible individual initiates a cascade of events, including activation of helper T-2 cells (T_H2 cells) and stimulation of IgE-secreting B cells. IgE then binds to FcεRI receptors on mast cells and basophils. After several episodes of exposure to the inciting allergen, a cross-linkage develops between the receptors by the allergen that triggers the mast cells to release mediators, including histamine, tryptase, tumor necrosis factor, and so on. These mediators then produce the serious manifestations of anaphylactic reaction in various organ systems such as the respiratory system (stridor, bronchospasm, hypoxia), cardiovascular system (hypotension, tachycardia, dysrhythmia), cutaneous system (erythema, pruritus, urticaria, angioedema), and gastrointestinal system (nausea, vomiting, diarrhea).[5]

Pregnant patients are thought to be predisposed to anaphylaxis as a result of alteration in cellular immunity, possibly due to increased level of progesterone.[6] Also, increased production of T_H2-type cytokine (which initiates the immediate hypersensitivity reaction) by maternal T cells at the fetomaternal interface and simultaneous inhibition of cytokine production from T_H1 cells (which normally play a role in allograft rejection) during pregnancy help to maintain the pregnancy and to prevent fetal loss.[7,8]

CAUSATIVE AGENTS

During anesthesia, neuromuscular blocking agents (succinylcholine, rocuronium), latex (gloves, tourniquet), and antibiotics (penicillins and other cephalosporins) are implicated as the most common agents in the etiology of anaphylactic reactions. Other less frequently involved agents include colloids, propofol, chlorhexidine, iodinated contrast media, local anesthetics, and so on.[9,10]

In one of the earliest reports, succinylcholine was implicated to be a causative agent for anaphylaxis in pregnant women.[11] Several other agents have since been implicated in obstetric patients, including muscle relaxants,[12] anesthetic induction agents,[13] bee stings,[14] latex,[15-18] latex and chlorhexidine,[19] synthetic colloid solutions,[20,21] ranitidine,[22,23] iron,[24] antivenin after snakebite,[25] laminaria (a hygroscopic cervical dilator prepared from seaweed),[26,27] and synthetic oxytocin.[28] However, one of the commonly reported agents to cause anaphylaxis are parenteral antibiotics including ampicillin,[29-32] penicillin,[33-35] and cephalosporins.[36-38] One epidemiologic study found that the β-lactam antibiotics were the most common causative agents of anaphylaxis during pregnancy.[4] Significant neurologic sequelae have been reported, especially with ampicillin.

CLINICAL MANIFESTATIONS

During anesthesia, a wide variety of clinical manifestations may commonly affect the cardiac (hypotension, bradycardia, asystole), cutaneous (urticaria, erythema), and respiratory (bronchospasm, difficulty to ventilate) systems. Anaphylaxis might also present with cardiovascular collapse, bronchospasm, or cutaneous symptoms.[39] Cutaneous manifestations may be absent or may be missed during anesthesia because patients are covered by surgical drapes. In the majority of cases during anesthesia, anaphylaxis occurs immediately after parenteral injection of the offending agent.[10]

Clinical signs of anaphylaxis are categorized into four grades[9,40]:

- Grade 1: involvement of skin and mucosa only (generalized erythema, urticarial, angioedema)
- Grade 2: moderate multiorgan system involvement (cardiovascular: hypotension, tachycardia; respiratory: bronchospasm; difficulty to ventilate; gastrointestinal: nausea)

- Grade 3: severe life-threatening symptoms (cardiac collapse, bradycardia, dysrhythmia, bronchospasm)
- Grade 4: cardiac and/or respiratory arrest

Selected published case reports involving anaphylaxis during pregnancy are detailed in Table 17-1. Cardiac manifestations, especially maternal hypotension, are the most common clinical manifestation during anaphylaxis among pregnant patients.

MANAGEMENT

Aggressive management of anaphylactic reaction immediately after suspicion is imperative to reduce morbidity and mortality of the mother and the unborn baby. The goals of management should be to inhibit the release of mediators and to modulate their actions. Peripheral vasodilation and capillary leakage, compounded by decreased venous return as a result of aortocaval compression from a gravid uterus, are important reasons for hypotension. Because fetal perfusion is directly proportional to uterine blood flow, maternal hypotension may cause ischemic damage to the vulnerable central nervous system of the baby infant. The magnitude and duration of the hypotension probably determine the extent of this injury.

Primary Management

Primary management[9,41-43] includes a quick evaluation of airway, breathing, and circulation (ABC); cessation of all possible offending agents; informing the obstetrician (or surgeon); maintaining the airway with 100% oxygen; left uterine displacement; administering epinephrine; aggressive fluid resuscitation (rapid infusion of 1 to 2 L of crystalloid solution); and consideration for emergency cesarean section, if warranted.

Epinephrine is the cornerstone in the primary management of anaphylaxis. It should be started early in titrated doses. Failure to administer epinephrine expeditiously, or administering it in inadequate doses, is a frequent reason for poor outcome during anaphylaxis.[10]

Epinephrine should not be administered during grade 1 anaphylaxis. In cases with grade 2 severity (hypotension, bronchospasm), initial dose of epinephrine should be 10 to 20 μg, to be titrated higher if needed. In grade 3 anaphylaxis, the initial dose should be 100 to 200 μg (may be repeated every 1-2 minutes if needed). If there is a need for repeated dosing, an intravenous infusion of epinephrine (1-4 μg/min) may be considered. During grade 4 reaction (cardiac arrest), cardiopulmonary resuscitation and aggressive volume resuscitation should accompany administration of epinephrine. The dose of epinephrine in grade 4 reaction should be 1 to 3 mg intravenously for 3 minutes, then 3 to 5 mg intravenously for 3 minutes, and then an infusion at 4 to 10 μg/min. The Advanced Cardiac Life Support algorithm should be followed in cases of pulseless electrical activity.

Table 17-1. Clinical Manifestations of Anaphylaxis During Pregnancy[a]

Author(s)	Offending Agent	Gestational Age at Onset	Therapeutic Management	Maternal Outcome	Neonatal Outcome
Sitarz (1974)[11]	Suxamethonium	41 weeks at CS	Noradrenaline, hydrocortisone, fluids, promethazine, ephedrine, Lasix	Hypotension, prompt resolution, good outcome	Delivery by CS in 45 min, good outcome
Baraka and Sfeir (1980)[13]	Propanidid	Term at CS	External cardiac massage, mechanical ventilation, epinephrine, hydrocortisone	Cardiac arrest, resolution in < 3 min, good outcome	Delivery by CS in 10 min, good outcome
Erasmus et al (1982)[14]	Bee sting	30 weeks	Hydrocortisone	Unconscious for 2 h, hypotension for > 4 h, good outcome	Vaginal delivery 5 weeks later, multicystic encephalomalacia
Entman and Moise (1984)[25]	Snakebite antivenin	28 weeks	Epinephrine, methylprednisolone, isoproterenol bolus and infusion, diphenhydramine	Hypotension > 3 h, good outcome	Decreased fetal movements, vaginal delivery 6 weeks later, depressed neonate, intracranial hemorrhage
Gallagher (1988)[29]	Ampicillin	36-37 weeks during labor	Diphenhydramine, methylprednisolone, intravenous epinephrine postpartum	Hypotension < 1 h, initial subendocardial ischemia, good outcome	Fetal bradycardia, vaginal delivery within 10 min, normal outcome
Heim et al (1991)[30]	Ampicillin	40 weeks during labor	Glucocorticoids, calcium, antihistaminics	Hypotension, prompt resolution, good outcome	Fetal heart rate 100/min, delivered by CS; time unclear, neurologic damage
Powell and Maycock (1993)[22]	Ranitidine	At term	Promethazine, hydrocortisone	Wheezing, facial and periorbital edema	Transient fetal bradycardia, vaginal delivery 4 h later, normal Apgar scores
Edmondson (1994)[12]	Suxamethonium	36 weeks during incision and drainage of pilonidal abscess	Hydrocortisone, adrenaline	Hypotension > 10 min, prompt resolution, good outcome	Fetal heart rate 100/min, delivered by CS; time unclear, neurologic damage

Reference	Allergen	Timing	Treatment	Maternal reaction/outcome	Fetal outcome
Konno and Nagase (1995)[36]	Cefazolin	36 weeks during labor	Ephedrine, methylprednisolone	Hypotension < 30 min, pre-disseminated intravascular coagulation, good outcome	Fetal bradycardia, delivered by CS in 30 min, normal outcome
Luciano et al (1997)[24]	Iron	27 weeks	Drugs used unclear	Severe cardiovascular collapse, resuscitation over 5 days	Vaginal delivery 10 weeks later, multicystic encephalomalacia
Porter et al (1998)[19]	Latex and chlorhexidine	39 weeks	Intravenous adrenaline	Shock, prompt resolution, good outcome	Delivered by CS 2 days later, normal outcome
Dunn et al (1999)[33]	Penicillin	35 weeks during labor	Ephedrine	Recurrent hypotension, disseminated intravascular coagulation, anuria, pneumonia, wound dehiscence	Fetal bradycardia, delivered by CS; time unclear, initial support, good outcome
Cole and Bruck (2000)[26]	Laminaria	21 weeks during elective abortion	Antihistaminics, corticosteroids β-agonist nebulizer	Respiratory distress, aspiration, convulsions, ventilatory support, good outcome	N/A
Chanda et al (2000)[27]	Laminaria	8-20 weeks elective abortions	Diphenhydramine, prednisone β-agonist nebulizer, subcutaneous epinephrine	Angioedema, respiratory distress, good outcome	N/A
Eckhout and Ayad (2001)[16]	Latex	32 weeks during preterm labor	Diphenhydramine, hydrocortisone ephedrine	Hypotension, respiratory distress, prompt resolution, good outcome	Fetal bradycardia, vaginal delivery weeks later, normal outcome
Gei et al (2003)[31]	Ampicillin	40 weeks during labor	Diphenhydramine, methylprednisolone, famotidine epinephrine infusion	Persistent hypotension, resolution with infusion	Fetal bradycardia < 5 min, vaginal delivery 5 h later, good outcome
Berardi et al (2004)[32]	Ampicillin	37 weeks during labor	Antihistaminics, steroids, etilefrine boluses	Severe hypotension	Persistent fetal bradycardia, delivered by CS; time unclear, neurologic damage
Jao et al (2006)[37]	Cefazolin	At term	Epinephrine, glucocorticoids	Hypotension, good outcome	Delivered by prompt CS, normal outcome

(continued)

Table 17-1. Clinical Manifestations of Anaphylaxis During Pregnancy[a] (Continued)

Author(s)	Offending Agent	Gestational Age at Onset	Therapeutic Management	Maternal Outcome	Neonatal Outcome
Draisci et al (2007)[17]	Latex (four patients)	? term at CS	Antihistaminics, steroids, (epinephrine and mechanical ventilation in one patient)	Hypotension (cardiovascular collapse in one patient), cutaneous signs, all good outcome	Delivered by CS, ?normal outcome
Sheikh (2007)[34]	Penicillin	During labor	Epinephrine	Dyspnea, malaise, severe hypotension	Delivered by CS, neonatal death
Sengupta(2008)[38]	Cefotaxime	During CS	Fluids, steroids	Cough, dyspnea	Fetal death
Chaudhuri et al (2008)[35]	Penicillin	During labor	Ephedrine, epinephrine	Erythema, hypotension	Significant neurologic injury
Turillazzi et al (2008)[18]	Latex	During CS	Fluids, inotropes	Bronchospasm, cardiorespiratory arrest, maternal death	Normal outcome
Karri et al (2009)[21]	Colloid	During CS	Epinephrine hydrocortisone, chlorpheniramine	Hypotension, difficulty in breathing	Normal outcome
Pant et al (2009)[28]	Syntocinon	During CS	Epinephrine, fluid, cardiopulmonary resuscitation	Hypotension, bronchospasm, pulseless electrical activity	

Abbreviations: S, fetal death; N/A, not available.
[a]Modified from Chaudhuri K, Gonzales J, Jesurun CA, et al.[35]

In patients who are resistant to epinephrine, which is often noted among patients on β-blocker therapy, intravenous glucagon (1-2 mg every 5 minutes) may be considered. The use of vasopressin (2-10 IU intravenously, may be repeated) or norepinephrine (0.05-0.1 μg/kg/min) is also suggested in patients with resistance to epinephrine.

Because the fetal central nervous system may suffer from serious permanent ischemic injury during prolonged hypotension, majority of adverse outcomes during these events frequently affect the neonates rather than mothers. Emergency cesarean section should be seriously considered if condition permits or if there is a cardiac arrest to facilitate maternal closed chest cardiac massage.

Secondary Management

Secondary management[9,41] of anaphylaxis includes inhalation of bronchodilators (albuterol) in cases of bronchospasm, antihistamines (25-50 mg diphenhydramine, a H_1 blocker), and corticosteroid (hydrocortisone 250 mg intravenously or methylprednisolone 80 mg intravenously). The roles of antihistamines and corticosteroid in the management of acute anaphylaxis have not been shown to have any proven value. Corticosteroids may help prevent the late phase of hypersensitivity reaction (in biphasic reaction), which may occur 4 to 6 hours after the acute reaction.

Further care includes transfer of the patient to a critical care unit in cases of grade 2 and above reactions, collection of blood samples to diagnose anaphylaxis, and performance of appropriate skin testing with suspected agents approximately 4 to 6 weeks after the incident.

Laboratory investigations during acute anaphylactic reactions include the measurement of serum histamine (peaks immediately after the reaction with a half-life of 20 minutes), serum tryptase (peak level is attained at 20 minutes with a half-life of 90 minutes), and specific immunoglobulin E assays of common offenders, such as β-lactam antibiotics, rocuronium, morphine, and so on.[9,43]

Skin prick tests and intradermal tests are available for several agents commonly responsible for perioperative anaphylaxis, including rocuronium, succinylcholine, penicillin, cephalosporins, and opioids.[9]

Although immediate-type hypersensitivity reactions are rare with amide local anesthetics, a history of allergy to these agents should be elicited from the pregnant patient. Provocative skin testing with local anesthetics in the mother with a possible prior reaction is discouraged due to increased sensitization during pregnancy and potential for fetal injury.[44] Allergy diagnostic testing should be considered only in select patients with definite and immediate therapeutic implications while ensuring that sufficient resources are available for aggressive management of anaphylaxis.[45]

Occurrence of immediate-type hypersensitivity reactions during anesthesia is usually underestimated, probably because of lack of confirmation of diagnosis and timely reporting. Because this complication during pregnancy has the potential to cause devastating damage to the baby, the knowledge, vigilance, and aggressive management immediately after the suspicion are imperative.

CASE STUDY

A 27-year-old G1, P0 patient at 40 weeks' gestation is admitted to the labor and delivery unit with a history of premature rupture of membranes. Past medical and surgical histories are unremarkable. She denies any history of allergy to any medication or any food. Her prenatal history has been uneventful. Because she did not receive any regular prenatal care, intravenous penicillin was started as chemoprophylaxis for chorioamnionitis against group B streptococcal infection. Within a few minutes after initiation of penicillin treatment, the patient develops generalized erythema and becomes tachycardic, with heart rate increasing to 160 to 170 beats/min. Her blood pressure drops to around 60 to 50/30 to 20 mm Hg, and she is breathing spontaneously without any obvious distress. You suspect that her symptoms are probably due to the effects of an immediate hypersensitivity reaction to penicillin.

Questions

1. Which of the following immunologic agents is primarily responsible in the pathogenesis of the immediate-type hypersensitivity reaction?
   A. Immunoglobulin M
   B. Helper T-1 (T_H1) cell
   C. Immunoglobulin E
   D. Immunoglobulin G

2. Which of the following agents are most frequently involved in maternal anaphylaxis?
   A. Muscle relaxants
   B. β-lactam antibiotics
   C. Latex
   D. Colloid solutions

3. How would you grade the severity of anaphylaxis in the patient described in this clinical scenario?
   A. Grade 1
   B. Grade 2
   C. Grade 3
   D. Grade 4

4. Which of the following will be the most important step in the initial management of this patient?
   A. Ephedrine 10 mg IV
   B. Diphenhydramine 25 mg IV
   C. Epinephrine 100 μg IV
   D. Epinephrine 1 mg IV

Answers

1. The answer is C. The primary mediator of the immediate-type hypersensitivity reaction (or anaphylaxis) is immunoglobulin E, or IgE. Following exposure to a specific allergen, the T_H2 cells become activated and stimulate the B cells to produce IgE. IgE cells, via FcεRI receptors, initiate the release of vasoactive mediators from the mast cells and basophils. Immunoglobulin M is thought to be involved in anaphylactoid reactions. Immunoglobulin G does not play any significant role in immediate type of hypersensitivity reactions.

2. The answer is B. Muscle relaxants, especially rocuronium, have been reported to be the most common offending agents in causing perioperative anaphylaxis. However, in pregnant patients, β-lactam antibiotics, penicillin, and ampicillin are the most common allergens. Latex and colloid solutions are also important agents for the immediate-type hypersensitivity reactions during anesthesia.

3. The answer is C. Anaphylactic reactions are classified into four grades. Involvement of two or more organ systems (cutaneous and cardiovascular) and severe life-threatening hypotension (50/20 mm Hg) in this patient should be classified as grade 3. Patients with grade 1 severity exhibit only cutaneous symptoms (erythema, urticaria); patients with grade 2 severity have more than one symptom with moderate degree of hypotension, tachycardia, and so on; and patients with grade 4 severity have cardiac and/or respiratory arrest as the primary manifestation.

4. The answer is C. Immediate management during acute anaphylaxis or immediate IgE-mediated hypersensitivity reaction includes assessment of ABC, cessation of the possible offending agent(s), administration of epinephrine and infusion of fluid bolus (1-2 L of crystalloid). Timely use of epinephrine in correct doses is important in managing patients with acute anaphylaxis. Epinephrine is not recommended for grade 1 anaphylaxis. In grade 2 severity with moderate degree of symptoms, the initial doses of epinephrine should be 10 to 20 μg and titrated according to response. In patients with grade 3 severity (severe hypotension, bradycardia, dysrhythmia, difficulties in ventilation), the initial dose of epinephrine should be 100 to 200 μg at a time. For patients with cardiac arrest, cardiopulmonary resuscitation should be initiated with epinephrine (1-3 mg) and fluid boluses.

REFERENCES

1. Cohen SG, Zelaya-Quesada M. Portier, Richet and the discovery of anaphylaxis: a centennial. *J Allergy Clin Immunol.* 2002;110(2):331-336.

2. Moneret-Vautrin DA, Morisset M, Flabbee J, Beaudouin E, Kanny G. Epidemiology of life-threatening and lethal anaphylaxis: a review. *Allergy.* 2005;60:443-451.

3. Lieberman P, Kemp SF, Oppenheimer J, Lang DM, Bernstein IL, Nicklas RA. The diagnosis and management of anaphylaxis: an updated practice parameter 2005. *J Allergy Clin Immunol.* 2005;115:S483-S523.

4. Mulla ZD, Ebraheim MS, Gonzalez JL. Anaphylaxis in the obstetric patients: analysis of a statewide hospital discharge database. *Ann Allergy Asthma Immunol.* 2010;104:55-59.

5. Abbas AK, Lichtman AH, eds. *Cellular and Molecular Immunology.* 5th ed. Philadelphia, PA: Saunders; 2003:432-452.

6. Meggs WJ, Pescovitz OH, Metcalfe D, et al. Progesterone sensitivity as a cause of recurrent anaphylaxis. *N Engl J Med.* 1984;311:1236-1238.

7. Wegmann TG, Lin H, Guilbert L, Mosmann TR. Bidirectional cytokine interactions in the maternal–fetal relationship: is successful pregnancy a TH2 phenomenon? *Immunol Today.* 1993;14:353-356.

8. Chaouat G., Meliani AA, Martal J, et al. IL-10 prevents naturally occurring fetal loss in the CBA X DBA/2 mating combination, and local defect in IL-10 production in this abortion-prone combination is corrected by in vivo injection of IFN-τ[1]. *J Immunol.* 1995;154:4261-4268.

9. Mertes PM, Tajima K, Regnier–Kimmoun MA, et al. Perioperative anaphylaxis. *Med Clin North Am.* 2010;94(4):761-794.

10. Krigaard M, Garvey LH, Gillberg L, et al. Scandinavian clinical practice guidelines on the diagnosis, management and follow-up of anaphylaxis during anesthesia. *Acta Anesth Scand.* 2007;51:655-670.

11. Sitarz L. Anaphylactic shock following injection of suxamethonium. *Anaesth Resus Intens Therap.* 1974;2:83-86.

12. Edmondson WC, Skilton RW. Anaphylaxis in pregnancy—the right treatment? *Anaesthesia.* 1994; 454-455.

13. Baraka A, Sfeir S. Anaphylactic cardiac arrest in a parturient: response of the newborn. *JAMA.* 1980;243:1745-1746.

14. Erasmus C, Blackwood W, Wilson J. Infantile multicystic encephalomalacia after maternal bee sting anaphylaxis during pregnancy. *Arch Dis Child.* 1982;57:785-787.

15. Deusch E, Reider N, Marth C. Anaphylactic reaction to latex during cesarean delivery. *Obstet Gynecol.* 1996;88:727.

16. Eckhout GV, Ayad S. Anaphylaxis due to airborne exposure to latex in a primigravida. *Anesthesiology.* 2001;95:1034-1035.

17. Draisci G, Nucera E, Pollastrini E, et al. Anaphylactic reactions during cesarean section. *Int J Obstet Anesth.* 2007;16: 63-7.

18. Turillazzi E, Greco P, Neri M, et al. Anaphylactic latex reaction during anesthesia: the silent culprit in a fetal case. *Foren Sci Int.* 2008;179:e5-e8.

19. Porter BJ, Acharya U, Ormerod AD, Herriott R. Latex/chlorhexidine–induced anaphylaxis in pregnancy. *Allergy.* 1998; 53:455-457.

20. Fanous LH, Gray A, Flemingham J. Severe anaphylactoid reaction to Dextran 70. *Br Med J.* 1977;2: 1189-1190.

21. Karri K, Raghavan R, Shahid J. Severe anaphylaxis to Volplex, a colloid solution during cesarean section: a case report and review. *Obstet Gynecol Int.* 2009;ID 374791.

22. Powell JA, Maycock EJ. Anaphylactoid reaction to ranitidine in an obstetric patient. *Anaesth Intensive Care.* 1993;21:702-703.

23. Kaneko K, Maruta H. Severe anaphylactoid reaction to ranitidine in a parturient with subsequent fetal distress. *J Anesth.* 2003;17:199-200.

24. Luciano R, Zuppa AA, Maragliano G, Gallini F, Tortorolo G. Fetal encephalopathy after maternal anaphylaxis. *Biol Neonate.* 1997;71:190-193.

25. Entman SS, Moise KJ. Anaphylaxis in pregnancy. *South Med J.* 1984;77:402.

26. Cole DS, Bruck LR. Anaphylaxis after laminaria insertion. *Am J Obstet Gynecol.* 2000;95:1025.

27. Chanda M, Mackenzie P, Day JH. Hypersensitivity reactions following laminaria placement. *Contraception.* 2000;62:105-106.

28. Pant D, Vohra VK, Pandey SS, Sood J. Pulseless electrical activity during caesarean delivery under spinal anaesthesia: a case report of severe anaphylactic reaction to Syntocinon. *Int J Obstet Anesth.* 2009;18:85-88.

29. Gallagher JS. Anaphylaxis in pregnancy. *Obstet Gynecol.* 1988;71:491-493.

30. Heim K, Alge A, Marth C. Anaphylactic reaction to ampicillin and severe complication in the fetus. *Lancet.* 1991;337:859-860.

31. Gei AF, Pacheco LD, Vanhook JW, Hankins GDV. The use of continuous infusion of epinephrine for anaphylactic shock during labor. *Obstet Gynecol.* 2003;102:1332-1335.

32. Berardi A, Rossi K, Cavalleri F, et al. Maternal anaphylaxis and fetal brain damage after intrapartum chemoprophylaxis. *J Perinat Med.* 2004;32:375-377.

33. Dunn AB, Blomquist J, Khouzami V. Anaphylaxis in labor secondary to prophylaxis against group B streptococcus: a case report. *J Reprod Med.* 1999;44:381-384.

34. Sheikh J. Intrapartum anaphylaxis to penicillin in a woman with rheumatoid arthritis who had no prior penicillin allergy. *Ann Allergy Asthma Immunol.* 2007;99:287-289.

35. Chaudhuri K, Gonzales J, Jesurun CA, et al. Anaphylactic shock in pregnancy: a case study and review of the literature. *Int J Obstet Anesth.* 2008;17:350-357.

36. Konno R, Nagase S. Anaphylactic reaction to cefazolin in pregnancy. *J Obstet Gynecol.* 1995;21:577-579.

37. Jao MS, Cheng PJ, Shaw SW, Soong YK. Anaphylaxis to cefazolin during labor secondary to prophylaxis for group B Streptococcus: a case report. *J Reprod Med.* 2006;51:655-658.

38. Sengupta A, Kohli JK. Antibiotic prophylaxis in cesarean section causing anaphylaxis and intrauterine fetal death. *J Obstet Gynaecol Res.* 2008;34(2):252-254.

39. Laxenaire MC, Mertes PM, et al. Anaphylaxis during anesthesia. Results of a two-year survey in France. *Br J Anaesth.* 2001;87:549-558.

40. Ring J, Messmer K. Incidence and severity of anaphylactoid reactions to colloid volume substitutes. *Lancet.* 1977;1:466-469.

41. Harper NJN, Dixon T, Dugue P, et al. Guidelines: suspected anaphylactic reactions associated with anaesthesia. *Anaesthesia.* 2009;64:199-211.

42. American Heart Association. Guidelines for cardiopulmonary resuscitation and emergency cardiovascular care. Part 10.6: Anaphylaxis. *Circulation.* 2005;112:IV(143–145).

43. Hepner DL, Castells M, Mouton-Faivre C, et al. Anaphylaxis in the clinical setting of obstetric anesthesia: a literature review. *Anesth Analg.* 2013;117:1357-1367.

44. Hepner D, Castells MC, Tsen L. Should local anesthetic allergy testing be routinely performed during pregnancy? (Letter to the Editor.) *Anesth Analg.* 2003;97:1852-1858.

45. Bernstein I, Storms WW. Practice parameters for allergy diagnostic testing. Joint task force on practice parameters for the diagnosis and treatment of asthma. The American Academy of Allergy Asthma and Immunology and the American College of Allergy, Asthma and Immunology. *Ann Allergy Asthma Immunol.* 1995;75(6 pt 2):543-625.

Section **4**

Obstetric Complications

Fever and Infection

18

James Brown and Joanne Douglas

INTRODUCTION

Control of Thermoregulation

Thermal homeostasis is controlled by the hypothalamus within a range of 36.5°C to 38°C. Fever is defined as a temperature greater than 38°C and is caused by resetting the thermoregulatory threshold of the hypothalamus (eg, by pyrogens released in response to infection), deregulation of heat production (eg, malignant hyperthermia), or dissipation. See Figure 18-1 for a schematic view of thermoregulation.

Causes of Fever in Pregnancy

There is a broad differential diagnosis for fever in the parturient, including infective and noninfective causes, which may or may not be directly related to the pregnancy (Table 18-1). Infective disease patterns, incidences, and outcomes vary significantly between more-developed and less-developed regions of the world.

Predisposition to Infection

Parturients are predisposed to infection for several reasons. These may be physiologic. Parturients may develop relative immunosuppression in order to tolerate fetal alloantigens and prevent fetal compromise and demise.[1,2] A pH change in vaginal epithelium may alter the environment for microorganism growth.[1] Alternatively, the reasons may be anatomic. Urinary tract dilation and urinary stasis, from a gravid uterus and progesterone, are risk factors for urinary tract infection (UTI).[1,2] Increased intra-abdominal pressure and upward diaphragm displacement by a gravid uterus increases basal atelectasis, potentially predisposing to pneumonia.[1]

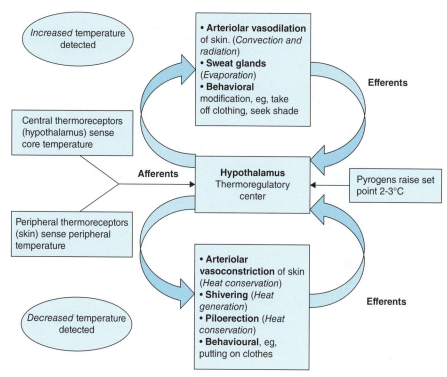

Figure 18-1. Schematic representation of thermoregulation.

Peripartum, there are additional risk factors:

- Premature rupture of membranes (PROM)
- Labor dystocia: prolonged labor and repeated vaginal examinations
- Use of immunosuppressive drugs (eg, steroids for preterm labor)
- Interventions, such as urinary catheterization

Consequences of Fever in Pregnancy

Maternal consequences include increased oxygen demand, increased use of antibiotics, increased assisted delivery rate, and increased cesarean delivery rate. Fetal consequences include increased oxygen demand, increased screening for sepsis,[3] increased use of prophylactic antibiotics,[3] admission to neonatal intensive care with separation from mother,[3] and possible increased incidence of hypoxic encephalopathy.[3,4]

Fetal temperature is dependent on maternal temperature and is commonly 0.5°C higher than maternal.[2] If maternal fever is infective in origin, there is the associated risk of vertical transmission of infection from mother to fetus.

Table 18-1. Causes of Fever in Pregnancy

		Pregnancy-Related Causes	**Non–pregnancy-Related Causes**
Infective	Bacterial	• Chorioamnionitis • Septic abortion • Infected cerclage suture • Postpartum endometritis • Wound infection (cesarean or episiotomy) • Retained products of conception	• Urinary tract infection (UTI) • Pyelonephritis • Community-acquired pneumonia • Cholestasis • Unrelated surgical infection (eg, appendicitis)
	Viral		• HIV • Herpes simplex virus • Rubella • Varicella zoster
	Other		• Malaria
Noninfective	Iatrogenic	• Ambient temperature of the labor room • Labor epidural	• Malignant hyperthermia • Drug administration (eg, prostaglandins, cocaine)
	Noniatrogenic	• Dehydration	• Inflammatory arthritis/connective tissue disease • Neoplasia (notably, lymphoma)

INFECTIVE CAUSES OF FEVER

In more developed regions of the world, the incidence of sepsis in the obstetric population is 0.3% to 0.6%.[1] The consequences of sepsis should not be underestimated. Failure to recognize the severity of sepsis is a major contributor to poor obstetric management and subsequent mortality. Sepsis has been implicated as the leading cause of direct maternal deaths in the United Kingdom, as demonstrated in Saving Mothers' Lives (CMACE 2006-2008).[5]

Obstetric sepsis is a concern not only at term. It can present in early pregnancy following fetal loss, or termination, or in the postpartum period (eg, from infected retained products of conception).

Exact sepsis terminology has been defined to facilitate research and communication between clinicians (Table 18-2). The physiologic changes associated with normal pregnancy (tachypnea and neutrophilia—up to 17,000 cells/mm^3 in the third trimester), and the sympathetic response to labor (tachycardia, tachypnea, and increases in temperature secondary to uterine muscle activity) often fulfill the criteria for systemic inflammatory response syndrome (SIRS) (Table 18-2). These factors contribute to the difficulty in assessing severity of illness. Therefore, an obstetric-specific physiologic warning score is recommended to detect early disease and monitor parturients.[6] Importantly, sepsis also can present with hypothermia, particularly in those women who have significant immunosuppression.

There is a paucity of specific evidence to support management of septic obstetric patients by algorithm, because they are often excluded from randomized

Table 18-2. Sepsis-Associated Definitions[a]

Term	Definition
Bacteremia	Presence of viable bacteria in blood
Infection	Inflammatory response to the presence of a microorganism
Systemic inflammatory response syndrome (SIRS)	Response to a variety of insults, characterized by two or more of the following:
	1. Temperature $< 36°C$ or $> 38°C$
	2. Heart rate > 90 beats/min
	3. Respiratory rate > 20 breaths/min
	4. White blood cell count of < 4000 cells/mm^3 or $> 12,000$ cells/mm^3
Sepsis	SIRS response to documented infection
Severe sepsis	Persistent hypotension from sepsis despite adequate fluid resuscitation
Septic shock	Sepsis-induced hypotension with a systolic blood pressure < 90 mm Hg

[a]Adapted from Bone RC, Balk RA, Cerra FB, et al. American College of Chest Physicians/Society of Critical Care Medicine Consensus Conference: Definitions for sepsis and organ failure and guidelines for the use of innovative therapies in sepsis. *Crit Care Med.* 1992;20:864-874.

controlled trials. Treatment is extrapolated, therefore, from the general population. Early goal-directed therapy aimed at restoring tissue perfusion, broad-spectrum antibiotics commenced within 1 hour of recognition of sepsis (to cover anaerobic as well as gram-positive and gram-negative bacteria), source control and supportive management, are the mainstays of treatment as recommended by the Surviving Sepsis Campaign guidelines.[7] Care is aimed at maximizing maternal physiology with consideration of fetal viability, depending on gestational age.[8] The guiding principle of caring for the sick parturient holds true here as well—optimizing the mother optimizes the fetus. The mother should be stabilized prior to surgery, which takes priority over an emergent cesarean delivery for neonatal indications.

Septic Shock

The definition of septic shock implies evidence of cardiovascular instability, impaired tissue oxygenation, and potential for coagulopathy. Septic shock in the parturient is associated with a relatively favorable prognosis when compared with the general population (less than 20% mortality compared with 30% to 60% in the general population).[1] There are multiple reasons to avoid neuraxial anesthesia in this setting as discussed below.

Specific Infections in Pregnancy

CHORIOAMNIONITIS

Chorioamnionitis is the infective inflammation of fetal membranes, commonly the result of bacteria ascending from the vagina. Diagnosis is clinical, and the condition is reported to occur in approximately 1% of all pregnancies.[9]

For diagnosis of chorioamnionitis,[3] a temperature over 38°C is necessary, with two of the following:

- Maternal tachycardia greater than 100 beats/min or fetal tachycardia greater than 160 beats/min for more than 5 minutes
- Uterine tenderness
- Offensive amniotic fluid
- Maternal leukocytosis greater than 16,000 cells/mm^3

Chorioamnionitis has an associated increased maternal and neonatal morbidity and mortality. Maternal risks include preterm labor, postpartum hemorrhage, postpartum endometritis, sepsis/severe sepsis/septic shock, pelvic thrombophlebitis, and death. Neonatal risks include pneumonia, meningitis, and increased rates of cerebral palsy.[2]

Treatment is with broad-spectrum antibiotics. There may be an increased cesarean delivery risk in these patients (46% in one study).[10]

GROUP B STREPTOCOCCAL INFECTION

Between 10% and 30% of parturients are colonized with group B *Streptococcus*; it is vertically transmitted at delivery to the fetus.[11] The organism can lead to infective complications in mothers (eg, UTI or chorioamnionitis), but of greater importance, it is the most common cause of neonatal infective morbidity and mortality.[11] The incidence of group B *Streptococcus* morbidity is decreasing due to screening (35-37 weeks) and antibiotic prophylaxis.

PARTURIENTS WITH SYSTEMIC INFECTION: IMPLICATIONS FOR ANESTHESIA

Neuraxial Anesthesia

Many anesthesiologists worry that neuraxial needle insertion in bacteremic parturients may cause bleeding and subsequent seeding of bacteria into the epidural or intrathecal space, potentially resulting in an epidural abscess or bacterial meningitis. Transient bacteremias are common in the peripartum period (around 9.9%)[1] but, fortunately, infective complications from neuraxial anesthesia are rare.[12,13]

Decisions concerning analgesic and anesthetic techniques in parturients with fever are based on risk-benefit assessment. Epidural analgesia offers advantages over other methods of labor analgesia, including:

- More effective analgesia
- Reduced stress response to labor in at-risk individuals (eg, a history of cardiac disease)
- An option for rapid conversion to anesthesia for cesarean delivery, thus avoiding the need for general anesthesia
- An option for improved postoperative analgesia

The final anesthetic plan should be made based on an informed discussion with the parturient and on a case-by-case basis. Factors to consider that may influence risk-benefit ratio of epidural analgesia include, the presence of risk factors for neuraxial infective complications (eg, diabetes, human immunodeficiency [HIV] or a history of illicit intravenous drug use), and the presence of factors increasing risks with general anesthesia (eg, morbid obesity, cardiovascular history).

Clinical evaluation of the parturient searching for a potential source of infection and assessing severity of disease is essential. Fever alone may be misleading, because pyrexia and leukocytosis are not predictive of bacteremia in the peripartum period.[10] Results of blood cultures will not be available immediately. In practice, most anesthesiologists are conservative about neuraxial procedures and would avoid insertion in parturients with high fever (temperature above 39°C) or those who have not responded to antibiotic therapy (persistent high fever or tachycardia). Presence of septic shock and cardiovascular compromise in the parturient should be considered an absolute contraindication to neuraxial anesthesia.[6]

Prevention remains the best treatment. The following are recommendations to reduce the risk of developing neuraxial infective complications:

- Strict asepsis for neuraxial procedures[14]
- Prophylactic antibiotics for at-risk individuals (eg, infective pyrexia, clinical evidence of bacteremia). This approach is supported by a study of lumbar puncture (LP) in bacteremic rats.[15]
- Methods that improve the success of neuraxial anesthesia (eg, use of epidural ultrasound) may reduce risk because technically difficult insertions, with multiple perforations of the epidural space, result in greater risk of hematoma, potentially increasing the infective complication rate.
- There is evidence suggesting that infective complication rates from combined spinal-epidural anesthesia (CSE) are greater and therefore should be avoided in at-risk individuals. In a large prospective audit that reviewed greater than 700,000 neuraxial procedures, CSEs represented 6% of the blocks performed but accounted for more than 13% of subsequent infective complications. The infective risks associated with spinal and epidural components of the technique appear to be cumulative for causing either bacterial meningitis or epidural abscess.[12]

EPIDURAL ABSCESS

Obstetric patients are typically younger and have fewer comorbidities relative to general surgical patients, and epidural catheters generally remain in-situ for less than 24 hours. For these reasons, epidural abscess rates are lower in the obstetric population.[12]

Theoretically, epidurals represent a greater infection risk than spinals. The larger needle increases the risk of bleeding and subsequent infective seeding in at risk women, while the catheter acts as a foreign body and nidus for infection.

Incidence The exact incidence of epidural abscess is difficult to quantify, with individual studies reporting incidences of between 0.2 and 3.7 in 100,000.[9] A meta-analysis of 13 studies involving 1.2 million parturients demonstrated an incidence of 0.9 in 100,000 obstetric epidurals.[13]

Presentation Of the traditional triad of symptoms, fever and backache usually precede neurologic dysfunction, but it is rare that all three will be present at the same time.[12,16] Most symptoms present within 2 weeks after epidural insertion but can be delayed up to 16 weeks.[12] Symptoms often are vague, especially in the early stages, so clinicians need to have a high index of suspicion. Later onset of symptoms can result in a delay in diagnosis, women may be under the care of a "generalist" by that time, and not a physician who would have a high index of suspicion, such as an anesthesiologist.

Diagnosis Magnetic resonance imaging is the neuroimaging technique of choice for diagnosis. Markers of infection (leukocytosis, C-reactive protein, erythrocyte sedimentation rate) add weight to the diagnosis but are nonspecific. Positive blood cultures provide a guide to antibiotic therapy.

Management Neurosurgery should be consulted urgently and treatment started promptly to preserve neurologic function. Options are: surgical decompression (usually posterior laminectomy), radiographic-guided drainage, or conservative management with systemic antibiotics.[16] All options require a prolonged course of antibiotics.

Outcome Outcome is related to duration of symptoms prior to treatment. Paralysis at presentation is a poor prognostic indicator.[16]

BACTERIAL MENINGITIS

Bacterial meningitis has been reported after epidural anesthesia, but there are more case reports following spinal anesthesia because of the intentional dural breach.

Incidence A national audit in the United Kingdom suggests that spinal meningitis occurs with an incidence of 0.5 in 100,000 (95% confidence interval of 0-3.5 in 100,000) in obstetric spinals.[12]

Presentation Headache is the most common presenting feature. Clinicians should have a high index of suspicion when reviewing patients with headache following neuraxial anesthesia and exclude meningitis as an alternate to more common diagnoses (ie, postdural puncture headache). Classic symptoms of meningeal irritation (neck stiffness, photophobia, and pyrexia) may be delayed.[12]

Diagnosis Diagnosis is based on clinical examination (ie, tachycardia, pyrexia, meningism [triad of nuchal rigidity, photophobia and headache] drowsiness), markers of infection, and bacterial cultures (blood cultures, LP).

Management If there are no signs of increased intracranial pressure (ie no new-onset seizures, papilledema, altered consciousness, or focal neurologic deficit), and history of central nervous system disease then a sepsis screen should be undertaken immediately (blood and cerebrospinal fluid culture [and cell count]). Steroids (dexamethasone) and broad-spectrum antibiotic therapy should be commenced immediately. If a computed tomography head scan is required prior to safely undergoing an LP, dexamethasone and antibiotic therapy should not be delayed.[17]

Outcome The majority of parturients with spinal-related bacterial meningitis make a full recovery. However, there are isolated cases of death in healthy parturients where recognition and treatment are delayed.[12,18]

Noninfectious Epidural Fever

Initially, there was uncertainty in the obstetric literature about whether labor epidurals cause noninfective fever, because many of the confounders that are common reasons prompting an epidural request are also risk factors for infection (eg, labor dystocia with frequent vaginal examinations). Subsequent randomized controlled trials have confirmed that epidurals are an independent risk factor causing fever in up to 33% of parturients.[4] Fever typically develops 5 hours postepidural insertion but may develop sooner.[4]

The exact cause of epidural-associated fever is unconfirmed, but several mechanisms have been proposed[4,19]:

- A direct effect on thermoregulation
- Increased heat production from epidural-associated shivering
- Reduced ability to dissipate heat resulting from the effects of the sympathetic blockade. Sweating is prevented in the lower half of the body. Vasodilation potentially leads to a fall in temperature as blood is redistributed from the core to the periphery. With time, normothermia is restored, but at this point skin vessels are still maximally dilated, and further heat dissipation by vasodilation is possible.
- The analgesic effect of the epidural reduces the respiratory rate, which is usually increased in response to labor pain. Heat loss through respiratory gas exchange, therefore, is reduced.
- A systemic inflammatory response to a catheter in situ in the epidural space.

Epidural-associated fever has the same potential consequences as pyrexia of other etiologies. It is an important diagnosis to make, to prevent unnecessary sepsis screening and antibiotic therapy in mother or neonate.[3]

Studies of treatments for epidural-associated fever have either been unsuccessful (acetaminophen) or have shown unacceptable side effects (steroid therapy). A proven effective intervention has not yet been determined.[4]

CASE STUDY

You are the resident covering the labor delivery ward. A nurse calls you about a 26-year-old healthy primiparous woman. She is 38 weeks' gestational age and was admitted to the antenatal ward for observation of PROM. Her labor is being induced with oxytocin, and she requests a labor epidural. The nurse mentions that maternal temperature is 38.8°C and heart rate is 120 beats/min.

Questions

1. What are your concerns with inserting a labor epidural in this patient?

2. Do you require any further information?

3. What incidence of risks would you describe in order to obtain informed consent for the procedure?

4. Are there any precautions you would take prior to inserting an epidural?

5. Does a labor CSE have the same risks as an epidural?

Answers

1. This woman has risk factors that raise concern for chorioamnionitis (eg, PROM), and may have a bacteremia. Concerns:
   - Increased risk of epidural abscess with a labor epidural
   - Sympathetic blockade from the epidural could potentially precipitate cardiovascular collapse in a septic patient with preexisting low systemic vascular resistance

2. Further information from history, physical examination, and investigation should address the following areas:
   - Specifically exclude additional maternal risk factors for immunosuppression and neuraxial infection, including:
     ◦ Diabetes
     ◦ HIV
     ◦ History of illicit intravenous drug use
   - Seek further evidence to support clinical diagnosis of chorioamnionitis:
     ◦ Uterine tenderness
     ◦ Offensive discharge/amniotic fluid
     ◦ Maternal leukocytosis greater than 16,000 cells/mm^3
   - Determine the obstetric plan.
   - Determine what treatment has been given, when, and the response (for example):
     ◦ Antibiotics
     ◦ Fluid resuscitation
   - Consider adjuncts to cardiovascular assessment:
     ◦ Clinical assessment, including central capillary refill
     ◦ Assessment of postural blood pressure drop
     ◦ Cardiovascular response to a fluid bolus
     ◦ Monitor hourly urine output
     ◦ Checking of blood lactate

   Additional considerations:
   - Potential for requiring emergent cesarean delivery, such as has the fetal heart rate been reassuring?
   - High-risk features associated with general anesthesia:
     ◦ Airway examination predictive of poor-grade laryngoscopy
     ◦ High body mass index
   - Maternal wishes, expectations, and attitude toward risks and available alternatives to labor analgesia

3. For all parturients, incidence of epidural abscess is approximately 1 per 100,000. Considering this case as high risk, a pessimistic estimate from the literature is 1 per 27,000.[9,13] A pessimistic estimate for bacterial meningitis would be 1 per 28,000.[12]

4. As a result you should:
   - Exclude cardiovascular instability.
   - Ensure broad-spectrum antibiotics have been administered prior to insertion of epidural and potentially wait for a response to treatment (eg, fall in temperature, reduction in heart rate).
   - Ensure informed consent from mother.
   - Insert epidural with strictest aseptic technique.
   - Review the patient regularly in the postpartum period.
   - Inform patient of potential postepidural symptoms that would cause concern, as epidural abscess may become symptomatic weeks after discharge from hospital. Instruct her to seek urgent medical opinion if she has:
     ○ Increasing lumbar tenderness or pain
     ○ Feeling unwell with fever
     ○ Numbness or weakness in her legs
     ○ Bladder or bowel disturbance
   - Consider reinforcing this guidance in writing.[12,16]

5. Evidence suggests increased infective complications with a CSE over those with an epidural, although the incidence is still low.[12]

REFERENCES

1. Fernandez-Perez ER, Salman S, Pendem S, Farmer C. Sepsis during pregnancy. *Crit Care Med*. 2005;33(10 suppl):S286-S293.
2. Kuczkowski KM, Reisner LS. Anesthetic management of the parturient with fever and infection. *J Clin Anesth*. 2003;15(6):478-488.
3. Apantaku O, Mulik V. Maternal intra-partum fever. *J Obstet Gynecol*. 2007;27(1):12-15.
4. Segal S. Labor epidural analgesia and maternal fever. *Anesth Analg*. 2010;111:1467-1475.
5. Centre for Maternal and Child Enquiries (CMACE). Saving Mothers' Lives. Reviewing maternal deaths to make motherhood safer: 2006-2008. *Br J Obstet Gynaecol*. 2011;118(suppl 1):1-203.
6. Cooper G, McClure J. Anaesthesia chapter from Saving mothers' lives; reviewing maternal deaths to make pregnancy safer. *Br J Anaesth*. 2008;100(1):17-22.
7. Dellinger R, Levy M, Carlet J, Bion J, Parker M, Jaeschke R. Surviving sepsis campaign: international guidelines for management of severe sepsis and septic shock. *Crit Care Med*. 2008;36(1):296-327.
8. Guinn D, Abel D, Tomlinson M. Early goal directed therapy for sepsis during pregnancy. *Obstet Gynecol Clin North Am*. 2007;34(3):459.
9. Loo CC, Dahlgren G, Irestedt L. Neurological complications in obstetric regional anaesthesia. *Int J Obstet Anesth*. 2000;9(2):99-124.
10. Goodman EJ, DeHorta E, Taguiam JM. Safety of spinal and epidural anesthesia in parturients with chorioamnionitis. *Reg Anesth*. 1996;21(5):436-441.
11. American College of Obstetricians and Gynecologists (ACOG). Prevention of early-onset group B streptococcal disease in newborns. ACOG Committee Opinion No. 485. *Obstet Gynecol*. 2011;117(4): 1019-1027.
12. Royal College of Anaesthetists. Major complications of central neuraxial block in the United Kingdom. *The Third National Audit Project of the Royal College of Anaesthetists*, 2009.
13. Ruppen W, Derry S, McQuay H, Moore A. Incidence of epidural hematoma, infection, and neurologic injury in obstetric patients with epidural analgesia/anesthesia. *Anesthesiology*. 2006;105(2):394-399.
14. Hebl J. The importance and implications of aseptic techniques during regional anesthesia. *Reg Anesth Pain Med*. 2006;31(4):311-323.
15. Carp H, Bailey S. The association between meningitis and dural puncture in bacteremic rats. *Anesthesiology*. 1992;76(5):739-742.

16. Grewal S, Hocking G, Wildsmith J. Epidural abscesses. *Br J Anaesth.* 2006;96(3):292-302.
17. Tunkel AR, Hartman BJ, Kaplan SL, et al. Practice guidelines for the management of bacterial meningitis. *Clin Infect Dis.* 2004;39(9):1267-1284.
18. Baer E. Post-dural puncture bacterial meningitis. *Anesthesiology* 2006;105(2):381-393.
19. Alexander JM. Epidural analgesia for labor pain and its relationship to fever. *Clin Perinatol.* 2005;32(3):777-787.

Embolic Disorders of Pregnancy and Amniotic Fluid Embolism

19

Laura Y. Chang

THROMBOEMBOLIC DISORDERS

Epidemiology

Pregnancy imparts a four fold to five fold increased risk of thromboembolism when compared to the nonpregnant state.[1] This risk rises to a 20-fold increase during the postpartum period and does not return to nonpregnant levels until approximately 6 weeks' postpartum.[1,2] The majority of thromboembolic events in pregnancy are venous in origin. The incidence of venous thromboembolism (VTE) in pregnant women is estimated to be 5 to 12 events per 10,000 pregnancies, evenly distributed between the time period from conception to delivery.[1] The mortality from pregnancy related VTE is 1.1 deaths per 100,000, an estimate of about 10% of all maternal deaths.[3]

Types of Venous Thromboembolism

Venous thromboembolism in pregnancy is commonly manifested as pulmonary embolism or as deep venous thrombosis (DVT). DVT accounts for 80% of thromboembolic cases, while pulmonary embolism is responsible for the remaining 20%.[4]

PULMONARY EMBOLISM

Pulmonary embolism (PE) is the leading cause of direct maternal deaths in developed countries, and it accounts for 20% of pregnancy-related deaths.[3] The incidence of PE is 0.01% to 0.05% of all pregnancies, and the risk is greater in the

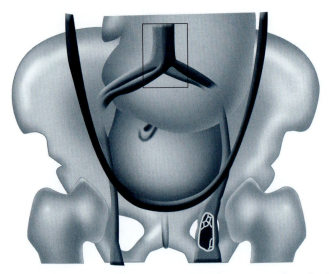

Figure 19-1. Mechanism for predilection for left leg deep venous thrombosis likely related to compression of the left iliac vein by the right iliac artery and the gravid uterus. (From Bourjeily G, Paidas M, Khalil H.[1], with permission.)

postpartum period, with 43% to 60% of pregnancy-related episodes occurring 4 to 6 weeks postpartum. PE after cesarean delivery is higher than after vaginal delivery by a factor of 2.5 to 20, and the incidence of fatal PE is higher by a factor of 10.[2]

DEEP VENOUS THROMBOSIS

The incidence of DVT is 0.02% to 0.36% of all pregnancies. A meta-analysis showed that two-thirds of cases of DVT occur antepartum and are equally distributed across trimesters.[5] Pregnancy-associated DVT is left sided in more than 85% of cases. The mechanism for this predilection for the left leg is probably related to compression of the left iliac vein by the right iliac artery and the gravid uterus (Figure 19-1).[1]

PELVIC VEIN THROMBOSIS

Isolated pelvic vein thrombosis (PVT) is more common in pregnancy. According to a multicenter prospective registry, 11% (6 of 53) of pregnant or postpartum women with DVT had isolated PVT compared with 1% (17 of 5451) of nonpregnant patients.[1] Ovarian vein thrombosis, a form of septic PVT, may complicate less than 0.05% of vaginal deliveries and up to 1% to 2% of cesarean deliveries. In 90% of cases, PVT occurs within 10 days' postpartum but can occur up to 10 weeks' postpartum. Symptoms include fever unresponsive to antibiotics (80%), pelvic pain (66%), and a palpable abdominal mass (46%).[6]

SUPERFICIAL VEIN THROMBOSIS

Superficial vein thrombosis (SVT) involving the lower extremity is occasionally noted during pregnancy. A retrospective study estimated the incidence of SVT during the peripartum period to be 47 out of 72,000 deliveries, with most occurring during the early postpartum period. Treatment for distal SVT includes compression and analgesia. Proximal SVT, however, is associated with an increased risk of deep vein extension and may necessitate anticoagulation.[7]

Etiology of Venous Thromboembolism

VIRCHOW'S TRIAD

The elements of Virchow's triad—venous stasis, vascular damage, and hypercoagulability—are all present during pregnancy and the postpartum period.

Venous Stasis Venous stasis begins in the first trimester and reaches a peak at 36 weeks' gestation. Compression of the pelvic veins by the enlarged uterus as well as progesterone-induced venodilation contributes to this stasis. By 25 to 29 weeks' gestation, venous flow velocity is reduced by approximately 50% in the legs and does not return to normal nonpregnancy flow velocity rates until around 6 weeks' postpartum.

Vascular Damage Local damage to pelvic veins may occur during vaginal and cesarean delivery. The separation of the placenta results in vascular trauma.

Hypercoagulable State Reduction in the anticoagulant activity of protein S and enhanced resistance to the anticoagulant activity of protein C are noted. Increased levels of procoagulant factors, including factors V, VII, IX, X, and fibrinogen lead to enhanced thrombin production. In addition, thrombus dissolution is reduced through decreased fibrinolysis as a result of decreased activity of tissue plasminogen activator.[1]

Thrombophilias are associated with a higher risk of venous thromboembolism during pregnancy. Approximately 50% of venous thromboembolic events in pregnancy are associated with inherited or acquired thrombophilia.[2] The prevalence and relative risk of thrombosis depend on the type of thrombophilia (Table 19-1).

ADDITIONAL RISKS OF VENOUS THROMBOEMBOLISM

In addition to the elements of Virchow's triad, identification of additional risk factors is useful for appropriate assessment on the need for thromboprophylaxis (Table 19-2).

Diagnosis of Venous Thromboembolism

CLINICAL

The most common signs of DVT are pain and tenderness of the leg, primarily in the left leg. Edema of thigh, erythema, palpable cord, and calf pain with passive dorsiflexion of thigh (Homans' sign) may be present. Because an accurate clinical diagnosis of PE in pregnancy is difficult (due to the overlap of signs and symptoms between physiologic changes of pregnancy and development of PE), it is an important diagnosis to rule out in patients with related symptoms. Symptoms of PE include dyspnea (62%), pleuritic chest pain (55%), cough (24%) with or without

Table 19-1. Relative Risk of Venous Thrombosis Depending on Type of Thrombophilia[a]

Thrombophilic Status	Relative Risk of Venous Thrombosis
Normal	1
Hyperhomocysteinemia, homozygous	2-4
Prothrombin gene mutation, heterozygous	3
Oral contraceptive (OCP) use	4
Antithrombin III deficiency, heterozygous	5
Protein S deficiency, heterozygous	6
Protein C deficiency, heterozygous	7
Factor V Leiden, heterozygous	5-7
Factor V Leiden, heterozygous plus OCP	30-35
Factor V Leiden, homozygous	80
Factor V Leiden, homozygous plus OCP	> 100
Prothrombin gene mutation, heterozygous plus OCP	16
Hyperhomocysteinemia, heterozygous plus factor V Lein, heterozygous	20

[a]Data from University of Illinois, Urbana/Champaign, Carle Cancer Center, Hematology Resources, Patient Resources, Factor V Leiden. http://www.med.illinois.edu/hematology/PtFacV2.htm.

hemoptysis, and diaphoresis (18%). Other clinical signs include tachycardia, tachypnea, hypoxemia, wheezing, decreased breath sounds, or fever. An accentuated second heart sound from right ventricular failure may be heard. With massive PE, defined as obstruction of more than 50% of the pulmonary circulation, hypotension, syncope, or cardiovascular collapse may be the presenting symptoms.[2]

Table 19-2. Risk Factors for Venous Thromboembolism in Pregnancy[a,b]

Risk Factors	Odds Ratio
Prior venous thromboembolism	24.8
Obesity (body mass index > 30)	2.65-5.3
Age > 35 years	1.3
Parity	1.5-4.03
Smoking	2.7
In vitro fertilization	4.3
Preeclampsia	2.9
Immobility	7.7-10.3
Multiple pregnancy	1.8-2.6
Cesarean delivery	3.6
Postpartum hemorrhage	9
Postpartum infection	4.1

[a]Adjusted odds ratios compared with women without the risk factor.
[b]Adapted from Gray G, Nelson-Piercy C.[44]

DIAGNOSTIC TOOLS

Evaluation of PE in pregnancy attempts to balance timely and accurate diagnostic approach while minimizing fetal exposure to ionizing radiation. Pregnancy must not interfere with using the most appropriate diagnostic imaging studies for suspected PE because of the significant risk of morbidity and mortality for both mother and the fetus (Figure 19-2).[2] The following studies may be useful:

- Compression ultrasound. This is the investigation of first choice in patients with suspected PE and positive signs of DVT, because it avoids the effect of radiation.

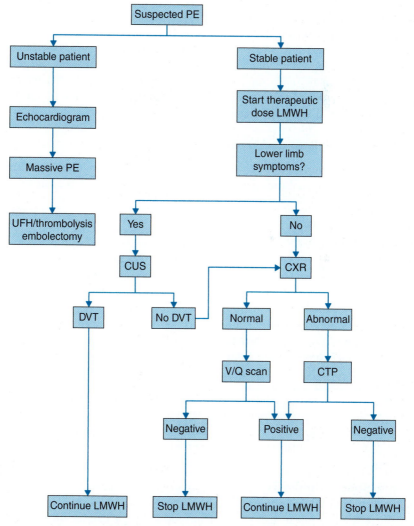

Figure 19-2. Proposed algorithm for diagnosis and treatment of pulmonary embolism in pregnancy. (From Gray G, Nelson-Piercy C,[44] with permission.)

- Chest x-ray. If signs of DVT are absent, this is used to rule out other diagnoses for symptoms (ie, pneumothorax, pleurisy) that may preclude further diagnostic imaging.[2]
- Ventilation-perfusion scan. In the setting of a normal chest x-ray, a ventilation-perfusion scan is recommended. Technetium-labeled albumin injected intravenously is trapped in the pulmonary capillary bed, depicting the distribution of pulmonary blood flow. This perfusion scan is coupled to a ventilation scan to enhance specificity. The Prospective Investigation of Pulmonary Embolism Diagnosis was a large, prospective, multicenter trial that examined the diagnostic use of the ventilation-perfusion scan. They found that the combination of clinical assessment and the ventilation-perfusion scan improved diagnostic accuracy.[8]
- Computed tomography with pulmonary angiography. This is used in the setting of a nondiagnostic ventilation-perfusion scan.
- D-dimer. D-dimer levels have a high negative predictive value when used to rule out PE in the nonpregnant population.[9] However, D-dimer levels increase gradually during pregnancy and drop in the immediate postpartum period to return to baseline by 6 weeks' postpartum. Therefore, D-dimer levels are not recommended for exclusion of PE in the pregnant population.[10]

Thromboprophylaxis and Treatment

The prevalence and severity of this condition during pregnancy and the peripartum period necessitates special consideration not only for management of acute thrombotic events but for prophylaxis of those at increased risk of thrombotic events.[4]

THROMBOPROPHYLAXIS

Recurrence rates of VTE in pregnant patients without thromboprophylaxis are higher than those in nonpregnant patients (10.9% versus 3.7%).[4] International societies such as the American College of Chest Physicians have recently published guidelines regarding use of antithrombotic agents in the management of VTE during pregnancy.[8] Anticoagulation prophylaxis during pregnancy is recommended in patients with a previous episode of VTE or with history of thrombophilia.[4] For most parturients, however, the benefits of anticoagulation do not outweigh the risk (2%) of bleeding complications from heparin or low-molecular-weight heparin.[5]

THERAPY

Anticoagulation is recommended for the treatment of established DVT or PE occurring during pregnancy and the postpartum period. Heparin, unfractionated or low molecular weight, is the anticoagulant of choice during pregnancy because it does not cross the placenta. Warfarin crosses the placenta and is considered teratogenic.

Deep Venous Thrombosis The current management approach for acute DVT during pregnancy is with unfractionated heparin (UFH) or low-molecular-weight heparin (LMWH). Advantages of UFH include a shorter half-life and ability to reverse with protamine sulfate. An advantage of LMWH is its more predictable dose-response, fewer bleeding episodes, lower risks of heparin-induced osteoporosis

and heparin-induced thrombocytopenia.[1] Dose adjustments are usually not necessary, and anti-Xa measurement does not need to be performed. Because UFH and
LMWH are metabolized by both the kidney and liver, additional precaution is
advised for those with renal or hepatic dysfunction. Current guidelines recommend
LMWH over UFH for anticoagulation during pregnancy and postpartum.[8]

Pulmonary Embolism Acute treatment includes prompt therapeutic anticoagulation with intravenous heparin, support of maternal circulation, and provision of adequate oxygenation. Because two-thirds of PE-related morbidity occurs
within 30 minutes of the acute event, if a patient has a strong clinical picture of
PE, anticoagulation should be initiated before diagnostic studies are performed.[2]
Treatment is usually initiated with a loading dose of 110 to 120 U/kg of heparin
intravenously, followed by a continuous infusion of 15 to 25 U/kg/h to maintain
the activated partial thromboplastin time (PTT) at two times the normal value.
If the patient requires delivery during the acute therapeutic treatment phase, full
anticoagulation is discontinued and reversed with protamine once in active labor
or in preparation for cesarean delivery.[2]

A vena cava filter is considered alongside anticoagulation if there is concern for
continuing embolism or solely, if anticoagulation is contraindicated. For pregnant
or postpartum patients, the filter should be placed in the suprarenal vena cava
rather than standard infrarenal position as the left ovarian vein empties into the
left renal vein.

Thrombolytic therapy is a relative contraindication in pregnancy. Its use should
be avoided close to time of delivery and shortly postpartum because of the risk
of hemorrhage. However, it may be appropriate and life saving for patients with
massive PE and hemodynamic instability. Urokinase, streptokinase, and tissue
plasminogen activator have been reported as successful thrombolytic agents in
pregnant patients.[11]

Surgical embolectomy is used when thrombolytic therapy is contraindicated
and PE is life threatening.

Anesthetic Management

Anticoagulated patients are at risk for bleeding complications associated with delivery. Management of anticoagulation near the time of delivery needs coordination
between the provider and the patient to minimize risk and to plan for the anticipated regional anesthesia during labor and delivery. Ideally, those on prophylactic
LMWH are switched to 5000 to 7500 units of UFH at least 1 to 2 weeks before
anticipated labor or admission for induction or cesarean delivery. The patient is usually instructed to avoid her next scheduled injection of heparin when regular uterine
contractions begin. On admission to labor, a clotting profile should be obtained.[3]

The American Society of Regional Anesthesia and Pain Medicine guidelines
recommend[12] that:

- Neuraxial anesthesia not be placed until 12 hours after the last dose of prophylactic and 24 hours after therapeutic LMWH dosing (enoxaparin 1 mg/kg every
  12 hours or enoxaparin 1.5 mg/kg daily).

- Patients receiving heparin for more than 4 days have a platelet count assessed before neuraxial block and catheter removal to rule out heparin-induced thrombocytopenia.
- Indwelling neuraxial catheters be removed 2 to 4 hours after the last heparin dose and the patient's coagulation status be assessed; heparin may be restarted 1 hour after catheter removal.
- The patient be monitored postoperatively to provide early detection of motor blockade, with considered use of minimal concentration of local anesthetics to enhance the early detection of a spinal hematoma.
- If on intravenous heparin, doses be stopped 6 hours before placement of a neuraxial block and a normal PTT be confirmed before proceeding with the block. If a cesarean section must be emergently carried out on patients without normalized PTT, the preferred method is general anesthesia.[2]

AMNIOTIC FLUID EMBOLISM

Amniotic fluid embolism (AFE) is a rare condition but responsible for a significantly high maternal mortality and morbidity.

Mechanism

EMBOLIC

AFE was initially thought to be the result of physical obstruction of the maternal pulmonary circulation by amniotic fluid. However, the absence of physical evidence of pulmonary vessel obstruction, a high degree of variability in clinical course, and failure to consistently reproduce the disease in animal models suggest that physical obstruction to the circulation is not the main mechanism of AFE.[13]

IMMUNOLOGIC

Hammerschmidt et al found that amniotic fluid could activate complement, which could contribute to the pulmonary collapse in this syndrome.[14] In 1993, Benson suggested that AFE might result from anaphylaxis to fetal material leaking into the maternal circulation, although a subsequent study did not support this hypothesis.[13] Another hypothesis is that amniotic fluid entering the circulation could result in activation of inflammatory mediators. These mediators—histamine, bradykinin, endothelin, and leukotrienes—can cause the physiologic derangements that characterize this syndrome. However, because of the low frequency of AFE, evidence has mainly been based on individual case reports, autopsy series, and uncontrolled case series.

Incidence

According to recent large population-based studies,[15-17] the incidence of AFE, which includes both fatal and nonfatal cases, ranges between 1.8 cases per 100,00 births in the United Kingdom[17] to 7.7 cases per 100,00 births in the United States.[2] The true incidence of AFE, however, is difficult to determine due

Table 19-3. Clinical Associations With Amniotic Fluid Embolism[a]

Maternal	Maternal age $\geq$ 35 years
	Preeclampsia/eclampsia
	Diabetes mellitus
Neonatal	Fetal macrosomia
	Fetal distress
Pregnancy related	Cesarean delivery
	Induction of labor
	Forceps delivery
	Vacuum delivery
	Placenta previa
	Placental abruption
	Chorioamnionitis
	Rupture of amniotic membrane
	Polyhydramnios
	Cervical laceration

[a]Data from Lewis G.[23]

to possible underreporting of nonfatal cases or to overdiagnosis, because the diagnosis is one of exclusion.[18]

The maternal mortality associated with AFE ranged from 0.5 to 1.7 deaths per 100,000 deliveries in developed countries, to 1.8 to 5.9 per 100,000 deliveries in developing countries. Currently, AFE accounts for 5% to 15% of all maternal deaths in developed countries and is the leading cause of maternal mortality in the United States.[19-21] Among cases of AFE, maternal fatality rate seems to have decreased from 86% in 1979 to 61% during 1988-1994,[22] with the most recent studies reporting 13% to 44%. This could be due to improved reporting, inconsistent case definitions, or improvements in treatment.[18]

Risk Factors

Population-based retrospective cohort studies[15,16] have examined the independent associations between AFE and potential risk factors after controlling for the effects of confounding variables (Table 19-3). Clinical associations found in both studies included maternal age of 35 years and older, cesarean delivery, forceps-assisted and vacuum-assisted vaginal deliveries, placenta previa, placental abruption, eclampsia, and fetal distress. Factors thought to be protective in both studies include maternal age less than 20 years and dystocia.

Signs and Symptoms

Most cases of AFE present during labor or immediately after vaginal or cesarean delivery.[18]

PREMONITORY SYMPTOMS

A report on maternal deaths in the United Kingdom stated that 11 out of 17 women who suffered AFE reported some or all of the following symptoms:

Table 19-4. Presenting Signs and Symptoms of Amniotic Fluid Embolism[a]

Hypotension
Pulmonary edema/acute respiratory distress syndrome
Cardiopulmonary arrest
Acute dyspnea
Cyanosis
Coagulopathy
Seizure
Acute agitation/anxiety
Fetal distress
Sudden tachycardia
Sudden desaturation on pulse oximeter
Loss of end-tidal carbon dioxide if intubated

[a]Used with permission from Dean LS, Rogers RP, Harley RA, et al.[24]

breathlessness, chest pain, feeling cold, lightheadedness, distress, panic, a feeling of pins and needles in the fingers, nausea, and vomiting. The time between onset of these symptoms and cardiovascular collapse ranged from almost immediately to more than 4 hours.[23]

PRESENTATION

The presenting signs and symptoms of AFE can vary from case to case. They can occur separately or in combination, and they can range in severity (Table 19-4).[24] The typical presentation of AFE includes sudden cardiovascular collapse with significant hypotension or cardiopulmonary arrest, pulmonary edema, acute dyspnea, cyanosis, seizure, and/or fetal distress.

COAGULOPATHY

The precise mechanism inducing disseminated intravascular coagulation (DIC) from AFE remains unclear. The current hypothesis is that the presence of tissue factor in amniotic fluid activates the extrinsic pathway by binding with factor VII, thereby triggering clotting via factors IX and X, with the subsequent development of a consumptive coagulopathy.[25] The development of abnormal coagulation can occur within a few hours of the initiating event. Whether this is due to a consumptive coagulopathy or to massive fibrinolysis is controversial. However, studies using thromboelastography analysis found no evidence of fibrinolysis, suggesting that the primary cause of bleeding in AFE is consumptive coagulopathy.[26]

Diagnosis

The first cases of AFE had large amounts of fetal material in the maternal pulmonary vasculature. This led to the presumption that finding any fetal material in the maternal circulation confirmed a diagnosis of AFE. There are many reports of amniotic fluid debris being aspirated from pulmonary arterial catheters of patients diagnosed with AFE.[27,28] On the contrary, fetal material has also been found in the maternal circulation in 21% to 100% of pregnant women without AFE.[29,30] The diagnosis of AFE continues to be one of exclusion.

LABORATORY

Although there are no tests that can reliably confirm the diagnosis of AFE in suspected cases, several tests have been suggested to increase the index of suspicion for this diagnosis. These include:

- Zinc coproporphyrin. A component of meconium was found to be increased in all four women with AFE but in only 1 of 50 control cases without the diagnosis of AFE.[31]
- Sialyl TN antigen (a fetal antigen present in meconium and amniotic fluid). Serum concentrations greater than 50 U/mL yielded sensitivities between 78% and 100% and specificities between 97% and 99%.[32]
- Tryptase (a marker of mast cell degranulation). This is controversial because this marker has been found in some studies[33] and have been found to be absent in others.[34]
- Complement factors. Decreased serum levels of C3 and C4 complement had sensitivities between 88% and 100% and a specificity of 100% for the diagnosis of AFE.[32]

RADIOGRAPHIC

The chief radiographic abnormalities in AFE are diffuse bilateral areas of increased opacity, which are indistinguishable from acute pulmonary edema from other causes.[29]

TRANSESOPHAGEAL ECHOCARDIOGRAPHY

During the early phase of AFE, transesophageal echocardiography (TEE) may demonstrate severe pulmonary vasoconstriction and acute right ventricular failure with right ventricular dilation. The late phase of AFE may show left ventricular failure secondary to myocardial ischemia.[35]

Anesthetic Management

Management is mainly supportive and directed toward the maintenance of oxygenation, circulatory support, and correction of any coagulopathy.

CARDIOPULMONARY RESUSCITATION

In the event of maternal cardiac arrest, cardiopulmonary resuscitation should be initiated immediately with left uterine displacement of the uterus. Cesarean section should be performed within 5 minutes of cardiovascular arrest regardless of gestational age if the gravid uterus is thought to interfere with maternal hemodynamics. Doing so increases the chance of neonatal neurologic recovery and overall maternal outcome. The best hope of fetal survival is maternal survival.[36]

MONITORING

Monitoring of patient with suspected AFE should include continuous cardiac telemetry monitoring (to detect and treat dysrhythmias), pulse oximetry, continuous blood pressure monitoring with arterial line, and possibly a pulmonary artery catheter. Central venous access will likely be necessary for fluid and blood product resuscitation. TEE may also be helpful to guide volume resuscitation and assess cardiac contractility.

LABORATORY

Initial laboratory data should include a complete blood count with platelets, type and cross-matching, arterial blood gases, and electrolytes. Coagulation studies, including prothrombin time, PTT, fibrin degradation products, D-dimer, and antithrombin III levels should also be obtained.

TRANSFUSIONS

Administration of blood components is considered the first line of treatment for correcting the coagulopathy associated with AFE. Packed red blood cells are often the first to be transfused because DIC is frequently associated with severe hemorrhage. Specific laboratory coagulation abnormalities are treated with transfusion of fresh frozen plasma, platelets, and/or cryoprecipitate. Cryoprecipitate contains fibronectin, which could facilitate removal of cellular and particulate matter, such as amniotic fluid debris from the blood via the monocyte/macrophage system.

Recombinant activated factor VIIa has been used to manage severe DIC resistant to conventional blood product replacement in women with AFE. However, recent review of case reports suggest worsened outcome.[37]

Less common therapeutic options include aprotinin[38] for DIC, uterine artery embolization for controlling severe postpartum hemorrhage,[39] cardiopulmonary bypass and pulmonary artery thromboembolectomy,[40] and continuous hemodiafiltration to eliminate amniotic fluid from the maternal blood stream.[41]

Hysterectomy may be required if uterine hemorrhage cannot be controlled.

Outcome/Complications

MATERNAL

Maternal death due to AFE is caused by sudden cardiac arrest, hemorrhage from coagulopathy, or development of acute respiratory distress syndrome and/or multisystem organ failure.[22] Although mortality rates for AFE have fallen, significant morbidity remains among those that survive. In 48 British survivors, four had neurologic injury, two had thrombotic events, one had renal failure, and another had septicemia.[42] In Clark et al's national registry,[22] among survivors, persisting neurologic impairment was reported in 61% of women. In the United Kingdom's registry,[20] of 31 women who survived, 6% had persisting neurologic impairment. The prognosis of a women experiencing AFE is improved with early diagnosis and prompt and aggressive treatment by a multidisciplinary team.[43]

FETAL

The morbidity and mortality for the fetus is also significant. If AFE occurs before delivery, the neonatal mortality rate is 10%.[44] In the British registry, among 15 women who died of AFE, 11 newborns also died. Among the 31 surviving women with known newborn outcomes, 9 newborns died or suffered serious injury.[21] In the national registry of Clark et al,[22] persistent neurological impairment was reported in 50% of the surviving infants. In the United Kingdom's registry,[20] among 33 infants who survived, 18% developed hypoxic ischemic encephalopathy and 6% developed cerebral palsy.

CONCLUSION

Most of the available literature on AFE is mainly based on case reports or case series. Although the understanding of AFE has improved over the last few decades, it continues to be associated with a high rate of maternal and perinatal morbidity and mortality. Early clinical suspicion of AFE and, therefore, early and aggressive treatment enhances both maternal and fetal survival.

CASE STUDY

A 38-year-old primigravida at 41 weeks' gestation underwent cesarean section because of a nonreassuring fetal heart tracing following an induction of labor for post dates. She had a history of gestational diabetes mellitus controlled with diet but was otherwise healthy. The patient had an epidural in situ for labor analgesia. She was given 18 mL of 2% lidocaine with epinephrine and 100 µg of fentanyl for surgical anesthesia, producing a bilateral T4 level. The cesarean section was performed uneventfully and a boy was delivered with an initial Apgar of 8.

Shortly after delivery of the placenta, the mother begins complaining of lightheadedness. This is followed almost immediately by loss of consciousness and convulsions. The SpO_2 falls to 78% and the next blood pressure measures 60/38 mm Hg.

Questions

1. What is the differential diagnosis?
2. What is your initial step?
3. What additional monitors will you utilize?
4. The obstetrician states that the bleeding from the uterus is uncontrollable and you notice that her IV sites are oozing. What can explain this clinical scenario and what should be done next?

Answers

1. The differential diagnosis for cardiovascular collapse and/or seizure in the setting of a cesarean section includes amniotic fluid emboli, air emboli, thrombotic pulmonary emboli, local anesthetic toxicity, high spinal anesthesia, eclampsia, septic shock, acute myocardial infarction, cardiomyopathy, anaphylaxis, aspiration pneumonitis, and cerebral hemorrhage. AFE is a diagnosis of exclusion but

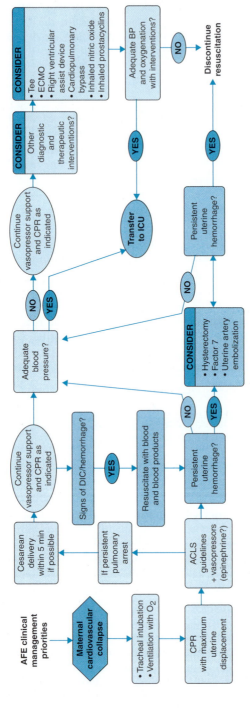

Figure 19-3. Flow chart depicting clinical management of amniotic fluid embolism. (From Dean LS, Rogers RP, Harley RA, et al[24] with permission.)

should be considered early in this scenario as early diagnosis and prompt and aggressive management enhances both maternal and fetal prognosis.[42]

2. Initial steps should include maintenance of oxygenation, ventilation, and circulatory support. A flow chart depicting clinical management of possible AFE is shown (Figure 19-3).[24]

3. The patient needs intravenous access, inclusive of large-bore peripheral lines as well as a central line for infusion of vasopressors and for monitoring central venous pressures. An arterial line will be necessary for continuous monitoring of blood pressures as well as access to frequent blood draws. If available, an early TEE may aid in diagnosis by showing pulmonary hypertension, with right ventricular dilation causing a leftward shift of the interventricular septum, obliterating the left ventricular space.[35] TEE may also be useful to guide resuscitation efforts.

4. Blood products should be replaced based on the clinical assumption of DIC, and laboratory values should be obtained. Because DIC is frequently associated with severe hemorrhage, transfusion of packed red blood cells is a priority. Specific laboratory coagulation abnormalities are treated with transfusion of fresh frozen plasma, cryoprecipitate, and platelets. Cell salvage and recombinant factor concentrations such as factor VII may be used for severe DIC resistant to conventional blood product replacement.[37] Hysterectomy may be required if uterine hemorrhage cannot be controlled.

REFERENCES

1. Bourjeily G, Paidas M, Khalil H. Pulmonary embolism in pregnancy. *Lancet*. 2010;375:500-512.
2. Brown HL, Hiett AK. Deep vein thrombosis and pulmonary embolism in pregnancy: diagnosis, complications and management. *Clin Obstet Gynecol*. 2010;53:345-359.
3. James AH. Prevention and management of venous thromboembolism in pregnancy. *Am J Med*. 2007;120:S26-S34.
4. James A. Practice bulletin no. 123: thromboembolism in pregnancy. *Obstet Gynecol*. 2011;118(3):718-729.
5. Benedetto C, Marozio L, Tavella AM, et al. Coagulation disorders in pregnancy: acquired and inherited thrombophilias. *Ann N Y Acad Sci*. 2010;1205:106-117.
6. Klima DA, Snyder TE. Postpartum ovarian vein thrombosis. *Obstet Gynecol*. 2008;111:431-435.
7. Kupelian AS, Huda MS. Pregnancy, thrombophlebitis and thromboembolism: what every obstetrician should know. *Arch Gynecol Obstet*. 2007;275:215-217.
8. Bates SM, Greer IA, Pabinger I, et al. Venous thromboembolism, thrombophilia antithrombotic therapy, and pregnancy: American College of Chest Physicians Evidence-Based Clinical Practice Guideline (8th ed.) *Chest*. 2008;133:844S-886S.
9. Mavromatis BH, Kessler CM. D-Dimer testing: the role of the clinical laboratory in the diagnosis of pulmonary embolism. *J Clin Pathol*. 2001;54:664-668.
10. Duran-Mendicuti A, Sodickson A. Imaging evaluation of the pregnant patient with suspected pulmonary embolism. *Int J Obstet Anesth*. 2011;20:51-59.
11. Harris T, Meek S. When should we thrombolyse patients with pulmonary embolism? A systematic review of the literature. *Emerg Med J*. 2005;22:766-771.
12. Horlocker TT, Wedel DJ, Rowlingson JC. Regional anesthesia in the patient receiving antithrombotic or thrombolytic therapy: American Society of Regional Anesthesia and Pain Medicine Evidence-Based Guidelines. *Regl Anesth Pain Med*. 2010;35:64-101.

13. Benson MD. A hypothesis regarding complement activation and amniotic fluid embolism. *Med Hypotheses*. 2007;68(5):1019-1025.

14. Hammerschmidt DE, Ogburn PL, Williams JE. Amniotic fluid activates complement—a role in amniotic fluid embolism syndrome? *J Lab Clin Med*. 1984;104:901-907.

15. Kramer MS, Rouleau J, Baskett TF, Joseph KS. Maternal health study group of the Canadian perinatal surveillance system: amniotic-fluid embolism and medical induction of labour: a retrospective, population-based cohort study. *Lancet*. 2006;368:1444-1448.

16. Abenhaim HA, Azoulay L, Kramer MS, et al. Incidence and risk factors of amniotic fluid embolisms: a population-based study on 3 million births in the united states. *Am J Obstet Gynecol*. 2008;199:49.

17. Knight M. Amniotic fluid embolism: active surveillance versus retrospective database review. *Am J Obstet Gynecol*. 2008;9:199.

18. Conde-Agudelo A, Romero R. Amniotic fluid embolism: an evidence-based review. *Am J Obstet Gynecol*. 2009:201(5).

19. Berg CJ, Callaghan WM, Syverson C, Henderson Z. Pregnancy-related mortality in the United States, 1998 to 2005. *Obstet Gynecol*. 2010;116(6):1302-1309.

20. Tuffnell DJ. United Kingdom amniotic fluid embolism register. *Br J Obstet Gynecol*. 2005;112(12): 1625-1629.

21. Oi H, Naruse K, Noguchi T, et al. Fatal factors of clinical manifestations and laboratory testing in patients with amniotic fluid embolism. *Gynecol Obstet Invest*. 2010;70(2):138-144.

22. Clark SL, Hankins GD, Dudley DA, et al. Amniotic fluid embolism: analysis of the national registry. *Am J Obstet Gynecol*. 1995;158:1167.

23. Lewis G. The confidential enquiry into maternal and child health (CEMACH). Saving mothers' lives: reviewing maternal deaths to make motherhood safer—2002-2005. CEMACH 2007.

24. Dean LS, Rogers RP, Harley RA, et al. Case scenario: amniotic fluid embolism. *Anesthesiology*. 2012;116:186-191.

25. Uszyński M, Zekanowska E, Uszyński W, et al. Tissue factor (TF) and tissue factor pathway inhibitor (TFPI) in amniotic fluid and blood plasma: implications for the mechanism of amniotic fluid embolism. *Eur J Obstet Gynecol Reprod Biol*. 2001;95:163-166.

26. Harnett MJ, Hepner DL, Datta S, et al. Effect of amniotic fluid on coagulation and platelet function in pregnancy: an evaluation using thromboelastography. *Anaesthesia*. 2005;60:1068-1072.

27. Duff P, Engelsgjerd B, Zingery LW, et al. Hemodynamic observations in a patient with intrapartum amniotic fluid embolism. *Am J Obstet Gynecol*. 1983;146:112-115.

28. Kuhlman K, Hidvegi D, Tamura RK, et al. Is amniotic fluid material in the central circulation of peripartum patients pathologic? *Am J Perinatol*. 1985;2(4):295-299.

29. Mulder JI. Amniotic fluid embolism: an overview and case report. *Am J Obstet Gynecol*. 1985;152(4): 430-435.

30. Lee W, Ginsburg KA, Cotton DB, et al. Squamous and trophoblastic cells in the maternal pulmonary circulation identified by invasive hemodynamic monitoring during the peripartum period. *Am J Obstet Gynecol*. 1986;155:999-1001.

31. Kanayama N, Yamazaki T, Naruse H, et al. Determining zinc coproporphyrin in maternal plasma—a new method for diagnosing amniotic fluid embolism. *Clin Chem*. 1992;38:526-529.

32. Benson MD, Kobayashi H, Silver RK, et al. Immunologic studies in presumed amniotic fluid embolism. *Obstet Gynecol*. 2001;97:510-514.

33. Nishio H, Matsui K, Miyazaki T, et al. A fatal case of amniotic fluid embolism with elevation of serum mast cell tryptase. *Foren Sci Int*. 2002;126:53-56.

34. Marcus BJ, Collins KA, Harley RA. Ancillary studies in amniotic fluid embolism: a case report and review of the literature. *Am J Foren Med Pathol*. 2005;26:92-95.

35. James CF, Feinglass NG, Menke DM, et al. Massive amniotic fluid embolism: diagnosis aided by emergency transesophageal echocardiography. *Int J Obstet Anesth*. 2004;13:279-283.

36. Vanden Hoek TL, Morrison LJ, Shuster M, et al. 2010 American Heart Association Guidelines for Cardiopulmonary Resuscitation and Emergency Cardiovascular Care Science. *Circulation*. 2010;122:5829-5861.

37. Prosper SC, Goudge CS, Lupo VR. Recombinant factor VIIa to successfully manage disseminated intravascular coagulation from amniotic fluid embolism. *Obstet Gynecol*. 2007;109:524-525.

38. Stroup J, Haraway D, Beal JM. Aprotinin in the management of coagulopathy associated with amniotic fluid embolus. *Pharmacotherapy.* 2006;26:689-693.

39. Goldszmidt E, Davies S. Two cases of hemorrhage secondary to amniotic fluid embolus managed with uterine artery embolization. *Can J Anaesth.* 2003;50:917-921.

40. Esposito RA, Grossi EA, Coppa G, et al. Successful treatment of postpartum shock caused by amniotic fluid embolism with cardiopulmonary bypass and pulmonary artery thromboembolectomy. *Am J Obst. Gynecol.* 1990;163:572-574.

41. Kaneko Y, Ogihara T, Tajima H, et al. Continuous hemodiafiltration for disseminated intravascular coagulation and shock due to amniotic fluid embolism: report of a dramatic response. *Intern Med.* 2001;40:945-947.

42. Knight M, Tuffnell D, Brocklehurst P, et al. Incidence and risk factors for amniotic-fluid embolism. *Obstet Gynecol.* 2010;115(5):910-917.

43. Tuffnell DJ. Amniotic fluid embolism. *Curr Opin Obstet Gynecol.* 2003;15;119-122.

44. Gray G, Nelson-Piercy C. Thromboembolic disorders in obstetrics. *Best Pract Res Clin Obstet Gynaecol.* 2012;26:53-64.

Management of Obstetric Hemorrhage

20

Ruth Landau, Christopher G. Ciliberto, and Pascal H. Vuilleumier

INTRODUCTION

Postpartum hemorrhage (PPH) remains a leading cause of maternal morbidity and mortality worldwide. Epidemiologic studies show an increasing frequency and severity of PPH in the past decade, due to an increase in uterine atony and placenta accreta, percreta, and increta. Management of PPH requires prompt and efficient multidisciplinary intervention to improve uterine tone; provide adequate fluid and hemodynamic resuscitation, administer blood products, and decide whether additional procedures such as interventional radiology or surgery are needed. Optimal management of PPH requires adequate communication between all team players (nurses, midwives, obstetricians, anesthesiologists, hematologists/ blood bank, surgeons, interventional radiologists, and intensive care unit staff). Teamwork is facilitated when protocols are in place to allow human allocation and tasks to be well defined along with adequate record keeping. Algorithms for the use of blood products, fibrinogen, recombinant activated factor VII (rFVIIa), tranexamic acid, blood cell salvage devices, and other conservative maneuvers (Bakri balloon, B-Lynch procedure, interventional radiology) should be in place to reduce the need for hysterectomy and massive transfusion. Adequate documentation, debriefing after clinical care, and audits should facilitate monitoring of the success of such protocols. Practice guidelines and recommendations established by national societies and organizations have flourished in the literature over the past 5 to 8 years to assist clinicians in the prevention and management of PPH, of which the practice bulletin of the American College of Obstetrics and Gynecology (ACOG) in 2006,[1] the International Confederation of Midwives, the International Federation of Gynecology and Obstetrics (FIGO) initiative in 2006,[2] the clinical practice guideline of the Society of Obstetricians and Gynaecologists of Canada (SOGC) in 2009,[3] the California Maternal Quality Care Collaborative (CMQCC) guide in 2010,[4] the Royal College of Obstetricians and Gynaecologists (RCOG) guidelines in 2011,[5] and the most updated World Health Organization (WHO) recommendations in 2012[6] are just a few examples.

The goal of this chapter is to present a practical and updated overview on current modalities and recommendations that are available, to improve the management of planned and unplanned obstetric hemorrhages, and to prevent fatal outcomes for both mothers and their infants.

DEFINITIONS AND TAXONOMY OF POSTPARTUM AND MAJOR OBSTETRIC HEMORRHAGES

The clinical estimation of blood loss during delivery is frequently inaccurate, in general underestimated, and the presence of amniotic fluid may be a confounding factor. It is important to bear in mind that healthy women will not become symptomatic before a significant amount of blood loss has occurred. In other words, by the time significant obstetric hemorrhage has been observed, women may already have lost 10% to 15% of their circulating blood volume. Nonetheless, whereas symptoms, hemodynamic parameters, a hematocrit value or the need for blood products would appear valuable to determine whether a hemorrhage is significant or not, the diagnosis is usually based solely on the estimated blood loss (Table 20-1).

- *PPH* is defined by ACOG as blood loss exceeding 500 mL after a vaginal delivery or 1000 mL after a cesarean delivery.[1] The WHO has defined PPH as a blood

Table 20-1. Definitions and Taxonomy of Postpartum Hemorrhage (PPH) and Major Obstetric Hemorrhage (MOH)

Hemorrhage	Blood Loss	Timing
PPH (ACOG[1])	> 500 mL after vaginal delivery	
	> 1000 mL after cesarean delivery	
Severe PPH (ACOG[1])	> 2000-2500 mL after delivery	
PPH (WHO[6])	> 500 mL after delivery	Within the first 24 hours after delivery
Severe PPH (WHO[6])	> 1000 mL after delivery	Within the first 24 hours after delivery
Antepartum	Bleeding from the vagina	As of 24 weeks' gestation
Primary PPH	Bleeding occurring at delivery	Within the first 24 hours after delivery
Secondary PPH	Any amount of excessive bleeding from the birth canal	24 hours after delivery and up to 6 weeks' postpartum
MOH	> 2000-2500 mL	Antenatal or postpartum

loss greater or equal to 500 mL within 24 hours after birth regardless of mode of delivery, and severe PPH is a blood loss greater or equal to 1000 mL in the first 24 hours postpartum.[6]

- *Severe PPH* is considered when blood loss is deemed to be greater than 2000 to 2500 mL.
- *Antepartum hemorrhage* is defined as bleeding, usually but not always manifested from the vagina after 24 weeks' gestation, and is associated with placenta previa, placental abruption, and uterine rupture or trauma.
- *Primary PPH* is defined as a bleeding that occurs before delivery (antepartum) and within the first 24 hours' postpartum.
- *Secondary PPH* is considered with any abnormal or excessive bleeding from the birth canal occurring between 24 hours' and up to 6 weeks' postpartum. The most common etiology of secondary PPH is retained placental tissue.
- *Major obstetric hemorrhage (MOH)* is the term typically used in the United Kingdom and Europe to describe major antenatal or postpartum hemorrhage. There is no consensus on what constitutes a major blood loss; blood loss exceeding 1500 mL, a hemoglobin decrease of more than 4 g/dL, or an acute transfusion requirement of more than 4 units of red blood cells are suggested criteria.

EPIDEMIOLOGY AND RISK FACTORS

The incidence of PPH has been steadily increasing in the last decade in the United States[7] and represents the second leading cause of maternal mortality after cardiovascular disorders. PPH complicates 2.9% of deliveries, is the second leading cause of intensive care unit admission among pregnant women and is associated with close to 20% of all in hospital maternal deaths after delivery in the United States. Atonic PPH is currently the leading cause of PPH irrespective of mode of delivery and accounts for up to 79% of all PPH.

The etiologies of PPH can be classified as follows (four *T*s):

1. **Tone:** abnormal uterine contractility or any condition that increases uterine distention, uterine muscle fatigue, uterine distortion or abnormality, chorioamnionitis, or pharmacologically induced uterine relaxation
2. **Tissue:** retained placental products or the morbidly adherent placenta that results in the abnormal placental detachment (eg, placenta accreta, percreta, increta) in the third stage of labor
3. **Trauma:** genital tract injury (laceration) or uterine injury (uterine rupture or inversion)
4. **Thrombin:** preexisting (eg, hemophilia, von Willebrand's disease [VWD]) or acquired abnormalities of coagulation (severe preeclampsia; hemolysis, elevated liver enzymes, low platelets [HELLP]; disseminated intravascular coagulation [DIC]) or anticoagulant therapies

A thorough antenatal screening may help identify risk factors for PPH and allow for some preparation if PPH is expected. In particular, identifying the risk for placenta accreta in the event of a repeat cesarean delivery with a placenta previa is critical. Other antenatal factors that substantially increase the risk for PPH include:

- Suspected or proven placental abruption
- Known placenta previa
- Multiple pregnancy
- Hypertensive disorders of pregnancy (preeclampsia)

Uterine Atony

Uterine atony is characterized by failure of the myometrium to contract after delivery, associated with excessive bleeding from the noncontracting placental implantation site. The rising rates of PPH in the last decades have been driven by the increasing incidence of atonic PPH, although specific explanations for these temporal trends are still under investigation.[8]

Unlike other causes of obstetric hemorrhage such as placental abnormalities that may be detected through antenatal screening, uterine atony may be difficult to predict, although risk factors for its occurrence after a vaginal delivery have been identified.

Demographic factors associated with uterine atony include:

- Advanced maternal age
- Obesity
- Ethnicity (Hispanic, Asian/Pacific Islander)

Obstetric factors associated with uterine atony include:

- Uterine overdistention (polyhydramnios, multiple gestation, macrosomia)
- Labor induction and prolonged exposure to oxytocin
- Prolonged labor and protracted second stage
- Chorioamnionitis
- Preeclampsia
- Previous PPH
- Pharmacologic agents relaxing the uterus (tocolytics, $MgSO_4$, halogenated anesthetics)

Active management of the third stage of labor is essential to facilitate placental separation and delivery, and promote contraction of the uterus to shorten the third stage of labor, prevent uterine atony and excessive bleeding. The duration of the third stage has been shown to correlate with the risk for PPH; a third stage of labor longer than 18 minutes is associated with a significant risk of PPH and the odds for PPH are 6 times higher if the third stage is longer than 30 minutes. The three key interventions of active management are presumed to be:

- Use of a prophylactic uterotonic agent (oxytocin at birth)[9]
- Early umbilical cord clamping, although evidence has emerged that it is not necessarily beneficial and no longer recommended[2]
- Controlled umbilical cord traction, although this has also been recently refuted

Pharmacologic management of uterine atony is essential, and oxytocin alone or in combination with other uterotonic agents is recommended based on the clinical situation and presence of contraindications to administrate second-line agents.

Retained Placental Products

Retained placental products (or products of conception) occurs in 0.1% to 3.3% of vaginal deliveries and is the second leading cause of PPH usually associated with uterine atony. Etiologies for a retained placenta include failure of the myometrium behind the placenta to contract resulting from an adherent placenta, a detached placenta trapped behind a closed cervix, or a placenta accreta. Given the entirely different etiologies and underlying pathologies, management should be based on the suspected diagnosis, which can be established with ultrasound imaging.

Sublingual or intravenous nitroglycerin along with controlled traction of the umbilical cord has been evaluated as an effective way to facilitate placental separation and removal, with mixed results. Studies evaluating the intraumbilical injection of oxytocin or other uterotonics also have yielded mixed results and do not seem to reduce the need for a manual removal of retained products.

Finally, anesthesia for manual removal of a retained placenta, requires a dense anesthetic block, via an indwelling epidural catheter or a de novo single shot spinal, with a T6 level to ensure maternal comfort and possibly the need for a uterine relaxant if the lower uterine segment is obstructing.[10]

Placental Abruption

Placental abruption is characterized by the premature separation of the placenta, which can be complete or partial, and is a serious obstetric complication that occurs in more than 1% of pregnancies. Placental abruption results in more than 50% preterm delivery. Overall perinatal mortality with placental abruption is high (119 in 1000 births), with 7% attributed to the abruption itself and a majority of deaths occurring in utero (77%). The etiology of placental abruption remains unclear but is thought to be the consequence of abnormal trophoblast invasion leading to the rupture of the spiral arteries causing premature separation of the placenta. Ultrasound imaging may show retroplacental clot(s) or bleeding but does not seem to predict the extent of placental abruption, and the diagnosis of abruption should be based on clinical criteria, which include vaginal bleeding with a nonreassuring fetal heart rate with or without tachysystole (uterine hypertonus), abdominal tenderness and pain.

More than 50 different risk factors or markers for placental abruption have been reported, with smoking (maternal and paternal), preeclampsia, and the history of a previous placental abruption being the strongest. Others include maternal age, chronic hypertension, cocaine use, hyperhomocysteinemia, inherited or acquired thrombophilia, abdominal trauma, premature rupture or membranes, and chorioamnionitis.

Placental abruption, particularly in the context of preeclampsia, can result in DIC, hemolysis, acute renal failure, and pulmonary edema, and serious maternal complications are not infrequent. Anesthetic management for an emergent cesarean delivery will depend on the urgency of the situation (fetal and maternal) and the maternal hemodynamic and coagulation status.

Placenta Previa

Placental previa occurs when there is an abnormally low attachment of the placenta, partially or totally covering the cervical os. Further distinctions can be made with regards to the distance of the placenta to the cervical os, as follows:

- Total previa: completely covering the cervical os
- Partial placenta previa: partially covering the cervical os
- Marginal placenta previa: close but not covering the cervical os
- Low-lying placenta: placental edge in close proximity to the cervical os (of note, 90% of placentas identified as low-lying in early pregnancy will resolve by the third trimester)

The incidence of placenta previa is 0.5%, but increases occur with multiparity, prior spontaneous and induced abortions, and smoking, as well as in Asian women.[11] Additional independent risk factors for placenta previa are prior cesarean delivery, advanced maternal age, and infertility treatments. The current rising trends for each of these factors contribute to the increasing incidence of placenta previa. In comparison with risk factors for placental abruption, placenta previa is associated with conditions that precede pregnancy, whereas placental abruption is more likely to be affected by conditions occurring during pregnancy.

Delivery options should be based on the distance between the lower edge of the placenta and the internal cervical os and, in the absence of antepartum bleeding, a cesarean delivery at term may be scheduled.

The anesthetic technique for a primary cesarean delivery need not be different from that otherwise planned for cesarean delivery in general (spinal or combined spinal-epidural anesthesia), with the exception that the potential blood loss may be greater, 1000 to 1500 mL, blood products should be available and adequate venous access ensured. Autologous blood salvage (cell saver) may be considered, particularly if the patient has a rare blood type or is refusing blood products (Jehovah's witness).

Other important considerations with a placenta previa are:

- Up to 3% of placenta previa are associated with a placenta accreta even in the absence of a previous cesarean delivery (or uterine scar). Therefore, specific ultrasound screening (and possibly magnetic resonance imaging [MRI]; see below) is essential.
- If a placenta accreta is suspected (with or without a previous cesarean delivery), a thorough multidisciplinary care plan is needed for the cesarean, including the possibility of hysterectomy (see under Placenta Accreta).

Placenta Accreta

Abnormal placentation can be life threatening because of the risk of massive hemorrhage at the time of delivery. In addition, maternal morbidity is significant because of the probable need for peripartum hysterectomy, transfusion of blood and blood products, damage to surrounding organs, and prolonged hospitalization, including intensive care unit admission. Clinically, placenta accreta becomes problematic during delivery when the placenta does not completely separate from the uterus and is followed by massive hemorrhage (typically 3-5 L of blood loss). The following definitions may be used:

- *Placenta accreta* is defined by the absence of a decidua basalis and is used to describe the clinical condition when part of the placenta, or the entire placenta, has invaded and is inseparable from the uterine wall.
- *Placenta increta* describes the situation when the chorionic villi invade into the myometrium.
- *Placenta percreta* describes the invasion through the myometrium and serosa, and possibility of adjacent organ invasion, such as the bladder.

The incidence of placenta accreta has been reported to be 1 in 533 pregnancies for the period 1982-2002,[12] which is significantly higher than previously reported and is likely paralleling the increase in cesarean deliveries. Numerous epidemiologic studies have demonstrated an increased incidence of accreta in women with a subsequent placenta previa and women with a history of previous cesarean delivery (with or without a placenta previa overlying the uterine scar). Indeed, the estimated rate of placenta accreta in women with a placenta previa undergoing a fourth or higher order repeat cesarean delivery is at least 60%. A recent study demonstrated that a primary elective cesarean delivery prior to labor is more likely to preserve fertility and result in subsequent pregnancy in women with placenta previa as compared with an urgent cesarean delivery performed when the parturient is in labor.[13] This study, suggesting that absence of labor at the time of the primary cesarean delivery, or in other words, that the uterine incision occurs in a thick quiescent myometrium, may modify the risk of future possibility of placenta accreta in subsequent pregnancies merits further investigation.

The recent ACOG Committee opinion on placenta accreta[14] emphasizes the following:

- The *diagnosis* of placenta accreta is usually established by prenatal ultrasonography and occasionally supplemented by MRI. In a study with sonographic and MRI findings that were each verified with the final diagnosis at delivery, ultrasonography had a sensitivity of 93% and specificity of 73%, while that of MRI was 80% and 65%, respectively (which was not significantly different).[15] A recent study to evaluate placental MRI in the diagnosis and surgical management of placenta accreta suggested that MRI may be more accurate than ultrasound to establish a precise topographic mapping of the invaded area, particularly in relation with the vascular anatomy and blood supply, which could be extremely useful to guide the surgical dissection during hysterectomy.[16]
- If there is a strong suspicion of an abnormal placental invasion, obstetricians and radiologists practicing at small hospitals or at institutions with insufficient blood bank supply or inadequate availability of subspecialty (hematologist, gynecologic oncology surgeons, urologists, intensivists, hematologists) and support personnel should consider *patient transfer to a tertiary perinatal care center.*

- The *timing* of delivery should be individualized. However, combined maternal and neonatal outcomes are optimized in stable patients with delivery at 34 weeks' gestation (even without an amniocentesis to demonstrate fetal lung maturation). The goal is for a planned delivery as greater blood loss, and complications have been shown to occur in emergent cesarean hysterectomies versus planned cesarean hysterectomies.

- For the *surgical approach*, the recommended management of suspected placenta accreta is planned preterm cesarean hysterectomy with the placenta left in situ because removal of the placenta is associated with significant hemorrhagic morbidity. However, alternative approaches may be considered for women who have a strong desire to preserve fertility. Generally, planned attempts at manual placental removal should be avoided. If hysterectomy becomes necessary, the standard approach is to leave the placenta in situ, quickly use a "whip stitch" to close the hysterotomy incision, and proceed with hysterectomy.

- *Blood loss* in women with a placenta accreta can be expected to be massive. In fact, blood loss was shown to exceed 5000 mL in 42% of women with a known diagnosis of placenta accreta, although there is no reliable individual predictor of blood loss.[17] Current recommendations for blood replacement are a 1:1:1 ratio of packed red blood cells (PRBCs) to fresh frozen plasma (FFP) and platelets, which should be available in the operating room from the start. Institutionally established massive transfusion protocols should be followed. Additional units of blood and coagulation factors should be infused quickly and as necessitated by the patient's vital signs and hemodynamic stability. It is helpful to perform multidisciplinary drills to prepare for hemorrhage.

- *Autologous blood salvage devices (cell saver)* are safe and valuable in the management of a MOH.

- Current evidence for *interventional radiologic procedures* prior to the cesarean delivery is insufficient to make a firm recommendation about the use of balloon catheter occlusion or embolization to reduce blood loss and improve surgical outcome. However, specific situations may warrant their use.

- *Methotrexate* has been proposed as an adjunct treatment for placenta accreta. However, there is insufficient evidence to recommend its use routinely, and although uterine conservation was initially achieved in some instances, patients may subsequently develop PPH requiring hysterectomy.

There is no consensus regarding the choice of anesthetic to adopt for the management of a cesarean delivery in a woman with a suspected placenta accreta. Nowadays, most obstetric anesthesiologists would opt for a continuous neuraxial anesthetic (combined spinal-epidural, or continuous epidural or spinal) to allow titration and redosing of local anesthetics in the event of prolonged surgical time. This also offers the advantage of allowing the patient to be awake for the delivery of the infant, the partner to be present if clinical conditions permits, and avoids a general anesthetic for both the mother and infant; another advantage of neuraxial techniques is that they can be used to manage postcesarean/hysterectomy analgesia with the indwelling catheter. If needed due to massive hemorrhage or discomfort, conversion to general anesthesia could be provided at a later stage.

Trauma

ANTENATAL ABDOMINAL TRAUMA

Pregnant women admitted because of an abdominal trauma require appropriate monitoring and management. Approximately 25% of patients, preterm labor, placental abruption, uterine rupture, or other circumstances may require a prompt delivery.

LACERATIONS OF THE CERVIX, VAGINA, OR PERINEUM

Vaginal and cervical lacerations during a vaginal delivery tend to occur more commonly with a precipitous delivery, with macrosomia, shoulder dystocia, an instrumental delivery, and an episiotomy (mediolateral in particular). Risk factors for cervical laceration specifically are young maternal age, induction of labor, cerclage, and vacuum extraction. Asian women appear to be at greater risk for vaginal and significant perineal tears (third-degree and fourth-degree) after a vaginal delivery.

Uterine Inversion

A uterine inversion is an extremely rare event but one that can result in serious adversity. It is usually associated with prolonged labor, grand multiparity, a fundal placenta, and third-stage manipulation using excessive cord traction, during which the internal surface of the uterus may be forced partially or completely through the uterine cervix. The incidence of acute uterine inversion has substantially decreased with the introduction of active management of third stage of labor protocols. Management of uterine inversion has two crucial components: the immediate restoring of the uterus to its normal position and treatment of the hemorrhagic shock. Immediate uterine reversion will prevent massive blood loss and hemodynamic instability but is not always successful. Nitroglycerin has been used to provide relaxation and enable uterine reversion because the lower uterine segment is often a mechanical obstacle. Regional anesthesia does not provide uterine relaxation but may be helpful by providing analgesia. In the past, case reports suggested the use of general anesthesia with volatile agents in order to replace the uterus. In the most resistant inversions, a surgical correction may be required; laparoscopic reduction has been reported.[18]

Uterine Rupture or Dehiscence

Uterine rupture is defined as a full-thickness separation of the uterine wall and overlying serosa. It is associated with uterine bleeding; fetal bradycardia (and other abnormalities of fetal heart rate); and protrusion or expulsion of the fetus, placenta, or both into the abdominal cavity. In contrast, uterine scar dehiscence constitutes separation of a preexisting scar that does not disrupt the overlying visceral peritoneum.

The incidence of complete uterine rupture is extremely low, and the most important risk factors are a previous uterine scar due to previous cesarean delivery, history of dilation and curettage, uterine polypectomy, endometrectomy, or an intrauterine device. Other risk factors include multiple previous cesarean deliveries, a short interpregnancy interval, a vertical uterine incision, and a locked single-layer uterine closure. To avoid catastrophic maternal and neonatal outcomes, women with a vertical uterine scar (postcesarean delivery or myomectomy) should have a planned cesarean delivery at 37 weeks' gestation.

The incidence of uterine rupture in women attempting a trial of labor after previous cesarean delivery (TOLAC) fluctuates and is estimated to range between 0.5% and 4%.[19,20] There is no available predictive model to estimate the risk of uterine rupture in women selecting a TOLAC, and although prostaglandins for induction of labor are considered to increase the risk of uterine rupture, the evidence is relatively scarce.[21] It has been suggested that the duration of labor, rather than the induction of labor per se, is the factor associated with the risk of rupture. A recent Cochrane review concluded that there is insufficient data to make any recommendations with regards to the optimal method of induction of labor in women with a previous cesarean delivery.

Uterine rupture is typically characterized by (1) a sudden constant abdominal pain that is recognizable because it persists in between contractions (although cessation of contractions can also occur), (2) a nonreassuring fetal heart rate tracing, and (3) antepartum bleeding (which may remain concealed). Pain is not usually masked by current regimens of low-dose epidural labor analgesia (ie, dilute concentrations of local anesthetics); however, frequent epidural dosing (top-ups for breakthrough pain) should raise suspicion for an impending uterine rupture[22] in women having a TOLAC as well as referred shoulder pain.

In 2010, after joint agreement by ACOG and American Society of Anesthesiologists (ASA), the ACOG statement on TOLAC includes the following: "Because the risks associated with TOLAC and uterine rupture may be unpredictable, the immediate availability of appropriate facilities and personnel (including . . . a physician capable of monitoring labor and performing cesarean delivery, including an emergency cesarean delivery) is optimal."[19] Issues surrounding the requirement of "immediate availability" have emerged,[23] because other emergent obstetric complications such as placental abruption or umbilical cord prolapse are equally catastrophic maternal and neonatal outcomes as uterine rupture, yet immediate availability is not mandated. ACOG supports the use of epidural for labor analgesia during TOLAC, because more women may opt for a trial of labor if they can benefit of adequate pain relief. As once believed, an epidural will neither mask the signs and symptoms nor delay the diagnosis of uterine rupture; changes in fetal heart rate and uterine patterns, and in particular bradycardia, are the most common signs of uterine rupture.

The ASA guideline recommendations published in 2007 state that "neuraxial techniques should be offered to patients attempting vaginal birth after previous cesarean delivery" and that "it is also appropriate to consider early placement of a neuraxial catheter that can be used later for labor analgesia or for anesthesia in the event of an operative delivery."[24]

As emphasized in a recent review on the role of the anesthesiologist during TOLAC[23]:

- Anesthesiologists should be involved in the antenatal counseling of women planning a TOLAC.
- A preanesthetic evaluation early in labor should be enabled.

- Women may have limited clear liquids; however, nothing-by-mouth is recommended if they have a potentially difficult airway, a nonreassuring fetal tracing, or if they are in active labor.
- Early neuraxial labor analgesia should be encouraged.
- A well-functioning epidural catheter may be used for cesarean delivery and may reduce the need for a general anesthetic, even in the event of an urgent cesarean delivery (general anesthesia has been shown to increase the risk of PPH[25]).

Preexistent or Acquired Coagulopathy

Coagulopathies that increase the risk of PPH may be inherited (eg, hemophilia, VWD, Glanzmann thrombasthenia) or may be acquired during pregnancy (severe preeclampsia, HELLP syndrome) and at the time of delivery (DIC). In addition, women with thrombophilias or other indications for anticoagulation or antithrombotic medication during pregnancy may be at increased risk for PPH.

Pregnancy is associated with a progressive increase in the levels of several coagulation factors including fibrinogen; factors VII, VIII, X, and XII; and von Willebrand's factor (VWF). The increase in these coagulation factors occurs gradually during pregnancy and accelerates in the third trimester. Factors II, V, IX, XI, and XIII levels are slightly elevated or unchanged during normal pregnancy. Similar changes may also be seen in women with inherited bleeding disorders, which may lead to normalization of the hemostatic defect in women with some bleeding disorders such as VWD or carriers of hemophilia A. In rare bleeding disorders, hemostatic abnormalities seem to persist throughout pregnancy, especially if the defect is severe.

When assessing the potential for bleeding in pregnant women with coagulopathies, a detailed bleeding history, family background, and obstetric history should be assessed, along with coagulation tests and factor levels. Having a severe bleeding disorder is not in itself an indication for a cesarean section delivery and, in most cases, normal vaginal delivery can be planned. In some cases, cesarean delivery may be deemed safer for obstetric indications. The management plan should be individualized, and a written multidisciplinary delivery plan should be established during the third trimester, one that is available to all of those involved in the patient's care (including the woman herself). Good communication between hematologists, obstetricians, anesthesiologists, midwives, and neonatologists is essential for the safe management of labor and delivery.

Neuraxial labor analgesia or neuraxial anesthesia for cesarean delivery has often been unjustifiably denied to women with bleeding disorders because of the potential risk of spinal/epidural hematoma formation with subsequent spinal cord compression. Epidurals or spinals can be offered to women with normalized factor levels during pregnancy or who have normal factor levels as a result of treatment, but women should be thoroughly informed about the risks and benefits of neuraxial techniques for labor analgesia and the availability of alternative modalities (N_2O and/or systemic opioids) as well as the risks of neuraxial anesthesia (spinals) for cesarean delivery. Factor levels also need to be maintained in the normal range at the time of epidural catheter removal. Neuraxial analgesia/anesthesia should not be used in situations in which hemostasis is not guaranteed, such as in patients with uncorrected severe deficiencies or in whom there is poor correlation between the bleeding risk and factor levels.

Several important points during management of labor and delivery include the following:

- If the fetus is at risk of having a bleeding disorder, invasive monitoring, such as fetal blood sampling, fetal scalp electrodes, and the use of vacuum extraction and midcavity forceps, should be avoided.
- Prolonged second stage of labor also increases the risk of neonatal hemorrhage. Therefore, in cases in which this is likely, an early recourse to cesarean delivery is suggested.
- Trauma to the maternal genital and perineal areas should be minimized during delivery.

Particular challenges will be faced by pregnant women with inherited coagulation factor deficiencies during the puerperium. Pregnancy care of women with such disorders should be managed by high-risk obstetric specialists, aided by a multidisciplinary team that includes a hematologist with expertise in hemostasis, anesthesia and, if appropriate, a pediatric hematologist, and the delivery should be planned in a hospital that has a hemophilia center. Factor levels should be checked antenatally, at 28 and 34 weeks' gestation, and certainly before invasive procedures Frequent follow-up may be required if prophylactic factor treatment is given during pregnancy. All women with factor deficiencies should deliver in a unit that has ready access to a blood bank and pathology service with the required factor treatments and laboratory tests. Specific targeted management to compensate for the deficient factor(s) according to the bleeding disorder will be required (and is not discussed in this chapter).[26,27]

Finally, at the time of delivery, placental abruption, amniotic fluid embolism, and retained placental products may result in acute intravascular activation of coagulation, which causes thromboembolic complications and consumption coagulopathy, resulting in severe hemorrhage.[28] The central underlying pathophysiologic perturbation in the coagulopathy associated with these syndromes is the release of tissue factor from the placenta and amniotic fluid into the circulation, in combination with low levels of physiologic anticoagulant factors during pregnancy. DIC is a catastrophic event, and rFVIIa has been suggested as an effective strategy,[29] although evidence to guide hematologic management of DIC is lacking.

MANAGEMENT OF PLANNED AND UNEXPECTED OBSTETRIC HEMORRHAGE

Pharmacologic Management

UTEROTONICS AGENTS (TABLE 20-2)

Oxytocinergics *Oxytocin* remains to date the first-line uterotonic agent in the prevention and management of uterine atony after vaginal deliveries as well as after cord clamping during cesarean deliveries.

Table 20-2. Uterotonic Agents

Agent	Dose	Cautions
Oxytocin (Pitocin)	10-20 IU/500 mL over 1-2 h IV *Lower doses are currently recommended*[31]: 3 UI/10 mL over 30 s + Two rescue doses 3 UI/10 mL over 30 s every 3 min + Maintenance infusion 3UI/L at 100 mL/h	Hypotension-tachycardia, ST-segment changes on ECG, pulmonary edema, water intoxication (large doses)
Ergometrine (Methergine)	0.2 mg IM (can be repeated q5min)	Contraindicated in patients with hypertension, coronary disease, preeclampsia
Carboprost (Hemabate)	0.25 mg IM (can be intramyometrial)	Gastrointestinal disturbance Contraindicated in patients with asthma, pulmonary hypertension
Misoprostol (Cytotec)	0.8 mg (four tablets) rectal, vaginal, PO	Gastrointestinal disturbance, shivering, pyrexia

For prevention of atony after a vaginal delivery, the timing, dosing, and mode of administration of oxytocin have all been studied. It has been advocated that it should be given as early as the delivery of the anterior shoulder of the infant; however, a recent Cochrane review concluded that administration of oxytocin before and after the delivery of the placenta does not significantly influence the incidence of PPH.[9] The intraumbilical injection of oxytocin has been suggested as a useful strategy to manage retained placenta and different dose regimens have been studied; however, routine administration via the umbilical cord is not currently recommended.

Recent studies have established that the intravenous dose achieving satisfactory uterine tone during elective cesarean deliveries, or even in laboring women undergoing an unplanned cesarean delivery, is substantially lower than the standard 5 to 10 UI (intravenous) that has become ubiquitous in clinical practice. Similarly, maintenance with an oxytocin infusion has only recently been evaluated, and current recommendations (including those of ACOG[1]) will need to be revised as the infusion of 20 UI intravenously every 4 to 6 hours, typically requested by obstetricians, is not substantiated by findings from dose-response clinical trials. In addition, desensitization of the oxytocin receptor has been demonstrated to occur as soon as 6 to 8 hours after oxytocin exposure during induction or augmentation of labor.

Awareness that oxytocin dosing may require a change in practice is increasing in the anesthesia literature.[30] The risk-to-benefit ratio of oxytocin administration during cesarean delivery has been elegantly reviewed and concluded that a dose of 3 UI intravenously followed by two rescue doses (3 UI intravenously) and then a maintenance infusion (3 UI/L, at 100 mL/h) as needed was sufficient.[31] The rationale to reduce the intravenous oxytocin dose lies in the fact that oxytocin-induced maternal hypotension and tachycardia are adverse side effects that occur in most, if not all, healthy normotensive women undergoing a cesarean delivery,[32] as well as in women with severe preeclampsia,[33] and that ST-segment depression has been correlated with higher oxytocin dosing.

Carbetocin, a synthetic analog of oxytocin, has a longer duration of action. Carbetocin (Duratocin or Pabal) is not commercially available in the United States but is used routinely in Europe and Canada as a first-line uterotonic agent during cesarean delivery. Carbetocin has been shown to be at least as effective as oxytocin in preventing PPH,[34] with similar hemodynamic profiles when comparing effects at relatively high dose of carbetocin (100 μg).[32] Studies are currently being conducted to define the effective dosing regimen, as doses lower than 100 μg have been shown to be effective.[35] Finally, one study has reported some intrinsic analgesic properties in women receiving carbetocin compared to those allocated to receive oxytocin.

Prostaglandins *Carboprost*, a synthetic prostaglandin analog of $PGF_2\alpha$ (15-methyl prostaglandin $F_2\alpha$) (Hemabate), stimulates myometrial contractions resembling labor contractions. It is primarily indicated for pregnancy termination in the second trimester of pregnancy and in the treatment of PPH due to uterine atony and not responding to conventional management. It is administered by intramuscular injection of 0.25 mg, with a time to peak concentration of 30 minutes. Absolute contraindications include asthma and cardiovascular adverse events (hypertension and pulmonary edema). Gastrointestinal side effects (diarrhea, nausea, and vomiting) have been reported.

Misoprostol, a synthetic prostaglandin E1-analog (Cytotec), is used as a non-steroidal anti-inflammatory drug–induced gastric ulcer prophylactic as well as to induce labor or abortion. Misoprostol has shown promising results compared to placebo as a uterotonic agent in different settings, because its formulation is thermostable (ie, does not require refrigeration); it is inexpensive; and its administration may be sublingual, oral, vaginal or rectal. Misoprostol may cause mild to moderate diarrhea, stomach cramps, and/or nausea, fever and shivering.

ERGOT DERIVATIVE

Methylergonovine maleate, a semisynthetic ergot alkaloid (Methergine), acts directly on the myometrium and increases the tone, rate, and amplitude of rhythmic contractions. It induces a rapid and sustained tetanic uterotonic effect, which shortens the third stage of labor and reduces blood loss. It is indicated for the prevention and management of PPH. The onset of action after an intramuscular dose of 0.2 mg is within 2 to 5 minutes. Methergine should not be given intravenously and is absolutely contraindicated in women with hypertension, preeclampsia, or cardiovascular disease because of the risk of myocardial ischemia and sudden hypertensive and cerebrovascular accidents. Drug interactions should be considered in women taking CYP3A4 inhibitors, and strong inducers of CYP3A4 are likely to decrease the pharmacologic action of Methergine.

FIBRINOGEN

Low fibrinogen levels have been shown to correlate with the severity of PPH and independently predict the need for an interventional procedure. Due to pregnancy's specific alterations of the coagulation profile, fibrinogen has a pivotal role in the context of PPH, which has been described in a recent review.[36] Several case series have reported on the benefits and apparent safety of early administration of fibrinogen concentrate,[37] and one nonrandomized trial compared fibrinogen and cryoprecipitate and found them to be equally efficacious in correcting hypofibrinogenemia.[38] The FIB-PPH trial is an ongoing placebo controlled randomized clinical trial to evaluate fibrinogen concentrate (2 g intravenously) to reduce by 33% the need for blood products, which should provide interesting results on the benefits of such therapy in the context of PPH.[39]

RECOMBINANT FACTOR VIIa

Management of PPH with rFVIIa (NovoSeven) in women without inherited coagulation disorders has been extensively reported for over 10 years. In 2007, recommendations for the use of rFVIIa in obstetrics as well as the results from the North European registry were published. Since then, some reports on the effectiveness and safety of rFVIIa for PPH management from the United States,[40] but mostly other countries, have reinforced its use (despite being off label).

Practical recommendations before starting rFVIIa therapy are to ensure the following[41]:

- Transfuse red blood cells to maintain a hemoglobin level of 9 to 10 g/L.
- Maintain a platelet count above 70×10^9/L.
- Transfuse FFP/fibrinogen/cryoprecipitate to maintain a fibrinogen level above 2 g/L.
- Transfuse FFP to maintain an activated partial thromboplastin time (aPTT) less than 1.5 times the norm.
- Avoid or correct hypothermia and acidosis.
- Correct low ionized calcemia.
- Rule out arterial bleeding.

There are no dose response studies for rFVIIa in the context of PPH, and most reports used a single dose ranging between 60 to 90 µg/kg. The French multicenter trial "Recombinant Human Activated Factor VII as Salvage Therapy in Women With Severe Postpartum Hemorrhage" (NCT00370877) randomized women with PPH to receive 60 µ g/kg of rFVIIa or standard management, and final findings of this trial are awaited.

TRANEXAMIC ACID

Early use of tranexamic acid is encouraged in the management of PPH and is part of all the current guidelines.

The first randomized trial to elucidate the efficacy of tranexamic acid in the management of PPH after vaginal delivery demonstrated that administration of a high dose of tranexamic acid (4 g given over 1 hour followed by 1 g/h for an additional 6 hours) at the time PPH was diagnosed resulted in reduced blood loss and fewer interventions.[42] The results of a large international trial to assess the benefits and safety of tranexamic acid (the WOMAN trial) will provide more insights on the benefits/safety/complications of tranexamic acid in the treatment of PPH.[43]

Most of the current published literature has focused on the prevention of PPH in healthy women. Tranexamic acid has been suggested as a prophylactic adjunct in the active management of the third stage of labor during vaginal delivery, and four placebo-controlled randomized trials in healthy women undergoing an elective cesarean delivery showed some benefits in reducing blood loss and oxytocin use. Tranexamic acid is usually given as an intravenous infusion of 1 to 2 g over 30 to 60 minutes.

Transfusion Therapies and Monitoring of Coagulation

Until recently, adequacy of resuscitation from hemorrhage was based on administration of crystalloids and PRBCs. However, this strategy results in dilutional coagulopathy, which will be complicated by hypothermia and acidosis, and further worsening the coagulopathy. Compelling evidence, recently accumulated from the non-pregnant trauma patients,[44] has resulted in most centers in the United States taking the following action. They have adopted massive transfusion protocols involving the use of high ratios of FFP to PRBCs and early use of rFVIIa, as emphasized in the California Toolkit to Transform Maternity Care.[4] Massive transfusion protocols to guide therapy have been shown to improve outcomes and potentially reduce the need for interventional therapies.[40,45]

BLOOD PRODUCTS

Current recommendations for resuscitation with blood bank products are as follows:

- Initiate a massive obstetric hemorrhage protocol (inform blood bank, send first blood sample for coagulation tests, receive "emergency blood products")
- Early "empiric" administration of blood products without waiting for laboratory tests
- Transfuse with a 1:1:1 ratio of PRBCs/FFP/platelets
- Reassess transfusion after first set of results is generated by the laboratory

AUTOLOGOUS BLOOD SALVAGE

Despite some initial concerns that amniotic fluid and other fetal cells contraindicated the use intraoperative autologous cell salvage, the cell saver has been deemed safe in the context of major obstetric hemorrhages once amniotic fluid has been suctioned and its recourse encouraged by all the national guidelines. Nonetheless, cell salvage should only be performed by a trained team with regular experience in intraoperative blood cell salvage, which is why its use may be limited if such conditions are not met. Advantages of intraoperative cell salvage are a reduction in the incidence of transfusion reactions and transfusion-related infection, as compared with allogenic transfusion. It may also be useful when there are difficulties with cross-matching (rare blood type) or if the patient is refusing a allogenic blood (some Jehovah's witnesses). Because the blood aspirated by the cannula during the cesarean delivery may include amniotic fluid and fetal cells, filtered blood should be washed (possibly twice) during the process and a leukocyte depletion filter should always be used. Several cases of severe hypotension and coagulopathy related to amniotic fluid embolism have been reported, which serve as a reminder that cell saver utilization is not trivial.

MONITORING TRANSFUSION REQUIREMENTS AND HEMOSTASIS

Prompt administration of blood products and correction of coagulopathy are essential steps in the management of PPH. In most cases, medical and transfusion therapy is not based on the actual coagulation status because standard laboratory test usually have limited value because of delays in the interval from obtaining the blood sample to receiving results. Also, conventional tests (aPTT, prothrombin time, and international normalized ratio) are poor predictors for transfusion requirements in the obstetric patient.[46,47] Nonetheless, knowing the etiology of the coagulopathy during massive blood loss is important as the imbalance between procoagulant, anticoagulant, profibrinolytic and antifibrinolytic activity develops. Identifying the degree of hemodilution versus consumption coagulopathy, particularly in the context of obstetrics where amniotic fluid embolism and placental abruption can precipitate DIC, can be critical to ensure a successful resuscitation. In addition, because of the speed with which massive blood loss occurs in the obstetric patient, frequent and timely monitoring is useful. Recent technologic developments make it possible to continuously monitor hemoglobin using pulse co-oximetry[48] as well as coagulation using point-of-care devices such as thromboelastography (TEG; Haemonetics Corp., Braintree, MA) and thromboelastometry (ROTEM; Tem International GmbH, Munich, Germany).[49] The major advantage of TEG/ROTEM over conventional coagulation tests is that they are performed on whole blood and not on plasma, and therefore they assess the process from coagulation initiation through to clot lysis, including clot strength and stability. These point-of-care devices have not been widely adopted in the context of MOH because they are currently no studies available in obstetrics patients with massive blood loss that assess normal reference values. Therefore, with the current lack of predefined target values, it is still premature to guide hemostasis management based on TEG/ROTEM results.[36,46]

Interventional Radiology

The role of interventional radiology in the management of PPH has increased tremendously over the past decade as a minimally invasive, fertility-preserving alternative to conventional surgical treatment.[50] Recommendations for its use were published by the RCOG in 2007.[51]

When abnormal placentation is suspected, or confirmed antenatally, planned preoperative bilateral internal iliac artery balloon catheter placement with inflation of the balloons immediately after delivery of the neonate is a procedure that some institutions have adopted. It is performed almost routinely in the radiology suite, where balloon catheter placement is then followed immediately with the cesarean delivery on the radiology table.[52] Theoretically, balloon inflation leads to bilateral vessel occlusion, limiting blood loss; such an approach, however, is controversial and the benefits versus complications rate remains unclear. Most complications are associated with embolization and balloon occlusion rather than catheterization alone. Studies have reported foot ischemia, small bowel ischemia, pseudoaneurysm, perforation of the internal iliac artery, deep vein thrombosis, thrombosis of the popliteal artery, thrombosis of the right common femoral artery, and various neuropathies The overall the role of interventional radiology to prevent major blood loss is still under debate.[53]

The RCOG suggested interventional radiology in the following emergency indications following delivery[51]:

- Uterine atony following prolonged labor, after a vaginal or cesarean delivery
- Surgical complications or uterine tears at the time of cesarean delivery
- Bleeding while in the post anesthesia recovery unit or in the postpartum floor following a vaginal or cesarean delivery
- Bleeding following hysterectomy

Surgical Interventions

In most instances, fertility-preserving surgical interventions will be attempted and hysterectomy will, at first, be avoided. Procedures that have been shown to be useful include the following:

- Intra-uterine balloon to provide internal tamponade (which can be inserted after vaginal delivery or during a cesarean delivery). The Bakri balloon, first described in 2001, has been shown to be very effective, and its addition in PPH protocols has reduced the need for interventional procedures. There have been very few reports of complications, although these have included migration of the catheter through unsuspected uterine ruptures.
- Uterine packing with chitosan-covered gauze is a novel approach that has been shown to be successful in reducing the need for hysterectomy in women with uterine atony. It can be inserted either intravaginally or via the hysterotomy in the case of a cesarean delivery.
- Surgical options that preserve fertility include the following:
  ◦ Bilateral uterine artery ligation seems to be effective and can be performed by obstetricians.
  ◦ Hypogastric ligation is an alternative surgical approach, but it requires a skilled surgeon.
  ◦ The B-Lynch procedure was first described in 1997 and is a suturing technique that has proved successful in managing uterine atony. Various versions of this technique have been described,[54] and it can be applied in combination with a Bakri balloon in a stepwise approach to avoid a hysterectomy.
- A hysterectomy may become unavoidable either after a vaginal delivery complicated by MOH in a patient too unstable to be transported to the radiology suite for embolization, or during a cesarean delivery in a planned or unplanned manner. Depending on the circumstances and whenever possible (urgency, coagulopathy, severity of blood loss), the anesthetic technique may be neuraxial (epidural if in place during labor or after delivery, combined spinal-epidural, or continuous spinal).[55]

ANESTHETIC CONSIDERATIONS

Managing PPH after a vaginal delivery includes the following:

- Establish etiology (based on the 4 *T*'s) and communicate with obstetricians, nurses, and blood bank.
- Ensure adequate venous access for fluid and blood resuscitation (two large-bore peripheral intravenous lines—14- or 16-gauge).
- Uterotonics (Pitocin, Methergine, Hemabate, Cytotec)
- Provide anesthesia if a manual removal of retained products or a dilation-curettage is needed (and ensure adequate monitoring, procedure should be performed in an operating room). There should be epidural redosing when appropriate or spinal anesthetic (achieving a T6 block).
- If bleeding is not rapidly controlled, activate massive hemorrhage protocol should be initiated.
  - Start transfusion according to protocol (empiric, 1:1:1 ratio); supplement low ionized calcium with calcium chloride as needed.
  - Consider alternatives (Bakri balloon, interventional radiology if available).
  - Consider tranexamic acid, fibrinogen, cryoprecipitate, and rFVIIa.
  - Transfer patient to radiology or operating room.
    - Arterial line
    - Vasopressors if needed (phenylephrine infusion 50-100 μg/min)
    - Warming devices (Bair Hugger, rapid infusion pumps)
    - Portable arterial blood gas analyzer
  - If surgery is decided (B-Lynch, arterial ligation, hysterectomy)
    - Anesthesia as indicated (neuraxial or general anesthesia—preferably with total intravenous anesthesia to avoid further uterine atony)
    - Cell saver
  - Consider intensive care unit for postoperative monitoring
    - Ensure postoperative analgesia (neuraxial analgesia or alternatives)

For a planned cesarean delivery with a suspected placenta accreta and possible need for hysterectomy, there should be a multidisciplinary approach to decide well in advance the feasibility and appropriateness of intravascular balloon placement or other preventative measures using interventional radiology. The optimal surgical team (obstetricians, gynecology/oncology surgeons, urologists) should be prepared in advance, and on the day of the surgery, hematology and blood bank, neonatology, and intensive care team, should be available. Optimal preparation in the operating room should include a perfusionist with a cell saver set-up:

Medication and blood products include:

- For neuraxial anesthesia (bupivacaine, fentanyl, Duramorph, lidocaine, clonidine)
- For sedation (midazolam, ketamine)
- For general anesthesia—preferably a totally intravenous anesthesia (propofol, remifentanil)
- Vasopressors (phenylephrine, vasopressin, epinephrine) and calcium
- Uterotonics (Pitocin, Methergine, Hemabate, Cytotec)

- Blood products in the operating room (Red Blood Cells [RPC], fresh Frozen Plasma [FFP], platelets, cryoprecipitate)
- Tranexamic acid, fibrinogen, rFVIIa

  Necessary equipment includes:

- Venous access (at least two large-bore peripheral lines)
- Arterial line
- Neuraxial anesthesia (combined spinal-epidural, continuous spinal)
- Bair Hugger
- Warmers for blood products
- Pumps for vasoactive agents
- Cell saver
- Arterial blood gas analyzer, other point-of-care monitoring if available (TEG/ ROTEM)
- Intensive care unit bed

Ideally, three obstetric anesthesiologists should be allocated to such a case, with preassigned tasks:

1. One overseeing the provision anesthesia (neuraxial, sedation, potentially, general anesthesia) and monitoring hemodynamics
2. Another in charge of the transfusion process (monitoring blood loss, deciding when to start cell salvage device, how much blood products to give, and continuously reassessing the situation with the obstetricians/surgeons, ordering more blood as needed, and deciding when and if rFVIIs is indicated after all other measures have been undertaken). Ongoing communication with blood blank and laboratory for optimal monitoring of transfusion requirements and hemostasis is essential.
3. Additional staff typically helping out with anesthesia and transfusion processes

Postoperatively, a debriefing of the case is always recommended, as part of a quality and improvement process. Such debriefings have been shown to be useful in addressing system issues that may be implemented with improved communication and education.[4]

CONCLUSIONS

Ideal management of PPH occurs when nurses/midwives, obstetricians, and anesthesiologists recognize early on the potential for excessive bleeding and trigger a "major obstetric hemorrhage protocol" that identifies specific tasks for each team player and an algorithm to be followed according to the etiology, circumstances, and time elapsed since delivery. The leading cause of PPH remains uterine atony, although the constant increase of women with prior uterine surgery and abnormal placentation (placenta accreta) is bound to also increase the incidence of massive hemorrhages at delivery.

It is necessary to identify all the steps that are required, from the implementation of algorithms and protocols for massive transfusion, describing all the tasks,

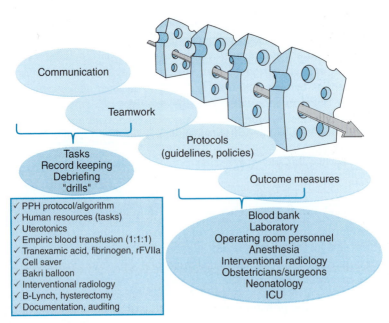

Figure 20-1. Applying the "Swiss cheese model" to ensure optimal management of obstetric hemorrhage.

improving communication processes, debriefing and audits, and recognizing the pivotal role of the anesthesia team throughout all the steps (Figure 20-1). Use of uterotonics, starting with oxytocin at appropriate dosing regimens as the first choice, followed by ergots derivatives and/or prostaglandins remains the key before other strategies become necessary. Transfusion guidelines have emphasized the need to start a "bleeding emergency protocol" prior to any laboratory results, and blood banks should provide sufficient amounts of blood products, given "empirically" following a 1:1:1 ratio. Fibrinogen, tranexamic acid and rFVIIa have been extensively used and are considered of great benefit. Cell saver, if available, can be useful and is particularly recommended if the bleeding is anticipated such as when a placenta accreta has been diagnosed antenatally. Conservative maneuvers to reduce the need for massive transfusion and hysterectomy include the Bakri balloon that creates an internal tamponade when inserted vaginally into the uterus. The B-Lynch procedure performed via Pfannenstiel or laparotomy has also been shown to reduce the need for hysterectomy, along with surgical uterine artery ligation or uterine artery embolization performed by interventional radiology. Finally, patients with major obstetric hemorrhages should be admitted to the intensive care unit for follow-up.

REFERENCES

1. American College of Obstetricians and Gynecologists (ACOG). ACOG Practice Bulletin No. 76. Postpartum hemorrhage. *Obstet Gynecol.* 2006;108:1039-1047.

2. Lalonde A, Daviss BA, Acosta A, Herschderfer K. Postpartum hemorrhage today: ICM/FIGO initiative 2004-2006. *Int J Gynaecol Obstet.* 2006;94:243-253.

3. Leduc D, Senikas V, Lalonde AB, et al. Active management of the third stage of labour: prevention and treatment of postpartum hemorrhage. *J Obstet Gynaecol Can.* 2009;31:980-993.

4. Bingham D, Melsop K, Main E. QMQCC Obstetric Hemorrhage Hospital Level Implementation Guide. The California Maternal Quality Care Collaborative (CMQCC) Stanford University, Palo Alto, CA; 2010.

5. Green Top Guidelines 52. 2009;52 http://www.rcog.org.uk/womens-health/clinical-guidance/prevention-and-management-postpartum-haemorrhage-green-top-52.

6. World Health Organization (WHO). WHO Recommendations for the Prevention and Treatment of Postpartum Haemorrhage. Geneva; 2012.

7. Bateman BT, Berman MF, Riley LE, Leffert LR. The epidemiology of postpartum hemorrhage in a large, nationwide sample of deliveries. *Anesth Analg.* 2010;110:1368-1373.

8. Mehrabadi A, Hutcheon J, Lee L, Kramer M, Liston R, Joseph K. Epidemiological investigation of a temporal increase in atonic postpartum haemorrhage: a population-based retrospective cohort study. *BJOG.* 2013;120:853-862.

9. Soltani H, Hutchon DR, Poulose TA. Timing of prophylactic uterotonics for the third stage of labour after vaginal birth. *Cochrane Database Syst Rev.* 2010:CD006173.

10. Adams L, Menon R, Dresner M. Anaesthetic protocol for manual removal of placenta. *Anaesthesia.* 2013;68:104-105.

11. Rao KP, Belogolovkin V, Yankowitz J, Spinnato JA II. Abnormal placentation: evidence-based diagnosis and management of placenta previa, placenta accreta, and vasa previa. *Obstet Gynecol Surv.* 2012;67:503-519.

12. Wu S, Kocherginsky M, Hibbard JU. Abnormal placentation: twenty-year analysis. *Am J Obstet Gynecol.* 2005;192:1458-1461.

13. Kamara M, Henderson J, Doherty D, Dickinson J, Pennell C. The risk of placenta accreta following primary elective caesarean delivery: a case-control study. *BJOG.* 2013;120:879-886.

14. American College of Obstetrics and Gynecology (ACOG). Placenta accreta. ACOG Committee Opinion No. 529. *Obstet Gynecol.* 2012;120:207-211.

15. Dwyer BK, Belogolovkin V, Tran L, et al. Prenatal diagnosis of placenta accreta: sonography or magnetic resonance imaging? *J Ultrasound Med.* 2008;27:1275-1281.

16. Palacios-Jaraquemada JM, Bruno CH, Martin E. MRI in the diagnosis and surgical management of abnormal placentation. *Acta Obstet Gynecol Scand.* 2013;92:392-397.

17. Wright JD, Pri-Paz S, Herzog TJ, et al. Predictors of massive blood loss in women with placenta accreta. *Am J Obstet Gynecol.* 2011;205:38.e1-38.e6.

18. Vijayaraghavan R, Sujatha Y. Acute postpartum uterine inversion with haemorrhagic shock: laparoscopic reduction: a new method of management? *BJOG.* 2006;113:1100-1102.

19. American College of Obstetrics and Gynecology (ACOG). Vaginal birth after previous cesarean delivery. ACOG Practice Bulletin No. 115 *Obstet Gynecol.* 2010;116:450-463.

20. National Institutes of Health (NIH). NIH Consensus Development Conference Statement. Vaginal birth after cesarean: new insights, March 8-10, 2010. *Semin Perinatol.* 2010;34:293-307.

21. Ophir E, Odeh M, Hirsch Y, Bornstein J. Uterine rupture during trial of labor: controversy of induction's methods. *Obstet Gynecol Surv.* 2012;67:734-745.

22. Cahill AG, Odibo AO, Allsworth JE, Macones GA. Frequent epidural dosing as a marker for impending uterine rupture in patients who attempt vaginal birth after cesarean delivery. *AmJ Obstet Gynecol.* 2010;202:355,e1-e5.

23. Hawkins JL. The anesthesiologist's role during attempted VBAC. *Clin Obstet Gynecol.* 2012;55:1005-1013.

24. American Society of Anesthesiologists Task Force on Obstetric Anesthesia. Practice guidelines for obstetric anesthesia: an updated report. *Anesthesiology.* 2007;106:843-863.

25. Chang CC, Wang IT, Chen YH, Lin HC. Anesthetic management as a risk factor for postpartum hemorrhage after cesarean deliveries. *Am J Obstet Gynecol.* 2011;205:462,e1-e7.

26. Chee YL, Townend J, Crowther M, Smith N, Watson HG. Assessment of von Willebrand disease as a risk factor for primary postpartum haemorrhage. *Haemophilia.* 2012;18:593-597.

27. Chow L, Farber MK, Camann WR. Anesthesia in the pregnant patient with hematologic disorders. *Hematol Oncol Clin North Am.* 2011;25:425-443, ix-x.

28. Levi M. Pathogenesis and management of peripartum coagulopathic calamities (disseminated intravascular coagulation and amniotic fluid embolism). *Thromb Res.* 2013;131 (suppl 1):S32-S34.

29. Franchini M, Manzato F, Salvagno GL, Lippi G. Potential role of recombinant activated factor VII for the treatment of severe bleeding associated with disseminated intravascular coagulation: a systematic review. *Blood Coag Fibrinolysis.* 2007;18:589-593.

30. Dyer RA, Butwick AJ, Carvalho B. Oxytocin for labour and caesarean delivery: implications for the anaesthesiologist. *Curr Opin Anaesth.* 2011;24:255-261.

31. Tsen LC, Balki M. Oxytocin protocols during cesarean delivery: time to acknowledge the risk/benefit ratio? *Int J Obstet Anesth.* 2010;19:243-245.

32. Rosseland LA, Hauge TH, Grindheim G, Stubhaug A, Langesaeter E. Changes in blood pressure and cardiac output during cesarean delivery: the effects of oxytocin and carbetocin compared with placebo. *Anesthesiology.* 2013.

33. Langesaeter E, Rosseland LA, Stubhaug A. Haemodynamic effects of oxytocin in women with severe preeclampsia. *Int J Obstet Anesth.* 2011;20:26-29.

34. Julie D, Elodie C, Anne D, Pauline S, Anne-sophie D, Damien S. Systematic use of carbetocin during cesarean delivery of multiple pregnancies: a before-and-after study. *Arch Gynecol Obstet.* 2013;287:875-880.

35. Cordovani D, Balki M, Farine D, Seaward G, Carvalho JC. Carbetocin at elective Cesarean delivery: a randomized controlled trial to determine the effective dose. *Can J Anaesth.* 2012;59:751-757.

36. Butwick AJ. Postpartum hemorrhage and low fibrinogen levels: the past, present and future. *Int J Obstet Anesth.* 2013;22:87-91.

37. Bell SF, Rayment R, Collins PW, Collis RE. The use of fibrinogen concentrate to correct hypofibrinogenaemia rapidly during obstetric haemorrhage. *Int J Obstet Anesth.* 2010;19:218-223.

38. Ahmed S, Harrity C, Johnson S, et al. The efficacy of fibrinogen concentrate compared with cryoprecipitate in major obstetric haemorrhage—an observational study. *Transfus Med.* 2012;22:344-349.

39. Wikkelsoe AJ, Afshari A, Stensballe J, et al. The FIB-PPH trial: fibrinogen concentrate as initial treatment for postpartum haemorrhage: study protocol for a randomised controlled trial. *Trials.* 2012;13:110.

40. Gutierrez MC, Goodnough LT, Druzin M, Butwick AJ. Postpartum hemorrhage treated with a massive transfusion protocol at a tertiary obstetric center: a retrospective study. *Int J Obstet Anesth.* 2012;21:230-235.

41. Ahonen J. The role of recombinant activated factor VII in obstetric hemorrhage. *Curr Opin Anaesth.* 2012;25:309-314.

42. Ducloy-Bouthors AS, Jude B, Duhamel A, et al. High-dose tranexamic acid reduces blood loss in postpartum haemorrhage. *Crit Care.* 2011;15:R117.

43. Cook L, Roberts I. Post-partum haemorrhage and the WOMAN trial. *Int J Epidemiol.* 2010;39:949-950.

44. Saule I, Hawkins N. Transfusion practice in major obstetric haemorrhage: lessons from trauma. *Int J Obstet Anesth.* 2012;21:79-83.

45. Shields LE, Smalarz K, Reffigee L, Mugg S, Burdumy TJ, Propst M. Comprehensive maternal hemorrhage protocols improve patient safety and reduce utilization of blood products. *Am J Obstet Gynecol.* 2011;205:368,e1-e8.

46. de Lange NM, Lance MD, de Groot R, Beckers EA, Henskens YM, Scheepers HC. Obstetric hemorrhage and coagulation: an update. Thromboelastography, thromboelastometry, and conventional coagulation tests in the diagnosis and prediction of postpartum hemorrhage. *Obstet Gynecol Surv.* 2012;67:426-435.

47. Stocks G. Monitoring transfusion requirements in major obstetric haemorrhage: out with the old and in with the new? *Int J Obstet Anesth.* 2011;20:275-278.

48. Butwick A, Hilton G, Carvalho B. Non-invasive haemoglobin measurement in patients undergoing elective Caesarean section. *Br J Anaesth.* 2012;108:271-277.

49. Macafee B, Campbell JP, Ashpole K, et al. Reference ranges for thromboelastography (TEG®) and traditional coagulation tests in term parturients undergoing caesarean section under spinal anaesthesia. *Anaesthesia.* 2012;67:741-747.

50. Rao AP, Bojahr H, Beski S, MacCallum PK, Renfrew I. Role of interventional radiology in the management of morbidly adherent placenta. *J Obstet Gynaecol.* 2010;30:687-689.

51. Royal College of Obstetricians and Gynaecologists. The role of emergency and elective interventional radiology in posptartum haemorrhage. Good Practice No. 6 2007. http://www.rcog.org.uk/womens-health/clinical-guidance/role-emergency-and-elective-interventional-radiology-postpartum-haem.

52. Jeffrey A, Clark V. The anaesthetic management of caesarean section in the interventional radiology suite. *Curr Opin Anaesth.* 2011;24:439-444.

53. Sadashivaiah J, Wilson R, Thein A, McLure H, Hammond CJ, Lyons G. Role of prophylactic uterine artery balloon catheters in the management of women with suspected placenta accreta. *Int J Obstet Anesth.* 2011;20:282-287.

54. Matsubara S, Yano H, Ohkuchi A, Kuwata T, Usui R, Suzuki M. Uterine compression sutures for postpartum hemorrhage: an overview. *Acta Obstet Gynecol Scand.* 2013;92:378-385.

55. Gallos G, Redai I, Smiley RM. The role of the anesthesiologist in management of obstetric hemorrhage. *Semin Perinatol.* 2009;33:116-123.

Section 5

Common Comorbidities During Pregnancy

Managing Cardiac Comorbidities During Pregnancy

21

Elsje Harker and Richard Smiley

With advances in medical and obstetric care, more and more women with cardiac disease are able to become pregnant and deliver a viable fetus. This chapter is divided into four main sections corresponding to four types of cardiac or cardiopulmonary disease that women may present with during pregnancy: valvular disease, congenital heart disease, cardiomyopathy, and pulmonary arterial hypertension. Although the incidence of ischemic/coronary heart disease may be increasing, we will not discuss it in this chapter, because there is much less experience and literature to guide therapeutic strategies in this area.

VALVULAR DISEASE

The prevalence of valvular disease in pregnant women is low and has decreased with the decline of rheumatic fever in developed countries. Although rare, clinically significant valvular disease increases the risk of adverse maternal, fetal, and neonatal outcomes. Risk to the pregnant patient and developing fetus depends on the severity of the valvular lesion and underlying cardiac function. Ideally, patients with known valvular heart disease should be evaluated prior to conception; this should include a detailed history and physical examination, 12-lead electrocardiogram (ECG), and an echocardiogram with Doppler study. Pregnancy outcome and complications in patients with valvular disease can be closely correlated to prepregnancy New York Heart Association (NYHA) functional status and further to any deterioration of NYHA status during the pregnancy. In general, stenotic lesions are much more poorly tolerated during pregnancy than regurgitant lesions, because pregnancy usually requires, or at least causes, an increase in cardiac output, a process impaired by stenotic lesions and potentially causing decompensation.

Mitral Stenosis

ETIOLOGY/RISK FACTORS

Mitral stenosis (MS) is the most commonly encountered valvular lesion in pregnancy.[1] Mitral stenosis usually occurs secondary to childhood rheumatic disease but may also be seen in association with congenital heart disease.

PATHOPHYSIOLOGY

The normal mitral valve area determined by echocardiography is 4 to 5 cm^2. A valve area of 1.5 to 2 cm^2 is classified as mild stenosis, 1 to 1.5 cm^2 as moderate, and less than 1 cm^2 as severe. Stenosis of the mitral valve impedes blood flow from the left atrium to the left ventricle, creating a pressure gradient across the valve. As left ventricular filling is restricted, longer diastolic filling time is necessary to maintain ventricular preload and cardiac output. Accordingly, the left atrium enlarges and pulmonary venous and arterial pressures increase, eventually leading to pulmonary edema and right-sided heart failure. Left atrial enlargement can result in atrial dysrhythmias, particularly fibrillation, which can lead to significant sudden hemodynamic decompensation from the loss of the contribution of atrial contraction to ventricular filling.

The pressure gradient across the stenotic mitral valve will generally increase with pregnancy-associated increases in heart rate and blood volume. Tachycardia reduces diastolic filling time, which limits left ventricular filling through the stenotic valve, thus decreasing stroke volume. Increases in blood volume may lead to pulmonary edema. Many patients with mitral stenosis become symptomatic for the first time during pregnancy, and a majority of women will demonstrate symptomatic deterioration, particularly those with high-order functional impairment as classified by NYHA class during pregnancy.[2] Symptoms include dyspnea, chest pain, palpitations, orthopnea, pulmonary edema, and decreased exercise capacity.

Parturients with mild stenosis (NYHA 1 or 2) tend to tolerate pregnancy well and have favorable outcomes. Those with moderate to severe stenosis experience a much higher incidence of morbidity, including development of dysrhythmias, heart failure, and the need to start and/or adjust medications, as well as the need for hospitalization. Whereas morbidity may be high, maternal mortality is rare in contemporary practice. Fetal risk, including preterm delivery and intrauterine growth retardation, is increased with moderate and severe stenosis.[2]

MANAGEMENT AND ANESTHETIC CONSIDERATIONS

Patients with severe mitral stenosis who are contemplating pregnancy should be offered percutaneous mitral balloon valvuloplasty or mitral valve replacement before conceiving. Management of the patient with mitral stenosis who is already pregnant should focus on control of heart rate (usually ≤ 80 beats/min) and left atrial pressure. Heart rate reduction is typically achieved with β-adrenergic receptor antagonists and restriction of physical activity. Digoxin may be necessary in patients with atrial fibrillation. Atrial fibrillation should be treated promptly with rate control or electrical cardioversion if the patient is hemodynamically unstable. Diuretics are used to treat volume overload but should be used cautiously to avoid hypovolemia and reduction of uteroplacental perfusion.[1]

For patients with severe symptoms despite maximal medical therapy, balloon mitral valvuloplasty may be necessary even during pregnancy, and it has been successfully performed. The risk of radiation exposure to the fetus can be reduced by minimizing fluoroscopy time, ensuring adequate abdominal and pelvic shielding of the mother and delaying the procedure until after the first trimester. The most common time for a parturient to undergo valvuloplasty is 28 to 32 weeks' gestation, both because this is the safest time for the fetus, with delivery a reasonable option if absolutely necessary, and because this is when many women with severe stenosis develop symptoms. Balloon valvuloplasty has been shown to be safe and effective for pregnant women and carries a decreased risk of fetal mortality compared to valve repair or replacement with cardiopulmonary bypass.[3,4]

Vaginal delivery is preferred over cesarean delivery, which is associated with more blood loss and larger fluid shifts, particularly during the postoperative period when vigilance may be decreased and fluid shifts may be exaggerated. Cesarean delivery is reserved for obstetric indications or in patients too hemodynamically unstable to tolerate labor. Outlet forceps or vacuum extraction may be used to shorten the second stage of labor and to help avoid sudden increases in venous return associated with bearing down.

Epidural anesthesia should be used for relief of labor pain using a dilute local anesthetic and opioid infusion. Small incremental boluses of 2% lidocaine or 3% 2-chloroprocaine may be necessary and desirable for planned instrumental delivery to control bearing-down reflex. Careful infusion of fluid and vasoconstrictors should be used to treat hypotension from sympathetic blockade.

In women with moderate to severe mitral stenosis and most other cardiovascular lesions that limit cardiac output and forward flow (eg, some congenital lesions, pulmonary hypertension, cardiomyopathy, aortic coarctation), a common strategy is to increase the "density" of epidural analgesia as the parturient approaches full dilation (5-10 mL 2% lidocaine, with or without additional fentanyl, occasionally 50-100 μg clonidine). This allows for the fetus to descend passively and deliver with outlet forceps while minimizing pushing (Valsalva) that can impair venous return. Reversible vasoconstriction with phenylephrine infusions, rather than fluid to treat hypotension from sympathetic blockade will prevent fluid overload, particularly after delivery of the infant. Epidural anesthesia (or combined spinal-epidural [CSE] anesthesia with a very low dose initial spinal) is also the preferred anesthetic for cesarean delivery, allowing for incremental titration of surgical blockade. Single-shot surgical spinal anesthesia should be avoided, because abrupt hypotension is poorly tolerated and may be more likely in these patients given their dependence on preload. If general anesthesia is necessary for cesarean delivery, a short-acting β-adrenergic receptor antagonist (esmolol) and/or opioid (remifentanil) are reasonable options during induction to limit sympathetic response to laryngoscopy and intubation.

The level of monitoring for labor or cesarean delivery depends on the severity of the lesion and symptoms. There should be a low threshold for continuous ECG monitoring in any laboring woman susceptible to dysrhythmias and a low threshold for arterial line placement during labor or cesarean delivery, because the benefits (even simply multiple blood draws) probably outweigh the risks in most women with significant mitral stenosis or other significant cardiac abnormalities. The indications, if any, for pulmonary artery (PA) catheters are unclear, as in most other clinical scenarios in obstetrics and elsewhere in medicine. If used at all, the PA catheter should probably be reserved for the most severely ill women undergoing cesarean delivery or those with severe pulmonary edema of unclear etiology. Many of these patents might benefit more from echocardiography rather than a PA catheter to clarify the pathophysiology leading to the hemodynamic abnormalities.

POSTPARTUM CARE

Patients with significant/symptomatic mitral stenosis are at risk for hemodynamic compromise and pulmonary edema due to peripartum blood loss and fluid shifts, irrespective of the mode of delivery. Mild to moderate pulmonary edema is often seen in the first few hours postpartum or postoperatively and usually responds to diuresis. Oxytocin, methylergonovine, and 15-methylprostaglandin F2α should be used with caution and with appreciation of their potential cardiovascular effects, because these agents can alter systemic and pulmonary vascular resistance. Patients with severe mitral stenosis should be monitored in an intensive care or similar high-dependency setting after delivery for 1 to 2 days, especially after cesarean delivery.

Aortic Stenosis

ETIOLOGY/RISK FACTORS

Aortic stenosis in pregnancy occurs most commonly secondary to congenitally stenotic aortic valves, including bicuspid aortic valve and supravalvular or subvalvular stenosis. Rheumatic aortic stenosis is much less common.

PATHOPHYSIOLOGY

Normal aortic valve area is 3 to 4 cm^2. As valve area decreases, pressure in the left ventricle increases, and the left ventricle hypertrophies to maintain cardiac output. With disease progression, stroke volume becomes relatively fixed, and alterations in cardiac output become dependent on heart rate. Symptoms, including angina, dyspnea, and syncope, are related to the degree of stenosis and are usually not present until late in the course of the disease. Severe aortic stenosis, defined as a valve area less than 1 cm^2, is rare in pregnancy.

Two decades ago, it was thought that the presence of aortic stenosis was a much more serious problem in pregnancy than mitral stenosis, but more recent reports suggest similar outcomes with either, dependent on severity. Patients with mild to moderate aortic stenosis tend to tolerate pregnancy reasonably well with close attention and follow-up. Patients with severe disease are often unable to accommodate the increase in blood volume and cardiac output associated with pregnancy. These patients are more likely to develop congestive heart failure and pulmonary edema. In addition, severe disease is associated with premature delivery and small-for-gestational age infants. Despite an increase in morbidity, mortality due to aortic stenosis in pregnancy is now rare.

MANAGEMENT AND ANESTHETIC CONSIDERATIONS

Ideally, patients with severe aortic stenosis should undergo balloon valvuloplasty or valve replacement before conceiving. Medical management of patients who become pregnant despite severe aortic disease includes diuretics and sometimes β-adrenergic blocking agents. Patients with severe symptoms despite optimal medical therapy may require termination of pregnancy or repair of the valve. As with mitral stenosis, valvuloplasty is associated with much lower risk to the fetus and is preferred over valve replacement.[1]

Goals in the management of the laboring patient with aortic stenosis include maintenance of normal heart rate and sinus rhythm, avoidance of hypotension and aortocaval compression, and maintenance of intravascular volume and venous return. Bradycardia may significantly decrease cardiac output in patients with aortic stenosis due to a fixed stroke volume. Tachycardia results in increased myocardial oxygen consumption and decreased diastolic perfusion time.

Vaginal delivery with an assisted second stage of labor as previously described with mitral stenosis is preferred over cesarean section. As with mitral stenosis, epidural anesthesia using a dilute local anesthetic and opioid infusion is recommended early for relief of labor pain. Cesarean delivery is reserved for obstetric indications or for patients too hemodynamically unstable to tolerate labor. Single-shot spinal anesthesia is contraindicated in women with severe aortic stenosis and relatively contraindicated in those with moderate disease. Many reports describe the successful use of incrementally dosed epidural or spinal catheters for cesarean delivery in patients with severe disease. Careful vasopressor (typically phenylephrine) infusion and intravenous fluids should be administered to avoid decreases in systemic vascular resistance (SVR) and preload. Local anesthetics without epinephrine are preferable because of the risk of severe tachycardia if injected intravascularly and mild tachycardia and hypotension when absorbed systemically. Many general anesthetic induction strategies have been suggested in the presence of aortic stenosis, typically involving moderate to high-dose rapid-acting opioids (fentanyl, alfentanil, remifentanil) to limit sympathetic activation and tachycardia with induction, intubation, incision, and delivery.

Blood pressure monitoring with an arterial line is recommended in patients with moderate to severe aortic stenosis. Use of pulmonary artery catheters is controversial and now rarely used; monitoring of central venous pressure (CVP) with a central line may be considered for monitoring volume status. The potential for hypovolemia is of greater concern than pulmonary edema in severe aortic stenosis, and CVP should be maintained at high-normal levels. Transesophageal echocardiography (TEE) should be considered in patients receiving general anesthesia.

POSTPARTUM CARE

Patients with aortic stenosis may be unable to accommodate the further increase in blood volume and cardiac output seen after delivery as the uterus involutes; this may lead to pulmonary edema requiring diuresis in the early postpartum period. Conversely, hypovolemia from postpartum hemorrhage is very poorly tolerated and should be managed aggressively; again, mild hypervolemia is probably preferable to hypovolemia. Patients with severe aortic stenosis or those with symptoms during the puerperium should be monitored in an intensive care setting after delivery for 1 to 2 days.

Mitral Regurgitation

ETIOLOGY/RISK FACTORS

Mitral regurgitation (MR) in women of reproductive age is usually due to myxomatous degeneration or rheumatic disease. In general, MR is well tolerated during pregnancy because the pregnancy-induced decrease in SVR tends to promote forward blood flow. Acute MR, usually caused by endocarditis or papillary muscle rupture, is much more problematic but is rarely seen in pregnancy.

PATHOPHYSIOLOGY

In acute MR, the left atrium experiences a sudden increase in volume load; this inhibits pulmonary venous return and leads to pulmonary congestion and edema. Cardiac output is decreased as a portion of the stroke volume flows backward through the incompetent mitral valve. If MR develops slowly over months to years (as is seen with myxomatous degeneration or rheumatic disease), the left atrium is able to gradually dilate to accommodate the increase in volume. Atrial dilation predisposes the patient to developing atrial fibrillation and thrombus formation. With disease progression, patients eventually develop left ventricular dysfunction and signs of congestive heart failure. Even if severe, MR is usually well tolerated unless the patient is symptomatic prior to pregnancy.

MANAGEMENT AND ANESTHETIC CONSIDERATIONS

Patients who are asymptomatic do not require medical therapy during pregnancy; those who develop heart failure usually benefit from diuretics and vasodilators (such as hydralazine). Angiotensin-converting enzyme (ACE) inhibitors or angiotensin receptor antagonists (commonly used for afterload reduction) are contraindicated during pregnancy due to teratogenicity.

General goals in anesthetic management include the following: (1) prevent increases in SVR, (2) maintain sinus rhythm and avoid bradycardia, and (3) maintain venous return. Epidural analgesia helps minimize pain-related increases in SVR and is strongly recommended. Epidural anesthesia and spinal anesthesia for cesarean delivery are usually tolerated well because decreases in SVR favor forward blood flow. However, decreases in venous return should be treated with careful titration of intravenous fluids and vasopressor (phenylephrine) infusion. Invasive monitoring is usually reserved for patients with severe, symptomatic MR.

POSTPARTUM CARE

As noted above, most patients do not require much more than fairly routine care. Symptomatic patients, or those with known dysrhythmias, may need a more monitored setting for 1 to 2 days.

Aortic Insufficiency

ETIOLOGY/RISK FACTORS

Aortic insufficiency (AI) is often due to rheumatic disease and may occur with mitral valve disease. Other causes include congenital abnormalities of the aortic valve, endocarditis, and collagen vascular disease.

PATHOPHYSIOLOGY

AI leads to a state of volume overload and progressive left ventricular dilation and hypertrophy. Disease progression leads to left ventricular failure. Symptoms, such as dyspnea, orthopnea, palpitations, and angina, are usually not seen until disease is severe. Pregnancy and labor are typically well tolerated in patients with AI. The decrease in SVR with pregnancy promotes forward blood flow, and the concomitant increase in heart rate reduces time for regurgitation across the incompetent valve during diastole.

MANAGEMENT AND ANESTHETIC CONSIDERATIONS

Goals in the management of AI during labor and delivery primarily consist of maintaining a normal to slightly elevated heart rate and avoiding increases in SVR. Epidural analgesia is recommended during labor to avoid pain-induced increases in SVR. As with MR, epidural anesthesia and spinal anesthesia are usually tolerated well for cesarean delivery; decreases in SVR promote forward blood flow. However, abrupt hemodynamic changes associated with spinal anesthesia may be poorly tolerated in patients with severe disease, and epidural anesthesia is usually a better choice for these patients. Bradycardia (eg, from thoracic levels of regional anesthesia) may lead to an increase in regurgitant fraction; this may be problematic and should be treated promptly. Invasive monitoring is typically not needed.

POSTPARTUM CARE

Increases in blood volume and changes in SVR after delivery may lead to volume overload and left ventricular failure. Aggressive diuresis and afterload reduction (with nitrates and/or hydralazine) may be required.

Mitral Valve Prolapse

Mitral valve prolapse (MVP) is a variant of mitral valve disease, occurring commonly in women of childbearing age. MVP is usually asymptomatic, but some women may experience chest pain or palpitations and a small percentage of women will develop progressive mitral regurgitation. In the absence of coexisting cardiovascular disease, analgesic and anesthetic management rarely needs to be altered.

Pulmonary Stenosis

Pulmonary stenosis (PS) is one of the more common congenital cardiac defects and many patients remain asymptomatic well into adult life. Although severe PS can lead to right ventricular failure, it is very rare during pregnancy. It is important to understand that these patients *do not* behave like women with pulmonary vascular disease (pulmonary arterial hypertension), who are at grave risk during pregnancy and delivery. Isolated PS is usually well tolerated in pregnancy and labor, and cesarean delivery should be reserved for patients with obstetrical indications. Anesthetic and obstetric management in a stable patient with isolated PS does not usually need to be altered.

Prosthetic Valves

Management of pregnant women with prosthetic heart valves is extremely challenging. These women are at high risk for both fetal and maternal complications. These complications include thromboembolism, valve failure, endocarditis, and fetal hemorrhage and teratogenicity due to anticoagulation. The advantage of bioprosthetic valves in young women is the reduced risk of thromboembolism and need for anticoagulation during pregnancy. However, these valves are less durable than mechanical valves.[5] Mechanical valves seldom require replacement but require lifelong anticoagulation, which can be difficult to maintain due to hypercoagulable state during pregnancy and may complicate hemorrhage of delivery.

Warfarin crosses the placenta and is associated with a higher risk of spontaneous abortion, stillbirth, and fetal hemorrhage. Although considered safe during the first 6 weeks of pregnancy and after the first trimester, a fetus exposed to warfarin during weeks 6 through 12 of gestation is at risk for warfarin embryopathy. Unfractionated heparin (UFH) does not cross the placenta and is generally considered safer for the fetus regarding risk of embryopathy and hemorrhage. However, the incidence of thromboembolic disease, including fatal valve thrombosis, is higher.[6] Low-molecular-weight heparin (LMWH) also does not cross the placenta, and it has a longer half-life and more predictable dose-response pattern. Although LMWH at relatively high doses is now frequently being used in more women with prosthetic heart valves, treatment failures have been reported.

According to the American College of Chest Physicians, there is no single accepted treatment option for pregnant women with mechanical prosthetic valves, and the decision as to which regimen to use should be made after discussing risks and options with the patient. Possible regimens include (1) warfarin throughout pregnancy with LMWH or UFH substitution close to term, (2) either LMWH or UFH between 6 weeks and 12 weeks and close to term only and warfarin at other times, (3) aggressive dose-adjusted UFH throughout pregnancy, or (4) aggressive adjusted dose LMWH throughout pregnancy.[7]

Anticoagulation therapy may be discontinued prior to, or during labor, but occasionally therapy will need to be continued during this period and increases the risk of postpartum hemorrhage. The use of neuraxial anesthesia may be contraindicated based on the type and timing of anticoagulation doses, prolonged activated partial thromboplastin time (aPTT), elevated international normalized ratio (INR), or thrombocytopenia associated with heparin administration.

CONGENITAL HEART DISEASE

In the United States, congenital heart disease (CHD) is the most common form of heart disease in pregnant women. The majority of women with CHD now reach childbearing age because of advances in medical and surgical management, and many of these women will desire pregnancy. In general, asymptomatic patients with mild defects, or who underwent definitive repair as children, will tolerate pregnancy and labor well; these patients can usually be managed with routine or moderately advanced care. Patients with uncorrected or partially corrected anomalies, and those with residual defects, are less likely to tolerate the physiologic changes of pregnancy and can pose challenges to the obstetrician and anesthesiologist.

In patients who underwent corrective or palliative surgery as children, it is extremely important to understand the patient's anatomy. A discussion with the patient's cardiologist may be invaluable, and recent echocardiography or cardiac catheterization records should be reviewed. It is surprising (and concerning) how often the physicians caring for such patients do not fully understand the current cardiac anatomy/function of the patient (ie, "where does the blood flow actually go?"). Knowledge of complex anatomy, residual defects, and current functional status can guide decision making regarding anesthetic technique and invasive hemodynamic monitoring.

Although maternal mortality during pregnancy is rare generally, many patients with CHD will experience adverse events. Risk factors for complications during pregnancy include the following[8,9]:

- NYHA functional class greater than II
- Cyanosis
- Left heart obstruction
- Prior cardiac event or dysrhythmia
- Systemic ventricular dysfunction

Specific congenital cardiac abnormalities to be discussed in this section include: left-to-right shunts, tetralogy of Fallot, single ventricle with Fontan physiology, transposition of the great vessels, coarctation of the aorta, and Marfan syndrome. Bicuspid aortic valve and pulmonic stenosis have been discussed in the "valve disease" section.

Left-to-Right Shunts (Atrial Septal Defect, Ventricular Septal Defect, and Patent Ductus Arteriosus)

Left-to-right shunts include atrial septal defect (ASD), ventricular septal defect (VSD), and patent ductus arteriosus (PDA). Large defects are associated with congestive heart failure and are typically detected and repaired in childhood.

Patients with small defects may be asymptomatic into adulthood and usually tolerate pregnancy well. ASDs account for about one-third of congenital heart defects in adults and occur more commonly in women.[10] ASDs typically do not spontaneously close and may be associated with other cardiac abnormalities (mitral valve prolapse, MR, partial anomalous pulmonary venous return). VSDs are the most common congenital heart defect and occur with similar frequency in males and females. Up to 40% of VSDs close spontaneously by 2 years of age, and 90% close spontaneously by 10 years of age. PDA accounts for about 10% of congenital heart defects; lesions that persist past infancy are unlikely to close spontaneously.

PATHOPHYSIOLOGY

The overall physiologic effect of an ASD is shunting of blood from the left atrium to the right atrium regardless of anatomic location of the defect (ostium primum, ostium secundum, or sinus venosus). Most ASDs are initially asymptomatic and may not be detected for years. The size of the defect ultimately determines the hemodynamic consequences of this lesion. Patients with small defects (less than 0.5 cm in diameter) typically remain asymptomatic and do not require closure. Those with moderate to large (greater than 2 cm in diameter) defects may have severe hemodynamic consequences that may not be apparent until the third to fourth decade of life.[10] With time, the increased blood flow to the right side of the heart leads to right atrial and ventricular dilation and pulmonary hypertension. Patients with an ASD are at risk of developing dysrhythmias and paradoxical embolism. Severe disease may lead to Eisenmenger syndrome, although the latter is rare and more likely to occur with VSD.

VSDs may occur in isolation or with other congenital heart defects, such as tetralogy of Fallot. VSDs may occur at various locations within the ventricular septum and are classified a: membranous, subpulmonic (outlet), atrioventricular canal (inlet), or muscular. As with ASD, the size of the defect determines the hemodynamic consequences of this lesion. Small defects lead to minimal increases in pulmonary blood flow. Large defects, however, lead to sizable increases in pulmonary blood flow and ultimately result in left ventricular volume overload and dilation. With time, pulmonary vascular resistance (PVR) increases. As PVR exceeds systemic resistance, reversal of flow across the defect and cyanosis results (Eisenmenger syndrome). Large VSDs rarely persist into adulthood without surgical intervention. Surgical closure typically is performed in childhood; this involves a right atrial or ventricular incision and can lead to significant conduction abnormalities.

PDA occurs when the ductus arteriosus fails to close shortly after birth. In the fetus, the ductus arteriosus connects the aorta and pulmonary artery allowing blood to bypass the lungs. Failure of the ductus to close after birth results in continued blood flow from the aorta to the pulmonary artery. As with a VSD, the resultant left-to-right shunt results in left ventricular volume overload and dilation. When uncorrected, pulmonary vascular changes may lead to reversal of flow and cyanosis. Infants with PDA are typically diagnosed with symptoms of heart failure or failure to thrive; rarely, uncorrected adults may present with heart failure or cyanosis.

MANAGEMENT AND ANESTHETIC CONSIDERATIONS

The balance between SVR and PVR determines the amount of shunt flow. Acute changes in either can alter amount or direction of flow. Early epidural anesthesia is recommended to avoid pain-induced increases in SVR during labor. An increase in SVR is likely to worsen left-to-right shunting and can lead to right ventricular failure. Large decreases in SVR should also be avoided, because direction of flow through the defect may reverse and create a right-to-left shunt and hypoxemia. Thus, incrementally dosed epidural anesthesia is favored over spinal anesthesia in patients with large defects requiring cesarean delivery. Increases in PVR should be avoided with the use of supplemental oxygen and avoidance of hypercarbia. Routine monitors include pulse oximetry and ECG. CVP and arterial line monitoring should be considered in symptomatic patients. PA catheters are typically not used and are often difficult or dangerous to position in the setting of left-to-right shunting.

Air embolism poses a particularly serious potential risk in these patients, and intravenous lines should be meticulously monitored and cleared of air. In addition, saline is recommended for loss of resistance during epidural placement, because paradoxical embolism can occur if air enters an epidural vein. Uterotonics that increase SVR, such as methylergonovine (Methergine), should be used cautiously or not at all.

Tetralogy of Fallot

Tetralogy of Fallot (TOF) accounts for 10% of CHD and is the most common cause of cyanotic CHD.[11] TOF is typically diagnosed prenatally or during infancy with manifestation of cyanosis. The majority of patients who have undergone corrective repair are asymptomatic, and the long-term survival rate at 35 years following repair is approximately 85%.[11]

PATHOPHYSIOLOGY

The defect consists of four parts: VSD, right ventricular outflow tract obstruction (RVOTO), right ventricular hypertrophy (RVH), and an "overriding" aorta. Obstruction of the right ventricular outflow tract leads to right-to-left shunting of blood across the VSD and results in cyanosis. The severity of RVOTO (which varies) and alterations in SVR determine the magnitude of shunting.

Traditionally, palliation was achieved with a systemic-to-pulmonary shunt (eg, Blalock-Taussig shunt) to improve pulmonary blood flow, and definitive repair was performed later in life. Problems with chronic hypoxia, shunt dysfunction, and other long-term sequelae led to a change in surgical practice. Corrective surgery is now typically completed during infancy. Complete surgical correction includes closure of the VSD and relief of RVOTO. Chronic complications of repaired TOF include ventricular dysrhythmias, right bundle branch block, pulmonary regurgitation, recurrent RVOTO, and residual VSD.[10] Although most patients with corrected TOF tolerate pregnancy well, changes in cardiac output, blood volume and SVR during pregnancy may unmask previously undetected residua. A moderate (8%) risk of cardiovascular events, most commonly dysrhythmias, has been reported in a recent series.[12]

MANAGEMENT AND ANESTHETIC CONSIDERATIONS

Echocardiography should be performed prior to and during pregnancy to assess cardiac function and identify residual defects. Heart failure and dysrhythmias may develop with changes in blood volume and cardiac output early in pregnancy. Continuous ECG monitoring during labor is reasonable given the increased risk of dysrhythmias. Otherwise, asymptomatic patients with corrected TOF can usually be managed routinely.

Patients with uncorrected TOF and those with residua are more challenging to manage. Large increases or decreases in SVR should be avoided; thus, early labor epidural analgesia is recommended to prevent pain-induced changes in SVR, and spinal anesthesia should be avoided because of a rapid and profound sympathectomy. Elevations in PVR should be minimized with use of supplemental oxygen and avoidance of hypercarbia and acidosis. Euvolemia should be maintained, and hypotension should be treated immediately. Phenylephrine, probably by infusion rather than intermittent bolus, should be used to increase SVR if right-to-left shunting develops. Invasive monitoring (at least an arterial line) should be used in patients who have demonstrated hemodynamic instability. Arterial lines should be placed in the opposite extremity of any surgically created systemic to pulmonary shunts.

Single Ventricle With Fontan Physiology

The Fontan procedure was initially introduced as a palliative procedure for patients with tricuspid atresia. It has since been utilized in patients with complex congenital defects in which biventricular repair is not possible, including double-inlet left ventricle, double-outlet right ventricle, and hypoplastic left heart syndrome.

PATHOPHYSIOLOGY

The Fontan procedure is performed as a staged repair and has multiple variations that ultimately result in the separation of pulmonary and systemic circulation. The Fontan circulation is unique in that systemic venous return is diverted directly into the pulmonary arteries. Pulmonary blood flow is entirely passive and dependent on high systemic venous pressure. Negative intrathoracic pressure during spontaneous respiration also aids in maintaining forward pulmonary blood flow. Cardiac output is derived from pulmonary venous return. Long-term complications of the Fontan procedure include atrial dysrhythmias, ventricular dysfunction, thromboembolic events, hepatic dysfunction, and protein-losing enteropathy.[13] Although long-term survival with Fontan circulation is significantly reduced and complications are common, many of these women will survive to adulthood and desire pregnancy. Small case series of pregnancies in patients with Fontan circulation have reported a high spontaneous miscarriage rate and increased incidence of cardiac complications (dysrhythmia and decreased functional status) but no maternal deaths have been reported.[14]

MANAGEMENT AND ANESTHETIC CONSIDERATIONS

Preload must be maintained, because pulmonary blood flow is passive and dependent on high systemic venous pressure. Hypovolemia and aortocaval compression can be deleterious and must be avoided. Any elevation in PVR will limit forward pulmonary blood flow; notably, hypercarbia and acidosis must be avoided, and supplemental oxygen should be administered. Early epidural anesthesia is recommended to avoid pain-associated alterations in hemodynamics, although any decrease in venous return can be very detrimental. Slow titration of dilute local anesthetic with opioid will minimize alterations in SVR and preload and allow time for treatment. Slow incremental dosing of epidural anesthesia is also recommended for cesarean delivery. Maintenance of preload, the main "driving force" for pulmonary blood flow in the absence of a right ventricle, is essential and will frequently require a vasopressor (phenylephrine or norepinephrine) support. An arterial line and central venous line may be useful both for monitoring rapid changes with changes in preload and for administering vasopressor agents rapidly and safely. Although the need for CVP monitoring is controversial, intra-arterial pressure monitoring in laboring (or cesarean) patients with Fontan physiology is useful because it enables the physician to titrate phenylephrine or norepinephrine more accurately and maintain the CVP at prelabor or preanesthesia baseline values (typically 15-20 mm Hg). A less invasive alternative is to simply treat any decrease in blood pressure with aggressive fluid loading and vasopressor support. Spinal anesthesia for cesarean or even analgesic doses for labor is a poor choice due to associated sympathectomy and decrease in preload in these patients who are dependent exclusively on preload. Given the increased risk of thromboembolic events in the Fontan state, in addition to the hypercoagulable state of pregnancy, many of these patients will be anticoagulated. As many of these patients also have chronic liver dysfunction from congestion, coagulation studies should be reviewed prior to administration of neuraxial anesthesia. Routine monitors should include pulse oximetry and continuous ECG monitoring. For cesarean delivery, spontaneous ventilation should be preserved (regional anesthesia) if possible, because negative intrathoracic pressure aids in maintaining forward pulmonary blood flow. All efforts should be made to avoid increases in PVR and preserve adequate function of the single ventricle.

Transposition of the Great Vessels

Transposition of the great vessels (TGV) is relatively rare, but women with congenitally corrected TGV and those with surgically corrected complete TGV will often reach childbearing age.

PATHOPHYSIOLOGY

Congenitally corrected TGV (L-TGV) is characterized by atrioventricular and ventriculoarterial discordance. Blood flows from the right atrium into the morphologic left ventricle and into the pulmonary artery to the lungs. Blood returns into the left atrium, flows into the morphologic right ventricle and out the aorta. L-TGV is associated with other defects, most commonly intracardiac shunts, but may occur in isolation (and the patient may not be symptomatic until adulthood). The morphologic right ventricle is ultimately at risk for hypertrophy and failure because it functions as the systemic ventricle.

Complete TGV (D-TGV) consists of two circulations in parallel. Systemic venous blood flows into the right atrium, right ventricle, and out the aorta, and pulmonary venous blood flows into the left atrium, left ventricle, and into the pulmonary artery. This defect requires a site for mixing of blood (PDA, ASD, or VSD) for survival to occur. Traditional atrial switch (Mustard or Senning) procedures involve the creation of baffles, which are conduits that route venous blood to the appropriate ventricle at the level of the atria. Problems with this procedure include baffle stenosis, dysrhythmias, and right ventricular failure (the right ventricle remains the systemic ventricle). The arterial switch or Jatene procedure involves switching the great vessels to the correct anatomic location and reimplantation of the coronary arteries.

Patients who have undergone successful arterial switch procedures should tolerate pregnancy well. Those with a systemic right ventricle are at risk for developing heart failure with expansion of blood volume and increase in cardiac output. Connolly et al. reported on 60 pregnancies in 22 women with L-TGV; pregnancy was well tolerated in all but 2 women. One woman experienced atrioventricular valve dysfunction requiring valve replacement in the postpartum period. The other woman, who had 11 previous pregnancies, suffered from multiple cardiac complications including congestive heart failure, endocarditis and a myocardial infarction.[15]

MANAGEMENT AND ANESTHETIC CONSIDERATIONS

Echocardiography should be performed prior to or early in pregnancy to evaluate valvular and systemic ventricular function and to assess baffle patency. Continuous ECG monitoring should be utilized during labor, because dysrhythmias are common in patients who have undergone cardiac surgery.

Patients with evidence of heart failure should be carefully monitored with an arterial line and central venous line during labor. Volume shifts are poorly tolerated, and invasive hemodynamic monitoring will help guide fluid administration. Early epidural analgesia will help limit pain-associated increases in SVR and cardiac output. Forceps may be used to shorten the second stage of labor and reduce stress on the heart. Vaginal delivery is associated with less hemodynamic alterations after delivery and is preferred over cesarean delivery.

Patients with successful arterial switch procedures in childhood are likely to tolerate pregnancy and labor well, and they should be treated as normal patients.

Coarctation of the Aorta

Coarctation of the aorta is present in 6% to 8% of patients with congenital heart disease and disproportionately affects men rather than women.[16] The diagnosis is usually made in infancy or childhood but occasionally it is not detected until adulthood. The most frequent association with coarctation is a bicuspid aortic valve, but VSD, PDA, mitral stenosis, and aneurysms of the circle of Willis may also be seen.[10]

PATHOPHYSIOLOGY

Coarctation of the aorta consists of a narrowing that typically occurs distal to the origin of the left subclavian artery, resulting in upper extremity hypertension.

Occasionally, the narrowing occurs proximal to the left subclavian artery, and hypertension is only seen in the right arm. Perfusion distal to the narrowing is achieved with extensive collateral circulation involving the internal thoracic, intercostal, subclavian, and scapular arteries. The diagnosis may be made in the neonatal period with poor feeding and failure to thrive; circulatory collapse and shock may be seen in severe cases. More commonly, the diagnosis is made in childhood with upper extremity hypertension, diminished lower extremity pulses, wide pulse pressure, and left ventricular hypertrophy on ECG. Those who are diagnosed as adults typically present with symptoms related to severe hypertension (headache), claudication, or heart failure.

Complications include left ventricular hypertrophy and failure, coronary artery disease, aortic dissection, infective endocarditis, and stroke.[10] Treatment includes balloon dilation or surgical repair, and surgery is considered for patients with a gradient of more than 30 mm Hg across the narrowing. Persistent hypertension is common when repair is not performed until adulthood.

Patients with coarctation (both corrected and uncorrected) tend to tolerate pregnancy well. In a series of 118 pregnancies in 50 women, Beauchesne et al. described fatal aortic dissection in one patient with previously repaired coarctation but no other serious cardiovascular complications. Hypertension was common and was related to the presence of hemodynamically significant coarctation gradients.[16]

MANAGEMENT AND ANESTHETIC CONSIDERATIONS

Blood pressure management during pregnancy and labor is challenging in patients with uncorrected or residual coarctation. Poorly controlled hypertension increases the risk of fetal growth retardation, placental abruption, premature delivery, heart failure, and aortic rupture or dissection. However, placental perfusion may depend on high pressures proximal to the coarctation if there is a large distal pressure drop and inadequate collaterals. β-Adrenergic blockade is utilized to decrease blood pressure and reduce hemodynamic stress on the aortic wall. Any antihypertensive must be titrated carefully to avoid compromising placental perfusion distal to the coarctation.

In general, vaginal delivery is associated with fewer hemodynamic alterations and fluid shifts than cesarean delivery and is preferred in patients with corrected or mild coarctation. Epidural anesthesia reduces hemodynamic stress and should be administered early. The second stage of labor may be shortened with forceps-assisted delivery. If cesarean delivery is necessary, local anesthetic and opioids should be titrated slowly to avoid large decreases in SVR and hypotension distal to the coarctation. Planned cesarean delivery may be safer in patients with severe uncorrected coarctation. Pain-associated alterations in hemodynamics during labor may increase the risk of aortic rupture or dissection, and decreases in SVR with labor epidural analgesia may compromise placental perfusion. General anesthesia with a preinduction upper extremity arterial line is usually preferred for cesarean delivery if the obstruction is severe enough to warrant this mode of delivery. Epidural anesthesia may be considered; slow dosing and judicious use of phenylephrine are necessary to avoid compromises in placental perfusion. In addition to an upper extremity arterial line, a lower extremity arterial line can be placed to measure perfusion pressure distal to the coarctation during epidural dosing, and continuous fetal monitoring should be utilized as another measure of adequate placental perfusion.

Marfan Syndrome

Marfan syndrome is a disorder of connective tissue inherited as an autosomal dominant pattern. Because of its considerable clinical variability, Marfan syndrome may remain undiagnosed before pregnancy and be recognized only after the development of complications.[17]

PATHOPHYSIOLOGY

A defect in fibrillin synthesis leads to a range of musculoskeletal, ocular, and cardiovascular abnormalities, with aortic dilation being the most serious defect. Mitral valve prolapse is common, and aortic insufficiency may be seen with dilatation of the aortic root.

Progressive aortic dilation may lead to dissecting aortic aneurysm or even aortic rupture. Pregnancy is associated with an increased risk of aortic dissection. This is likely due to hormonally mediated histologic changes in the aortic wall in addition to the hemodynamic changes seen with pregnancy.[18] Dissection occurs when a tear in the intima allows blood to flow in a false lumen between the intima and media or adventitia in the aortic wall. Severe chest or back pain is the most common symptom. Patients at increased risk include those with aortic root diameter exceeding 40 mm, rapid aortic dilation, or previous dissection.[17] Aortic dissection in pregnancy is associated with a high mortality rate, and aortic rupture is almost always fatal.

MANAGEMENT AND ANESTHETIC CONSIDERATIONS

All women with Marfan syndrome should be evaluated prior to pregnancy by a cardiologist, with echocardiographic evaluation of aortic diameter and valvular function. Prophylactic aortic repair before pregnancy is recommended in women with ascending aortic dilation exceeding 50 mm, evidence of rapid dilatation, a family history of premature aortic dissection, or the presence of more than mild aortic insufficiency. Medical management consists of β-blocker therapy to limit shear stress and slow the growth of the aortic root and to reduce the rate of cardiovascular complications. Serial echocardiography should be performed during pregnancy to monitor for aortic root growth.

There is no consensus regarding the most optimal mode of delivery in patients with Marfan syndrome. Women with no significant cardiovascular disease and a normal size and nonexpanding aorta tend to tolerate pregnancy and labor well. Epidural analgesia should be utilized early to reduce pain-associated cardiovascular stress, and forceps may be utilized to shorten the second stage of labor. However, there is strong tendency toward recommending cesarean delivery for patients at perceived higher risk for dissection (as outlined above) to avoid the cardiovascular stress associated with prolonged labor and expulsive efforts, and this is one of the few disease entities that some regard as a cardiovascular indication for cesarean delivery. It may well be that most patients with diagnosed Marfan syndrome deliver by cesarean; however, it is not clear if cesarean delivery is truly safer in those with a dilated aorta. Epidural anesthesia is the preferred anesthetic for cesarean delivery, avoiding increases in heart rate and blood pressure associated with laryngoscopy and intubation. If general anesthesia is necessary, significant efforts should be made to attenuate the sympathetic response to laryngoscopy, and transient hypotension or bradycardia would seem to be less concerning than a short period of tachycardia/hypertension. Maintenance of β-blockade and control of blood pressure and heart rate are the centerpieces of hemodynamic management. Short-acting vasodilators and β-adrenergic blocking agents should be readily available to treat hypertension and tachycardia, and an arterial line should be in place for continuous blood pressure monitoring to facilitate rapid therapy.

Postpartum Care of Women With Congenital Heart Disease

It is difficult to make general recommendations for postpartum care of women with CHD given the wide variability in the nature and severity of disease, because decisions about the nature and location of care of these women are based on the severity of disease and the course of labor and delivery. For uncomplicated cases of ASD or VSD, completely routine postpartum observation and management may be warranted. Simply increased vigilance may be all that is needed for most women with CHD who have had relatively uneventful courses. For patients with more severe disease, especially those who have had complications (heart failure, dysrhythmias) during pregnancy or labor and delivery, observation in a high-risk unit or intensive care unit for 1 or 2 days is warranted.

Pharmacologic diuresis is frequently needed in the first hours to day 1 or 2 in patients with impaired myocardial function. As a general rule, any invasive monitoring indicated and used during a cesarean delivery or labor should almost always be continued for 24 to 48 hours. This time period is associated with significant hemodynamic alterations, especially volume overload, and the possibility of hemorrhage, either of which may be poorly tolerated in compromised patients.

CARDIOMYOPATHY

Peripartum Cardiomyopathy

Peripartum cardiomyopathy (PPCM) is a pregnancy-associated form of heart failure in women without known cardiovascular disease. The European Society of Cardiology Working Group on PPCM recently proposed the following definition of PPCM: "Peripartum cardiomyopathy is an idiopathic cardiomyopathy presenting with heart failure secondary to left ventricular (LV) systolic dysfunction towards the end of pregnancy or in the months following delivery, where no other cause of heart failure is found. It is a diagnosis of exclusion. The LV may not be dilated but the ejection fraction (EF) is nearly always reduced below 45%."[19] Historical criteria for diagnosis include the onset of heart failure in the last month of pregnancy, or within 5 months of delivery. This strict time cutoff may lead to underdiagnosis of PPCM, as it is not uncommon for women to present earlier in pregnancy.[20]

EPIDEMIOLOGY

The true incidence of PPCM is unknown. Existing single-center case series suggest that PPCM is more common in certain areas of the world (Haiti, South Africa, West Africa), but prospective, population-based, epidemiologic studies are needed.[19] Recent studies of PPCM in the United States suggest an incidence of approximately 1:3200 deliveries, with a higher incidence in African-American women.[20] PPCM has also been associated with increased maternal age, hypertensive disease, multiparity, and multiple gestation. Maternal mortality due to cardiomyopathy may be increasing, whereas other causes of cardiac mortality are tending to decline.

ETIOLOGY

The etiology of PPCM is unknown. Theoretical causes include viral myocarditis, abnormal autoimmune or inflammatory response to pregnancy, abnormal response to the hemodynamic burden of pregnancy, and malnutrition. Recent experimental studies suggest a mechanism involving enhanced oxidative stress and cleavage of prolactin into an antiangiogenic and proapoptotic prolactin fragment that leads to impaired myocardiocyte function[21] and some intriguing relationships and similarities between the pathophysiologic mechanisms of PPCM and preeclampsia.[22]

PATHOPHYSIOLOGY

Heart failure usually develops during the last month of pregnancy or in the first 5 months after delivery. Many of the signs and symptoms of early heart failure (shortness of breath, fatigue, and peripheral edema) are also seen toward the end of a normal pregnancy, and diagnosis can be delayed. Cough, chest pain, elevated jugular venous pressure, new murmurs of mitral and tricuspid regurgitation, and rales on chest examination should raise the suspicion for heart failure. Diagnosis of PPCM relies on the exclusion of other causes of cardiomyopathy and echocardiographic evidence of reduced left ventricular function. Left ventricular dilation is typical but not uniform, and left ventricular thrombosis is not uncommon in patients with an EF less than 35%. The prognosis in PPCM varies geographically. In the United States, approximately 50% of women will show recovery of left ventricular function at 6 months. The rate of recovery appears to be lower in African-American women and in those with EF less than 30% at time of diagnosis. Although many patients recover, PPCM is associated with severe complications, including progressive heart failure, cardiogenic shock, thromboembolic complications and death. Mortality rates in the United States vary between 0% and 19%, with heart transplant rates ranging between 6% and 11%.[20]

MANAGEMENT AND ANESTHETIC CONSIDERATIONS

Rapid treatment of acute heart failure in pregnancy is essential. Management is similar to that of heart failure from other causes and includes supplemental oxygen, diuretics, and afterload reduction (ACE inhibitors are contraindicated during pregnancy but are a mainstay of therapy after delivery). Inotropic agents may be necessary in patients with evidence of hypoperfusion. In the setting of rapid deterioration despite medical therapy, placement of an intra-aortic balloon pump or left ventricular assist device may be necessary as a bridge to recovery or transplant. Delivery of the fetus should be expedited in the hemodynamically unstable patient. The fetus is unlikely to thrive in the setting of hypoperfusion and delivery allows for more aggressive treatment of the woman. Anticoagulation (with UFH or enoxaparin during pregnancy and warfarin after delivery) is recommended from the time of diagnosis until left ventricular function recovers (EF greater than 35%) because of the high risk of thromboembolic events.

Invasive hemodynamic monitoring, including arterial and PA catheters, is usually required for patients with severe, symptomatic PPCM, similar to therapy in other patients with severe end-stage heart failure undergoing intensive hemodynamic stress (in this case, delivery). Pain management with epidural anesthesia for vaginal delivery should attenuate heart rate increases and gently lower SVR. Epidural anesthesia should be utilized early, and the second stage of labor should be shortened with use of forceps or vacuum. A slow, incrementally dosed epidural anesthetic is also recommended for cesarean delivery if time is available. General anesthesia may be necessary in the setting of sudden, severe decompensation (eg, severe pulmonary edema unresponsive to diuresis); high-dose, short-acting opioids (remifentanil) may be the best option to avoid myocardial depression. TEE should be strongly considered if general anesthesia is necessary in order to evaluate cardiac function and for therapeutic and diagnostic/prognostic reasons.

POSTPARTUM CARE

Autotransfusion of blood from the contracted uterus may increase preload, and additional diuresis may be needed. Methylergonovine should be avoided if possible because it is likely to increase SVR. Medical management after delivery includes fluid restriction, diuretics, ACE inhibitors, β-blockers, and anticoagulation. In general, women have a high risk of relapse of PPCM in subsequent pregnancies. Patients with an EF less than 25% at diagnosis and those who have not returned to normal cardiac function are generally advised against subsequent pregnancy.

Hypertrophic Cardiomyopathy

Hypertrophic cardiomyopathy (HCM) is a genetic cardiovascular disorder resulting in left ventricular hypertrophy (LVH) and dynamic left ventricular outflow tract obstruction (LVOTO). Diagnosis is made with cardiac imaging (typically echocardiography) and genetic testing.

EPIDEMIOLOGY

HCM appears to be a global disease with a prevalence of 0.2%.[23] The disorder is not commonly seen in clinical practice, implying that most affected individuals are asymptomatic and never diagnosed. However, HCM is the leading cause of sudden cardiac death in young patients.[24]

ETIOLOGY

HCM is inherited in an autosomal dominant pattern and involves mutation of genes that encode sarcomere proteins. Children of a parent with HCM have a 50% chance of inheriting the disease. Genetic screening of family members is important to identify those with unrecognized disease.

PATHOPHYSIOLOGY

Patients with HCM typically have LVH with asymmetric hypertrophy of the septum. LVOTO is variable; approximately one-third of patients have obstruction at rest, one-third have no obstruction at all, and one-third have labile obstruction.[23] The degree of LVOTO depends on loading conditions and contractility of the left ventricle; increased contractility, decreased ventricular volume, and decreased SVR tend to worsen obstruction. Hypertrophy and stiffness of the left ventricle commonly lead to diastolic dysfunction, and ischemia may occur due to mismatch of oxygen supply and demand. Unpredictable ventricular tachydysrhythmias may result in sudden cardiac death.

Pregnancy tends to be well tolerated among women with HCM, although the decrease in SVR and increase in contractility associated with pregnancy may exacerbate LVOTO and worsen symptoms in some patients. The volume increase may be of some benefit. Autore et al studied 199 pregnancies in 100 women with HCM; although maternal mortality was increased in patients with HCM compared to the general population, absolute maternal mortality was low. As is common in the epidemiology and prognosis of cardiac disease of all types, morbidity was more common in women who were symptomatic prior to pregnancy.[25]

MANAGEMENT AND ANESTHETIC CONSIDERATIONS

Medical treatment consists of decreasing cardiac contractility, maintaining intravascular blood volume, and avoiding decreases in SVR. β-Blockers and calcium channel blockers are used to decrease cardiac contractility and increase diastolic filling time; these should be continued during pregnancy. Diuretics and vasodilating medications should be avoided. Septal reduction therapy may be considered in patients who remain symptomatic despite optimal medical therapy. Anesthetic goals include maintaining intravascular volume, avoiding decreases in SVR, and preventing increases in heart rate and contractility. Neuraxial anesthesia (epidural or CSE) may be used for labor. Decreases in preload (ie, ventricular volume) are problematic, but excess sympathetic stimulation form pain in labor can also increase LVOTO, so the best plan, as with many other syndromes discussed in this chapter, is analgesia with attention paid to maintenance of preload. Phenylephrine is clearly preferred over ephedrine given its pure vasoconstrictive effect; contractility will worsen outflow tract obstruction. The combination of β-blockade and α-1 agonism is commonly used to keep the left ventricular outflow tract "open." Cesarean delivery is typically reserved for obstetric indications. Epidural anesthesia (or perhaps low-dose CSE) is preferred over single-shot spinal for cesarean delivery due to the profound sympathectomy associated with the latter. If general anesthesia is necessary, short-acting β-blockers and opioids may be used to decrease the response to laryngoscopy and intubation. Regardless of anesthetic technique, phenylephrine should be used to maintain SVR. Invasive lines are usually only necessary for those patients with severe or worsening symptoms.

POSTPARTUM CARE

Autotransfusion from uterine involution is likely to improve symptoms in the postpartum period, and hypovolemia from postpartum hemorrhage is poorly tolerated and should be aggressively treated with intravenous fluids and phenylephrine. On balance, mild volume overload is better than hypovolemia. Oxytocin should be administered slowly because it may cause vasodilation; methylergonovine would be the preferred uterotonic agent—the SVR increase is well tolerated and perhaps beneficial.

PULMONARY HYPERTENSION

EPIDEMIOLOGY

Idiopathic pulmonary hypertension is a rare disease, with an estimated annual incidence of 4 cases per million, and it is traditionally regarded as a disease that affects young females. The incidence of pulmonary hypertension associated with cardiac and respiratory disorders is likely to be much higher.[26] Although rare, pulmonary vascular disease in pregnancy is associated with an extremely high maternal mortality rate between 30% and 50%.[27]

ETIOLOGY/RISK FACTORS

Pulmonary hypertension is defined by a mean pulmonary artery pressure greater than 25 mm Hg with a mean pulmonary capillary wedge pressure (PCWP) less than 15 mm Hg. There are five main categories of pulmonary hypertension with shared pathologic and clinical features: (1) pulmonary arterial hypertension (PAH), which can be idiopathic, heritable, or associated with congenital heart disease or connective tissue disease; (2) pulmonary hypertension secondary to left heart disease; (3) pulmonary hypertension in association with lung disease and/or hypoxia; (4) chronic thromboembolic pulmonary hypertension; and (5) a miscellaneous group.[28,29] Patients with PCWP greater than 15 mm Hg typically have pulmonary hypertension secondary to heart disease.

PATHOPHYSIOLOGY

Pulmonary hypertension is associated with a reduction in vascular nitric oxide and prostacyclin synthesis together with an increase in endothelin and thromboxane production. Histologically, the pulmonary arteries in pulmonary hypertension are characterized by intimal fibrosis, medial hypertrophy, adventitial proliferation, and obliteration of small arteries. Hypertrophy and fibrosis of the pulmonary vasculature result in increases in PVR. As PVR increases, the right ventricle hypertrophies, dilates, and eventually results in right ventricular dysfunction. As right-sided cardiac pressures increase, the intraventricular septum paradoxically bows to the left during systole, impairing left ventricular filling. The combination of impaired left ventricular filling and right ventricular dysfunction leads to decreases in cardiac output. This can lead to myocardial ischemia and worsening of right and left ventricular function. Hypoxemia from low cardiac output and pulmonary blood flow further increases PVR. As the disease progresses, PVR continues to increase, cardiac output continues to fall, and right ventricular failure ultimately leads to death.

The normal cardiovascular changes seen in pregnancy are poorly tolerated in patients with pulmonary hypertension. Pregnancy is associated with a 40% to 50% increase in cardiac output, a 50% increase in blood volume, and a 20% increase in oxygen consumption. The impaired right ventricle often cannot accommodate these changes. Previously undiagnosed patients may present with progressive dyspnea, palpitations, and chest pain due to right ventricular ischemia, fatigue, and presyncope or syncope. The hypercoagulable state of pregnancy combined with the decreased output and flow from the pressure-overloaded right ventricle can lead to pulmonary embolus and thrombus formation. Platelet activity is enhanced, and thrombosis is often found in pulmonary arterioles of patients with pulmonary hypertension.[30] Even "subclinical" pulmonary embolism may be significantly deleterious in patients with an already compromised pulmonary circulation. Of note, pulmonary pressures are often assessed by echocardiography during pregnancy in women in whom pulmonary hypertension is suspected; these measurements have been shown to be very unreliable and may not correlate at all with directly measured pressures.[31]

MANAGEMENT AND ANESTHETIC CONSIDERATIONS

Women with pulmonary hypertension are frequently counseled to avoid or terminate pregnancy. A multidisciplinary team, including high-risk obstetricians, anesthesiologists, cardiologists, and hematologists, should manage patients who do become pregnant; frequent visits throughout pregnancy are necessary. Detailed plans for timing and mode of delivery, early hospitalization, and targeted therapy may facilitate safer delivery.

Anesthetic and hemodynamic goals during labor and delivery include (1) prevention of increases in PVR by avoiding hypoxemia, acidosis, and hypercarbia; (2) maintenance of intravascular volume and venous return; (3) avoidance of aortocaval compression; (4) maintenance of adequate SVR; and (5) avoidance of myocardial depression during general anesthesia. The goals are not easy to accomplish, and no consensus exists on optimal management despite recent advances in pharmacologic therapy of PAH.

The optimal mode of delivery for women with PAH is controversial. Vaginal delivery is associated with smaller hemodynamic fluctuations as well as fewer bleeding and clotting complications, although a recent series reported excellent outcomes with elective cesarean delivery.[28] It is often difficult to compare series and outcomes due to significant differences in severity of disease. Although pulmonary pressures are not the only variable denoting severity, it is clear that a woman with PA pressures of 110/70 mm Hg is at higher risk than the women with pressures of 60/30 mm Hg, both clearly fulfill the criteria for PAH, however. In labor, early epidural placement would seem essential, and instrumental delivery may be beneficial to avoid increases in PVR associated with pain and bearing down.

Intrathecal opioids may produce effective analgesia without sympathectomy for early first-stage labor pain, allowing more careful titration of blockade as labor proceeds. Although oxytocin infusion can lower SVR and increase PVR, it has been used to induce labor without hemodynamic compromise in several reports.

Although operative delivery has been associated with increased mortality in women with pulmonary hypertension, Kiely et al. described improved survival using a strategy of early introduction of targeted pulmonary vascular therapy and early planned cesarean delivery under regional anesthesia.[28] Cesarean delivery avoids a prolonged second stage of labor and the hemodynamic effects of bearing down, but the potential for hypovolemia from excessive blood loss or hypervolemia from rapid uterine contraction after delivery remains a concern. Single shot spinal anesthesia is contraindicated due to profound decreases in SVR, but slowly titrated epidural anesthesia with fluid or pharmacologic agents to help maintain venous return is usually well tolerated.

General anesthesia is generally poorly tolerated in patients (pregnant or not) with pulmonary hypertension. Positive pressure ventilation impairs venous return, stimulation from laryngoscopy and intubation can increase pulmonary pressures and volatile agents depress cardiac contractility and decrease SVR. An opioid-based technique for induction can minimize the sympathetic response to laryngoscopy and intubation at the cost of long-term ventilation. Nitrous oxide increases PVR and should be avoided. In general, elevation in PVR due to hypoxia, hypercarbia, hypothermia, acidosis, high ventilation pressures, and sympathomimetic agents should be avoided. One advantage of general anesthesia is the ability to administer nitric oxide, particularly in patients known to be sensitive/responsive. Arterial and central venous pressure monitoring are frequently utilized regardless of mode of delivery. PA catheter placement enables continuous monitoring of pulmonary pressures and cardiac output but is associated with serious, possible fatal complications such as pulmonary artery rupture and thrombosis. Oxygen saturation and cardiac rhythm should be continuously monitored in all patients with PAH. TEE should be strongly considered in patients receiving general anesthesia.

The vasculature in PAH typically remains responsive to vasodilators, whereas Eisenmenger syndrome is characterized by an unresponsive vasculature. PAH therapies include endothelin-receptor antagonists, prostacyclin and prostacyclin analogs, phosphodiesterase inhibitors, calcium channel blockers, and inhaled nitric oxide. Only a minority of patients respond to calcium channel blockers and endothelin-receptor antagonists are contraindicated in pregnancy due to risk of teratogenicity.[26] Anticoagulation with LMWH is recommended because of the hypercoagulable state of pregnancy and risk of thromboembolic events. There are no large studies investigating PAH treatment in pregnancy, but several case reports of successful use of prostacyclin analogs exist. Epoprostenol, a naturally occurring vasodilator, is administered by continuous infusion, whereas Iloprost, a prostacyclin analog, is administered via nebulizer multiple times daily. In addition to acting as a potent vasodilator, prostacyclin has an inhibitory effect on platelet aggregation. Inhaled nitric oxide is a selective pulmonary vasodilator and has been used successfully during labor and delivery in a number of reports.

POSTPARTUM CARE

Patients tend to deteriorate during the second trimester of pregnancy when most hemodynamic changes occur, but the majority of deaths due to pulmonary hypertension occur in the first month postpartum, with the first week postpartum posing the greatest mortality risk.[27] All women with significant pulmonary hypertension should be monitored closely in an intensive care unit setting for 48 to 72 hours, in a unit where pulmonary vasodilator therapy can be titrated in accordance with postpartum changes in cardiac output and SVR and where there will be pharmacologic and mechanical hemodynamic support available. Possible rescue measures at this time include extracorporeal membrane oxygenation, cardiopulmonary bypass, and heart-lung transplantation.

Women with significant pulmonary hypertension are probably the most high-risk pregnant women an anesthesiologist will see, with mortality in the 50% range. Multidisciplinary, highly coordinated care utilizing all contemporary modalities including inhaled prostaglandins; nitric oxide; and perhaps even "standby" cardiopulmonary bypass is critical, preferably at a tertiary care referral center.

SUMMARY

Most women with diagnosed cardiac disease who become pregnant are at low risk for cardiac complications. They are best served by an anesthesiologist who can consult with them and mostly reassure them that their risk of complications is small and will require little, if any change in routine monitoring and management. A smaller group with moderate disease (eg, mitral and aortic stenosis, impaired myocardial function, uncorrected or partially corrected congenital disease) are at moderate risk and often best managed with a strategy of vaginal delivery with early and effective analgesia, careful hemodynamic management based on the lesion with special attention to preload, good analgesia in the second stage to minimize pushing efforts and time, and an assisted delivery. Women at very high risk, especially those with pulmonary hypertension, end-stage heart failure, or critical symptomatic stenotic lesions, need an aggressive multidisciplinary care team at a center with experience in advanced cardiovascular care and therapy, and they must be counseled that a good outcome cannot be guaranteed or anticipated.

CASE STUDY

A 30-year-old woman, G3,P2 (vaginal deliveries 8 and 10 years prior), with primary pulmonary hypertension (PPH) diagnosed 3 years earlier, presented with worsening symptoms (shortness of breath at rest or minimal exertion) and intermittent contractions at 26 weeks' gestation. Evidence of right-sided heart failure (peripheral edema, enlarged liver, jugular venous distention) was apparent. She had been advised to terminate the pregnancy at 6 weeks' gestation due to the PPH but declined. Her PA pressures 2 years prior to admission had been 65/40 mm Hg but were thought to have probably become worse either before or during her pregnancy based on symptomatology. She was now NYHA class 3. She was receiving (before admission) continuous prostacyclin infusion, furosemide 40 twice daily, nasal oxygen at night and was started on enoxaparin 40 mg twice daily on admission. The obstetric anesthesiology team consulted and followed the patient. The patient was the subject of two multidisciplinary conferences involving her cardiologist, a specialist in right ventricular failure and PPH, maternal-fetal medicine physicians, obstetric anesthesiology, and labor and delivery nursing to discuss management options.

At 30 weeks' gestation, she was admitted to labor and delivery with moderate contractions and a worsening room air SpO_2 of 93%. The decision was made not to treat her with terbutaline or magnesium in an attempt to stop the contractions for fear of adverse hemodynamic consequences and limited chance of success, and the decision was made for delivery, with the preference being a vaginal delivery, especially given her multiparous status. Cervix was 3 cm dilated with painful contractions every 4 to 6 minutes. Blood pressure was 120/70 mm Hg (cuff and radial arterial line in agreement), and heart rate was 105 beats/min. A PA catheter was placed, revealing a PA pressures of 100/50 mm Hg and CVP of 28 mm Hg. The last dose of enoxaparin had been about 10 hours prior. The decision was made that the benefits of placing an epidural catheter to manage pain, stress, and hemodynamics greatly outweighed any bleeding risk. The catheter was placed uneventfully. Three milliliters 0.25% bupivacaine was administered, followed by 10 mL 0.125% bupivacaine with 50 μg fentanyl in two 5-mL doses. The CVP decreased to 12 mm Hg over 15 minutes, and the systemic blood pressure was now 95/45 mm Hg, with no change in PA pressures. She was treated with 500 mL lactated Ringer's with an increase in the CVP to 18 mm Hg and systemic blood pressure to 110/55 mm Hg. Thermodilution cardiac output (CO) was 3.0 L/min. Transaminase levels came back from the laboratory greater than 300 U/L with prothrombin time 19 seconds and INR 1.45 (these had been normal 3 days prior).

An attempt was made to increase CO because 3 L/min was not thought to be sufficient for a successful labor. Dobutamine 5 μg/min was administered, with no change in CO (now 2.8 L/min), but PA pressures increased to 150/100 mm Hg. Dobutamine was discontinued with hemodynamics returning to baseline, and milrinone was started without a bolus/loading dose. PA pressures again increased, to 135/100 mm Hg, with no improvement in CO.

With no response to "inodilators," evidence of worsening right-sided heart failure and low CO in labor, and the patient probably being remote from delivery, the decision was made to deliver by cesarean. General anesthesia was decided on despite the presence of an indwelling, apparently functional epidural catheter because of the possibility of administering nitric oxide (NO) by endotracheal tube and the opinion of the cardiologist that the patient would need this in any case postoperatively (eg, intubation and NO).

General anesthesia was induced over a few minutes with 1.5 mg fentanyl, 2 mg midazolam, and 100 mg rocuronium, and the patient was ventilated. No cricoid pressure was used in order to maximize the ability to maintain easy ventilation. Over the induction period, blood pressure fell to 60/40 mm Hg, PA pressure was also 60/40 mm Hg, and CVP was 10 mm Hg (all approximately 50% of preinduction pressures). Because the perception was that cardiac arrest might be imminent, and difficult intubation was not anticipated, the obstetricians were advised to make the skin incision even before the patient was intubated. The patient was rapidly and easily intubated and ventilated with 100% oxygen and 40 ppm NO, and ephedrine 25 mg × 2, phenylephrine 240 μg, and a "wide-open" vasopressin infusion was started, and, Her blood pressure increased to 170/95 mm Hg, with PA pressure 95/50 mm Hg and CVP 14 mm Hg. Uterine incision was 6 minutes after induction and delivery occurred 1 minute later (Apgar scores of 5 and 9 at 1 and 5 minutes, respectively). At the moment of delivery, maternal hemodynamics were blood pressure 120/70 mm Hg, PA pressure 95/50 mm Hg, CVP 15 mm Hg, and heart rate 80 beats/min, and she was receiving 0.25% isoflurane along with oxygen and NO at 40 ppm. Immediately at delivery of placenta (20 to 30 seconds after delivery of fetus), maternal systolic blood pressure decreased to 40 mm Hg and then quickly to no arterial or PA tracing. ECG was sinus at approximately 110 beats/min at that time. A diagnosis of pulseless electrical activity was made, cardiopulmonary resuscitation (CPR) and Advanced Cardiac Life Support (ACLS) protocols were instituted, but no perfusing rhythm was ever obtained, and resuscitation efforts were stopped at 25 minutes.

Questions

1. What should the patient have been told by the obstetric anesthesia team (and obstetric team) about her morbidity/mortality risks predelivery?

2. Why did the dobutamine and milrinone cause an increase in PA pressures?

3. What do you think was the cause of the cardiac arrest during the cesarean delivery?

4. Are there any ways the cardiac arrest could have been prevented?

5. Was it justified to *not* perform a rapid sequence induction and start the cesarean delivery before intubation?

Answers

1. She was informed that her mortality risk was 30% to 60% for the predelivery period, and that the team members believed that a vaginal delivery would put her on the lower end of this risk range.

2. It appears that both "inodilators" functioned more as inotropic agents than pulmonary dilators, perhaps because her pulmonary vasculature was "fixed" in a constricted state and not responsive to these agents. If the drugs increased right ventricular inotropy without any significant pulmonary vasodilation, one might see this as an increase in PA pressure with little or no change in output. At the time, clinicians were concerned that she "needed" more CO in labor because normal labor is reported to result in a doubling of CO, often to the 10 to 12 L/min range and she was showing signs of right ventricular failure (eg, increasing liver function tests). In retrospect (and discussed at the time), it is not completely clear that the team's attempts to increase her CO above 3.0 L/min were necessary, because fetal status was acceptable at all times.

3. Of course one cannot be sure, but patients with PPH or other causes of pulmonary arterial hypertension are exquisitely sensitive to changes in preload. The right ventricle needs high preload (CVP) to pump against the high PA pressure, but too much volume/pressure may distend the stressed right ventricle beyond the point where effective forward flow can occur. In addition, it is *very* difficult to perform effective CPR/ACLS in patients with PPH once an arrest has occurred because the high pulmonary pressures make it very difficult to get blood from right to left across the lungs with chest compressions. The possible causes here could have been bleeding postdelivery leading to sudden *decrease* in preload, or the "autotransfusion" phenomenon postdelivery leading to an *increase* in preload. The suddenness of the event at delivery of the placenta led the team to conclude that this was most likely some kind of embolic phenomenon. The leading diagnosis was an air embolus, which is common at cesarean (perhaps in > 75% of women), especially under general anesthesia. These are usually of no great consequence in normal patients, but in this patent with extremely high pulmonary resistance, it may have led to a sudden further increase and essentially stopped any right ventricular ejection. Another possibility is a thromboembolus, because thrombosis in these patients are common due to the low flow state, and it is conceivable that the delivery of the fetus or surgical manipulation in general could have dislodged part of a pelvic thrombus. This, too, in a compromised patient such as this could lead to irreversible cardiac arrest.

4. If this was an air embolism, perhaps, because air embolism is probably more common under general anesthesia; a regional anesthetic might have made this less likely. Extroversion of the uterus, or any other manipulation that makes air entry more likely by raising the site higher than the heart will increase risk. The team now delivers such extremely high-risk patients in slight "reverse Trendelenburg" position and tries to avoid extroversion of the uterus. All of the above is quite speculative, and most other possible causes would appear quite difficult to avoid or treat much differently than was actually done, especially considering that at the time of delivery the woman's hemodynamic "numbers" were just about "perfect."

5. The team believes that a standard rapid sequence induction for cesarean section with something like 150 mg propofol and succinylcholine would have been a very poor choice and quite likely led to an immediate arrest from decreased preload and contractility. Even the "careful, opioid-based induction" caused a 50% decrease in blood pressure requiring massive vasopressor support. The team thought that the benefits of a slower induction, with the goal (if not the perfect outcome) of less hemodynamic alteration was clearly the preferred choice. One could even make a case for maintenance of spontaneous ventilation because positive pressure ventilation can be (and may have been in this case) a major problem in patients with severe pulmonary hypertension because it decreases right ventricular preload acutely. The point is that when patients are at this level of risk, it may be completely appropriate to take actions that would be viewed as unusual or inappropriate in normal pregnant women. Luckily for clinicians and their patients, such patients are relatively rare.

REFERENCES

1. Elkayam U, Bitar F. Valvular heart disease and pregnancy part I: native valves. *J Am Coll Cardiol.* 2005;46(2):223-230.
2. Hameed A, Karaalp IS, Tummala PP, et al. The effect of valvular heart disease on maternal and fetal outcome of pregnancy. *J Am Coll Cardiol.* 2001;37(3):893-899.
3. de Souza JA, Martinez EE Jr, Ambrose JA, et al. Percutaneous balloon mitral valvuloplasty in comparison with open mitral valve commissurotomy for mitral stenosis during pregnancy. *J Am Coll Cardiol.* 2001;37(3):900-903.
4. Esteves CA, Munoz JS, Braga S, et al. Immediate and long-term follow-up of percutaneous balloon mitral valvuloplasty in pregnant patients with rheumatic mitral stenosis. *Am J Cardiol.* 2006;98(6):812-816.
5. Elkayam U, Bitar F. Valvular heart disease and pregnancy: part II: prosthetic valves. *J Am Coll Cardiol.* 2005;46(3):403-410.
6. Castellano JM, Narayan RL, Vaishnava P, Fuster V. Anticoagulation during pregnancy in patients with a prosthetic heart valve. *Nat Rev Cardiol.* 2012;9:415-424.
7. Bates SM, Greer IA, Pabinger I, et al. Venous thromboembolism, thrombophilia, antithrombotic therapy, and pregnancy: American College of Chest Physicians Evidence-Based Clinical Practice Guidelines (8th Edition). *Chest.* 2008;133(6 suppl):844S-86S.
8. Jastrow N, Meyer P, Khairy P, et al. Prediction of complications in pregnant women with cardiac diseases referred to a tertiary center. *Int J Cardiol.* 2011;151(2):209-213.
9. Siu SC, Sermer M, Colman JM, et al. Prospective multicenter study of pregnancy outcomes in women with heart disease. *Circulation.* 2001;104(5):515-521.
10. Brickner ME, Hillis LD, Lange RA. Congenital heart disease in adults. First of two parts. *N Engl J Med.* 2000;342(4):256-263.
11. Lovell AT. Anaesthetic implications of grown-up congenital heart disease. *Br J Anaesth.* 2004;93(1):129-139.
12. Balci A, Drenthen W, Mulder BJ, et al. Pregnancy in women with corrected tetralogy of Fallot: occurrence and predictors of adverse events. *Am Heart J.* 2011;161(2):307-313.
13. Walker F. Pregnancy and the various forms of the Fontan circulation. *Heart.* 2007;93(2):152-154.
14. Drenthen W, Pieper PG, Roos-Hesselink JW, et al. Pregnancy and delivery in women after Fontan palliation. *Heart.* 2006;92(9):1290-1294.
15. Connolly HM, Grogan M, Warnes CA. Pregnancy among women with congenitally corrected transposition of great arteries. *J Am Coll Cardiol.* 1999;33(6):1692-1695.
16. Beauchesne LM, Connolly HM, Ammash NM, Warnes CA. Coarctation of the aorta: outcome of pregnancy. *J Am Coll Cardiol.* 2001;38(6):1728-1733.
17. Goland S, Elkayam U. Cardiovascular problems in pregnant women with marfan syndrome. *Circulation.* 2009;119(4):619-623.
18. Meijboom LJ, Drenthen W, Pieper PG, et al. Obstetric complications in Marfan syndrome. *Int J Cardiol.* 2006;110(1):53-59.
19. Sliwa K, Hilfiker-Kleiner D, Petrie MC, et al. Current state of knowledge on aetiology, diagnosis, management, and therapy of peripartum cardiomyopathy: a position statement from the Heart Failure Association of the European Society of Cardiology Working Group on peripartum cardiomyopathy. *Eur J Heart Fail.* 2010;12(8):767-778.
20. Elkayam U. Clinical characteristics of peripartum cardiomyopathy in the United States: diagnosis, prognosis, and management. *J Am Coll Cardiol.* 2011;58(7):659-670.
21. Karaye KM, Henein MY. Peripartum cardiomyopathy: a review article. *Int J Cardiol.* 2011.
22. Patten IS, Rana S, Shahul S, et al. Cardiac angiogenic imbalance leads to peripartum cardiomyopathy. *Nature.* 2012;485(7398):333-338.
23. Gersh BJ, Maron BJ, Bonow RO, et al. 2011 ACCF/AHA Guideline for the Diagnosis and Treatment of Hypertrophic Cardiomyopathy: a report of the American College of Cardiology Foundation/American Heart Association Task Force on Practice Guidelines. Developed in collaboration with the American Association for Thoracic Surgery, American Society of Echocardiography, American Society of Nuclear Cardiology, Heart Failure Society of America, Heart Rhythm Society, Society for Cardiovascular Angiography and Interventions, and Society of Thoracic Surgeons. *J Am Coll Cardiol.* 2011;58(25):e212-e260.

24. Maron BJ. Contemporary insights and strategies for risk stratification and prevention of sudden death in hypertrophic cardiomyopathy. *Circulation.* 2010;121(3):445-456.

25. Autore C, Conte MR, Piccininno M, et al. Risk associated with pregnancy in hypertrophic cardiomyopathy. *J Am Coll Cardiol.* 2002;40(10):1864-1869.

26. Madden BP. Pulmonary hypertension and pregnancy. *Int J Obstet Anesth.* 2009;18(2):156-164.

27. Weiss BM, Zemp L, Seifert B, Hess OM. Outcome of pulmonary vascular disease in pregnancy: a systematic overview from 1978 through 1996. *J Am Coll Cardiol.* 1998;31(7):1650-1657.

28. Kiely DG, Condliffe R, Webster V, et al. Improved survival in pregnancy and pulmonary hypertension using a multiprofessional approach. *Br J Obstet Gynaecol.* 2010;117(5):565-574.

29. Simonneau G, Robbins IM, Beghetti M, et al. Updated clinical classification of pulmonary hypertension. *J Am Coll Cardiol.* 2009;54(1 suppl):S43-S54.

30. Blaise G, Langleben D, Hubert B. Pulmonary arterial hypertension: pathophysiology and anesthetic approach. *Anesthesiology.* 2003;99(6):1415-1432.

31. Penning S, Robinson KD, Major CA, Garite TJ. A comparison of echocardiography and pulmonary artery catheterization for evaluation of pulmonary artery pressures in pregnant patients with suspected pulmonary hypertension. *Am J Obstet Gynecol.* 2001;184(7):1568-1570.

Hypertension of Pregnancy

22

Migdalia H. Saloum and Dimitrios Kassapidis

TOPICS

Hypertensive disorders seriously complicate approximately 2% to 8% of all pregnancies.[1] Indeed, 19% of pregnancy-related maternal mortality is due to complications related to hypertensive disorders.[2] Hypertensive disorders during pregnancy involve a variety of clinical entities, including gestational hypertension, preeclampsia, eclampsia, chronic hypertension, superimposed preeclampsia on chronic hypertension, and *h*emolysis, *e*levated *l*iver enzymes, *l*ow *p*latelets (HELLP) syndrome.[3] The normal physiologic changes of pregnancy result in a net reduction of systolic, diastolic, and mean arterial blood pressure by midpregnancy because of decreased systemic vascular resistance and the presence of a low resistance to flow placenta. At the end of term pregnancy, the blood pressure returns to baseline prepregnant level.[4]

Gestational hypertension occurs when a pregnant woman without a previous history develops isolated hypertension (greater than 140/90 mm Hg) after 20 weeks' gestation. It is not associated with significant proteinuria or other symptoms and signs of preeclampsia and resolves within 12 weeks' postpartum.

Preeclampsia is diagnosed when a pregnant woman develops new onset hypertension (greater than 140/90 mm Hg) after 20 weeks' gestation often in conjunction with proteinuria (greater than 300 mg in a 24-hour collection). In 2013, the American College of Obstetricians and Gynecologists (ACOG) updated its diagnostic criteria of preeclampsia-eclampsia and eliminated the dependence on proteinuria for diagnosis. To reflect the syndromic nature of preeclampsia, in the absence of proteinuria, it is diagnosed as hypertension in association with thrombocytopenia, impaired liver function, renal insufficiency, pulmonary edema, or cerebral or visual disturbances.[5] Preeclampsia may be classified as severe based on *any* of the following:

- Systolic blood pressure greater than or equal to 160 mm Hg, or diastolic blood pressure greater than or equal to 110 mm Hg

- Thrombocytopenia (platelet count less than or equal to 100,000/mm^3)

- Impaired liver function as indicated by elevated liver enzymes (to twice normal levels) and/or severe persistent right upper quadrant pain

- Renal insufficiency as indicated by serum creatinine concentration greater than 1.1 mg/dL or a doubling of the serum creatinine

- Pulmonary edema

- New-onset cerebral or visual disturbances

The most recent report of ACOG's task force on hypertension in pregnancy has eliminated proteinuria greater than 5 g from the diagnostic criteria for severe preeclampsia for the reason that there is a minimal relationship between the quantity of urinary protein and pregnancy outcome.[5]

Eclampsia is defined by new-onset seizures or impaired mental state (ie, coma) in a preeclamptic woman. It is not a separate entity from preeclampsia but rather signifies a continuum of severity. Eclampsia carries a high maternal morbidity and mortality rate. Intracerebral hemorrhage/stroke, pulmonary aspiration, cardiopulmonary arrest, acute renal failure, and death are major complications of seizures. In addition, there is significant potential for fetal jeopardy.[6]

HELLP syndrome is considered a variant of preeclampsia. Aside from hemolysis, elevated liver enzymes, and low platelets, associated symptoms may include hypertension, proteinuria, right upper quadrant/epigastric pain, nausea and vomiting, and headache. Clinical presentation can be variable, and patients may initially be normotensive or without proteinuria. HELLP may devolve rapidly to various maternal complications, including disseminated intravascular coagulation (DIC), placental abruption, renal failure, and cerebral and liver hemorrhage. It is associated with a 70% preterm delivery rate. HELLP is an indication for stabilization and delivery, especially at 34 weeks' gestation or later.[7]

Chronic hypertension is diagnosed when blood pressure levels are greater than or equal to 140 mm Hg systolic or greater than or equal to 90 mmHg diastolic before pregnancy or before 20 weeks' of gestation, or when elevated blood pressures fail to resolve 12 weeks' postpartum. The pathophysiology of chronic hypertension is much better understood than that of preeclampsia. *Chronic hypertension with superimposed preeclampsia* occurs when pregnant women who have a history of chronic hypertension before pregnancy develop preeclampsia. The diagnosis is made in the presence of new-onset proteinuria or a sudden increase in proteinuria and/or hypertension, or when other manifestations of severe preeclampsia appear. Maternal and perinatal morbidity is higher with superimposed preeclampsia than it is with preeclampsia alone.

The goal of classifying hypertensive disorders during pregnancy by blood pressure, proteinuria, seizures, and organ system involvement is to allow management decisions to be made about the timing of delivery and the initiation of therapies. The only definitive treatment of preeclampsia is delivery of the neonate and placenta.

PREECLAMPSIA

Preeclampsia is a leading cause of maternal and perinatal morbidity and mortality. Even in developed countries with low maternal mortality rates, preeclampsia/eclampsia remains a leading cause of maternal morbidity and mortality.[1] Maternal complications from hypertensive disorders include placental abruption, eclampsia, cerebrovascular accidents, multisystem organ failure, and DIC. Maternal deaths are due mostly to intracranial hemorrhage, cerebral infarction, acute pulmonary edema, and hepatic rupture or failure. Preeclampsia also results in fetal complications such as preterm birth, intrauterine growth retardation, and fetal/neonatal death.[8]

Preeclampsia is a multisystem disease that is typically diagnosed when new-onset hypertension occurs with proteinuria after 20 weeks' gestation (Table 22-1). Preeclampsia can evolve during its course, and complications could be avoided if clinicians stay vigilant for the progression of the disease. Diagnosis and interventions are sometimes delayed because of the absence of proteinuria.[5] Some women may have an atypical presentation of preeclampsia, where signs and symptoms may vary and would not fit into the classical definition. Atypical preeclampsia can present

Table 22-1. Criteria for Diagnosis of Preeclampsia[a]

BLOOD PRESSURE
≥ 140 mm Hg systolic or ≥ to 90 mm Hg diastolic on two occasions at least 4 hours apart at 20 weeks' gestation
≥ 160 mm Hg systolic or ≥ 110 mm Hg diastolic; hypertension can be confirmed within a short interval (minutes)
AND
PROTEINURIA
> 300 mg per 24-hour urine collection *OR* protein-creatinine ratio > 0.3 mg/dL
Dipstick reading of 1+ (used only if other methods are not available)

OR in the absence of proteinuria, new-onset of any of the following:	
Thrombocytopenia	Platelet count < 100,000/mm³
Renal insufficiency	Serum creatinine concentrations > 1.1 mg/dL or a doubling of serum creatinine
Impaired liver function	Elevated serum concentrations of liver transaminases to twice normal levels
Pulmonary edema	
Cerebral or visual symptoms	

[a]Adapted from Roberts JM, August PA, Bakris G, et al.[5]

before 20 weeks' gestation, without proteinuria, or as proteinuria only.[9] Edema was previously a part of the diagnostic criteria but has been excluded because edema is a common physical finding in many pregnant women and is therefore nonspecific. Preeclampsia usually presents near term or during the intrapartum period. It can also manifest in the postpartum period, usually within 7 days post-delivery. Risk factors include nulliparity, age greater than 40 years, obesity, previous preeclampsia, multiple gestation, diabetes mellitus, preexisting kidney disease or chronic hypertension, sickle cell disease, and in vitro fertilization (possibility of multiple pregnancies).

Depending on the time of presentation, preeclampsia is classified into early-onset (develops before 34 weeks' gestation) and late-onset (develops at or after 34 weeks' gestation) types. Women with early-onset disease usually develop more severe disease.[10] Severe preeclampsia, characterized by blood pressure greater than 140/90 mm Hg and proteinuria greater than 5 g/24 hours, is associated with a higher maternal morbidity and mortality because patients are at higher risk for HELLP syndrome, DIC, cerebrovascular accidents, pulmonary edema, renal failure, placental abruption, and eclampsia than women with mild preeclampsia.

Serum uric acid levels are often elevated early in the disease process, and this has been used as a sentinel marker of the disease. However, hyperuricemia has poor correlation with severity of disease and maternal/fetal complications.[11]

HELLP Syndrome

HELLP syndrome complicates 10% to 20% of cases of severe preeclampsia. The diagnostic criteria of HELLP syndrome include hemolysis with elevated serum lactate dehydrogenase level (greater than 600 IU/L), increased serum aspartate aminotransferase level (greater than 70 IU/L), and decreased platelet count (less than 100,000/mm^3). Hemolysis is defined as the presence of microangiopathic hemolytic anemia and is confirmed by visualizing Burr cells (contracted red blood cells with spikes) and schizocytes (fragmented) on a peripheral blood smear.[7]

Eclampsia

Eclampsia is the occurrence of seizures and/or coma in a patient with preeclampsia. In the United States, the incidence of eclampsia is relatively low, ranging from 0.03% to 0.7%. Eclamptic seizures are of tonic-clonic type and in majority of patients, convulsions appear during the antepartum period. Eclamptic convulsion also may appear during the postpartum period, within 7 days after delivery of the infant. Associated neurologic complications in patients with eclampsia include cortical blindness, aphasia, hemiparesis, facial nerve palsy, postpartum psychosis, and cerebrovascular accidents. Unlike hypertensive encephalopathy, focal neurologic deficits and papilledema are not commonly noted in eclampsia.[12]

Management of eclamptic seizure includes termination of the convulsion, protection and maintenance of the airway, adequate oxygenation, establishment of intravenous access, and monitoring of fetal well-being.

Pathophysiology of Preeclampsia

The placenta is the pathogenic focus of preeclampsia. The exact mechanism in which the abnormal placenta leads to multisystem effects which characterize preeclampsia is not well understood. Currently, the most widely accepted theory is that the placenta fails to embed adequately into the myometrium, which leads to poor placental perfusion. As a consequence, the placenta becomes hypoxic and releases factors into the circulation that damage the maternal endothelium and give rise to the multisystem effects of preeclampsia. In normal pregnancy, the villous cytotrophoblast invades the inner third of the myometrium, and the spiral arteries lose their endothelium and most of their muscle fibers. The spiral arteries are then structurally modified into low-resistance vessels that are unresponsive to vasoactive stimuli. In preeclampsia, there is defective invasion of the spiral arteries by the cytotrophoblast and impaired spiral artery remodeling, which results in abnormal placentation and development of high-resistance vessels that are hyperresponsive to vasomotor stimuli. Increased uterine arterial resistance leads to decreased placental perfusion and placental infarcts. This chronic placental ischemia causes fetal intrauterine growth restriction. In addition, substances such as free radicals, oxidized lipids, cytokines, and endothelial growth factors may be released into the maternal circulation in response to the chronic hypoxia, which create widespread maternal endothelial dysfunction. Necrotic injury of syncytiotrophoblast due to placental hypoxia releases antiangiogenic factors, such as soluble form of the vascular endothelial growth factor receptor and soluble endoglin. Normal endothelium is responsible for preventing platelet activation, keeping fluid in the intravascular compartment, and buffering the response to pressors. In preeclampsia, the endothelium becomes hyperpermeable and thrombogenic, and vascular tone is increased.[13,14]

Clinical Manifestations of Preeclampsia

Manifestations of severe preeclampsia occur in all organ systems as a result of widespread endothelial dysfunction.

CENTRAL NERVOUS SYSTEM

Central nervous system (CNS) symptoms of preeclampsia/eclampsia include severe persistent headaches, visual disturbances, hyperreflexia, seizures, and coma. CNS manifestations are a result of loss of cerebral autoregulation. Breakdown of autoregulation and disruption of the blood-brain barrier due to a rapid rise in blood pressure and forced dilation of the cerebral vessels may result in cerebral edema, similar to the changes seen in hypertensive encephalopathy.[15] Eclampsia, which is defined as new-onset seizures during pregnancy, most commonly occurs in the intrapartum period or within 48 hours of delivery.

PULMONARY

Preeclampsia is reported to be one of the important causes of pulmonary edema in pregnant women. Endothelial injury, combined with decreased colloid osmotic pressure, is the primary underlying mechanism for increased leakage of intravascular fluid into the lungs.[16]

CARDIOVASCULAR

The physiologic changes in the cardiovascular system during normal pregnancy involve a state of high cardiac output, primarily due to increased stroke volume, and decreased systemic vascular resistance. However, in patients with preeclampsia, changes in the cardiovascular system reverse to a state of low cardiac output with high systemic vascular resistance. However, myocardial contractility remains unaffected.[17] Increased vascular tone and sensitivity in preeclampsia is responsible for these changes, manifested by hypertension, vasospasm, and end-organ ischemia. Sustained increases in blood pressure and systemic vascular resistance can dramatically reduce intravascular volume with severe disease. Acute elevations in blood pressure, especially if severe, may render the patient at risk for hypertensive encephalopathy, cerebrovascular hemorrhage, myocardial ischemia, and congestive heart failure.

HEMATOLOGIC

Thrombocytopenia is the most common hematologic abnormality, occurring in 15% to 20% of preeclamptic patients. Platelet count less than $100,000/mm^3$ are typically seen in patients with severe disease or HELLP syndrome and correlate with severity of disease or the occurrence of severe placental abruption. DIC can occur in women with preeclampsia but is more common with HELLP syndrome. DIC is characterized by uncontrolled activation of the coagulation system and depletion of coagulation factors and fibrinogen. In severe cases, spontaneous hemorrhage can result. In cases where the platelet count is greater than $100,000/mm^3$, further coagulation testing is not required, because clinically significant impaired coagulation is rarely present. However, with a platelet count less than $100,000/mm^3$, coagulopathy is more likely and further coagulation studies (prothrombin time [PT], partial thromboplastin time [PTT], INR, fibrinogen levels) are warranted.[18]

HEPATIC

Hepatic involvement in preeclampsia ranges from mild hepatic dysfunction to HELLP syndrome and can be associated with subcapsular hematoma or rupture. Subcapsular hepatic rupture is rare but it is a surgical emergency that can be associated with shock and carries a 32% mortality rate. Preeclampsia is associated with periportal hemorrhages and fibrin deposition in hepatic sinusoids. Signs and symptoms of HELLP syndrome include right upper quadrant/epigastric pain (from liver capsule involvement), nausea, vomiting, headache, hypertension, and proteinuria. Diagnosis of HELLP can be challenging because the clinical presentation tends to vary and hypertension is not a prominent feature. Indeed, 12% to 18% of women may be normotensive or have no proteinuria. Because of the high mortality rate and incidence of maternal complications, HELLP is an indication for stabilization and delivery beyond 34 weeks' gestation or in the presence of associated complications such as DIC, liver hemorrhage, placental abruption, or nonreassuring fetal heart rate. Before 34 weeks in the setting of HELLP without complications, there is debate as to the optimum timing of delivery.[10]

RENAL

Proteinuria is a defining element of preeclampsia. The mechanism for proteinuria involves changes in the endothelium of the glomerulus that results in altered filtration and impaired proximal tubular reabsorption. During normal pregnancy, glomerular filtration rate (GFR) normally increases, which results in decreased blood urea nitrogen (BUN), creatinine, and uric acid. In preeclampsia, GFR is approximately 30% lower than in normal pregnancy Therefore, a preeclamptic woman may have a BUN and creatinine in the normal range in relation to a nonpregnant woman; relative to pregnancy, this is abnormally high. Hyperuricemia is a strong early marker for possible preeclampsia. The mechanism for hyperuricemia is most likely related to impaired renal clearance. Oliguria is a late manifestation of severe preeclampsia and correlates with the severity of the disease. Acute renal failure, rare in patients with severe preeclampsia, is usually related to acute tubular necrosis. In rare circumstances, renal failure may occur due to bilateral renal cortical necrosis, which has a high morbidity and mortality.[19]

Management of Preeclampsia

The primary strategies for management of patients with preeclampsia include continuous assessment and monitoring of the clinical condition, management and prevention of severe hypertension, management and prevention of eclamptic seizures, and avoidance of aggressive fluid administration.

ANTIHYPERTENSIVE TREATMENT

Most guidelines recommend lowering blood pressure to 140 to 150 mm Hg systolic and 90 to 100 mm Hg diastolic, particularly if hypertension has been severe. Currently, national guidelines recommend treatment of hypertension at a threshold of 160 mm Hg systolic or 110 mm Hg diastolic.[5] Often, it may be necessary to attain rapid control of blood pressure, which is most commonly achieved with hydralazine and labetalol; sometimes, nifedipine or nitroprusside are required. Antihypertensive medications should be carefully titrated to avoid hypotension that could adversely reduce uteroplacental perfusion and oxygen delivery to the fetus.[20]

Hydralazine, a direct vasodilator, has been a popular agent for decades, because it is effective and relatively safe during pregnancy. It is a direct nitric oxide donor that relaxes both arteriolar and venous smooth muscle. It can have untoward maternal side effects such as tachycardia, palpitations, nausea, and headache. When used intravenously, hydralazine, in comparison to labetalol and nifedipine, has been reported to have more side effects, including maternal hypotension and association with placental abruption.[21] The recommended dose of hydralazine is 5 mg intravenously, then 5 to 10 mg every 20 to 40 minutes.

Labetalol, a combined α- and β-adrenergic blocker (ratio of 1:7) has emerged as the primary choice of antihypertensive in treatment of preeclamptic hypertension. When compared to hydralazine, use of labetalol results in a lower incidence of maternal hypotension. The recommended dose of labetalol is 20 mg intravenously, with additional doses every 20 to 30 minutes up to 220 mg. Labetalol should be avoided in women with severe asthma.

Nifedipine, a calcium channel blocker and arterial vasodilator, is also an effective antihypertensive agent, but caution must be exercised because it can have adverse interactions with magnesium sulfate. Magnesium sulfate is also calcium inhibitor as well, and when combined with calcium channel blockers can have synergistic effects. Severe hypotension and neuromuscular block have been reported in the mother with concurrent use of both drugs. Nonreassuring fetal status has also been reported with combined use of both medications.

Sodium nitroprusside, a direct vasodilator, is used as an antihypertensive of last resort or where there must be fine tuning of blood pressure, such as during laryngoscopy and intubation. The potential for cyanide toxicity and excessive vasodilation are concerns with its use. However, the drug has been used safely at recommended doses (ie, intravenous infusion of 0.25-5 µg/kg/min).

MAGNESIUM SULFATE

Magnesium sulfate has a long history of use in obstetrics. It was originally used as a tocolytic agent for its ability to inhibit smooth muscle contractions. Magnesium sulfate is now widely used for prophylaxis and treatment of eclamptic seizures. The exact mechanism by which it prevents seizures is not fully understood, but there is clear evidence of its effectiveness. Studies show that magnesium sulfate is superior to phenytoin, nimodipine, or diazepam for prevention of eclamptic seizures. Magnesium sulfate is a nonspecific calcium channel antagonist that affects vascular smooth muscle, causing vasodilation. There are several theories as to how magnesium sulfate works to prevent seizures, including acting as a peripheral and cerebral vasodilator to relieve cerebral vasoconstriction, protecting the blood-brain barrier to reduce cerebral edema formation and suppressing glutamate-mediated epileptogenesis as an N-methyl-D-aspartate receptor antagonist. The role of magnesium in preventing seizures via its vasodilator action is not completely understood. Eclamptic seizures were previously thought to occur as a result of cerebral vasospasm, which supported the theory that magnesium sulfate, at least in part, prevented seizures by acting as a vasodilator. However, more recent evidence suggests that eclamptic seizures are a result of abrupt, sustained blood pressure elevation that forces dilation of cerebral vessels, causing hyperperfusion, increased blood-brain barrier permeability, and cerebral edema. If magnesium acted as a vasodilator, it would in effect worsen cerebral hyperperfusion and edema. The protective mechanism of magnesium sulfate may then be more closely related to peripheral vasodilation and lowering of systemic blood pressure which in turn may decrease cerebral perfusion pressure.[22,23] The disadvantage to using magnesium sulfate is the risk of systemic toxicity. Because magnesium is a competitor of calcium, it decreases calcium availability in the myocytes for muscle contraction and can produce profound muscle relaxation (paresis). At high doses, respiratory depression and cardiac arrest can occur as a result of its muscle relaxant properties.

Normal serum magnesium (Mg^{2+}) concentrations are 1.7 to 2.4 mEq/L. Magnesium levels considered therapeutic for the prevention of seizures are 3.5 to 7 mEq/L.[19] Usually a loading dose of 4 to 6 g of magnesium sulfate intravenously is given, followed by an infusion of 1 to 2 g/h. Side effects of magnesium include chest pain, palpitation, nausea/vomiting, blurred vision, sedation, hypotension, and pulmonary edema. Magnesium blood levels are frequently assessed to make certain that a therapeutic level is maintained. Because magnesium sulfate is eliminated by the kidneys, patients with renal insufficiency are at higher risk of reaching toxic levels. Deep tendon reflexes are used to clinically monitor hypermagnesemia. At 8 to 12 mEq/L, loss of patellar deep tendon reflexes can be reliably observed, and at greater than 13 mEq/L, respiratory depression can occur. Respiratory arrest occurs at levels 15 to 20 mEq/L, and cardiac arrest at levels greater than 25 mEq/L. In the event of a cardiac arrest from hypermagnesemia, the magnesium infusion should be immediately stopped and calcium gluconate 1 g over 10 minutes should be given.

ANESTHESIA FOR LABOR AND DELIVERY

Adequate assessment of a preeclamptic woman must involve the airway, blood pressure control, coagulation status, and fluid balance. There are several benefits to regional analgesia in preeclamptic women either with combined spinal-epidural (CSE) or with epidural placement.

- Early placement of an epidural/CSE can provide a means to avoid general anesthesia in emergency situations and reduce the risk of airway complication.

- Regional analgesia will prevent the exaggerated responses in blood pressure and catecholamine secretion related to painful uterine contractions.

- Regional analgesia provides effective analgesia without administration of systemic medications, such as opioids, that may obtund maternal airway reflexes.

- Uteroplacental perfusion is improved with sympathectomy related to regional anesthesia.[24]

As previously discussed, preeclamptic patients are at an increased risk for thrombocytopenia or coagulation abnormalities (DIC). Thrombocytopenia and coagulopathy are more common with severe preeclampsia or HELLP syndrome than with mild preeclampsia. When the platelet count is less than 100,000/mm³, other coagulation abnormalities (ie, PT, PTT, INR, fibrinogen) may be present and thus should be assessed. In a mild preeclamptic with a platelet count above 100,000/mm³, further coagulation testing is not required. Many obstetric anesthesiologists consider a platelet count above 75,000/mm³ to be adequate for placement of neuraxial anesthesia. A rapidly falling platelet count is more concerning because the nadir in the platelet count cannot be identified prospectively. Platelet counts obtained within 6 hours of neuraxial anesthesia placement are adequate for stable platelet counts, but for rapidly falling platelets a platelet count every 1 to 3 hours may be necessary. Most anesthesiologists agree that a platelet count less than 50,000/mm³, which coincides with the potential for surgical bleeding, precludes the placement of neuraxial anesthesia. With a platelet count between 50,000 and 75,000/mm³, clinical judgment must be made, weighing the risks of general anesthesia against potential neurologic compromise. The risk of epidural hematoma formation exists not only during placement of an epidural catheter but also during removal. An epidural catheter should not be removed until an acceptable platelet count with a rising trend is present. The same criteria apply to platelet counts for removal of the catheter. There is controversy whether a single shot spinal or an epidural is preferable where there is the potential for coagulopathy. Anesthesiologists have speculated that there may be lower risk to a single-shot spinal with a small-gauge needle as compared to a larger epidural needle and subsequent threading of a catheter. Indeed, reported risk of spinal hematoma with placement of spinals is 1 per 220,000 as compared to 1 per 150,000 with epidurals.[25]

Fluid preloading prior to neuraxial anesthesia has been used to mitigate hypotension related to sympathectomy. In current clinical practice, fluid preloading has lost its prominence partly because of a change in practice with the use of lower concentrations of local anesthetics, which may produce less profound sympathectomy. Indeed, studies have shown that there is no *clinically important* difference in the severity, timing, or duration of hypotension following spinal blockade in patients who do not receive fluid preloading compared to those that do.[26] In severely preeclamptic patients, however, varying degrees of volume contraction may be present and there is a greater risk of hypotension from the sympathectomy. Coloading, a technique where intravenous fluid is given concomitant with the start of regional blockade, has been shown to be more effective than preloading.[27] Fluid administration should be closely monitored in severe preeclamptics as they are more likely to develop pulmonary edema.

Anesthesia for Cesarean Section

Neuraxial anesthesia is preferred over general anesthesia for cesarean section because it avoids the potential risk of difficult intubation secondary to airway edema, as well as the fluctuations in hemodynamics that can occur with general anesthesia. Of particular concern is the hypertensive response that can occur in an already hypertensive, severely preeclamptic patient during laryngoscopy and intubation. The leading cause of death in women with severe preeclampsia remains intracranial hemorrhage.

In the past, an epidural was the technique of choice to provide regional anesthesia for a cesarean section. Spinal anesthesia was avoided because of concern that the almost instantaneous sympathectomy would result in rapid and severe hypotension. Nonetheless, spinal anesthesia is an alternative to general anesthesia, particularly in emergency situations, because it provides a quick and effective induction block for operative delivery, avoiding the risk of airway manipulation. This is important because the case fatality rate directly attributed to anesthesia was as much as 17 times greater with general anesthesia compared to regional anesthesia. More recent studies and clinical experience have shown that the concern for profound hypotension after spinal anesthesia in severely preeclamptic women has been overstated in modern day practice so long as the patient has been adequately prepared. In a retrospective study, the lowest mean blood pressure measurements did not differ between severely preeclamptic women given spinal or epidural anesthesia for cesarean section.[28] Only one prospective study showed that severely preeclamptic women who received subarachnoid block had more incidence of hypotension than those receiving epidurals; however, the hypotension was short lived and the patients responded to ephedrine as effectively as the epidural group.[29] However, this was a multisite study, and the incidence of hypotension with spinal as compared to epidural anesthesia was two to three times greater in two hospitals as compared to the other three, casting some doubt as to the universality of these findings. Even though an epidural may provide a more hemodynamically stable neuraxial block, spinal anesthesia is useful in severely preeclamptic patients in an emergent situation to avoid the risks associated with general anesthesia.[30]

There are instances when general anesthesia is preferred in a severely pre-eclamptic woman (eg, in the case of a severe coagulopathy or thrombocytopenia, a fetus in severe jeopardy [placental abruption], or in severe hemorrhage where a sympathectomy would be undesirable). Of primary importance is airway management in preeclamptic patients due to the potential for airway edema. Even in the face of a normal airway examination, there can be significant upper airway edema and narrowing, which can make visualization of airway landmarks difficult in addition to passing an endotracheal tube. Edema can also make the airway prone to traumatic bleeding with repeated intubation attempts. Endotracheal tubes of various sizes should be available, as well as difficult intubation equipment including a video laryngoscope. Laryngeal mask airway (LMA) insertion should be considered early in the management of a difficult airway to secure the airway and to avoid any further trauma before the airway irretrievably lost. In a dire situation when LMA is not available, mask ventilation through cricoid pressure has been used. Further, there may be hemodynamic instability associated with rapid-sequence intubation in a severely preeclamptic patient that leads to life-threatening hypertension and may put the patient at risk for cerebral hemorrhage or pulmonary edema. Vigilance of blood pressure is paramount, and an arterial line may be warranted. The medications that have been successfully used to blunt the hypertensive response to laryngoscopy and intubation include labetalol, esmolol, nitroglycerin, sodium nitroprusside, and remifentanil. The goal of antihypertensive therapy is to decrease the blood pressure to approximately 140/90 mm Hg before induction of general anesthesia. Labetalol is commonly used because it is effective, easy, and relatively safe to use. Labetalol crosses the placenta and can cause fetal bradycardia and/or hypoglycemia but to a lesser extent than other β-blockers. Esmolol is an ideal agent because it is a short-acting drug with an ultra-rapid onset; however, many concerns about its safety in terms of the fetus (disproportionate bradycardia) have made it a less popular choice. Most of these studies used esmolol as an infusion, and a more recent study has shown that short-term administration of esmolol is safe for the fetus in this clinical setting.[31,32] Nitroglycerin is also a rapid and short-acting agent that is safe for the mother and fetus. It is a direct vasodilator and has been used effectively to blunt the hypertensive response. Sodium nitroprusside is an effective vasodilator as well, although infusions should be used only for in the short term to avoid cyanide toxicity in the fetus. Remifentanil is rapidly metabolized by the mother and fetus, and therefore it has also been used to blunt the hypertensive response. It is effective, has a rapid onset and short duration of action when compared to other opioids, but still has the potential to cause respiratory depression in the neonate.[33]

Severely preeclamptic patients who have received prolonged magnesium sulfate infusions are at increased risk for muscle weakness and uterine atony. Muscle paralysis provided by nondepolarizing muscle relaxants can be prolonged in the presence of magnesium therapy. Careful titration and smaller doses of nondepolarizing muscle relaxants should be used in these patients, as well as administration of full reversal with cholinesterase inhibitors. A neuromuscular monitor should be used. Uterotonics should be readily available in these cases for the potential risk of uterine atony. Methylergonovine should be avoided as it is a potent vasoconstrictor and can cause severe hypertension in an already hypertensive patient.

SUMMARY

Hypertensive disorders of pregnancy are varied, perhaps the most common being preeclampsia. Careful attention to fluid status, hemodynamics, and coagulopathy are required. In most cases, regional anesthesia is preferred for labor and cesarean delivery. General anesthesia may be required in rare instances related to severe coagulopathy, hemorrhage, or immediate fetal jeopardy.

REFERENCES

1. Ghulmiyyah L, Sibai B. Maternal mortality from pre-eclampsia/eclampsia. *Semin Perinatol.* 2012;36(1):56-59.
2. Chang J, Elam-Evans LD, Berg CJ, et al. *MMWR Surveill Summ.* 2003;52(2):1-8.
3. American College of Obstetricians and Gynecologists (ACOG). ACOG Practice Bulletin No. 33. *Int J Gynecol Obstet.* 2002;77:67-75.
4. Clark SL, Cotton DB, Lee W, et al. Central hemodynamic assessment of normal term pregnancy. *Am J Obstet Gynecol.* 1989;161:1439-1442.
5. Roberts JM, August PA, Bakris G, et al. Executive summary: hypertension in pregnancy. American College of Obstetricians and Gynecologists. *Obstet Gynecol.* 2013;122:1122-1131.
6. Mackay AP, Berg CJ, Atrash HK. Pregnancy-related mortality from preeclampsia and eclampsia. *Obstet Gynecol.* 2001;97:4.
7. Sibai BM, Ramadan MK, Usta I, et al. Maternal morbidity and mortality in 442 pregnancies with hemolysis, elevated liver enzymes, and low platelets (HELLP syndrome). *Am J Obstet Gynecol.* 1993;169:1000-1006.
8. Lewis G. The confidential enquiry into maternal and child health (CEMACH). Saving mother's lives: reviewing maternal deaths to make motherhood safer. 2003–2005. The seventh report on confidential enquiries into maternal deaths in the United Kingdom. London: CEMACH 2007.
9. Sibai BM, Stella CL. Diagnosis and management of atypical preeclampsia-eclampsia. *Am J Obstet Gynecol.* 2009;200(5):481.
10. Sibai BM. Diagnosis and management of gestational hypertension and preeclampsia. *Obstet Gynecol.* 2003;102:181-192.
11. Thangaratinam S, Ismail KM, Sharp S, et al. Accuracy of serum uric acid in predicting complications of pre-eclampsia: a systematic review. *Br J Obstet Gynaecol.* 2006;113:369-378.
12. Okanloma KA, Moodley J. Neurological complications associated with the pre-eclampsia/eclampsia syndrome. *Int J Gynaecol Obstet.* 2000;71:223-225.
13. Granger JP, Alexander BT, Bennett WA, et al. Pathophysiology of pregnancy-induced hypertension. *Am J Hyperten.* 2001;14:1785-1855.
14. Steegers EA, von Dadelszen P, Duvekot JJ, Pijnenborg R. Pre-eclampsia. *Lancet.* 2010;376:631-644.
15. Cipolla MJ. Cerebrovascular function in pregnancy and eclampsia. *Hypertension.* 2007;50:14-24.

16. Bendetti TJ, Kates R, Williams V. hemodynamic observations in severe pre-eclampsia complicated by pulmonary oedema. *Am J Obstet Gynecol.* 1985;152:330-334.

17. Hibbard JU, Shroff SG, Lang RM. Cardiovascular changes in preeclampsia. *Semin Nephrol.* 2004;24:580-587.

18. Leduc L, Wheeler JM, Kirshon B, et al. Coagulation profile in severe preeclampsia. *Obstet Gynecol.* 1992;79:14-18.

19. Moran P, Lindheimer MD, Davison JM. The renal response to preeclampsia. *Semin.* 2004;24:588-595.

20. Dennis AT. Management of preeclampsia: issues for anaesthetists. *Anaesthesia.* 2012;67:1009-1020.

21. Magee LA, Cham C, Waterman EJ, et al. Hydralazine for treatment of severe hypertension in pregnancy: meta-analysis. *BMJ.* 2003;327:955-960.

22. Euser AG, Cipolla MJ. Magnesium sulfate treatment for the prevention of eclampsia: a brief review. *Stroke.* 2009;40(4):1169-1175.

23. Belfort MA, Varner MW, Dizon-Townson DS, et al. Cerebral perfusion pressure, and not cerebral blood flow, may be the critical determinant of intracranial injury in pre-eclampsia: a new hypothesis. *Am J Obstet Gynecol.* 2002;187:626-634.

24. Jouppila P, Jouppila R, Hollmen A, et al. Lumbar epidural analgesia to improve intervillous blood flow during labor in severe preeclampsia. *Obstet Gynecol.* 1982;59:158-161.

25. Vandermuelen EP, Aken VH, Vermylen J, et al. Anticoagulants and spinal-epidural anesthesia. *Anesth Analg.* 1994;9:1165-1177.

26. Rout CC, Rocke DA, Levin JM, et al. A reevaluation of the role of crystalloid preload in the prevention of hypotension associated with spinal anesthesia for elective cesarean section. *Anesthesiology.* 1993:79(2):262-269.

27. McDonald S, Fernando R, Ashpole K. Maternal cardiac output changes after crystalloid or colloid coload following spinal anesthesia for elective cesarean delivery: a randomized controlled trial. *Anesth Analg.* 2001;113(4);803-810.

28. Hood DD, Curry R. Spinal versus epidural anesthesia for cesarean section in severely preeclamptic patients: a retrospective survey. *Anesthesiology.* 1999;90:1276-1282.

29. Visalyaputra S, Rodanant O, Somboonviboon W, et al. Spinal versus epidural anesthesia for cesarean delivery in severe preeclampsia: a prospective, randomized, multicenter study. *Anesth Analg.* 2005;101:862-868.

30. Santos AC. Spinal anesthesia in severely preeclamptic women: when is it safe? *Anesthesiology.* 1999; 90:1252-1254.

31. Fairley CJ, Clarke JT. Use of esmolol in a parturient with hypertrophic obstructive cardiomyopathy. *Br J Anaesth.* 1995;75:801-804.

32. Bansal S, Pawar M. Haemodynamic responses to laryngoscopy and intubation in patients with pregnancy-induced hypertension: effect of intravenous esmolol with or without lidocaine. *Int J Obstet Anesth.* 2002;11:4-8.

33. Ngan Kee WD, Khaw KS, Ma KC, Wong AS, Lee BB, Ng FF. Maternal and neonatal effects of remifentanil at induction of general anesthesia for cesarean delivery: a randomized, double-blind, controlled trial. *Anesthesiology.* 2006;104:14-20.

Anesthetic Management of Diabetes During Pregnancy

23

A. Fedson Hack

Diabetes mellitus is associated with the significant risks of developmental defects and stillbirth for the fetus, organ dysfunction for the mother during pregnancy, and increased lifetime likelihood for developing hypertensive disease, dyslipidemias, and progressive glucose intolerance. Physicians who care for pregnant women must be aware of the interplay between the physiologic changes of pregnancy and diabetes in order to optimize outcomes for both parturient and neonate.

EPIDEMIOLOGY AND ETIOLOGY OF DIABETES

Diabetes mellitus is a heterogeneous group of endocrine disorders characterized by elevated glucose levels, caused by a deficiency of insulin secretion or insulin resistance in peripheral tissue. Diabetes occurs in approximately 11% of the US population, with an additional 35% exhibiting symptoms of prediabetes. The prevalence has increased by 128% from 1988 to 2008, largely due to soaring rates of obesity.[1,2] The incidence of preexisting diabetes during pregnancy grew from 10% to 21% between 1999 and 2005.[3]

Insulin is a peptide hormone secreted by the β cells in the pancreatic islets of Langerhans that binds to insulin cell surface receptors in the liver, skeletal muscle, and adipose tissue. Insulin binding causes a conformational change in the α portion of the receptor, which activates kinase domains on its intracellular β subunits. Autophosphorylation of tyrosine residues initiates a series of signaling events that increases translocation of glucose transporter type 4 (GLUT4) from storage vesicles to the cell membrane. Insulin is critical in modulating maternal glucose, fat, and protein metabolism. Normal glucose metabolism represents a balance between insulin and the counteractive effects of glucagon, cortisol, epinephrine, and growth hormone.

PATHOPHYSIOLOGY AND RISK FACTORS FOR DIABETES IN PREGNANCY

Diabetes that is diagnosed before pregnancy is described by the standard classification as either type 1 or type 2. A third type, gestational diabetes, refers to a glycemic disorder discovered during pregnancy in the absence of preexisting metabolic disease. Individuals who have impaired fasting glucose (IFG) are referred to as having prediabetes, and they have a higher risk of developing future diabetes. As expected, IFG and impaired glucose tolerance (IGT) are associated with obesity, particularly abdominal obesity, dyslipidemia, and hypertension.

Type 1 Diabetes

Patients with type 1 diabetes (T1D) account for approximately 5% to 10% of those with the disease. This term includes patients previously referred to as insulin-dependent diabetes mellitus, or juvenile-onset diabetes mellitus. T1D is due to an absolute deficiency of insulin secretion following the cell-mediated autoimmune destruction of the β cells of the pancreas. Biomarkers of this immune destruction include autoantibodies to islet cells, insulin itself, glutamic acid decarboxylase, and tyrosine phosphatases IA-2 and IA-2β. One or more of these autoantibodies is present when fasting hyperglycemia is initially detected. There is also a strong association with human leukocyte antigen (HLA) types linked to DQA and DQB genes and influenced by DRB genes. These HLA-DR/DQ alleles can be either predisposing or protective.[4] Approximately 15% of those with autoimmune diabetes also have other autoimmune disorders such as Graves disease, Hashimoto thyroiditis, Addison disease, vitiligo, celiac sprue, autoimmune hepatitis, myasthenia gravis, and pernicious anemia.[4]

In infants and children, destruction of 85% of β cells can lead to hyperglycemia, whereas in adults as little as a 40% reduction by the age of 20 years is sufficient for development of the disease.[5] Although autoimmune destruction of β cells is more common in childhood and adolescence, it can occur at any age. It is thought to have multiple genetic predispositions and is believed to be related to poorly understood environmental factors.[6,7] T1D may initially present with ketoacidosis or with a long-standing fasting hyperglycemia that worsens in the presence of infection or other stressors. Some forms of T1D have no known etiology. In these cases, there are episodes of ketoacidosis and varying degrees of insulin deficiency but no immunologic evidence of β cell autoimmunity and the known HLA associations.[8]

Type 2 Diabetes

Type 2 diabetes (T2D) is caused by a combination of a resistance to insulin action and an inadequate insulin secretion to compensate for surges in glucose levels. The prevalence of T2D in pregnant women has increased as global obesity rates have soared. In the United States, approximately two-thirds of people are overweight or obese. Among pregnant women, 40% are either overweight or obese.[9-11] There are substantial perinatal risks associated with obesity including hypertensive disease, gestational diabetes, fetal macrosomia, induction of labor, cesarean section, and postpartum hemorrhage.[12,13] The risks associated with obesity increase with each elevation in the body mass index.

Diagnosis of preexisting T2D occurs at the patient's initial examination in the first trimester. A hemoglobin A1c (HbA1c) greater than 6.5%, fasting glucose greater than 126 mg/dL (6.99 mmol/L), a 2-hour plasma glucose greater than 200 mg/dL (11.1 mmol/L) after a 75-g glucose load, or a random plasma glucose greater than 200 mg/dL, indicate that the patient has T2D rather than gestational diabetes.[4,8]

The hyperglycemia of T2D may evolve in several ways, depending on the underlying disease process. IFG and/or IGT can exist without meeting the criteria for a diagnosis of diabetes. Some patients can achieve adequate glucose control with weight loss, exercise, nutritional management, and/or oral hypoglycemic agents. Others may require medications such as metformin or exogenous insulin for glucose control. Although the precise causes of T2D are not known, autoimmune destruction of β cells is not involved. Most of these patients are obese, and increased weight confers a degree of insulin resistance that cannot be compensated for by normal insulin secretion. Although insulin resistance may improve with pharmacologic management or weight loss and exercise, it seldom disappears or resolves completely.[4,8]

In addition to T1D and T2D, other rare types of diabetes can affect pregnant women. These include genetic defects of the β cell, abnormalities in insulin action (as is found in mature-onset diabetes of the young), diseases of the exocrine pancreas, endocrinopathies, drug-induced diabetes, and those caused by infections such as rubella. Other congenital syndromes, such as Down syndrome, can be associated with an elevated risk of diabetes. Finally, there are uncommon syndromes of immune-mediated diabetes, such as Stiff Person syndrome (SPS) syndrome and diabetes caused by anti-insulin receptor antibodies (known in the past as type B insulin resistance).[4,8]

Gestational Diabetes

Pregnancy exerts complex changes on maternal physiology and metabolism. During pregnancy, there is a progressive increase in peripheral resistance to insulin at the receptor and postreceptor level due to an increase in counterregulatory hormones, such as placental lactogen, placental growth hormone, cortisol, and progesterone.[14] Gestational diabetes (GDM) occurs when the increase in insulin resistance is not met by augmented pancreatic β cell mass and insulin secretion.[15,16] GDM is defined as hyperglycemia that is newly diagnosed during pregnancy. GDM is now found in 2% to 17.8% of pregnant women, depending on the diagnostic criteria used and the population studied.[17] It is the most common medical complication of pregnancy and is increasing worldwide. Pregnant women with GDM or pre-GDM are at elevated risk of significant neonatal and obstetric complications, morbidity, and mortality.[18,19]

For many years, the criteria used to diagnose GDM included any degree of glucose intolerance, regardless of whether its onset occurred in pregnancy. These criteria did not take into account whether the hyperglycemia persisted after pregnancy and did not exclude the possibility that unrecognized glucose intolerance may have preceded or begun concomitantly with the pregnancy. In addition, the criteria varied among countries, making international comparisons of the incidence of diabetes in pregnancy and treatment protocols difficult.[20]

Although the association between a history of previous stillbirth, fetal macrosomia, and diabetes was recognized as early as in the 1950s, the precise nature of the relationship between maternal glucose levels and poor pregnancy outcomes remains obscure to this day.[21] The Hyperglycemia and Adverse Pregnancy Outcome study was designed to evaluate the relationship between a 75-g glucose load in a 2-hour oral glucose tolerance test (OGTT) and poor pregnancy outcomes.[22] This study demonstrated a continuous relationship between OGTT serum glucose values below those that are diagnostic for diabetes and several perinatal outcomes. The International Association of Diabetes in Pregnancy Study Groups (IADPSG) study was organized to identify OGTT plasma glucose levels that correspond to an increased risk of fetal macrosomia, neonatal adiposity, and fetal hyperinsulinemia (all greater than 90th percentile). The IADPSG recommended either testing all pregnant women or only those with risk factors (depending on background frequency of abnormal glucose metabolism in the population and local circumstances) using a single 75-g, 2-hour OGTT with cutoffs at an odds ratio of 1.75.[23] The diagnosis of GDM is made when the fasting plasma glucose values are at least 92 mg/dL (5.1 mmol/L), a 1-hour value of at least 180 mg/dL (10.0 mmol/L), and a 2-hour value of at least 153 mg/dL (8.5 mmol/L). Please refer to Table 23-1.[23]

Table 23-1. International Association of Diabetes and Pregnancy Study Groups (IADPSG) Recommendations for Gestational Diabetes Screening[a]

At initial first trimester visit, obtain blood sample
Preexisting diabetes criteria:
Fasting plasma glucose (FPG) ≥ 126 mg/dL (≥ 6.99 mmol/L)
HbA1c ≥ 6.5% (≥ 48 mmol/mol)
Random plasma glucose ≥ 200 mg/dL (≥ 11.1 mmol/L) (confirmed by FPG or HbA1c)
Gestational diabetes criteria:
FPG ≥ 92 mg/dL (≥ 5.11 mmol/L) and < 126 mg/dL (≤ 6.99 mmol/L)
At 24-28 weeks' gestation, perform 75-g, 2-hour oral glucose tolerance test
Gestational diabetes criteria:
FPG ≥ 92 mg/dL (≥ 5.11 mmol/L)
1-hour plasma glucose ≥ 180 mg/dL (≥ 9.99 mmol/L)
2-hour plasma glucose ≥ 153 mg/dL (8.49 mmol/L)

[a]Adapted from the (IADPSG) Consensus Panel.[26]

These criteria have been shown to be cost-effective compared with current standard of care.[24] The American Diabetes Association (ADA) has adopted these criteria, although the American College of Obstetricians and Gynecologists (ACOG) still advocates testing all pregnant women with a 50-g, 1-hour test at 24 to 28 weeks and relying on the result of a 100-g, 3-hour OGTT.[8,25]

Risk factors for developing GDM include advanced maternal age, obesity, polycystic ovary disease, a family history of T2D, and a previous history of gestational diabetes, stillbirth, fetal malformation or macrosomia. Obesity increases the overall risk of GDM by a factor of 3.76.[26] Perinatal mortality and an increase in congenital malformations are also strongly correlated with maternal obesity in patients with T2D.[27]

Diabetes during pregnancy has historically been classified using the system proposed by Priscilla White in 1949 based on a case series of women with T1D at the New England Deaconess Hospital in Boston, Massachusetts.[28] In this study, she found significant associations among the onset of diabetes, its duration, and the degree of vasculopathy, to adverse outcomes of pregnancy. These criteria were later modified to make clear that class A diabetes should include only those women with pre-GDM.[29] The ongoing relevance of the White classification to assess pregnancies at risk for elevated perinatal morbidity and mortality has been eroded by the increasing prevalence of T2D.[30,31] Currently, 90% of pregnant diabetic patients have GDM, and T1D and T2D account for the remaining 10% of cases.

ACUTE MATERNAL COMPLICATIONS OF DIABETES

During pregnancy, women with diabetes experience both acute and chronic diabetic complications related to glycemic control, as well as the risks associated with their higher prevalence of preeclampsia. Acute complications include diabetic ketoacidosis (DKA), hyperosmolar hyperglycemia state (HHS), and hypoglycemia. The underlying mechanism for both DKA and HHS is reduction in the effective action of insulin and the elevation of the counterregulatory hormones such as glucagon, cortisol, growth hormone, and catecholamines.

Diabetic Ketoacidosis

DKA can occur in patients with T1D and in those with T2D who develop further insulin resistance following trauma or severe infection.[32,33] DKA is characterized by hyperglycemia, metabolic acidosis, and increased ketone formation.[32] Although the incidence of DKA during pregnancy has declined significantly over the years, it remains a medical emergency; historically fetal mortality rates of 30% to 90% and maternal mortality rates of 5% to 15% have been reported.[33-35]

DKA occurs in approximately 1% to 2% of pregnancies complicated by diabetes, and it is rare in patients with gestational diabetes.[32,34-36] Although improved glycemic control in pregnant diabetics has decreased the incidence of DKA in those with known diabetes, up to 30% of cases occur in those women who are unaware they have diabetes.[34,36] DKA is also more common as further insulin resistance develops in the second and third trimesters.[37,38]

Several triggers have been reported to precipitate DKA in pregnancy. Cessation of insulin therapy and infection account for 40% and 20% of cases, respectively, and in 30% of cases acidosis has been the initial presentation of undiagnosed diabetes.[39,40] Risk factors that predispose pregnant patients to DKA include infection, vomiting, diabetic gastroparesis, the use of corticosteroids (such as betamethasone given to accelerate fetal lung maturation) and β-sympathomimetic drugs used for uterine tocolysis. In one case series, vomiting and the use of β-mimetic drugs accounted for up to 57% of cases of DKA.[41] During an episode of DKA, a patient may experience nausea, vomiting, abdominal pain, tachypnea, hypotension, tachycardia, and stupor, and he or she may have a sweet-scented breath from exhaled ketones.

DKA is a result of inadequate insulin action and the failure of glucose utilization at the cellular level. Hormones, such as glucagon, catecholamines, cortisol, and growth hormone, enable cellular metabolism of carbohydrates, proteins, and lipids. An increase in gluconeogenesis and glycogenolysis in the liver and decreased peripheral glucose utilization leads to hyperglycemia. Free fatty acids are released from adipose tissue and converted into ketones, acetoacetate, and β-hydroxybutyrate. Ketones dissociate at physiologic pH and are neutralized by bicarbonate. The compensated respiratory alkalosis of pregnancy, however, reduces patient's buffering capacity and renders patients more susceptible to metabolic acidosis at lower glucose levels.

Glucose resorption in the renal tubules reaches a maximum threshold of about 240 mg/dL (13.3 mmol/L), beyond which glucosuria develops. With increasing hyperglycemia, an osmotic diuresis occurs leading to total body water depletion, hypovolemia, hyperosmolarity, and electrolyte depletion.[42] Maternal acidosis, hyperglycemia, severe volume depletion, and electrolyte abnormalities contribute to the high rates of fetal loss. The consequences of maternal DKA for the fetus are discussed below.

The greater susceptibility to develop ketosis during pregnancy is reflected in the likelihood that overt DKA can occur at lower blood glucose levels.[43,44] While euglycemic ketoacidosis is rare, it has been reported in pregnancies complicated by gestational diabetes.[45,46] In euglycemic (or normoglycemic) ketoacidosis, the patient has a metabolic acidosis in the absence of elevated serum glucose, a process that is thought to be due to accelerated starvation and near total depletion of hepatic glycogen stores.[45-48]

Hyperosmolar Hyperglycemic State

Previously known as hyperosmolar nonketotic coma or hyperosmolar hyperglycemic nonketotic syndrome, HHS is a severe complication of uncontrolled hyperglycemia. It develops predominantly in patients with T2D.[49] In one study of HHS patients diagnosed in an emergency department, 30% to 40% were unaware of their underlying diabetes.[50] Typically, patients become increasingly hyperglycemic without increasing their fluid intake to compensate for their polyuria. As a result, they develop severe osmotic dehydration, increasing hyperosmolarity, and moderate azotemia without ketosis or significant acidosis. Mental status changes may be followed by somnolence, coma, and seizures.[51]

Treatment of Diabetic Ketoacidosis and Hyperosmolar Hyperglycemia State

Initial laboratory evaluation for suspected hyperglycemic associated DKA and HHS should include determination of plasma glucose, blood urea nitrogen, creatinine, serum ketones, electrolytes (with calculation of the anion gap), chemistry profile, osmolality, urinalysis, urine ketones, arterial blood gas, complete blood count and differential.[37] Diagnostic criteria for DKA include a serum glucose greater than 250 mg/dL (13.9 mmol/L), arterial pH less than 7.3, serum bicarbonate less than 18 mEq/L, and moderate ketonuria or ketonemia.[52] For HHS, the diagnostic criteria include a serum glucose greater than 600 mg/dL (33.3 mmol/L), arterial pH greater than 7.3, serum bicarbonate greater than 15 mEq/mL, and minimal ketonuria or keturia. HHS develops over several days to weeks, but the time course for acute DKA in T1D and T2D is shorter. Although both DKA and HHS are often precipitated by infection, altered mental status is more common with HHS due to the hyperosmolality, and vomiting, dehydration, and abdominal pain are more characteristic of DKA.

Successful management of DKA and HHS requires resolution of dehydration, hyperglycemia, electrolyte abnormalities, precipitating factors, and close monitoring. The goal of fluid resuscitation is to expand the intravascular and extravascular volume and restore renal perfusion. Typically, 1 to 1.5 L isotonic saline (0.9% NaCl) should be infused over the first hour. Additional fluid replacement is guided by volume status, glucose-corrected serum sodium levels, and urine output. Fluid replacement should aim to correct deficits within the first 24 hours.

The average fluid deficit in a nonpregnant patient with HHS may be up to 9 L.[50] A general guideline is to replace half of the fluid deficit in the first 12 hours and the remaining deficit in the next 12 to 24 hours, with frequent monitoring of the serum sodium. Serum osmolality should not be decreased by more than 3 mOsm/kg per hour to reduce the risk of developing cerebral edema.[32]

Regular insulin has usually been the insulin treatment of choice. In the absence of hypokalemia, an intravenous bolus of 0.1 U/kg is initiated followed by a continuous infusion of 0.1 U/kg per hour. If the blood glucose does not decrease at a rate of 50 to 75 mg/dL per hour (2.7-4.2 mmol/L per hour), the insulin rate should be increased. When the plasma glucose decreases to 200 mg/dL (11.1 mmol/L) in DKA or 300 mg/dL (16.6 mmol/L) in HHS, the rate of insulin infusion can be decreased to 0.05 to 0.1 U/kg per hour and a 5% dextrose drip initiated to maintain blood glucose levels.[52] Subsequent management involves adjusting of the rate of insulin and dextrose infusions to maintain glucose levels until the acidosis in DKA resolves or the hyperosmolality in HHS clears.

Administering bicarbonate to treat the metabolic acidosis in DKA is controversial. Bicarbonate use may be associated with paradoxical central nervous system acidosis, hypokalemia, hypertonicity, and cerebral edema.[41,53] Electrolyte abnormalities necessitate continuous electrocardiographic (ECG) monitoring, and patients should be treated in an intensive care unit setting with continuous fetal monitoring and assessment of fetal well-being with a biophysical profile.

Studies have evaluated the efficacy of the rapid-acting insulin analogs, such as Lispro, given subcutaneously for patients in diabetic ketosis.[54,55] Although these regimens permit treatment of noncomplicated DKA in general wards or in the emergency department, their use in pregnancy has not been evaluated.

Other Complications

HYPOGLYCEMIA

Hypoglycemia is the greatest limitation to insulin therapy in T1D and to tight glucose control in T2D.[56,57] It occurs in 33% to 71% of those with T1D, and in these patients, severe hypoglycemia is three to five times more frequent than T2D during early pregnancy.[58] Severe hypoglycemia is the most common adverse event in pregnant women who use insulin. There are no data, however, which suggest that treated episodes of hypoglycemia contribute to poor pregnancy outcomes.[59]

Hypoglycemia is most common in the first trimester, although it can occur in subsequent trimesters and can be asymptomatic at night. Insulin requirements increase during pregnancy because of a progressive insulin resistance in periphery. At term, insulin needs are 1.0 U/kg per day compared with 0.7 U/kg per day prior to pregnancy.[60] The risk of hypoglycemia in diabetic pregnancy also may be related to fetal use of maternal glucose during periods of maternal fasting. As blood glucose levels drop, patients initially experience adrenergic symptoms of palpitations, perspiration, and hunger, which signify physiologic efforts to restore carbohydrate levels. With further decreases in blood glucose levels, patients experience neurologic symptoms of altered behavior, mood swings, and finally diminished consciousness and convulsions.[61]

Severe hypoglycemia in pregnant diabetics has been implicated as a cause for maternal traffic accidents and even death.[61-63] In a patient who has severe low blood sugar and is able to swallow, oral carbohydrates must be given promptly. In those who are obtunded and who do not have intravenous access, 1 mg of glucagon can be given intramuscularly.[52,64]

PREECLAMPSIA

Pregnant women with diabetes are at higher risk for developing preeclampsia, which is characterized by hypertension and proteinuria after 20 weeks of pregnancy. Those with severe disease may develop the syndrome known as HELLP (hemolysis, elevated liver enzymes, low platelets) or eclampsia.[65-67] Although the topic of hypertensive disease of pregnancy is discussed in detail elsewhere, it is important to note that preeclampsia and cesarean delivery are both more common in undiagnosed GDM and may be prevented with treatment of even mild hyperglycemia.[68]

NONACUTE AND LONG-TERM MATERNAL COMPLICATIONS OF DIABETES

Hyperglycemia causes changes at the cellular level that result in accelerated microvascular and macrovascular disease. Elevated glucose levels are associated with oxidative stress, decreased nitric oxide availability, oxidation of low-density

Table 23-2. Complications of Chronic Diabetes

Macrovascular
  Coronary
  Cerebrovascular
  Peripheral vascular
Microvascular
  Diabetic retinopathy
  Nephropathy
Neuropathy
  Autonomic
    Cardiovascular
    Gastrointestinal
  Somatic
    Peripheral

lipoproteins, and activation of procoagulants.[60,69] In general, the occurrence of chronic complications is related to the duration of diabetes and degree of glycemic control (see Table 23-2). Whereas the long-term complications of T1D are typically microvascular angiopathies, affecting the retina, kidneys, and the autonomic nervous system, those for T2D are macrovascular and affect the heart, central nervous system, and peripheral vascular system. Tight glucose control can lessen the severity and/or progression of these microvascular complications.[70-72]

Infection

Patients with diabetes have greater susceptibility to infection through increased inflammation and decreased cell-mediated immunity. During pregnancy women are at elevated risk for urinary tract infections that can develop into pyelonephritis and septicemia. Candidal infections, such as oral thrush and vulvovaginal yeast infections, are also more prevalent. Gingival inflammation is common in pregnancy and can lead to oral infections in diabetics. Among pregnant patients, obesity and diabetes are independent risk factors for infection following cesarean section.[73]

Diabetic Nephropathy

Renal disorders complicate approximately 5% of pregnancies in women with pre-existing diabetes, especially those with T1D, and may progress in those with poorly controlled hypertension and worsening glomerular filtration rates. Intensive glycemic control and aggressive treatment of hypertension can attenuate progression of nephropathy.[74] Women with diabetes often have progressive proteinuria during pregnancy (protein excretion can double or triple in the third trimester), and this can cause confusion with the diagnosis of preeclampsia. Those with normal serum creatinine levels may have no further decline in kidney function or impairment of long-term survival.[74] Women with creatinine levels higher than 1.5 mg/dL have the greatest risk of perinatal complications. Approximately 50% will deliver before term, 50% will develop preeclampsia, and 15% will have fetuses with intrauterine growth restriction (IUGR).[75] Strict glycemic control and intensive antihypertensive treatment are essential in these patients.[76]

Diabetic Retinopathy

The prevalence of retinopathy in women with pre-GDM of both types is 10% to 36%. These rates increase in patients with T1D, and 57% to 62% are diagnosed with retinopathy during their initial eye examination during pregnancy. In patients with T2D, retinopathy is found in 17% to 28%. In T1D retinopathy often worsens during pregnancy, but this occurs less frequently in T2D.[77] Neither the long-term risk of retinopathy nor its progression appears to worsen with pregnancy itself.[78] Although rare, diabetic retinopathy has also been reported in GDM.[79]

Microvascular changes in the eye may be caused by diabetes, by pregnancy itself, or by rapid improvement in glycemic control when diabetes is discovered in pregnancy. Fluid retention, vasodilation, and augmented blood flow during pregnancy are thought to accelerate the loss of autoregulation in the retinal capillary bed. All patients with retinopathy should have their baseline level of ophthalmologic disease level established by a specialist after their first visit to the obstetrician. Laser photocoagulation treatment of retinopathy is effective in pregnancy and should not be delayed until after delivery.

Factors associated with the progression of retinopathy include the duration of T1D, degree of hyperglycemia, level of glycemic control at conception, stage of disease at the onset of pregnancy, and presence of chronic hypertension or preeclampsia.[80-82] Rapid reduction in HbA1c has been associated with worsening of diabetic retinopathy.[78] Although there are no controlled studies of whether the Valsalva maneuver during the second stage of labor can induce vitreous hemorrhages in patients with diabetic retinopathy, the ADA still recommends use of epidural anesthesia with an assisted second stage or cesarean delivery in these patients.[82]

Diabetic Neuropathy

Pregnant diabetics may experience several forms of diabetic neuropathy, but they have not been well studied. In patients with evidence of diabetes-induced cardiovascular autonomic dysfunction, hypotension must be avoided. In nonpregnant patients, the corrected QT interval (QTc) has been noted to correspond to the severity of autonomic neuropathy.[83] It is not known whether the same association is seen in pregnant diabetics. Cardiovascular autonomic neuropathy can be evaluated by looking for diminished heart rate variability (such as with time domain analysis of R-R interval to paced breathing and Valsalva maneuvers) and decreased blood pressure on standing.[84-86] Lack of heart rate variability in nonpregnant patients with a history of GDM is indicative of cardiac autonomic neuropathy and is related to glycemic control, not insulin sensitivity.[86]

A short-term increase in sensorimotor distal symmetric polyneuropathy (DPN) may develop during pregnancy and later resolve. Acute sensory neuropathy is rare, tends to result from poor glycemic control, and can follow acute changes in metabolic management. The neuropathy is typically worse at night, with few neurologic findings on physical examination. DPN is more common in T1D and in patients with long-standing T2D; it is rare in GDM.

Gastroparesis occurs when damage to the ganglia in the gastrointestinal tract inhibits gastric motility and delays intestinal transit time. Recent work indicates that gastric motility is directly influenced by glucose levels and that diminished autonomic nervous function is not the sole cause of gastroparesis diabeticorum.

Women with gastroparesis may experience more protracted nausea and vomiting during pregnancy, and those with severe gastroparesis may require inpatient nutritional therapy and antiemetic therapy to prevent fetal losses.[87-89] Gastroparesis is a diabetic complication that carries with it a significant risk of morbidity and poor pregnancy outcome, which is second only to coronary heart disease.[90-92] Autonomic neuropathy is a complication of long-standing T1D, but it does not appear that pregnancy itself is a risk factor for the deterioration of autonomic nervous function.[93-95]

Cardiovascular Disease

Although macrovascular diseases are more often found in T2D patients, coronary artery disease is not commonly seen in women of childbearing age, and only case reports have been published. Nonetheless, pre-GDM was associated with the risk of an acute coronary event with an odds ratio of 4.3 (2.3-7.9).[90-92] Atypical and "silent" manifestation of coronary ischemia remain a concern, although improvements in care have reduced maternal mortality rates to 7.3% to 11%.[90-92]

A pregnancy with diabetes has significant health consequences for women in later life. Postpartum metabolic syndrome in patients with GDM is well described.[96-101] Elevated plasma total cholesterol, low-density lipoprotein, and triglyceride concentrations are also found in women with GDM.[102] In these patients, the increased lifetime risk of developing T2D may be as high as sevenfold.[103] Women with GDM also exhibit higher elevations in plasma fibrinogen, thrombin-antithrombin complexes, and lower levels of coagulation inhibitors than those with normal pregnancies.[69,104]

Although the occurrence of hypertensive disease in pregnancy increases in the presence of diabetes, the relationship between the two is not well understood. Transient hypertension of pregnancy, which is diagnosed after 20 weeks' gestation and not accompanied by proteinuria, is known to be associated with a higher risk of essential hypertension and glucose intolerance in later life. Interestingly, an abnormal glucose-loading test during pregnancy is a predictor of the development of preeclampsia in a subsequent pregnancy and future hypertension.[97] Pregnant women with diabetes and those with gestational hypertension also have an elevated risk of cardiovascular disease, particularly those with a family history of T2D.[98,99]

ACUTE PHYSIOLOGIC AND METABOLIC ABNORMALITIES OF THE FETUS AND NEONATE

Maternal DKA has substantial effects on the fetus as a result of its effects on oxygen transport. Hyperglycemia results in covalently bound glycosylated hemoglobin, which in turn alters the interaction between the β chains of the hemoglobin molecule. As a result of elevations in glycosylated hemoglobin, maternal red blood cells transfer less oxygen to the fetal hemoglobin molecules and may contribute to fetal hypoxia.[105,106] Additionally, as maternal ketone bodies dissociate, the hydrogen ions and organic anions cross the placenta and cause fetal acidosis. A leftward shift of the oxyhemoglobin dissociation curve, with decreased 2,3-diphosphoglycerate levels, increases maternal hemoglobin affinity for oxygen, thus decreasing overall oxygen delivery to the fetus.

Fetal blood flow has been observed to redistribute during episodes of DKA, and treatment of maternal acidosis reverses abnormal blood flow.[107,108] A fetal heart rate tracing that lacks variability, or has variable or late decelerations, such as an indeterminate category II tracing, is not an indication for immediate delivery until the metabolic condition is corrected.[109] Emergency cesarean section in the setting of decompensated DKA could worsen maternal outcomes. β-Hydroxybutyrate is known to cross the placenta, and fetuses can thus acquire ketoacidosis. Bilateral basal ganglia infarctions have been noted in a case report of a neonate born during an episode of DKA.[110]

Perinatal hypoxia and birth asphyxia also occur in infants whose mothers have poorly controlled diabetes (primarily T1D), vascular disease, and nephropathy. In these cases, extreme hyperglycemia and ketosis reduce uterine and placental blood flow, which increases the risk of fetal hypoxia. Elevated fetal glucose concentrations also lead to increased placental glucose consumption, contributing to further lactate production and glycogen deposition.

Transient hypoglycemia in the immediate postnatal period is normal for all infants but occurs more quickly and to lower levels in infants of diabetic mothers, particularly in the setting of unstable maternal glucose levels. Neonatal hypoglycemia occurs in 5% to 12% of infants born of pre-GDM or GDM mothers.[111] Early feeding or a glucose infusion started at 4 to 6 mg/min per kilogram body weight can be used to stabilize plasma glucose levels until the infant can take adequate oral nutrition.

Other acute physiologic abnormalities occur in infants of diabetic mothers (IDMs). Neonatal hypocalcemia and hypomagnesemia occurs in one-half of IDMs within 72 hours of birth. Hypocalcemia is likely to be a result of slow transition from fetal parathyroid to neonatal parathyroid control. Neonatal hypomagnesemia may be related to the same parathyroid issues but may also be worsened in cases of maternal hypomagnesemia with severe renal disease.[112]

Respiratory distress is often found in premature infants but occurs with even greater frequency in term infants born to women with GDM because hyperglycemia is thought to delay fetal lung maturation.[112,113] In addition, the elevated risk of cesarean delivery leads to increased rates of transient tachypnea of the newborn and neonatal persistent pulmonary hypertension.[114,115] See Table 23-3.

Table 23-3. Fetal Complications of Maternal Diabetes

Acute
  Hypoglycemia
  Hyperglycemia
  Hypocalcemia
  Hypomagnesemia
  Iron deficiency
  Hypoxia
  Acidosis
  Transient tachypnea of the newborn
  Persistent pulmonary hypertension
  Thrombocytopenia
  Polycythemia
  Hyperbilirubinemia
  Preeclampsia
  HELLP syndrome
  Eclampsia
  Emergency cesarean section
Chronic
  Growth abnormalities
    Macrosomia/large-for-gestational age
    Intrauterine growth restriction
    Polyhydramnios
  Birth trauma
    Erb palsy (C5-7)
    Klumpke paralysis (C7-C8)
    Diaphragmatic paralysis (C2-C5)
    Recurrent laryngeal nerve damage (T1-T2)
  Congenital anomalies
    Central nervous system
      Neural tube defects
    Cardiovascular
      Transposition of the great vessels
      Persistent truncus arteriosus
      Visceral heterotaxia
      Asymmetrical septal hypertrophy
      Transient hypertrophic subaortic stenosis
      Ventricular septal defects
      Myocardial hypertrophy
      Single ventricle
      Coarctation of the aorta
      Single umbilical artery

(Continued)

Table 23-3. Fetal Complications of Maternal Diabetes (*Continued*)

Pulmonary
  Surfactant deficiency
Renal
  Fetal hydronephrosis
  Renal agenesis
  Ureteral duplication
Gastrointestinal
  Situs anomalies
  Meconium plug syndrome
  Duodenal atresia
  Anorectal atresia
Skeletal
  Polydactyly
  Syndactyly
  Focal femoral hypoplasia
  Caudal regression syndrome
  Syringomyelia

Polycythemia can develop as a result of chronic fetal hypoxia and increased fetal erythropoietin. Heightened secretion of insulin and insulin-like growth factors also increases red blood cell production, as do high concentrations of β-hydroxybutyrate, a metabolic product of ketosis.[116] The fetal expansion of red cells may occur at the expense of platelet formation causing thrombocytopenia and may lead to hyperbilirubinemia.[112] Furthermore, hyperviscosity from polycythemia and decreased cardiac output related to common cardiac anomalies increase the risk of developing blood clots.

Up to 65% of infants of diabetic mothers have abnormalities in iron metabolism with ferritin concentrations found in the majority. The severity of iron abnormalities is related to maternal glycemic control.[117] Perinatal iron deficiency can put these infants at higher risk for acute and chronic hypoxemia and at risk for perinatal brain injury.[112]

NONACUTE AND LONG-TERM COMPLICATIONS IN INFANTS OF DIABETIC MOTHERS

Despite advances in perinatal care, IDMs remain at risk for chronic complications (Table 23-3). Polyhydramnios, growth derangements, and congenital anomalies contribute to increased infant morbidity. Rates of perinatal mortality can be 3 to 10 times higher than they are in unaffected pregnancies for a given gestational age. Congenital anomalies are now the leading cause of perinatal mortality and infants of diabetic mothers have congenital malformation rates that are 4 to 10 times higher than their normal peers.[118,119] Clinical studies have demonstrated that poor glycemic control (HbA1c greater than 6.4%) during preconception and organogenesis is linked to a fourfold elevation in the risk of congenital abnormalities (brain, heart, kidney, intestinal, and skeletal) and stillbirth.[71,119-121]

Growth Abnormalities

IDMs suffer accelerated fetal growth and macrosomia (birth weight greater than 4000 g and/or greater than the 90th percentile for gestational age) as a result of unstable elevations in maternal glucose.[122,123] Pulsatile hyperglycemia creates surges in fetal insulin secretion and production of fat from glucose and other fuel sources. Hepatomegaly, splenomegaly, and cardiomegaly (from intraventricular septal hypertrophy) are common.[112]

The primary risk of macrosomic, or large-for-gestational age (LGA) infants, is injury to the nerves of the fetal brachial plexus during a vaginal delivery. Shoulder dystocia is the most common event and can produce an Erb palsy (nerve roots C5-C7), Klumpke paralysis (roots C7-C8), diaphragmatic paralysis (roots C3-C5), and recurrent laryngeal nerve damage (roots T1-T2).[113] The use of forceps or vacuum extractor can also cause fetal injuries, such as subarachnoid hemorrhage, or elevated risk for intraventricular hemorrhage. Cephalopelvic disproportion in LGA infants also is an independent cause for cesarean deliveries or birth trauma for the mother.[124]

Although macrosomia is the more common growth anomaly in IDMs, some infants develop IUGR as a consequence of maternal vascular disease. Placental vascular insufficiency results in protein-energy malnutrition, leading to fetal growth deceleration and restricted oxygen delivery with fetal polycythemia. These pregnancies often end in preterm deliveries and neonatal intensive care unit admissions.

Congenital Abnormalities

The incidence of major anomalies in diabetic pregnancies is estimated at 6% to 10%.[112,125] The malformations usually are multiorgan, with cardiac abnormalities being the most common, followed by those of the central nervous system. The anomalies are thought to develop during organogenesis in the face of unstable glucose levels. They have long been associated with maternal diabetic vascular complications.[126] The triad of fetal hypoxia, cardiomyopathy, and tissue iron deficiency is often found in macrosomic fetuses and can impair the fetal response to the stresses of delivery.[112]

The majority of cardiac malformations occur in infants whose mothers have had poorly controlled T1D. Elevated maternal HbA1c levels during the first trimester have been associated with an increased potential for these abnormalities.[127] Half of these are vascular conotruncal anomalies (transposition of the great vessels, persistent truncus arteriosus, visceral heterotaxia, and single ventricle). Other cardiac disorders are found in infants with maternal T1D and T2D, including asymmetric septal hypertrophy, transient hypertrophic subaortic stenosis from ventricular septal defects, and myocardial hypertrophy.[128] Septal hypertrophy is common and occurs in 25% to 75% of IDMs.[129]

Central nervous system abnormalities such as neural tube defects (myelomeningoceles, spina bifida, encephaloceles) are more common in neonates of mothers with poorly controlled T1D. The fetal and newborn central nervous system can be affected by fetal hypoxia, glucose abnormalities, polycythemia, and birth asphyxia.[112]

Other organ systems at risk for congenital anomalies in IDMs include the pulmonary (delay in development of type II alveolar cells and surfactant deficiency), renal (hydronephrosis, agenesis, ureteral duplication), cardiovascular (cardiomyopathy, singular umbilical artery, ventricular and atrial septal defects, and coarctation of the aorta), gastrointestinal (situs anomalies, meconium plug syndrome, small left colon syndrome, duodenal, anorectal atresia) and skeletal (caudal regression, syringomyelia, polydactyly, syndactyly, focal femoral hypoplasia) systems.[112,113]

Like their diabetic mothers, neonates experience long-term consequences of maternal hyperglycemia. Higher rates of childhood obesity, IGT in adolescence, hypertension, and dyslipidemia have been linked to IDMs.[130-134] Infants of mothers with GDM have a 61% higher risk of being overweight at age 7 years compared with their peers.[135] Another study found that 3-year-old children were twice as likely to be obese if exposed in utero to maternal glucose concentrations of at least 130 mg/dL (7.2 mmol/L) rather than less than 100 mg/dL (5.5 mmol/L).[136]

IDMs are at elevated risk for delayed motor and cognitive development which may become manifest later in life.[137] These long-term delays can be related to acute perinatal events or changes in brain development related to abnormalities in the intrauterine environment. Adverse neurologic outcomes are related to glucose, calcium, and magnesium metabolism, fetal hypoxia, polycythemia, and tissue iron deficiency; and a history of birth trauma and asphyxia.[112,138]

Exposure to hyperglycemia and hyperinsulinemia may disturb epigenetic, structural, and functional adaptive responses that are crucial for developmental programming.[138-141] Embryos exposed to maternal diabetes have altered gene expression, and this plays an important role in the pathogenesis of diabetes-induced disease programming and appears to be permanent.[139] There also appears to be epigenetic regulation of gene expression in fetal growth retardation often found in pregnant diabetics.[142]

GLYCEMIC MANAGEMENT DURING PREGNANCY AND DELIVERY

Strict glycemic control is critical to prevent fetal abnormalities in women with diabetes and forestall progression of diabetic comorbidities. Pregnant women should frequently check their capillary blood sugar levels to determine whether adjustments in diet or insulin therapy are needed. Control of hyperglycemia is of particular importance in the first trimester during fetal organogenesis.

During the typical pregnancy, insulin requirements increase in the second and third trimester. Total insulin requirements average approximately 0.9 U/kg per day in the first trimester, 1 U/kg per day during the second trimester, and 1.2 U/kg per day in the third trimester. For women with T2D, insulin requirements during the second and third trimesters may reach 1.2 U/kg per day and 1.6 U/kg per day, respectively.[8]

Insulin treatment can be divided into basal requirements, prandial, and correction doses. The basal dose of insulin is approximately 50% to 60% of the total daily amount, with the remainder given in prandial doses. The intent of the basal dose is to control hepatic glucose production between meals and during fasting, while prandial insulin doses reduce elevations in glucose levels due to meals. Correction doses are given to treat premeal or intermeal hyperglycemia.[143] A fasting blood glucose concentration between 60 and 95 mg/dL (3.3-5.3 mmol/L) is thought to be optimal, but tight control is accompanied by a risk of maternal hypoglycemia.

Therapeutic insulin exists in several forms. Historically, insulin production involved converting isolates obtained from pigs and cattle into human insulin. The more recent development of recombinant insulin has enabled women to have greater flexibility in dosing and improved quality of life. Lispro and Aspart insulin have been shown to be a safe and effective treatment in pregnancy. Compared with regular insulin, these rapid-acting analogs reach twice the maximum concentration of insulin in half the time. As a result, patients experience fewer episodes of hyperglycemia between meals.

During the first trimester, patients with T2D are usually switched from oral hypoglycemic agents to insulin because of concerns about the safety of oral agents for the fetus.[144] Patients who develop GDM are usually diagnosed later in pregnancy (eg, at 24-28 weeks). Because the risks of teratogenicity at this stage are minimal, treatment with glyburide (a second-generation sulfonylurea) or metformin (a biguanide) may be initiated instead of insulin therapy.[145] These agents offer greater convenience and comfort for the patient, although they may not fully suppress hyperglycemia.[146,147]

Long-acting or oral hypoglycemic agents should be discontinued 1 to 2 days prior to a scheduled cesarean delivery or stopped once the patient begins to labor. During labor and delivery, glycemic control must be maintained. Glucose levels should remain between 70 and 90 mg/dL (3.9 and 5.0 mmol/L) during delivery to prevent fetal hypoxemia and acidosis. Maternal hyperglycemia results in glycosylation of fetal hemoglobin, reducing its oxygen carrying capacity and increasing the risk of fetal acidosis. Plasma glucose values greater than 126 mg/dL (7.0 mmol/L) have been shown to increase the risk of neonatal hypoglycemia.[143] All patients should have glucose levels monitored during labor at time intervals appropriate to their disease status (eg, at 30- to 60-minute intervals).

Typically, in insulin-dependent patients who are scheduled for cesarean delivery, the morning dose of intermediate-acting insulin is omitted. When the patient arrives at the hospital, a normal saline infusion is initiated and used for bolus infusions and maintenance. Lactated Ringer's is generally not used because it contains sodium lactate, which can be oxidized to a gluconeogenic precursor and elevate blood glucose levels.[148] Boluses of 5% dextrose cause fetal acidosis, and glucose infusions should be placed on a pump.[149] The trauma of a cesarean section will lead to increasing demand for glucose. If the patient's glucose level falls, a 5% dextrose infusion is started with a separate intravenous line and a regular insulin drip initiated to maintain fasting blood glucose levels.

Women who are planning a vaginal delivery should be instructed not to take their basal or long-acting insulin when in labor or on the day labor is induced. In T1D women, labor has a glucose-lowering effect and reduces insulin requirements, and to prevent hypoglycemia and ketosis, a glucose infusion is given. Starvation-induced ketosis during labor has adverse fetal effects, including fetal ketonemia, hypoxia, and fetal lactic acidosis. The fetus has limited glycogen stores and rapidly secretes insulin in response to hyperglycemia. During the first stage of active labor when maternal insulin needs are reduced, a glucose infusion rate of 2.55 mg/kg per minute is required to maintain a glucose level of 70 to 90 mg/dL (3.9-5.0 mmol/L). The increased need for insulin in the second stage of labor remains unaffected by epidural analgesia or Pitocin-augmentation and glycemic adjustments may not be required.[150]

Following delivery, insulin needs to be decreased to 60% of the prepregnancy dose due to the loss of counterregulatory hormones produced by the placenta. Once patients have resumed eating, they can be restarted on lower doses of short-acting and intermediate-acting insulin on their first postpartum day. Insulin requirements return to prepregnancy levels within several weeks following delivery. However, because glucose levels in T1D patients fluctuate during breastfeeding, there is a risk of hypoglycemia, and glycemic control should be loosened.[72,151]

ANESTHETIC MANAGEMENT DURING LABOR AND DELIVERY

There have been no prospective, randomized trials evaluating the efficacy or safety of various anesthetic techniques in pregnant diabetics.[148,152] Individual clinical decisions must be made with an understanding of the relationship of anesthetic techniques to the physiologic changes in pregnancy and the pathophysiology of diabetes. The preanesthetic history and physical evaluation should focus on identifying the chronic and acute complications of diabetes, particularly as they relate to the patient's pregnancy.[152-155] Anesthetic interventions that might cause placental insufficiency, fetal hypoxia, and acidosis must be avoided.

The use of neuraxial anesthesia in pregnancy has resulted in decreased maternal morbidity and mortality. By reducing circulating maternal catecholamines, epidural analgesia increases placental perfusion and decreases fetal acidosis. In diabetic patients with suspected autonomic dysfunction, it is especially important to avoid hypotension to ensure good perinatal outcomes.[156] Although symptoms of autonomic neuropathy can be obscured by physiologic changes in pregnancy, the potential must be considered, particularly in those with T1D. In these patients, slow initiation of epidural anesthesia may be preferable to allow for slower compensatory hemodynamic mechanisms.

If a general anesthetic is required, etomidate might be preferable to thiopental or propofol to avoid postinduction hypotension. Any hypotension requires prompt treatment with vigorous volume expansion using a nondextrose solution and vasopressors. Autonomic neuropathy in pregnant diabetics can also produce abnormalities in temperature regulation. During cesarean section, inappropriate regulation of peripheral vasoconstriction can lead to hypothermia due to excessive heat losses, so passive warming may be indicated.[157]

During elective or emergency intubation, decreased gastric motility renders the patient at higher risk for aspiration. In these patients, aspiration prophylaxis should include a nonparticulate antacid administered approximately 30 minutes before surgery.[158] Metoclopramide may be necessary to enhance gastric emptying and gastroesophageal sphincter tone. The administration of a histamine-2 receptor antagonist such as ranitidine may further reduce gastric acidity.

Intubation of pregnant diabetics can be complicated by stiff joint syndrome. The mechanism for the reduction in joint mobility is not well understood, although there is speculation that abnormal glycosylation of collagen contributes to the process of joint stiffening. Limitation in atlanto-occipital joint extension can also cause difficulty with intubation.[159-161]

Some have suggested that restrictions in small joint mobility can be discerned by evaluating the hands of patients. Patients with stiffening in the interphalangeal joint have incomplete phalangeal prints when they "print" their hands. Some have correlated these partial prints with difficult laryngoscopy.[160-163] In one study, however, an inability to fully approximate the palmar surfaces of interphalangeal joints ("prayer sign") was found not to predict difficult intubation.[164] In the morbidly obese, the extended Mallampati score (when the patient's craniocervical junction is extended rather than remaining neutral) and diabetes were statistically significant predictors of difficult laryngoscopy, but an elevated body mass index was not.[165]

The increasing prevalence of obesity in pregnancy and its association with GDM and T2D raises additional concerns.[166,167] Although a full review of the anesthetic management of obesity in pregnancy is beyond the scope of this chapter, diabetic patients who are obese may be difficult to intubate. For emergency and elective procedures, they should be placed in a "ramped" position on the operating table. This is achieved by placing blankets underneath the patient's body until a horizontal plane is established between the external auditory meatus and the sternal notch.[168] This position has been shown to facilitate direct laryngoscopy and intubation.[169]

During the preoperative anesthetic evaluation, the patient's blood glucose level should be evaluated, and blood samples sent for HgA1c, electrolytes, serum glucose, creatinine, and typing and cross-matching. Urine should be evaluated for glucose and protein and a culture should be sent to the clinical laboratories. In a patient with long-standing diabetes, an ECG should be evaluated for decreased R-wave variability indicative of autonomic neuropathy. Evaluation of orthostatic blood pressure changes, time-domain heart rate responses to deep breathing, and Valsalva maneuver (except in those without retinopathy) may reveal abnormalities in vascular tone.[96] The anesthesiologist must perform a physical examination, with particular attention paid to a careful airway examination. If there are findings that indicate laryngoscopy might be difficult (eg, inability to visualize structures in the posterior pharynx or decreased thyromental distance), then early epidural placement should be strongly considered.

Neuraxial analgesia should be considered early in labor, particularly in the obese diabetic patient. Reducing maternal catecholamines may facilitate glucose regulation in the mother and improve perinatal outcomes. There is some evidence that the clearance of lidocaine and its metabolite may be reduced in patients with GDM, which suggests that it affects CYP1A2/CYP3A4 enzyme isoforms responsible for its metabolism. Further studies are needed to determine whether this is clinically relevant.[170]

If an epidural anesthetic is to be relied on for emergency cesarean section, the catheter must be carefully secured to the patient's back so it will not migrate out of the epidural space. The distance to the epidural space is shallower when the patient is in a sitting position; when the patient assumes a left uterine displacement position, the catheter can inadvertently come out of the epidural space.[171,172] In obese patients, the change in tissue depth from sitting to lateral decubitus or left uterine displacement position is more pronounced. Furthermore, any epidural catheter that provides inadequate analgesia during labor and needs frequent supplemental boluses of medication should be promptly replaced. If rapid epidural anesthesia is required for urgent cesarean section, a surgical level of pain relief can be achieved with 3% 2-chloroprocaine.

Strict asepsis must be maintained, because wound infections remain an important cause of morbidity and increased length of stay in diabetic patients, particularly in those who are obese.[81,173] Administration of prophylactic antibiotics prior to skin incision is critical to help reduce postoperative wound infections.[174,175] Successful postoperative pain management is important to decrease catecholamine levels, and this can be achieved with neuraxial opiates, parenteral or oral narcotics, or nonsteroidal inflammatory agents, depending on individual patient attributes such as renal insufficiency or obesity.

CONCLUSION

Every pregnant diabetic patient is at risk for serious harm to herself and to her fetus and newborn. Careful attention must be paid to the risks of poorly controlled maternal glucose levels before and throughout the pregnancy; most morbidities are closely linked to fetal hyperglycemia and hyperinsulinemia. Any preexisting diabetes-related organ dysfunction must be recognized because it could affect anesthetic management during delivery. Although there have been substantial improvements in pregnant diabetic care, the global epidemic of obesity guarantees that diabetes in pregnancy will become increasingly prevalent. Thoughtful consultation with an anesthesiologist before the time of delivery can help ensure optimal outcomes for both the mother and her infant.

REFERENCES

1. American Diabetes Association (ADA). ADA diabetes statistics. http://www.diabetes.org/diabetes-basics/diabetes-statistics/.
2. American Diabetes Association (ADA). ADA National Diabetes Fact Sheet. http://www.diabetis.org/in-my-community/local-offices/miami-florida/assets/files/national-diabetes-fact-sheet.pdf.
3. Lawrence JM, Contrearas R, Chen W, Sachs DA. Trends in the prevalence of preexisting diabetes and gestational diabetes mellitus among a racially/ethnically diverse population of pregnant women, 1999-2005. *Diabetes Care.* 2008;31:899-904.
4. American Diabetes Association. Diagnosis and classification of diabetes mellitus. *Diabetes Care.* 2010;33(suppl 1):S62-S69.

5. Klinke DJ. Extent of beta cell destruction is important but insufficient to predict the onset of type 1 diabetes mellitus. *PLoS ONE*. 2008;e1374.

6. Herold KC, Vignali DAA, Cooke A, Bluestone JA. Type 1 diabetes: translating mechanistic observations into effective clinical outcomes. *Nat Rev Immunol*. 2013;13:243-256.

7. Landin-Olsson M, Hillman M, Erlanson-Albertsson C. Is type 1 diabetes a food-induced disease? *Med Hypoth*. 2013; http://www.dx.doi.org/10.1016.j.mehy.2013.03.046.

8. American Diabetes Association. Diagnosis and classification of diabetes mellitus. *Diabetes Care*. 2013;36(suppl):S67.

9. Kim SY, Dietz PM, England L, et al. Trends in pre-pregnancy obesity in nine states, 1933-2003. *Obesity (Silver Springs)*. 2007;15:986-993.

10. Ogden CL, Carroll MD, Cutin LR, et al. Prevalence of overweight and obesity in the United States. 1999-2004. *JAMA*. 2006;295:1549-1555.

11. Ehrenberg HM, Dierker L, Milluzzi C, et al. Prevalence of maternal obesity in an urban center. *Am J Obstet Gynecol*. 2002;198:1189-1193.

12. Scott-Pillai R, Spence D, Cardwell C, Hunter A, Holmes V. The impact of body mass index on maternal and neonatal outcomes. A retrospective study in a UK obstetric population, 2004-2011. *Brit J Obstet Gynecol*. 2013. DOI: 10.1111/1471-0528.12193.

13. Mission JF, Marshall NE, Caughey AB. Obesity in pregnancy: a big problem and getting bigger. *Obstet Gynecol Surv*. 2013;68:389-399.

14. Langer O. Management of gestational diabetes. *Clin Obstet Gynecol*. 2000;43:106-115.

15. Rieck S, Kaestner KH. Expansion of beta-cell mass in response to pregnancy. *Trends Endocrinol Metab*. 2010;21:151-158.

16. Buchanan TA, Xiang A, Kjos SL, Watanabe R. What is gestational diabetes? *Diabetes Care*. 2007;30(suppl 2):S105-S111.

17. Negrato CA, Mattar R, Gomes MB. Adverse pregnancy outcomes in women with diabetes. *Diabetol Metabolic Syndr*. 2012;11:41.

18. Coustan DR. Clinical chemistry review: gestational diabetes mellitus. *Clin Chem*. 2013. DOI:10.1313/clinchem.2013.203331.

19. Landon MB, Gabbe SG. Gestational diabetes mellitus. *Obstet Gynecol*. 2011;118:1379-1393.

20. Houshman A, Møller Jensen D, Mathiesen ER, Damm P. Evolution of diagnostic criteria for gestational diabetes mellitus. *Acta Obstet Gynecol Scand*. 2013;19. DOI:10.111.aogs.12152.

21. Jackson WPU. Studies in pre-diabetes. *Br Med J*. 1952;3:690-696.

22. Metzger BE, Lowe LP, Dyer AR, Trimble ER, Chaovarindr U, et al, for the HAPO Study cooperative Research Group. Hyperglycemia and adverse pregnancy outcomes. *N Engl J Med*. 2008;358:1991-2002.

23. International Association of Diabetes and Pregnancy Study Groups (IADPSG) Consensus Panel. The IADPSG recommendations on the diagnosis and classification of hyperglycemia in pregnancy. *Diabetes Care*. 2010;33:676-682.

24. Werner EF, Pettker CM, Zuckerwise L, Reel M, Funai EF, et al. Screening for gestational diabetes mellitus: are the criteria proposed by the International Association of the Diabetes and Pregnancy Study Groups cost-effective? *Diabetes Care*. 2012;35:529-535.

25. American College of Obstetricians and Gynecologists (ACOG). ACOG Committee Opinion No. 504. September 2011.

26. Torloni MR, Beltran AP, Horta BL, et al. Pre-pregnancy BMI and the risk of gestational diabetes: a systematic review of the literature with meta-analysis. *Obes Rev*. 2009;10:194-204.

27. Sathyapalan T, Mellor D, Atkin SL. Obesity and gestational diabetes. *Semin Fetal Neonatal Med*. 2010;15:89-93.

28. White P. Pregnancy complicating diabetes. *Am J Med*. 1949;7:609-616.

29. Hare JW, White P. Gestational diabetes and the White classification. *Diabetes Care*. 1980;3:394-396.

30. Cormier CM, Martinez CA, Refueurzo JS, Monga M, Ramin, SM, et al. White's classification of diabetes in pregnancy in the 21st century: is it still valid? *Am J Perinatol*. 2010;27:349-352.

31. Sachs DA, Metzger BE. Classification of diabetes in pregnancy: time to reassess the alphabet. *Obstet Gynecol*. 2013;121:345-348.

32. Kitabachi AE, Umpierrez GE, Miles JM, Fisher JN. Hyperglycemic crisis in adult patients with diabetes. *Diabetes Care.* 2009;32:1335-1343.

33. Newton CA, Raskin P. Diabetic ketoacidosis in type 1 and type 2 diabetes mellitus: clinical and biochemical differences. *Arch Intern Med.* 2004;164:1924-1931.

34. Pitteloud N, Binz K, Caulfield A, Philippe J. Ketoacidosis during gestational diabetes. *Diabetes Care.* 1998;21:1031-1032.

35. Parker JA, Conway DL. Diabetic ketoacidosis in pregnancy. *Obstet Gynecol Clin North Am.* 2007;34:533-543.

36. Pinto ME, Villena JE. Diabetic ketoacidosis during gestational diabetes. A case report. *Diab Res Clin Pract.* 2011;93:e92-e94.

37. Schneider MB, Umpierrez GE, Ramsey RD, Mabie WC, Bennett KA. Pregnancy complicated by diabetic ketoacidosis. Maternal and fetal outcomes. *Diabetes Care.* 2003;26:958-959.

38. Ramin K. Diabetic ketoacidosis in pregnancy. *Obstet Gyncecol Clin North Am.* 1999;26:481-488.

39. Montoro MN, Meyers VP, Mestman JH, et al. Outcome of pregnancy in diabetic ketoacidosis. *Am J Perinatol.* 1993;10:17-20.

40. Sills IN, Rappaport R. New onset IDDM presenting with diabetic ketoacidosis in a pregnant adolescent. *Diabetes Care.* 1994;17:904-905.

41. Rodgers BD, Rodgers DE. Clinical variables associated with diabetic ketoacidosis during pregnancy. *J Reprod Med.* 1991;36:797-800.

42. Carroll MA, Yeomans ER. Diabetic ketoacidosis in pregnancy. *Crit Care Med.* 2005;33(suppl):S347-S353.

43. Madaan M, Aggrawal K, Sharma R, Trivedi SS. Diabetic ketoacidosis occurring with lower blood glucose levels in pregnancy: a report of two cases. *J Reprod Med.* 2012;57:452-455.

44. Guo RX, Yang LZ, Li LX, Zhao XP. Diabetic ketoacidosis in pregnancy tends to occur at lower blood glucose levels: case-control study and a case report of euglycemic ketoacidosis in pregnancy. *J Obstet Gynaecol Res.* 2009;34:324-0.

45. Clark JD, McConnell A, Hartog N. Normoglycemic ketoacidosis in a woman with gestational diabetes. *Diabet Med.* 1991;8:388-389.

46. Darbhamulla S, Shah N, Bosio P. Euglycemic ketoacidosis in a patient with gestational diabetes. *Eur J Obstet Gynecol Reprod Biol.* 2012;163:117-122.

47. Chico M, Levin SN, Lewis DR. Normoglycemic diabetic ketoacidosis in pregnancy. *J Perinatol.* 2008;28:310-312.

48. Franke B, Carr D, Hatem MH. A case of euglycaemic diabetic ketoacidosis in pregnancy. *Diabet Med.* 2011;18:858-859.

49. Nayak S, Lippes HA, Lee V. Hyperglycemia hyperosmolar syndrome (HHS) during pregnancy. *J Obstet Gynaecol.* 2005;25:599-601.

50. Nugent BW. Hyperosmolar hyperglycemic state. *Emerg Med Clin North Am.* 2005;23:629-648.

51. Gonzalez HM, Edlow AG, Silber A, Elovitz MA. Hyperosmolar hyperglycemic state of pregnancy with intrauterine fetal demise and preeclampsia. *Am J Perinatol.* 2007;24:541-544.

52. American Diabetes Association. Hyperglycemic crises in diabetic adults. *Diabetes Care.* 2006;29:2739-2748.

53. Chua HR, Schneider A, Bellomo R. Bicarbonate in diabetic ketoacidosis: a systemic review. *Ann Intensive Care.* 2011;1:23; DOI: 10.1186/2110-5820-1-23.

54. Vincent M, Nobécourt E. Treatment of diabetic ketoacidosis with subcutaneous insulin lispro: a review of the current evidence from clinical studies. *Diabetes Metab.* 2013; http://dx.doi.org/10/1016/j.diabet.2012.12.003.

55. Barski L, Kezerle L, Zeller L, Zekster M, Jotkowitz A. New approaches to the use of insulin in patients with diabetic ketoacidosis. *Eur J Intern Med.* 2013;24:213-6; DOI: 10.1016/j.ejim.2013.01.014.

56. Zammitt NN, Frier BM. Hypoglycemia in type 2 diabetes: pathophysiology, frequency and effects of different treatment modalities. *Diabetes Care.* 2005;28:2948-2961.

57. Rosenn BM, Miodovnik M, Holcberg G, Khoury, J, Siddiqi TA. Hypoglycemia: the price of intensive insulin therapy for pregnancy women with insulin-dependent diabetes mellitus. *Obstet Gynecol.* 1994;85:417-422.

58. Nielsen LR, Pedersen-Bjergaard U, Thorsteinsson B, et al. Hypoglycemia in pregnant women with type 1 diabetes: predictors and role of metabolic control. *Diabetes Care.* 2008;31:9-14.

59. Confidential Enquiry into Maternal and Child Health. Diabetes in pregnancy: are we providing the best care? Findings of a national enquiry: England, Wales, and Northern Ireland. London: CEMACH, 2007.

60. de Valk HW, Visser GHA. Insulin during pregnancy and labor. *Best Pract Res Clin Obstet Gynecol.* 2011;25:65-76.

61. Kimmerle R, Heinemann L, Delecki A, Berger M. Severe hypoglycemia incidence and predisposing factors in 85 pregnancies of type 1 diabetic women. *Diabetes Care.* 1992;15:1034-1037.

62. Leinon PJ, Hiilesmaa VK, Kaaja RJ, Teramo KA. Maternal mortality in type 1 diabetes. *Diabetes Care.* 2001;24:1501-1502.

63. Confidential Enquiry into Maternal and Child Health. Why Mothers Die 2000-2002: The Sixth Report of the Confidential Enquiries into Maternal Death in the United Kingdom. London: RCOG Press, 2004.

64. American Diabetes Association, American Diabetes Working Group on Hypoglycemia. Defining and reporting hypoglycemia in diabetes. *Diabetes Care.* 2005;28:1245-1249.

65. Negrato AN, Jovanovic L, Tambascia MA, et al. Association between insulin resistance, glucose intolerance, and hypertension in pregnancy. *Metabol Syndr Rel Disord.* 2009;7:53-59.

66. Howarth C, Gazis, J, James D. Association of type 1 diabetes mellitus, maternal vascular disease, and complications of pregnancy. *Diabet Med.* 2007;24:1229-1234.

67. Guerci B, Bohme P, Kearney-Schwartz A, et al. Endothelial dysfunction and type 2 diabetes. *Diabetes Metab.* 2001;27:436-447.

68. Jovanovic R, Jovanovic L. Obstetric management when normoglycemia is maintained in diabetic pregnant women with vascular compromise. *Am J Obstet Gynceol.* 1984;149:617-623.

69. Bellart J, Gilabert R, Fontcubera J, Carreras E, Miralles RM, Cabrero L. Coagulation and fibrinolysis parameters in normal pregnancies and in gestational diabetes. *Am J Perinatol.* 1998;15:479-486.

70. Mathiensen ER, Vaz JA. Insulin treatment in diabetic pregnancy. *Diabetes Metab Res Rev.* 2008;24 (suppl 2):S3-S20.

71. Crowther CA, Hiller JE, Moss JR, Mcphee AJ, Jeffries WS, Robinson JS. Australian carbohydrate intolerance study in pregnant women (ACHOSIS) trial group. Effect of treatment of gestational diabetes on pregnancy outcomes. *N Engl J Med.* 2005;352:2477-2486.

72. Landon MB, Spong CY, Thom E, et al; Eunice Kennedy Shriver National Institute of Child Health and Human Development Maternal-Fetal Medicine Units Network. A multicenter, randomized trial of treatment for mild gestational diabetes. *N Engl J Med.* 2009;361:1339-1348.

73. Leth RA, Uldbjerg N, Nørgaard M, Møller JK, Thomsen RW. Obesity, diabetes, and the risk of infections diagnosed in hospital and post-discharge infections after cesarean section: a prospective cohort study. *Acta Obstet Gynecol Scand.* 2011;90:501-509.

74. Rossing K, Jacobsen P, Hommel E, et al. Pregnancy and progression of diabetic nephropathy. *Diabetologia.* 2002;45:36-41.

75. Gordon M, Landon MB, Samuels P, Hirsch S, Gabbe SG. Perinatal outcome and long-term follow up associated with modern management of diabetic nephropathy (class F). *Obstet Gynecol.* 1996;87:401-440.

76. Mathiesen ER, Ringholm L, Feldt-Rasmussen B, Clausen P, Damm P. Obstetric nephropathy: pregnancy in women with diabetic nephropathy—the role of antihypertensive treatment. *Clin J Am Soc Nephrol.* 2012;7:2081-2088.

77. Rosen B, Miodovnik M, Kranias G, et al. Progression of diabetic retinopathy in pregnancy. *Am J Obstet Gynecol.* 1992;166:1214-1218.

78. Errera, M, Kohly, RP, daCruz L. Pregnancy associated retinal diseases and their management. *Surv Opthamol.* 2013;58:127-142.

79. Hagay Z, Schachter M, Pollack A, et al. Development of proliferative retinopathy in a gestational diabetes patient following rapid metabolic control. *Eur J Obstet Gyncecol Reproduc Biol.* 1994;57:211-213.

80. Lovestam-Adrian M, Agardh DH, Aberg A, Agardh E. Preeclampsia is a potent risk factor for deterioration of retinopathy during pregnancy in type 1 diabetic patients. *Diabetes Med.* 1997;14:1059-1065.

81. Gordon D, Jaaja R, Forsblom C, Hillesmaa V, Teramo K, Groop PH. Pre-eclampsia and pregnancy-induced hypertension are associated with severe diabetic retinopathy in type 1 diabetes later in life. *Acta Diabetol.* 2012; DOI 10.1007/s00592-012-0415-0.

82. The Diabetes Control and Complications Trial Research Group. Effect of pregnancy on microvascular complications in the diabetes control and complications trial. *Diabetes Care.* 2000;23:1084-1091.

83. Veglio M, Chinaglia A, Borra M, Perin PC. Does abnormal QT interval prolongation reflect autonomic dysfunction in diabetic patients? QTc interval measure versus standardized tests in diabetic autonomic neuropathy. *Diabetes Med.* 1995;12:302-306.

84. Vinik AI, Maser RE, Mitchel BD, Freeman R. Diabetic autonomic neuropathy. *Diabetes Care.* 2003;26:1553-1579.

85. Voulgari C, Tentolouris N, Stefanadis C. The ECG vertigo in diabetes and cardiac autonomic neuropathy. *Exp Diabetes Res.* 2011; DOI:10.1155/2011/687624.

86. Gasic S, Winzer Ch, Bayerle-Eder M, Roden A, Pacini G, Kautzky-Willer A. Impaired cardiac autonomic function in women with prior gestational diabetes mellitus. *Eur J Clin Invest.* 2007;37:42-47.

87. Lavin JP, Gimmon Z, Miodovnik M, von Meyenfeldt M, Fischer JE. Total parenteral nutrition in a pregnant insulin-requiring diabetic. *Obstet Gynecol.* 1982;59:660-664.

88. Macleod AF, Smith SA, Sönksen PH, Lowy C. The problem of autonomic neuropathy in diabetic pregnancy. *Diabetes Med.* 1990;7:80-82.

89. Hare JW. Diabetic complications of diabetic pregnancies. *Semin Perinatol.* 1994;18:41-58.

90. Roth A, Elkayam V. Acute myocardial infarction associated with pregnancy. *J Am Coll Cardiol.* 2008;52:171-180.

91. Ladner, HE, Danielsen B, Gilbert WM. Acute myocardial infarction in pregnancy and puerperium: a population-based study. *Obstet Gynecol.* 2005;105:480-484.

92. Jones TB, Savasan ZA, Johnson Q, Bahado-Smith R. Management of pregnant patients with diabetes with ischemic heart disease. *Clin Lab Med.* 2013;33:243-256.

93. Hawthorne G. Maternal complications in diabetic pregnancy. *Best Prac Res Clin Obstet Gynaecol.* 2011;25:77-90.

94. Airaksinen KE, Samela PI. Pregnancy is not a risk factor for a deterioration of autonomic nervous function in diabetic women. *Diabetes Med.* 1993;10:540-542.

95. Straug RH, Zietz B, Palitzsch KD, Schölmerich J. Impact of disease duration on cardiovascular and pupillary autonomic nervous function in IDDM and NIDDM patients. *Diabetes Care.* 1996;19:960-967.

96. Lauenborg J, Mathiesen E, Hansen T, et al. The prevalence of the metabolic syndrome in a Danish population of women with previous gestational diabetes mellitus is three-fold higher than in the general population. *J Clin Endo Metab.* 2005;90:4004-4010.

97. Verma A, Boney CM, Tucker R, Vohr BR. Insulin resistance in women with a prior history of gestational diabetes mellitus. *J Clin Endo Metab.* 2002;87:3227-3235.

98. Retnakaran R, Qi Y, Connelly PW, Sermer M, Zinman B, Hanley AJ. Glucose intolerance in pregnancy and postpartum risk of metabolic syndrome in young women. *J Clin Endo Metab.* 2010;95:670-677.

99. Gunderson EP, Jacobs DR Jr, Chiang V, et al. Childbearing is associated with higher incidence of the metabolic syndrome among women of reproductive age controlling for measurements before pregnancy: the CARDIA study. *Am J Obstet Gynecol.* 209;201:177.e1-177.e9.

100. Brewster S, Zinman B, Retnakaran R, Floras JS. Cardiometabolic consequences of gestational dysglycemia. *J Am Coll Card.* 2013; DOI:10.1.16/j.jacc2013.01.080.

101. Colstrup M, Mathiesen ER, Damm P, Jensen DM, Ringholm L. Pregnancy in women with type 1 diabetes: have the goals of St. Vincent declaration been met concerning fetal and neonatal complications? *J Matern Fetal Neonatal Med.* 2013; DOI: 10.3109/14767058.2013.794214.

102. Retnakaran R, Qi Y, Connelly PW, Sermer M, Hanley AJ, Zinman B. The graded relationship between glucose tolerance status in pregnancy and postpartum levels of low-density-lipoprotein cholesterol and apolipoprotein B in young women: implications for future cardiovascular risk. *J Clin Endo Metab.* 2010;95:4345-4353.

103. Shah BR, Retnakaran R, Booth GL. Increased risk of cardiovascular disease in young women following gestational diabetes mellitus. *Diabetes Care.* 2008;31:1668-1669.

104. Gader AMA, Khashoggi TY, Habib F, Awadallah SBA. Haemostatic and cytokine changes in gestational diabetes mellitus. *Gynecol Endo.* 2011;27:356-360.

105. Madsen H, Ditzel J. Changes in red blood cell oxygen transport in diabetic pregnancy. *Am J Obstet Gynecol.* 1982143:421-424.

106. Madsen H, Ditzel J. Blood-oxygen transport in first trimester of diabetic pregnancy. *Acta Obstet Gynecol Scand.* 1984;63:317-320.

107. Takahashi Y, Kawabata I, Shinohara A, et al. Transient fetal blood flow redistribution induced by maternal diabetic ketoacidosis diagnosed by Doppler ultrasonography. *Prenat Diagn.* 2000;20: 524-525.

108. Hagay ZJ, Weissman A, Lurie S, et al. Reversal of fetal distress following intensive treatment of maternal diabetic ketoacidosis. *Am J Perinatol.* 1994;11:430-432.

109. Macones GA, Hankins GD, Spong CY, Hauth J, Moore T. The 2008 National Institute of Child Health and Human Development workshop report on electronic fetal monitoring: update on definitions, interpretation, and research guidelines. *Obstet Gynecol.* 2008;12:661-666.

110. Stenerson MB, Collura CA, Rose CH, Lteif AN, Carey WA. Bilateral basal ganglia infarctions in a neonate born during maternal diabetic ketoacidosis. *Pediatrics.* 2011;128:e707; DOI: 10.1542/peds.2010-3597.

111. Durnwald CP, Landon MB. Insulin analogues in the management of the pregnancy complicated by diabetes mellitus. *Curr Diab Rep.* 2011;11:28-34.

112. Nold, JL, Georgieff MK. Infants of diabetic mothers. *Pediatr Clin North Am.* 2004;51:619-637.

113. Hay WHH Jr. Care of the infant of the diabetic mother. *Curr Diab Rep.* 2012;12:4-15.

114. de Luca AK, Nakazawa CY, Azevedo BC, et al. Influence of glycemic control on fetal lung maturity in gestations affected by diabetes or mild hyperglycemia. *Acta Obstet Gynecol Scand.* 2009;88: 1036-1040.

115. Storme L, Aubrey E, Rakza T, et al. Pathophysiology of persistent pulmonary hypertension of the newborn: impact of perinatal environment. *Arch Cardiovasc Dis.* 2013;106:169-177.

116. Cetin H, Yalaz M, Akisu M, Kultursay N. Polycythaemia in infants of diabetic mothers: β-hydroxybutyrate stimulates erythropoietic activity. *J Int Med Res.* 2011;39:815-821.

117. Verner AM, Manderson J, Lappin TR, McCance DR, Halliday HL, Sweet DG. Influence of maternal diabetes mellitus on fetal iron status. *Arch Dis Child Fetal Neonatal Ed.* 2007;92:F399-401. E-pub 2006.

118. Jacobsen JD, Cousins LA. A population-based study of maternal and perinatal outcome in patients with gestational diabetes. *Am J Obstet Gynecol.* 1989;61:981-986.

119. Jenson DM, Damm P, Moelsted-Pedersen L, et al. Outcomes in type 1 diabetic pregnancies: a nationwide, population-based study. *Diabetes Care.* 2004;27:2819-2823.

120. Casson F, Clarke CA, Howard CV, et al. Outcomes of pregnancy in insulin dependent diabetic women: results of a five year population study. *Br Med J.* 1997;315:275-278.

121. Mathiesen ER, Ringholm L, Damm P. Stillbirth in diabetic pregnancies. *Best Pract Res Clin Obstet Gynecol.* 2011;25:105-111.

122. Sacks DA. Etiology, detection and management of fetal macrosomia in pregnancies is complicated by diabetes mellitus. *Clin Obstet Gynecol.* 2007;50:980-989.

123. Stotland NE, Caughey AB, Breed EM, Escobar GJ. Risk factors and obstetric complications associated with macrosomia. *Int J Gynecol Obstet.* 2004;87:220-226.

124. Miailhe G, Le Ray C, Timsit J, Lepercq J. Factors associated with urgent cesarean delivery in women with type 1 diabetes mellitus. *Obstet Gynecol.* 2013;121:983-989.

125. Reece EA, Homko CH. Diabetes-related complications of pregnancy. *J Natl Med Assoc.* 1993;85: 537-545.

126. Pedersen LM, Tygstrup I, Pedersen J. Congenital malformations in newborn infants of diabetic women: correlation with maternal diabetic vascular complications. *Lancet.* 1964;1:1124-1126.

127. Starikov R, Bohrer J, Goh W, et al. Hemoglobin A1c in pregestational diabetic gravidas and the risk of congenital heart disease in the fetus. *Pediatr Cardiol.* 2013; DOI 10.10.1007/s00246-013-0704-06.

128. Lisowski LA, Verheijen PM, Copel JA. Congenital heart disease in pregnancies complicated by maternal diabetes mellitus. An international clinical collaboration, literature review, and meta-analysis. *Herz.* 2010;35:19-26.

129. Huang T, Kelly A, Becker SA, Cohen MS, Sanley CA. Hypertrophic cardiomyopathy in neonates with congenital hyperinsulinism. *Arch Dis Child Fetal Neonatal Ed.* 2013;98:F351-F354.

130. Hillier TA, Pedula KL, Schmidt MM, Mullen JA, Charles MA, Pettit DJ. Childhood obesity and metabolic imprinting: the ongoing effects of maternal hyperglycemia. *Diabetes Care.* 2007;30: 2287-2292.

131. Silverman BL, Metzger BE, Cho NH, Loeb CA. Impaired glucose tolerance in adolescent offspring of diabetic mothers: relationship to fetal hyperinsulinism. *Diabetes Care.* 1995;18:611-617.

132. Dabiela D. Crume T. Maternal environment and the transgenerational cycle of obesity and diabetes. *Diabetes.* 2011;60:1849-1855.

133. Pettitt DJ, Baird HR, Aleck KA, Bennett, PH, Knowler WC. Excessive obesity in offspring of Pima Indian women with diabetes during pregnancy. *N Engl J Med.* 1983;308:242-245.

134. Baptiste-Roberts K, Nicholson WK, Brancati FL. Gestational diabetes and subsequent growth patterns of offspring: the National Collaborative Perinatal Project. *Matern Child Health J.* 2012;16:125-132.

135. Vohr BR, McGarvey ST. Growth patterns of large-for-gestational-age and appropriate-for-gestational-age infants of gestational diabetic mothers and control mothers at age 1 year. *Diabetes Care.* 1997;20:1066-1072.

136. Deierlein AL, Sigea-Riz AM, Chantala K, Herring AH. The association between maternal glucose concentration and child BMI at age 3 years. *Diabetes Care.* 2011;4:480-484.

137. Rizzo TA, Metzger BE, Dooley SL, Cho NH. Early malnutrition and child neurobehavioral development: insights from the study of children of diabetic mothers. *Child Dev.* 1997;68:26-38.

138. Georgieff MK. The effect of maternal diabetes during pregnancy on the neurodevelopment of offspring. *Minn Med.* 2006;89:44-47.

139. Pinney SE, Simmons RA. Metabolic programming, epigenetics, and gestational diabetes mellitus. *Curr Diab Rep.* 2012;12:67-74.

140. Pavlinkova, G, Salbaum HM, Kappen C. Maternal diabetes alters transcriptional programs in the developing embryo. *BMC Genomics.* 2009;10:274.

141. Tenenbaum-Gavish K, Hod M. Impact of maternal obesity on fetal health. *Fetal Diagn Ther.* 2013; DOI: 10.1159/000350170.

142. Simmons RA, Templeton LJ, Gertz SJ. Intrauterine growth retardation leads to the development of type 2 diabetes in the rat. *Diabetes.* 2001;50:2279-2286.

143. Mathiesen ER, Ringholm L, Damm P. Therapeutic management of diabetes before and during pregnancy. *Exp Opin Pharmacother.* 2011;12:779-785.

144. Feldman DM, Fang YMV. Use of oral hypoglycemic and insulin agents in pregnant patients. *Clin Lab Med.* 2013;22:235-242.

145. Langer O, Conway DL, Merkus MD, et al. A comparison of glyburide and insulin in women with gestational diabetes. *N Engl J Med.* 2000;343:1134-1138.

146. Rowan JA, Hague WM, Gao W, et al. Metformin versus insulin for treatment of gestational diabetes. *N Engl J Med.* 2008;358:2003-2015.

147. Nicholson W, Bolen S, Witkop CT, et al. Benefits and risk of oral diabetes agents compared with insulin in women with gestational diabetes: a systematic review. *Obstet Gynecol.* 2009;113:193-205.

148. Tsen LC. Anesthetic management of the parturient with cardiac and diabetic diseases. *Clin Obstet Gynecol.* 2003;46:700-710.

149. Phillipson EH, Kalhan SC, Riha MM, Pimentel R. Effects of maternal glucose infusion on fetal acid-base status in human pregnancy. *Am J Obstet Gynecol.* 187;157:866-873.

150. Jovanovic L, Peterson CM. Insulin and glucose requirements during the first stage of labor. *Am J Med.* 1983;75:607-612.

151. Ringholm L, Mathiesen ER, Kelstrup L, Damm P. Managing type 1 diabetes in pregnancy—from planning to breastfeeding. *Nat Rev Endocrinol.* 2012;8:659-667.

152. Pani N, Mishra SB, Rath SK. Diabetic parturient—anaesthetic implications. *Indian J Anaesth.* 201054:387-393.

153. Kadoi Y. Anesthetic considerations in diabetic patients. Part I: preoperative considerations of patients with diabetes mellitus. *J Anesth.* 2010;24:739-747.

154. Kadoi Y. Anesthetic considerations in diabetic patients. Part II: intraoperative and postoperative management of patients with diabetes mellitus. *J Anesth.* 2010;24:748-756.

155. Moitra VK, Meiler SE. The diabetic surgical patient. *Curr Opin Anaesthesiol.* 2006;19:339-345.

156. Datta S, Kitzmiller JL, Naulty JS, Osteheimer GW, Weiss JB. Acid-base status of diabetic mothers and their infants following spinal anesthesia for cesarean section. *Anesth Analg.* 1982;61:662-665.

157. Kitamura A Hoshino T. Patients with diabetic neuropathy are at risk of greater intraoperative reduction in core temperature. *Anesthesiology.* 2000;92:1311.

158. O'Sullivan GM, Bullingham RES. The assessment of gastric acidity and antacid effect in pregnant women by a non-invasive radiotelemetry technique. *Br J Obstet Gynaecol.* 1984;91:973-978.

159. Salzarulo HH, Taylor LA. Diabetic "stiff joint syndrome" as a cause of difficult endotracheal intubation. *Anesthesiology.* 1986;64:366-368.

160. Reissell E, Orko R, Maunuksela EL, Lindgren L. Predictability of difficult laryngoscopy in patients with long-term diabetes. *Anesthesia.* 1990;45:1024-1027.

161. Hogan K, Rusy D, Springman SR. Difficult laryngoscopy and diabetes mellitus. *Anesth Analg.* 1988;67:1161-1165.

162. Nadal JL, Fernandez BG, Escobar IC, Black M, Rosenblatt WH. The palm print as a sensitive predictor of difficult laryngoscopy in diabetics. *Acta Anaesthesiol Scand.* 1998;42:199-203.

163. Vani V, Kamath SK, Naik LD. The palm print as a sensitive predictor of difficult laryngoscopy in diabetics: a comparison with other airway indices. *J Postgrad Med.* 200046:75-79.

164. Erden V, Basarangoglu G, Delatioglu H, Hamzaoglue NS. Relationship of difficult laryngoscopy to long-term non-insulin dependent diabetes and hand abnormality detected using the "prayer sign." *Br J Anesth.* 2003;91:159-160.

165. Mashour GA, Kheterpal S, Vanasharam V, et al. The extended Mallampati score and a diagnosis of diabetes mellitus are predictors of difficult laryngoscopy in the morbidly obese. *Anesth Analg.* 2008;107:1919-1923.

166. Soens MS, Birnbach DJ, Ranasinghe JS, van Zundert A. Obstetric anesthesia for the obese and morbidly obese patient: an ounce of prevention is worth more than a pound of treatment. *Acta Anesthesiol Scand.* 2008;52:6-19.

167. Mace HS, Paech MJ, McDonell NJ. Obesity and obstetric anesthesia. *Anaesth Intensive Care.* 2011;39:559-570.

168. Collins JS, Lemmens HJ, Brodsky JB, et al. Laryngoscopy and morbid obesity: a comparison of the "sniff" and "ramped" positions. *Obes Surg.* 2004;14:1171-1175.

169. El-Orbany M, Woehlck H, Salem MR. Head and neck position for direct laryngoscopy. *Anesth Analg.* 2011;113:103-109.

170. Moisés ECD, Duarte LB, Cavalli R, et al. Pharmacokinetics of lidocaine and its metabolite in peridural anesthesia administered to pregnant women with gestational diabetes mellitus. *Eur J Clin Pharmacol.* 2008;64:1189-1196.

171. Hamza J, Smida M, Benhamou D, Cohen SE. Parturient's posture during epidural puncture affects the distance from skin to epidural space. *J Clin Anesth.* 1995;7:1-4.

172. Hamilton CL, Riley Et. Cohen SE. Changes in the position of epidural catheters associated with patient movement. *Anesthesiology.* 1997;86:778-784.

173. Tipton AM, Cohen SA, Chelmow D. Wound infection in the obese pregnant woman. *Semin Perinatol.* 2011;35:345-349.

174. Young BC, Hacker MR, Dodge LE, Golen TH. Timing of antibiotic administration and infectious morbidity following cesarean delivery: incorporating policy change into workflow. *Arch Gynecol Obstet.* 2012;285:1219-1224.

175. Costantine MM, Rahman M, Ghulmiyah L, et al. Timing of perioperative antibiotics for cesarean delivery: a meta-analysis. *Am J Obstet Gynecol.* 2008;199:301.e1-6; DOI: 10.1016/j.ajog.2008.06.077.

Hematologic Disorders and Coagulopathies

24

Michaela K. Farber and Lorraine Chow

INTRODUCTION

The management of pregnant women with hematologic disorders or coagulopathy requires a multidisciplinary approach involving hematologists, obstetricians, anesthesiologists, and possibly blood banks. Management of these patients requires the recognition of intrinsic or acquired hematologic disease in pregnancy, knowledge of the pharmacokinetics of antithrombotic medication, and an individualized approach to prevention of blood loss and use of blood products, if necessary, in the peripartum period.

COAGULATION TESTS

The evaluation of coagulation test results during pregnancy must be in the context that pregnancy is associated with hypercoagulable changes (Table 24-1).

Platelets

Platelet counts decrease in normal pregnancy due to enhanced turnover and hemodilution from plasma volume expansion. The American Society of Anesthesiologists (ASA) does not recommend obtaining a platelet count prior to neuraxial blockade in healthy parturients with no bleeding risk.[1,2] However, in some at risk patients, a platelet count of less than 70×10^9/L may be indicative of disease such as

Table 24-1. Interpretation of Abnormal Coagulation Tests in Pregnancy

Test	Range in Pregnancy Compared to Nonpregnancy	Abnormality	Differential
Platelet count	Normal to decreased ($100\text{-}150 \times 10^9/L$)	Decreased ($< 70 \times 10^9/L$)	HELLP, preeclampsia, disseminated intravascular coagulation, idiopathic thrombocytopenic purpura
Prothrombin time	Shortened (11-13 s)	Prolonged	Deficiency in factors II, V, VII, X, or fibrinogen; nutritional/liver disease
Activated partial thromboplastin time	Shortened (23-37 s)	Prolonged	Deficiency in factors VIII, IX, XI, or XII; heparin, antiphospholipid syndrome (false positive)
Thromboelastography	Maximum amplitude increased (range undefined)	Maximum amplitude decreased	Platelet or fibrinogen dysfunction, antiplatelet (eg, Plavix)
	Reaction time shortened range undefined	Reaction time prolonged	Factor deficiency, warfarin

Abbreviation: HELLP, hemolysis, elevated liver enzymes, low platelets.

hemolysis, elevated liver enzymes, low platelet (HELLP) syndrome, disseminated intravascular coagulation (DIC), or immune thrombocytopenic purpura (ITP).[2]

Prothrombin Time

The PT and its derived measure, international normalized ratio (INR), evaluate the function of coagulation factors II, V, VII, X, and fibrinogen.[2] Prothrombin time (PT) is shortened during pregnancy because of a hormone-related increase in procoagulant factors.[2]

Activated Partial Thromboplastin Time

Activated partial thromboplastin time (aPTT) evaluates the function of coagulation factors VIII, IX, XI, and XII. The effect of unfractionated heparin can prolong aPTT. A patient with antiphospholipid syndrome and antiphospholipid antibody can have a prolonged aPTT, which represents a false positive test in this prothrombotic subset of patients.[2]

Thromboelastography

Thromboelastography (TEG) is a bedside test of global coagulation and fibrinolysis. Maximum amplitude is reflective of clot strength and is decreased if platelet function or fibrinogen activity is decreased. The reaction time is prolonged in the setting of a clotting factor deficiency (Table 24-1). TEG is a useful test for dynamic global coagulation, but its widespread use in obstetric centers has been limited by difficulty in standardization of results in the literature.

ANEMIA

Dilutional Anemia of Pregnancy

The physiologic changes of normal pregnancy cause a disproportionate increase in plasma volume (50%) compared to red blood cell mass (30%), resulting in a dilutional anemia in pregnant women.[3]

EPIDEMIOLOGY

Anemia, defined as a hemoglobin concentration of less than 10 g/dL, occurs in 18% of pregnant women in the developed countries. In contrast, this value is as high as 35% to 75% of pregnant women in developing countries.[4] This is likely due to superimposed iron deficiency anemia compounding the physiologic anemia of pregnancy.[4]

PATHOPHYSIOLOGY

Increased maternal blood volume and cardiac output during gestation are thought to occur primarily as a result of placentally elaborated estrogen and activation of the renin-angiotensin-aldosterone system, which leads to renal sodium reabsorption and water retention.[3] The presence of low-resistance circuit, the uteroplacental unit, further augments the need for increased maternal blood volume.

MANAGEMENT AND ANESTHETIC CONSIDERATIONS

The hemodynamic consequences of physiologic anemia and increased plasma volume observed during pregnancy may have an impact on the management of patients with hematologic disease, bleeding risk, or active hemorrhage, as follows:

1. Patients with preexisting pathologic causes of anemia (sickle cell disease, thalassemia) may experience exacerbation of their underlying disease and worsening anemia during pregnancy.
2. In patients at high risk of peripartum bleeding, the detection of underlying anemia may prompt earlier transfusion.
3. The physiologic changes during pregnancy can mask the clinical signs of hypovolemia associated with bleeding, potentially delaying the identification and management of postpartum hemorrhage. A high degree of vigilance for the detection of abnormal bleeding at the time of vaginal or cesarean delivery is important.

Sickle Cell Disease

Sickle cell disease (SCD) is an autosomal recessive disorder involving abnormal hemoglobin (HbS); the most severe form is homozygous. Milder clinical variants occur with coinheritance of other abnormal hemoglobin such as HbC or β-thalassemia.

EPIDEMIOLOGY

SCD is the most common inherited condition worldwide, affecting more than 300,000 children born each year, predominantly in patients of African ancestry and, less frequently, Mediterranean and Middle East populations.[5] In the United States, SCD occurs in about 1 in 500 African-American births, and SCD affects about 100,000 Americans. Sickle cell trait occurs among about 1 in 12 African Americans.[5]

ETIOLOGY/RISK FACTORS

SCD results from inheritance of a mutant version of the β-globin gene (βA) on chromosome 11. The mutant β-allele (βS) codes for variant hemoglobin S; 70% of Americans with SCD are homozygous for βS, whereas others have sickle cell C disease or sickle-thalassemia. The clinical manifestation of SCD is heterogeneous and depends on multiple possible genotypes from hemoglobin alleles and variant regulation of gene expression. SCT is the clinically benign heterozygous carrier state persistent in evolution for its protective advantage against infection by the malarial parasite *Plasmodium falciparum*.[6]

PATHOPHYSIOLOGY

SCD manifests clinically as a continuum of chronic hemolytic anemia, recurrent episodic vaso-occlusive crises (VOCs) with severe pain, and progressive end-organ damage.[6] The tendency for HbS to sickle when it is in the deoxygenated state exacerbates chronic endothelial dysfunction and vascular inflammation. Acute ischemia, vaso-occlusion, and infarction cause VOCs, and these events occur more frequently in perioperative states of dehydration, acidosis, hypothermia, and increased oxygen demand.[6]

MANAGEMENT AND ANESTHETIC CONSIDERATIONS

Preconception counseling of women with SCD can identify comorbidities such as hypertension, renal dysfunction, pulmonary hypertension, retinopathy, or iron overload from chronic transfusion requirement, that may be optimized.[7] In the setting of chronic anemia, SCD patients can have high-output cardiac failure. An echocardiogram can evaluate baseline cardiac function and delineate the degree of pulmonary hypertension, a known contributor to morbidity and mortality in pregnancy. Iron chelation therapy is contraindicated during pregnancy but may be recommended prior to gestation. Genetic counseling about the risk of inheritance of SCD and screening of partners is important for women with SCD as well as for women with sickle trait. Neonates afflicted with the disease do not develop SCD symptoms until later in life due to the presence of fetal hemoglobin, which contains γ hemoglobin chains in place of β sickle hemoglobin chains.[6]

Parturients with SCD have a higher incidence of spontaneous abortion, intrauterine growth restriction (IUGR), premature labor, antepartum hospitalization, and postpartum infection.[6] The frequency of VOCs increases as pregnancy progresses and reaches a maximum during the third trimester; however, the frequency of VOCs does not correlate with fetal distress, uteroplacental insufficiency, or fetal outcome.

Preanesthesia assessment should focus on the potential for vasculopathy and associated organ dysfunction, with particular attention to transfusion history, stroke history, acute chest syndrome or pulmonary hypertension, VOC frequency, and chronic requirement of pain medication. Principles of anesthetic management include maintaining oxygenation, hydration, normothermia and acid-base neutrality.[6]

A parturient with SCD may require blood transfusion for symptomatic anemia, acute chest syndrome, or acute stroke.[7] Early cross-matching of blood on admission for labor and delivery is important due to the increased risk (8%-50%) of alloimmunization and the presence of atypical antibodies in patients who have received multiple transfusions.[6] The presence of atypical antibodies can delay cross-matching of blood products by several hours.

The use of epidural analgesia during labor in women with SCD should be encouraged to prevent increase metabolic demands related to pain.[7] The use of epidural analgesia as part of the therapy of a vaso-occlusive pain crisis during labor has also been described.[8] Epidural anesthesia for cesarean delivery is preferable to general anesthesia in SCD patients to reduce the risk of hypoxemia, hypotension, and hypothermia, all of which could precipitate a sickling crisis. Adequate lateral tilt position is critical to prevent vena caval compression by the gravid uterus and resulting venous stasis that may contribute to sickling.[9]

POSTPARTUM CARE

Patients with SCD have a higher potential for infection and risk of VOCs in the puerperium. The reported incidence of complications is 14% to 19% following dilation and curettage and 11% to 17% after cesarean delivery or hysterectomy.[10] The use of regional anesthesia may reduce pain-induced respiratory splinting and improve oxygenation in these patients.[6] Vigilant management of volume status to avoid dehydration and acid-base imbalance is paramount.

COMMON THROMBOPHILIAS

Thromboembolic disease is the leading cause of maternal mortality in the United States and occurs more frequently in women with underlying thrombophilias.[11]

EPIDEMIOLOGY

Inherited Thrombophilias

The most common inherited thrombophilias include factor V Leiden heterozygosity, prothrombin gene mutation, plasminogen activator inhibitor (PAI-1) gene mutation homozygosity, and methylenetetrahydrofolate reductase mutation with hyperhomocysteinemia.[12] The factor V Leiden mutation or homozygous prothrombin gene mutation is present in 5% to 9% and 2% to 3% of white European populations, respectively, but rare in Asian and African populations.[12] Up to 40% and 17% of thromboembolic events in pregnant women have been attributed to factor V Leiden or prothrombin gene mutations, respectively. A homozygous mutation in PAI-1 causing an increase in circulating PAI-1 is relatively common but causes more modestly increased risk of thromboembolism, fetal loss, IUGR, preeclampsia, and preterm delivery compared to other thrombophilias.

Acquired Thrombophilias

The most common cause of acquired thrombophilia during pregnancy is antiphospholipid syndrome (APS), an immune-mediated multisystem disorder strongly associated with poor obstetric outcome.[13] The prevalence of APS is approximately 2% to 4%, with more than 50% of affected individuals having a primary form of APS. Generally speaking, 30% of patients with systemic lupus erythematosus (SLE) will develop secondary APS. The most clinically significant antiphospholipid antibodies associated with recurrent pregnancy loss and thromboembolic disease are anticardiolipin antibodies and lupus anticoagulant.[13]

ETIOLOGY/RISK FACTORS

Inherited or acquired thrombophilias impart increased clotting risk during pregnancy as a result of the background hypercoagulable changes associated with pregnancy—resistance to activated protein C; a decrease in protein S activity; an increase in fibrinogen and factors II, VII, VIII, and X; and an increase in fibrinolysis inhibitors PAI-1 and PAI-2.[12] If a woman with a prior history of venous thromboembolic events in the absence of nonrecurrent risk factors (eg, fractures, surgery, prolonged immobilization) is found to have a thrombophilia, then the recurrence risk of venous thromboembolic events is 16% if untreated during pregnancy.[14]

PATHOPHYSIOLOGY

Thrombophilias are associated with maternal thromboembolic disease during pregnancy, stillbirth, IUGR, abruption, and severe preeclampsia.[14] Each of the inherited or acquired thrombophilias affects the balance between prothrombotic and antithrombotic factors in the coagulation pathway. Factor V Leiden mutation impairs the ability of protein C and protein S to inactivate factor Va. Pregnancy-induced reduction in protein S enhances the prothrombotic risk of this mutation.[12]

MANAGEMENT AND ANESTHETIC CONSIDERATIONS

Women are screened for inherited or acquired thrombophilia by their obstetrician based on the following circumstances: a personal history of venous thromboembolism in the absence of nonrecurrent risk factors, or a first-degree relative with a history of high-risk thrombophilia or venous thromboembolism before the age of 50 years.[15] Thrombophilia testing in other situations, such as recurrent fetal loss, IUGR, placental abruption, or history of preeclampsia, is not routinely recommended due to the lack of clinical evidence that anticoagulation therapy prevents occurrence of these complications. Anticoagulation with low-molecular-weight heparin (LMWH) during pregnancy is increasingly recommended for patients with factor V Leiden or prothrombin gene mutations due to emerging evidence that LMWH prophylaxis lowers the risks of fetal loss or thrombotic complications in these women.[16]

The American Society of Regional Anesthesia and Pain Medicine (ASRA) recently published the third edition of evidence-based guidelines regarding the use of regional anesthesia in patients receiving antithrombotic or thrombolytic therapy (Table 24-2).[17]

Providing epidural anesthesia for labor or delivery in women treated with prophylactic or therapeutic unfractionated heparin or LMWHs is no longer uncommon, providing the timing is appropriate. Nonetheless, these patients may have a higher risk of developing neuraxial hematoma and this should be included in the discussion of informed consent.[2]

POSTPARTUM CARE

Thrombotic risk is highest in the postpartum period, and prophylactic heparin during pregnancy should be continued for up to 6 weeks' postpartum.[18] Women on therapeutic-dose anticoagulation for a history of prior thrombosis may require anticoagulation for life. The need for lifelong anticoagulation depends on the underlying

Table 24-2. American Society of Regional Anesthesia and Pain Medicine Guidelines for the Timing of Neuraxial Anesthesia in Patients Receiving Anticoagulant and Antithrombotic Drugs

Medication	Before[a]	After[b]
Antiplatelet agents		
Aspirin/nonsteroidal anti-inflammatory drugs	No contraindication	No contraindication
Thienopyridines	7 days (clopidogrel); 14 days (ticlopidine)	
GPIIb/IIIa inhibitors		
Abciximab	48 hours	Unknown
Tirofiban, eptifibatide	8 hours	Unknown
Unfractionated heparin		
Subcutaneous	aPTT	1 hour
Intravenous	2-4 hours; aPTT	1 hour
Low-molecular-weight heparin		
Prophylactic	10-12 hours	6-8 hours
Therapeutic	24 hours	24 hours
Warfarin	INR < 1.5	Restart after catheter withdrawal
Fondaparinux	Unknown	Unknown
Direct thrombin inhibitors		
Hirudins, argatroban	Unknown	Unknown
Fibrinolytics	Not recommended	

Abbreviations: INR, international normalized ratio; PTT, activated partial thromboplastin time.
[a]Time interval before neuraxial block or catheter withdrawal.
[b]Time interval after neuraxial block catheter withdrawal before anticoagulation should be reinitiated.

inherited or acquired thrombophilia, in conjunction with a history of a thrombosis or stroke, fetal death, or recurrent pregnancy loss. Prevention strategies can range from no treatment at all to daily aspirin or more aggressive anticoagulation. Close coordination with the obstetric team is required to ensure that epidural catheters are removed prior to resumption of anticoagulation. Furthermore, if an inadvertent dural puncture has occurred peripartum, the risk of postdural puncture headache and potential benefit from an epidural blood patch can be discussed with the obstetric team prior to resumption of anticoagulation. Heparin, LMWH, and warfarin are minimally secreted into breast milk and are therefore safe to use during breastfeeding.[2]

THROMBOCYTOPENIA

Thrombocytopenia affects 6% to 10% of pregnancies. The most common causes include gestational thrombocytopenia, preeclampsia, disseminated intravascular coagulation (DIC), and idiopathic thrombocytopenic purpura (ITP).[19]

Gestational Thrombocytopenia

Gestational thrombocytopenia should be a diagnosis of exclusion. It is more likely to be the diagnosis if the degree of thrombocytopenia is mild to moderate (greater than $70 \times 10^9/L$), there is no history of symptomatic bleeding, there is no pregestational history of low platelets, and the platelet count returns to normal 2 to 12 weeks' postpartum.[19]

EPIDEMIOLOGY

Gestational thrombocytopenia has been attributed as the cause of thrombocytopenia in 81% of cases in pregnant patients.[2]

ETIOLOGY/RISK FACTORS

The cause of gestational thrombocytopenia is likely related to accelerated platelet consumption and possibly dilution related increased plasma volume during pregnancy.[2]

PATHOPHYSIOLOGY

Following injury to blood vessels, platelets initiate a hemostatic plug and subsequent activation of the coagulation cascade. A low platelet count may impair surgical hemostasis, leading to increased risk of hemorrhage and increased risk of anesthetic complications such as neuraxial hematoma.[2]

MANAGEMENT AND ANESTHETIC CONSIDERATIONS

A platelet count should be checked in a parturient with a history of menorrhagia, epistaxis, prolonged bleeding following dental procedures, or unexpected transfusion requirement with prior surgery. The physical examination may be significant for mucocutaneous bleeding, splenomegaly, petechiae, ecchymoses, or excessive bleeding around peripheral intravenous sites. Multiple medications can affect platelet function such as nonsteroidal anti-inflammatory drugs, aspirin, antibiotics, herbal medications, and others, and may compound bleeding risk in the setting of thrombocytopenia.[20] Pregnant women may report epistaxis, bleeding gums, and easy bruising, symptoms that warrant concern only if there is an associated coagulation abnormality.

The safe lower limit of platelet count for neuraxial anesthetic techniques is controversial, but a platelet count between 70×10^9/L and 100×10^9/L in an otherwise healthy patient should not contraindicate neuraxial anesthesia.[2] The American Society of Anesthesiologists (ASA) practice guidelines for obstetric anesthesia do not define a minimal platelet count for neuraxial anesthesia.[1] A single-shot spinal technique imparts less bleeding risk than an epidural because of the avoidance of proximity to the epidural venous plexus with a larger gauge needle and epidural catheter.[21] The risk of epidural hematoma is equal at the time of placement and catheter removal, and equal consideration and appropriate coagulation testing should occur at both periods.

Idiopathic Thrombocytopenic Purpura

EPIDEMIOLOGY

ITP accounts for 3% of all cases of thrombocytopenia during pregnancy.[19]

ETIOLOGY/RISK FACTORS

ITP is an autoimmune disorder resulting in platelet destruction. The presence of antiplatelet immunoglobulin (IgG) is common but not detectable in all patients with clinical ITP.[19]

PATHOPHYSIOLOGY

Patients produce IgG antiplatelet antibodies to their own platelet membrane glycoprotein, causing splenic sequestration and destruction of platelets.[19] Autoimmune-mediated thrombocytopenia can often be differentiated from gestational thrombocytopenia by the fact that it typically occurs earlier in gestation, and usually the decrease in platelet count is more severe as compared to gestational thrombocytopenia.[19]

MANAGEMENT AND ANESTHETIC CONSIDERATIONS

Patients with ITP are treated with oral steroids, which usually increase platelet counts within 1 week of initiation. If there is an inadequate response to steroid treatment, intravenous immunoglobulin (IV IgG) is effective within 6 to 72 hours and has a duration of effect up to 1 month.[19] Platelet function in ITP is usually normal; a platelet count of 50×10^9/L is typically acceptable for vaginal delivery. Higher platelet counts (greater than 70×10^9/L) are warranted for operative delivery or neuraxial anesthesia or in the presence of active bleeding. Transfused platelets are only a temporizing measure as they will be actively destroyed; the typical increase of 10×10^9/L after transfusing six units of pooled platelets will not occur in these patients. Patients who fail steroid and IV IgG therapy may require splenectomy, a surgery that carries increased risk to the fetus with advancing gestational age.[19]

Maternal IgG crosses the placenta and can cause fetal thrombocytopenia and a risk of melena, ecchymosis, and intracranial hemorrhage (ICH) in the neonate.[19] Serial neonatal platelet counts are required. The risk of ICH does not correlate with mode of delivery, therefore operative deliveries should occur only for obstetric indications.[19]

POSTPARTUM CARE

Patients with ITP during pregnancy have often been diagnosed with ITP prior to pregnancy. The course in these patients is chronic, and the response to the above therapies is of variable duration. ITP generally improves within 2 weeks' postpartum. The goal is to maintain a platelet count adequate for hemostasis; lower levels of platelets are acceptable when the potential for postpartum hemorrhage is no longer a concern.

FACTOR DEFICIENCIES

Von Willebrand Disease

Von Willebrand Disease (vWD) is an inherited bleeding disorder associated with a deficiency of von Willebrand factor (vWF), a multimeric protein required for platelet adhesion.[22]

EPIDEMIOLOGY

vWD is the most frequent inherited bleeding disorder, affecting 1% of the population.[2] It can be categorized by a qualitative (types I, II) or quantitative (type III) defect in vWF with a concomitant reduction in factor VIII activity.

ETIOLOGY/RISK FACTORS

vWD has a variable inheritance pattern; types I and II are typically inherited as an autosomal dominant trait and type III as an autosomal recessive trait. vWD can also be acquired with lymphoproliferative disorders, plasma-cell dyscrasias, and autoimmune disorders such as SLE.[22]

PATHOPHYSIOLOGY

vWF is a multimeric protein that binds to and stabilizes factor VIII. Dysfunctional interaction with vWF increases degradation of factor VIII, leading to impaired hemostasis. Diagnosis of vWD typically involves quantitative testing (vWF antigen [vWF:Ag], factor VIII levels) or qualitative testing (ristocetin cofactor [RiCoF] activity, ristocetin-induced platelet activity).[23] Most women with type I vWD have an increase in their factor VIII and vWF levels to within normal range during the course of pregnancy due to hormone-mediated changes in coagulation. For this reason, the initial diagnosis and classification of vWD may be inaccurate during pregnancy. Recommendations for peripartum administration of 1-desamino-8-arginine vasopressin (DDAVP) or vWF and factor VIII concentrate (Humate P) are generally based on the patient's individual bleeding history, response to DDAVP in prior surgery, and coagulation workup prior to pregnancy.

MANAGEMENT AND ANESTHETIC CONSIDERATIONS

Factor VIII activity, RiCoF activity and vWF: Ag levels should be within the normal range prior to spinal or epidural needle placement.[23] The goal is to maintain vWF:Ag and RiCoF assay levels at greater than 50 IU/L. If normalization of vWF:Ag and factor VIII levels cannot be accomplished, avoidance of regional anesthesia is generally recommended.

Pharmacotherapy for vWD depends on the disease subtype. DDAVP is generally effective for the treatment of mild forms, types I and IIa, and works by enhancing release of stored vWF from endothelial cells. More severe subtypes of types II and III require treatment with Humate P, which consists of factor VIII and vWF concentrates. Cryoprecipitate is a reasonable alternative to Humate P. vWD type IIb is associated with thrombocytopenia, which may worsen if DDAVP is administered.

Epidural analgesia or anesthesia has been performed without prior DDAVP treatment and with no reported bleeding complications.[24,25] However, patients with a bleeding history who have responded to DDAVP in the past should receive DDAVP 30 minutes prior to needle placement to protect against the risk of epidural hematoma.

POSTPARTUM CARE

The hypercoagulable state of pregnancy subsides postdelivery; thus, an indwelling epidural catheter should be removed shortly after delivery unless postpartum obstetric bleeding is a concern.[24] Close monitoring for the risk of postpartum hemorrhage is warranted, and postpartum administration of DDAVP or Humate P, depending on disease subtype, should be discussed with the obstetric team in patients at higher risk of bleeding.

Other Factor Deficiencies/Carrier States

EPIDEMIOLOGY

Hemophilias A and B are X-linked recessive bleeding disorders caused by mutations in the genes for factors VIII and IX, respectively. Factor XI deficiency is a rare inherited bleeding disorder predominantly occurring in the Ashkenazi Jewish population.

ETIOLOGY/RISK FACTORS

Due to pregnancy-induced physiologic increases in procoagulant factors, a female hemophilia carrier typically has factor VIII or IX levels of 50% or greater during pregnancy. However, factor levels should be confirmed by serologic testing prior to any invasive procedure or in the setting of bleeding.[23] Factor VIII levels increase more in pregnancy than factor IX among hemophilia carriers.[2]

PATHOPHYSIOLOGY

Hemophilias A and B are rare in females due to their X-linked recessive pattern of inheritance. However, occasionally lionization of the normal X chromosome can result in low factor level states in carriers.[2]

MANAGEMENT AND ANESTHETIC CONSIDERATIONS

Factor levels should be monitored early in pregnancy and again in the third trimester. In a patient with hemophilia, or a known carrier of hemophilia, neuraxial anesthesia can safely be performed if factor levels are greater than 50 IU/L and the remaining coagulation profile is normal. If factor levels are less than 50 IU/L, factor replacement should be considered prior to neuraxial anesthesia and delivery. Epidural analgesia has been utilized in obstetric patients with hemophilias A and B without neuraxial bleeding complications.[26] The bleeding risk in patients with factor XI deficiency correlates to a greater degree with a family bleeding history than with actual factor XI levels, and uneventful neuraxial anesthesia has been reported in parturients with factor XI deficiency with no bleeding history.[27] Women with severe factor XI deficiency and prolonged aPTT can be managed with fresh frozen plasma (FFP) transfusion (10-20 mL/kg) before neuraxial anesthesia.[27]

POSTPARTUM CARE

Parturients with factor deficiency should be managed with vigilance in the postpartum period, because the protective hypercoagulable pregnancy changes diminish. Management of postpartum bleeding may require specific factor replacement, but more common etiologies (eg, retained placenta, uterine atony) should not be overlooked.

DISSEMINATED INTRAVASCULAR COAGULATION

DIC is an acquired syndrome that involves overstimulation of the coagulation system, leading to fibrin deposition, end-organ damage, and bleeding secondary to the depletion clotting factors and platelets.[28]

EPIDEMIOLOGY

The incidence of DIC in the obstetric population is dependent on the characteristics of the referral center reporting. An estimated 1% to 5% of patients with DIC in the United States have a peripartum emergency as the underlying cause, and the frequency is thought to be much higher in developing countries.[29] DIC is a hematologic emergency and accounts for up to 27% of acquired bleeding disorders.

ETIOLOGY/RISK FACTORS

Obstetric causes of DIC include amniotic fluid embolism, intrauterine fetal demise, HELLP syndrome, preeclampsia/eclampsia, placental abruption, placenta previa, septic abortion, intrauterine infection, acute fatty liver of pregnancy, or massive transfusion for any reason.[28]

PATHOPHYSIOLOGY

The normal coagulation response begins with exposure to tissue factor and binding to factor VIIa. Factor VIIa causes activation of factor X to factor Xa, which subsequently converts prothrombin to thrombin. Thrombin generation is amplified to ultimately cleave fibrinogen to fibrin for clot formation.[30] DIC involves the pathologic generation of thrombin, leading to excessive fibrin deposition that damages end-organs from microvascular thrombosis and ischemia. As a result, massive bleeding can result from the depletion of platelets and coagulation factors.[28]

MANAGEMENT AND ANESTHETIC CONSIDERATIONS

DIC never occurs in isolation, and the aggressive treatment of the underlying cause is the cornerstone of management. Diagnosis of DIC involves identifying those at risk for developing DIC, along with coagulation test abnormalities that include, in decreasing frequency: thrombocytopenia, elevated fibrin degradation products, prolonged PT, prolonged aPTT, and low fibrinogen.[29] A low platelet count results from thrombin-induced platelet aggregation and consumption. Worsening thrombocytopenia correlates with ongoing pathologic thrombin formation. Fibrin degradation products (eg, D-dimer) can be nonspecific, and difficulty standardizing D-dimer assays has precluded its routine use to diagnose or monitor DIC. PT and aPTT may be normal, lengthened, or prolonged depending on the dynamic evolution of DIC. Fibrinogen is a useful tool for monitoring DIC but can be normal in up to 57% of patients with DIC; sequential measurements can be helpful.

Active bleeding from DIC should be managed with appropriate blood component therapy, including platelets; FFP; cryoprecipitate; and fibrinogen concentrate (RiaSTAP). Cryoprecipitate and fibrinogen concentrate are reserved for more fulminant cases of DIC. Equivalent doses of FFP, cryoprecipitate, and fibrinogen concentrate are four units FFP, 10 donor units cryoprecipitate, and 3 g fibrinogen concentrate.[29] There are no randomized clinical trials to confirm safety or efficacy of hematologic therapy such as unfractionated heparin, LMWH, antithrombin, activated protein C, protease inhibitor, antifibrinolytics, or activated factor VII (aFVII) for the treatment of DIC in pregnancy. The use of aFVII can be deleterious for increasing thrombotic risk in conditions that involve high levels of circulating tissue factor such as amniotic fluid embolism, and its use should be limited to cases of refractory bleeding despite aggressive component transfusion.[23] The use of activated protein C increases bleeding risk, and it should be reserved for patients with severe sepsis and DIC without coincident bleeding or thrombocytopenia.[30] Antifibrinolytics such as tranexamic acid should be avoided in patients with DIC unless there is a primary hyperfibrinolytic state such as malignancy, with associated DIC and severe bleeding.

POSTPARTUM CARE

Coagulopathy from DIC usually resolves once the inciting cause is removed. Supportive hemodynamic and transfusion management is required until obstetric intervention eliminates the cause of the coagulopathy.

CONCLUSION

An algorithmic, multidisciplinary approach can optimize the management of patients who have hematologic disease in pregnancy (Table 24-3). The challenges of anesthetic management of a parturient with hematologic disease include recognition, prevention, and management of peripartum bleeding from inherited,

Table 24-3. Algorithm for the Management of Obstetric Patients With Hematologic Problems

History and Physical Manifestations	Laboratory Values	Likely Cause	Differential Diagnosis	Additional Tests	Additional Considerations Prior to Neuraxial Technique
Normal	Hemoglobin 12-15 g/dL; platelets > 150 × 10⁹/L	Normal pregnancy			
Pallor	Hematocrit < 30%	Anemia of pregnancy	Iron deficiency, sickle cell disease, thalassemias, occult bleeding	Iron, total iron-binding capacity, hemoglobin electrophoresis Clinical correlation	
Easy bleeding, bruising, petechiae, transfusion history	Platelets ≥ 150 × 10⁹/L	vWD	Hemophilia A, B	vWD panel, factor levels	DDAVP, Humate P, factors ≥ 50%
	Platelets 100-150 × 10⁹/L	Gestational thrombocytopenia	ITP	Anti-platelet IgG	Platelets ≥ 70 × 10⁹/L
	Platelets < 70 × 10⁹/L	ITP	DIC, HELLP syndrome, preeclampsia, vWD type 2B	Fibrinogen, liver function tests, haptoglobin, pregnancy 0ubduced hypertension laboratory tests, vWD panel	Contraindicated

Obstetric bleeding			Clinical correlation	
Fibrinogen > 200 mg/dL	Uterine atony, retained placenta	Early DIC		Coagulation panel, hemodynamic stability
Fibrinogen < 200 mg/dL	DIC	Hypofibrinogenemia		Coagulation panel, hemodynamic stability
Thrombotic history				
On LMWH prophylactic dose	Thrombophilia		Anti-Xa not recommended	10-12 hours after last dose
On LMWH therapeutic dose				24 hours after last dose
On subcutaneous heparin				After Normal PTT
On intravenous heparin				4-6 hours; after normal PTT
On warfarin				5-7 days; after normal INR

Abbreviations: DDVAP, 1-desamino-8-D-arginine vasopressin; DIC, disseminated intravascular coagulation; HELLP (syndrome), hemolysis, elevated liver enzymes, low platelets; INR, international normalized ratio; ITP, idiopathic thrombocytopenic purpura; LMWH, low-molecular-weight heparin; PTT, prothrombin time; vWD, von Willebrand disease.

obstetric, or iatrogenic causes. Clinical care of patients with hematologic disorders involves recognition of underlying comorbidities and understanding how pregnancy-induced coagulation changes affect the preexisting disease.

Minimizing the risk of neuraxial hematoma requires recognition and management of inherited or acquired coagulopathy prior to needle placement. The use of neuraxial anesthesia may be increasingly challenging as more patients with thrombophilia risk are anticoagulated during pregnancy.

CASE STUDY

A 24-year-old G2, P1 (5'9," 190 lb), is admitted to the hospital in early labor at 39 weeks' gestation. She has a history of vWD, although she is not sure what type of vWD she has. A vWD laboratory panel was sent by her obstetrician during her second trimester, and all values were completely normal.

Questions

1. In a nonpregnant individual with vWD, all of the following would be expected to be abnormal *except*:
   A. Ristocetin cofactor level
   B. Factor V level
   C. Factor VIII level
   D. vWF level

2. The following is true about DDAVP *except*:
   A. It should be given 30 minutes prior to surgery or neuraxial technique
   B. It enhances release of vWF and factor VIII from endothelial cells
   C. vWD types I and IIa typically improve after DDAVP treatment
   D. vWD type III typically improves after DDAVP treatment

3. Side effects of DDAVP include all of the following *except*:
   A. Facial flushing
   B. Hyperkalemia
   C. Hyponatremia
   D. Nausea

Answers

1. The answer is B. You obtain a complete medical history of this patient for more information. She reports that she required a transfusion after her gallbladder surgery in 2006 but not after her first vaginal delivery in 2009. She was told that she was a "DDAVP responder" and that her obstetrician gave her DDAVP around the time of her last delivery.

2. The answer is D.

3. The answer is B.

REFERENCES

1. American Society of Anesthesiologists. Practice guidelines for obstetric anesthesia. *Anesthesiology*. 2007; 106(4):843-863.

2. Thornton P, Douglas J. Coagulation in pregnancy. *Best Pract Res Clin Obstet*. 2010;24:339-352.

3. Bernstein IM, Ziegler W, Badger GJ. Plasma volume expansion in early pregnancy. *Obstet Gynecol*. 2001;97:669-672.

4. Sekhavat L, Davar R, Hosseinidezoki S. Relationship between maternal hemoglobin concentration and neonatal birth weight. *Hematology*. 2011;16(6):373-376.

5. Centers for Disease Control and Prevention (CDC). Sickle cell disease: health care professionals: data and statistics. CDC, Department of Health and Human Services. http://www.cdc.gov/NCBDDD/ sicklecell/data.html. Accessed January 25, 2012.

6. Firth PG, Head CA. Sickle cell disease and anesthesia. *Anesthesiology*. 2004;101(3):766-785.

7. Howard J, Oteng-Ntim E. The obstetric management of sickle cell disease. *Best Pract Res Clin Obstet Gynaecol*. 2012;26(1):25-36.

8. Finer P, Blair J, Rowe P. Epidural analgesia in the management of labor pain and sickle cell crisis—a case report. *Anesthesiology*. 1988;68:799-800.

9. Dunn A, Davies A, Eckert G, et al. Intraoperative death during caesarian section in a patient with sickle-cell trait. *Can J Anaesth*. 1987;34(1):67-70.

10. Firth PG. Anesthesia and hemoglobinopathies. *Anesthesiol Clin*. 2009;27:321-336.

11. Chang J, Elam-Evans LD, Berg, CJ, et al. Pregnancy-related mortality surveillance—United States, 1991-1999. Centers for Disease Control and Prevention. http://www.cdc.gov/mmwr/preview/ mmwrhtml/ss5202a1.htm. Accessed January 30, 2012.

12. Lockwood CJ. Inherited thrombophilias in pregnant patients: detection and treatment paradigm. *Obstet Gynecol*. 2002;99:333-341.

13. Lim W. Antiphospholipid antibody syndrome. *Hematology Am Soc Hematol Educ Prog*. 2009: 233-239.

14. Kujovich JL. Thrombophilia and pregnancy complications. *Am J Obstet Gynecol*. 2004;191:412-424.

15. American College of Obstetricians and Gynecologists (ACOG). Inherited thrombophilias in pregnancy. ACOG Practice Bulletin No. 124. *Obstet Gynecol*. 2011;118:730-740.

16. Tormene D, Grandone E, De Stefano V, et al. Obstetric complications and pregnancy-related venous thromboembolism: the effect of low molecular weight heparin on their prevention in carriers of factor V leiden or prothrombin G20210A mutation. *Thromb Haemost*. 2012;107(3):1-8.

17. Horlocker TT, Wedel DJ, Rowlingson JC, et al. Regional anesthesia in the patient receiving antithrombotic or thrombolytic therapy: American Society of Regional Anesthesia and Pain Medicine Evidence-Based Guidelines (Third Edition). *Reg Anesth Pain Med*. 2010;35:64-101.

18. Ramires de Jesus GR, Cunha dos Santos F, Oliveira CS, Mendes-Silva W, Ramires de Jesus N, Levy RA. Management of obstetric antiphospholipid syndrome. *Curr Rheumatol Rep*. 2012;14:79-86.

19. Levy JA, Murphy LD. Thrombocytopenia in pregnancy. *J Am Board Fam Pract*. 2002;15:290-297.

20. Chow L, Farber MK, Camann WC. Anesthesia for pregnant women with hematologic disorders. *Hematol Oncol Clin North Am*. 2011;25(2):425-443.

21. Cook TM, Counsell D. Major complications of central neuraxial block: report on the third national audit project of the Royal College of Anaesthetists. *Br J Anaesth*. 2009;102(2):179-190.

22. Cuker A, Connors JM, Katz JT, Levy BD, Loscalzo J. A bloody mystery. *N Eng J Med*. 2009;361(19): 1887-1894.

23. McLintock C, Repke JT, Bucklin B. Hematologic disease in pregnancy. In: Powrie RO, Greene MF, Camann W, eds. *De Swiet's Medical Disorders in Obstetric Practice*. 5th ed. Chichester: Wiley-Blackwell; 2010:48-81.

24. Milaskiewicz RM, Holdcroft A. Epidural anaesthesia and von Willebrand's disease. *Anaesthesia*. 1990; 45(6):462-464.

25. Stedeford JC, Pittman JA. Von Willebrand's disease and neuraxial anaesthesia. *Anaesthesia*. 2000; 55(12):1228-1229.

26. Kadir RA, Economides DL, Braithwaite J, Goldman E, Lee CA. The obstetric experience of carriers of haemophilia. *Br J Obstet Gynecol*. 1997;104:803-810.

27. Singh AJ, Harnett MJ, Connors MJ, Camann WT. Factor XI deficiency and obstetrical anesthesia. *Anesth Analg.* 2009;108(6):1882-1885.

28. Martí-Carvajal AJ, Comunián-Carrasco G, Peña-Martí GE. Hematological interventions for treating disseminated intravascular coagulation during pregnancy and postpartum. *Cochrane Database Syst Rev.* 2011;3:CD008577.

29. Levi M. Disseminated intravascular coagulation (DIC) in pregnancy and the peri-partum period. *Thromb Res.* 2009;123(suppl 2):S63-S64.

30. Thachil J, Toh CH. Disseminated intravascular coagulation in obstetric disorders and its acute hematological management. *Blood Rev.* 2009;23(4):167-176.

Anesthetic Management of the Parturient With Neurologic/Neuromuscular Disease

25

Natesan Manimekalai, Joana Panni, and Moeen Panni

Neurologic and neuromuscular disorders can significantly complicate the clinical management of the obstetric patient. These disorders may have an impact on the course of pregnancy and/or lead to substantial challenges in the delivery of the parturient. A thorough assessment of the patient in collaboration with the neurology and obstetric services is necessary to provide optimum care. This chapter outlines the anesthetic considerations in women with common neurologic and neuromuscular disorders. Although the discussion is by no means exhaustive, the selected disorders may have significant impact on the anesthetic and obstetric management of parturients.

NEUROLOGIC DISORDERS

Multiple Sclerosis

EPIDEMIOLOGY

Multiple sclerosis (MS) belongs to a group of disorders characterized by abnormalities in the myelin sheath from either defective synthesis or loss of myelin postneuronal development. MS is the most common demyelinating disorder, with a prevalence of greater than 1 million individuals affected worldwide. Of these, 400,000 reside in the United States. Women are more commonly affected than men, with a mean onset age of 30 years. As a result, MS may occur during reproductive age. MS does not affect the peripheral nervous system and usually does not have a negative impact on fertility or pregnancy outcome. Indeed, most MS patients can maintain a high level of function for many years after initial diagnosis.

Etiology/Risk Factors

The clinical course of MS is highly variable and is characterized by either exacerbating-remitting or chronic progressive patterns of disability. Clinical symptoms depend on the location of the demyelinating lesions and may include muscle weakness, visual disturbances, paresthesia, loss of balance, fatigue, bowel or bladder dysfunction, cognitive impairment, and cerebellar manifestations (such as ataxia, slurred speech, and intention tremors). Severe respiratory complications can also occur from respiratory and bulbar muscle weakness.[1]

Diagnosis is based on the clinical presentation as well as diagnostic testing, such as magnetic resonance imaging (MRI) (Figure 25-1), computed tomography (CT), visual evoked potentials, and lumbar puncture for cerebrospinal fluid (CSF) testing for elevated immunoglobulin levels and specific oligoclonal bands of immunoglobulin G (IgG). The detection of plaques on MRI due to focal loss of myelin in white matter can confirm the diagnosis but may not always correlate with the severity of the disease (Figure 25-1).[2]

Although the cause of MS is still not known, several genetic factors, environmental factors, viral or infectious exposure, and autoimmune etiologies have been proposed. The disease is thought to develop from a complex interplay between genetic and environmental risk factors. Ethnicity and genetic risk factors, such

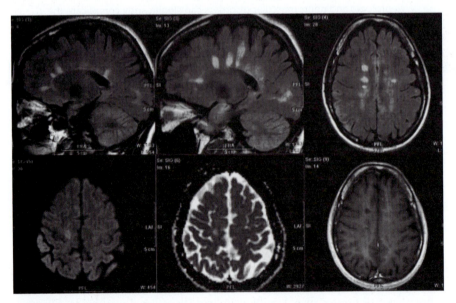

Figure 25-1. Magnetic resonance imaging scans include white matter plaques in multiple sclerosis. (Permission granted for Lövblad KO, Anzalone N, Dörfler A, et al. MR imaging in multiple sclerosis: review and recommendations for current practice. *AJNR Am J Neuroradiol.* 2010;31(6):983–989 © by American Society of Neuroradiology.)

as certain human leukocyte antigen (HLA) patterning, have been associated with the risk for developing the disease. The strongest environmental risk factors for MS identified so far include Epstein-Barr virus infection, smoking, and vitamin D deficiency. Certain conditions such as infection, fever, surgery, and emotional stress may adversely influence the clinical course of the disease.[3]

PATHOPHYSIOLOGY

MS is a chronic, progressive, degenerative disease of the central nervous system characterized by focal or segmental demyelination, resulting in axonal damage and loss, with gliosis in the brain and spinal cord. Demyelination leads to conduction blockade that fluctuates, resulting in varying clinical symptoms with relapses and remissions.

MANAGEMENT

There is at present no cure for MS. Treatment strategies focus on symptom control and slowing disease progression by using immunosuppressive and anti-inflammatory drugs. The management options include corticosteroids, interferon β-Ia, interferon β-Ib, glatiramer acetate, methotrexate, and mitoxantrone, several of which are contraindicated for pregnancy, especially during the first trimester (all of which are at least pregnancy category C).[4]

Many MS patients are able to reduce or stop their usual MS therapy during pregnancy because pregnancy itself may lead to immunosuppression. There is no significant increase in spontaneous abortion rate, or other major obstetric or neonatal complications for MS parturients, as compared to women without MS. However, there is an approximately 10% increase in premature delivery and a less significant increase in instrumental delivery and cesarean section in women with MS as compared to parturients without the disease.[5] Glucocorticoids are recommended for treatment of acute relapses during pregnancy and parturition.

ANESTHETIC CONSIDERATIONS

Parturients with MS should be evaluated for the chronology and pattern of MS symptoms, medications, and adequacy of respiratory function. Regardless of the anesthetic technique selected, frequent monitoring of body temperature is essential, because a single-degree rise in temperature may cause relapse or worsen existing symptoms. Thus, even mild temperature elevation should be aggressively treated with antifebrile agents. Regional anesthesia has not been reported to adversely affect the disease and may even be beneficial by mitigating the stress response during labor and delivery. However, controversy exists as to whether exposure to local anesthetics negatively impact demyelinated neurons. Based on this, the recommendation is that the lowest effective concentration of local anesthetic be used, combined with opioids, and that patient temperature be monitored, with any elevations treated aggressively. This is important because there has been conflicting evidence that epidural analgesia during labor may result in small temperature increases. In the past, small retrospective and observational studies suggested that any type of neuraxial anesthesia for labor and delivery would result in a 30% relapse rate of MS in the puerperium. However, in 2004, a large prospective study found that the relapse rate among woman with MS was 30% 3 months postpartum; regardless of anesthetic technique, or even if no anesthetic was administered.[6]

Cesarean delivery should be reserved for obstetric indications only. Epidural or combined spinal-epidural anesthesia may be safely used for cesarean section in parturients with MS. However, additional precautions need to be taken when general anesthesia is used. Succinylcholine should be avoided, with its potential to cause hyperkalemia, particularly if there are muscle-wasting symptoms present. Parturients with MS, particularly those on baclofen, may exhibit abnormal responses to nondepolarizing muscle relaxants. Accordingly, dosing of nondepolarizing muscle relaxants should be guided by neuromuscular monitoring.

POSTPARTUM CARE

MS patients require careful monitoring postdelivery, including monitoring of body temperature and hemodynamic variables. In addition, careful attention to pain relief will reduce stress and play a part in preventing exacerbations. There may be a risk of airway compromise, hypoventilation, and atelectasis if the bulbar or respiratory musculature is affected by MS. Residual neuromuscular blockade must be treated aggressively. A complete neurologic evaluation should be performed at intervals in the immediate and 3 months' postpartum period to assess any exacerbation of the MS. The patient should be restarted, as soon as possible, on her prepregnancy MS drug regimen. Exacerbations should be treated as described earlier, including intravenous immunoglobulin and steroids. There are no data to prevent or recommend breastfeeding with respect to the course of MS.[5] In some cases, it may not be recommended to breast feed when drugs that may affect the neonate are secreted in the breast milk.

Guillain-Barré Syndrome

EPIDEMIOLOGY

Guillain-Barré syndrome (GBS) can be an acute or subacute inflammatory demyelinating peripheral polyneuropathy, which is typically triggered by an acute infection. It initially presents with distal paresthesias and weakness, progressing to ascending paralysis. GBS incidence is reported to be 1.7 cases per 100,000 of the population[7] and fortunately is relatively rare during pregnancy.

ETIOLOGY/RISK FACTORS/PATHOPHYSIOLOGY

GBS is diagnosed by clinical presentation, CSF analysis (elevated CSF protein concentration occurs in 80% of cases), and electrodiagnostic tests such as nerve conduction studies. Many patients with GBS have an antecedent viral infection, such as cytomegalovirus, Epstein-Barr virus, and varicella zoster (most common), or a bacterial infection, such as with *Campylobacter jejuni*, *Mycoplasma pneumoniae*, or *Haemophilus influenzae*. The proposed mechanism is that infectious agents

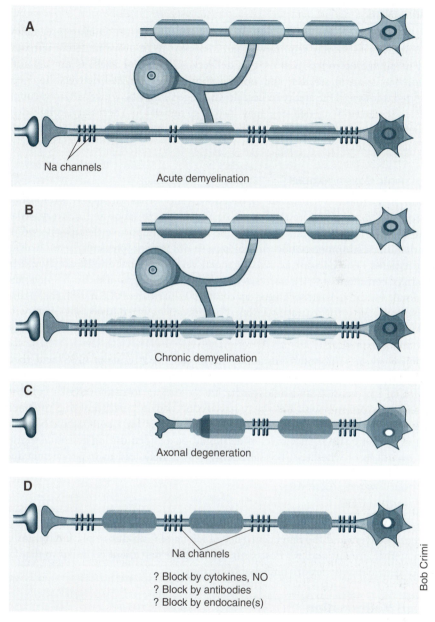

Figure 25-2. Mechanisms of dyemyelination. (Reprinted by permission from Macmillan Publishers Ltd: Waxman SG. Do "demyelinating" diseases involve more than myelin? *Nat Med.* 2000;6(7):738–739. Copyright 2000.)

induce autoantibody production that cross-react with peripheral nerve myelin components, such as specific gangliosides and glycolipids (Figure 25-2).[8] In its most severe form, the disease may result in life-threatening complications by affecting the respiratory muscles or the autonomic nervous system.

MANAGEMENT

There is no cure for GBS, and treatment is supportive. During pregnancy, patients with GBS may require ventilator support to improve maternal outcome and maximize uteroplacental oxygen delivery. GBS, in of itself, is not an indication for cesarean section, and normal spontaneous vaginal delivery has been reported. However, the ability to bear down (stage 2) may be weakened, so vacuum-assisted extraction at delivery may prove beneficial or necessary. High-dose intravenous pooled IgG plasmapheresis may be useful and is not contraindicated during pregnancy.

ANESTHETIC CONSIDERATIONS

Parturients with GBS usually are managed with supportive therapy. It is important to consider that an incremental acute strain, related to labor and delivery, in an otherwise stable patient may intensify the need for supportive therapy, including ventilation. Thromboembolic prophylaxis is important particularly in bedridden patients. The decision to select general versus regional anesthesia should be carefully considered in all patients with respiratory compromise. Both spinal and epidural anesthesia have been used successfully in parturients with GBS for vaginal delivery as well as for cesarean section. There is one reported case of a woman with GBS having worsening neurologic symptoms that was temporally related to an epidural anesthetic.[9]

Furthermore, autonomic instability may occur as a result of GBS, and there is the potential for local anesthetic–induced sympathectomy, which can result in profound hypotension and bradycardia, rarely leading to cardiovascular collapse. In addition, patients with GBS may have reduced pain perception due to denervation and thus require lower doses of local anesthetic for a comparable block to women without GBS. Succinylcholine should be avoided during general anesthesia, regardless of whether GBS has resolved, as it may lead to hyperkalemia and potential progression to cardiac arrest.[7]

POSTPARTUM CARE

Obstetric outcome is generally good, although there may be an increased risk of preterm delivery and the rare occurrence of neonatal GBS due to placental transfer of maternal autoantibodies.[9] Postpartum care of the parturient is similar to that for other demyelinating lesions and should be supportive.

Chiari Malformation

EPIDEMIOLOGY

Chiari malformation (CM) is a congenital anomaly where there is a downward displacement of the cerebellar tonsils through the foramen magnum (Figure 25-3). The incidence of CMs (types I and II) is estimated to occur in 1% of all live births. The actual incidence could be higher, because patients with type I CM can be asymptomatic or have few subtle symptoms for many years prior to diagnosis.

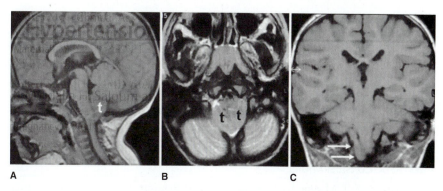

Figure 25-3. Magnetic resonance images showing Chiari malformation. Sagittal T1-weighted image A demonstrates herniation of the cerebellar tonsils (t) through the foramen magnum into the cervical spinal canal. Axial T2-weighted image B shows crowding of the foramen magnum due to the presence of the tonsils (t) associated with thinning of subarachnoid spaces. In coronal T1-weighted image C, tonsillar ectopia is asymmetric with low position of the right (arrows). (Permission granted for Chiapparini L, Saletti V, Solero CL, Bruzzone MG, Valentini LG. Neuroradiological diagnosis of Chiari malformations. *Neurol Sci.* 2011;32(suppl 3):S283-S286. With kind permission from Springer Science and Business Media.)

ETIOLOGY/RISK FACTORS/PATHOPHYSIOLOGY

The underlying cause of CM is unknown, with possible risk factors identified as vitamin/nutrient deficiencies, hazardous chemical exposure, infection, drug use, or alcohol consumption during pregnancy. The condition is classified into four types based on progressive degrees of severity.[10] Type I, the least severe form, presents with symptoms in young adults and 25% of cases have syringomyelia. Type II (also known as Arnold-Chiari malformation) presents in infancy. The defect includes a downward displacement of the cerebellar vermis, brainstem, and fourth ventricle, with formation of hydrocephalus and myelomeningocele. Multiple surgeries may be required and these children will likely have developmental delay as well as physical disabilities. Tragically, there is a 50% mortality in early childhood. Type III and Type IV are rare malformations with very poor prognoses, due to herniation and cervical myelomeningocele with fourth ventricle hydrocephalus or cerebellar hypoplasia without herniation, respectively.

The common symptoms associated with CM are severe occipital headache, numbness, tingling in the neck and arms, pain, syncope, dizziness, vertigo, tinnitus, nystagmus, and fatigue. Syringomyelia is an abnormal expanded cystic cavity within the spinal cord filled with CSF, which leads to disruption of neural tissue function. Symptoms of syringomyelia include weakness, burning pain in the neck or back, extremity paresthesia, and referred chest pain. There is also involvement of paraspinal muscles causing weakness, kyphoscoliosis, restrictive pulmonary function, and vocal cord abductor paresis. Autonomic dysfunction manifests as delayed gastric emptying, urinary bladder dysfunction, and impaired thermoregulation. MRI is the preferred diagnostic test, in concert with patient history and neurologic examination. Surgery may be necessary for posterior fossa decompression and duraplasty, particularly in patients with progressively worsening symptoms, hydrocephalus, or syringomyelia. In cases where progressive hydrocephalus occurs, shunts may be required.[11]

MANAGEMENT

Pregnancy itself does not have an influence on the course of the disease; however, parturients with CM and/or syringomyelia should be counseled carefully regarding the possible risk of increased intracranial pressure (ICP) during pregnancy and labor.

ANESTHETIC CONSIDERATIONS

Parturients with CM type I should be evaluated for signs of increased intracranial pressure (ICP) and neurologic deficits. Factors that may increase ICP, such as coughing, hypercapnia, and pushing with prolonged straining during the second stage of labor, should be minimized because they may cause increased risk of herniation or worsening of symptoms.[12] For those parturients with normal ICP and no other neurologic symptoms at the time of delivery, epidural analgesia has been safely administered. It is prudent to avoid transmitted increases in ICP by slowly administering local anesthetic to avoid sudden distention of the epidural space and avoiding sudden drops in arterial pressure if the patient has autonomic neuropathy. Epidural, spinal, and general anesthesia have all been used successfully for cesarean delivery in patients with CM who have normal ICP.[13]

Spinal anesthesia should be avoided in parturients who have CM with coexisting syringomyelia, regardless of ICP. For those women with symptoms of increased ICP, the mode of delivery should be either by planned cesarean delivery or a controlled labor with an abbreviated second stage culminating in assisted vaginal delivery. In patients with elevated ICP, dural puncture, either from spinal or accidental dural puncture from an epidural needle, may lead to herniation of the brain due to sudden excessive loss of CSF. Other forms of analgesia, such as lumbar sympathetic blocks, or intravenous patient controlled analgesia, should be considered, even if they are less effective than neuraxial techniques.[13] For cesarean delivery, general anesthesia should be considered in those women with elevated ICP, but precautions should be taken, such as hyperventilation, adequate depth of anesthesia during laryngoscopy/intubation, arterial line placement to monitor swings in blood pressure, and careful attention to head positioning to avoid neck hyperextension. In the presence of neurologic symptoms, there may be an increased sensitivity to succinylcholine administration with a potential altered response, and conversely, resistance to nondepolarizing muscle relaxants. Therefore, neuromuscular blockade should be monitored at all times and the need for postoperative ventilation considered.[14]

POSTPARTUM CARE

The goal of postpartum care is to prevent increases in ICP. Monitoring of neurologic status is essential in the immediate postpartum period, effective pain relief is required to prevent wide fluctuations in blood pressure that can impact ICP.[15]

Seizure Disorders

EPIDEMIOLOGY

More than 1 million women of reproductive age in the United States suffer from a seizure disorder; approximately 20,000 of whom give birth each year. Preexisting epilepsy is the most common cause of seizures during pregnancy, with eclamptic seizures the second. Less common causes include traumatic brain injury, brain tumor, stroke, electrolyte/metabolic abnormalities, and drug withdrawal. Epilepsy is a disease in which the patient develops recurrent seizures in the absence of an identifiable cause. The incidence of epilepsy in the general population is approximately 1% to 2% and has been reported to affect up to 0.7% of pregnancies.[16]

ETIOLOGY/RISK FACTORS

Seizures are grouped into two categories: generalized seizures (grand mal) and partial seizures (petit mal). Generalized seizures are produced by abnormal electrical impulses involving and spreading to the entire brain, whereas partial seizures involve just a focal area. Grand mal seizures are characterized by loss of consciousness, followed by "tonic" and "clonic" convulsions and then a "post-ictal" phase. The underlying cause of epilepsy is unknown, but it is likely due to a combination of environmental and genetic factors. Genetics may also influence the efficacy of antiepileptic drug.

PATHOPHYSIOLOGY

Seizures are characterized by abnormal, hyperexcitable neuronal firing, leading to hypersynchrony within the brain, which can affect motor control, sensory perception, behavior, and/or autonomic function. Defects in neuronal function, such as mitochondrial dysfunction, glia-mediated excitation, inflammation, and blood-brain barrier impairment have been implicated in the pathophysiology of epilepsy.[17]

MANAGEMENT

Although there are several drugs available to treat seizures, many patients suffer from refractory symptoms and/or have reduced quality of life due to side effects of anticonvulsant medications. Pregnancy can have a variable effect on seizure frequency; in some woman there may be up to a 30% increased frequency of seizures while pregnant. However, the likelihood of seizures may be lower during pregnancy if the woman was without seizures in the year leading up to pregnancy.[18] Serum levels of anticonvulsants may be reduced during pregnancy due to vomiting, delayed intestinal absorption, altered protein binding, folic acid supplementation, alterations in pharmacokinetics, and increased renal clearance. Higher estrogen concentration during pregnancy and the potential for alkalosis secondary to hyperventilation can lower the seizure threshold. There may be decreased maternal compliance in adherence to anticonvulsant regimens out of concerns for teratogenicity or other adverse fetal effects. Due to physiologic changes associated with pregnancy that may affect drug disposition, pregnant women require close monitoring of therapeutic anticonvulsant levels.

Some anticonvulsants have the potential for teratogenicity, particularly those with antifolate properties. When pregnancy is anticipated, it is prudent to convert to accepted anticonvulsant monotherapy that is not associated with teratogenicity. Administration of folate prior to conception and during pregnancy has been recommended to reduce the risk of fetal neural tube defects in woman taking anticonvulsants.[19]

There is controversy as to whether anticonvulsant drugs increase the risk of spontaneous hemorrhage in newborns due to increased vitamin K metabolism. Accordingly, oral vitamin K 10 to 20 mg recommended for pregnant women taking anticonvulsant drugs and 0.5 to 1 mg of vitamin K intramuscularly for newborns, immediately after delivery.[20]

Seizures during pregnancy may result in maternal and fetal risk. Generalized tonic-clonic seizures are especially dangerous to the developing embryo and fetus, because the potential for maternal hypoxia and hypercapnia during periods of apnea, can result in intrauterine fetal asphyxia. A generalized tonic-clonic seizure can also cause trauma, spontaneous abortion or placental abruption, fetal intracranial bleeding, fetal heart rate changes, and even intrauterine fetal death. Seizures occurring in a pregnant woman should be treated rapidly, with special care given the potential for aspiration, oxygenation and ventilation to prevent maternal hypoxia, left uterine displacement, and termination of the seizure with a small dose of rapidly acting anticonvulsant.

ANESTHETIC MANAGEMENT

Parturients with epilepsy have a higher risk of pregnancy-related hypertension, preeclampsia, preterm labor, bleeding in pregnancy, and an increased risk of cesarean delivery compared to nonepileptic parturients. All epileptic parturients should have an anesthesiology consultation early in the course of their pregnancy. Anticonvulsant medication levels should be assessed and if the serum drug level is inadequate, patients should be given supplemental doses of anticonvulsant or administered parenteral agents (eg, phenytoin) (to avoid unpredictable gastric absorption during labor).

Some anticonvulsant drugs have potential interactions with anesthetic medications. Phenytoin and phenobarbital induce hepatic microsomal enzymes, which increase the metabolism and breakdown of opioids, nondepolarizing muscle relaxants, and volatile anesthetic agents. Meperidine and ketamine can lower the seizure threshold and should be avoided if feasible. Neuraxial analgesia or anesthesia may be administered safely in epileptic parturients.[21] Epidural analgesia is indicated for vaginal delivery to decrease the requirement for systemically administered drugs and narcotics, relieve pain, reduce hyperventilation from uterine contractions, and reduce physical and emotional stress and fatigue; all of these may decrease the seizure threshold.

Cesarean delivery should be performed exclusively for obstetric indications. For elective cesarean delivery, both spinal and epidural anesthesia can be used successfully. General anesthesia may be necessary if the patient is in status epilepticus (intractable seizures either as a continuous seizure or a lack of full recovery between seizures (postictal stage). In these situations, it is important to protect the airway; ensure oxygenation and ventilation; and treat seizures pharmacologically with benzodiazepines, phenytoin, or phenobarbital. The fetus must be monitored and if there is a nonreassuring fetal status, there should be attempts at intrauterine resuscitation. In most cases, return of maternal oxygenation and ventilation, as well as cessation of the seizures, will usually result in improving fetal status. Rarely, an emergent cesarean delivery must be attempted. Some anesthetic agents, such as ketamine, meperidine, etomidate, methohexital, and phenothiazines should be avoided, because they are epileptogenic, particularly in the presence of hypocapnia. Certain volatile agents (sevoflurane more than isoflurane) are epileptogenic, whereas others, such as nitrous oxide, may suppress seizure-like activity. Thus, a combination of isoflurane and nitrous oxide may be a preferred combination when general anesthesia is required.[22] Because phenytoin and phenobarbital increase the metabolism and breakdown of nondepolarizing muscle relaxants, their doses needs to be adjusted accordingly.

POSTPARTUM CARE

Postdelivery, anticonvulsant medications should be continued with monitoring of therapeutic levels as indicated. There may also be an increased risk of postpartum bleeding.[16] Epidural morphine for postpartum pain relief should be used with caution because there are reports of seizure activity following its use.[23] Parturients with epilepsy may breastfed, and newborns should be monitored for any acute changes in behavior, such as lethargy/poor feeding. If these occur, serum anticonvulsant levels should be checked. There may be an increased risk of respiratory distress in neonates from mothers taking antiepileptic drugs.[24]

Spinal Cord Injury

EPIDEMIOLOGY

In the United States, approximately 2000 new spinal cord injuries (SCIs) occur in young women each year,[21] some of whom may be pregnant. In addition, improved medical care and survival have resulted in a higher number of women with SCIs who present for obstetric care.

ETIOLOGY/RISK FACTORS

The most common cause of SCIs include motor vehicle collisions (40%), diving accidents, gunshot wounds, MS, spinal cord hematomas, and transverse myelitis.[25] Spinal cord injuries above the T1 level result in paralysis of all four extremities (quadriplegia), whereas injuries below T2 usually cause paralysis of only the lower extremities (paraplegia).

Immediately after SCI, spinal shock can occur as a result of sympathetic denervation below the level of the injury, which then leads to generalized peripheral vasodilation, severe hypotension, and flaccid paralysis, with loss of tendon and autonomic reflexes. For lower level SCIs, reflex tachycardia can occur, in response to hypovolemia and hemodynamic instability in quadriplegic patients, with significant circulatory collapse developing in the absence of brainstem regulation of vasomotor tone. Alternatively there may be paradoxical bradycardia and there is often altered temperature regulation, sweating, and piloerection, which can last for 1 to 3 weeks after the injury due to loss of vasomotor tone. During spinal shock any slight change in position, Valsalva maneuver, or tracheal suctioning, can produce profound hypotension and bradycardia as a result of unopposed vagal stimulation.

Over time, SCI patients can maintain blood pressure through enhanced activation of the renin–angiotensin–aldosterone system, which may later play a role in the development of autonomic dysreflexia (ADR), a potentially life-threatening complication of SCI.[25]

PATHOPHYSIOLOGY

Brain and spinal cord tissue are very susceptible to traumatic injury with little or no ability to regenerate and repair. There are two major phases to SCI. Initially, in the acute phase, the injury leads to necrotic cell death, edema, and ischemia. Subsequently, a second injury cascade consisting of inflammation, release of free radicals and cytotoxic levels of excitatory amino acids (Figure 25-4).[26] The loss of white matter is a primary cause of neurologic dysfunction and is a major focus of research for therapeutic targets, many of which are geared to preventing the secondary excitatory damage phase and then promoting regenerative function that remains in the neuronal tissue.

MANAGEMENT

There is no current cure for SCI, and most SCI patients have significant disability. However, much research is focused on restoring function using multifactorial strategies, such as stem cell therapies.[26] Current treatment options include surgery to decompress and stabilize the injury, prevention and management of secondary complications, and rehabilitation.

Autonomic dysreflexia (ADR) or hyperreflexia is a serious, life-threatening complication of SCI. The onset of ADR following SCI is variable, affecting up to 85% of patients with an injury above the T6 level. ADR can be triggered by any stimulus, including bladder or bowel distention, pressure sores, or labor pain, any of which can lead to extreme sympathetic hyperactivity and severe systemic hypertension. In patients with SCI at T6 or below, there can be a compensatory reflex parasympathetic response, leading to bradycardia and vasodilation above the level of the injury, but injuries above T6 have insufficient autoregulatory mechanisms to compensate for the severe hypertension that may develop. The most common sequelae for ADR include severe systemic hypertension, hyperthermia, piloerection, increased extremity spasticity, respiratory distress, loss of consciousness, convulsions, intracranial hemorrhage, dysrhythmias, myocardial infarction, and in some cases mortality.[27] Immediate diagnosis and treatment can be life saving. Management includes ceasing the noxious stimulus, if feasible, and the use of rapid onset and shorter acting antihypertensive agents such as sodium nitroprusside, sublingual nitroglycerin, nifedipine, and/or hydralazine to control cardiovascular manifestations. Labetalol may be a more preferable choice for parturients. All these antihypertensive medications must be used judiciously because of the potential to cause acute hypotension that could diminish fetal blood flow.

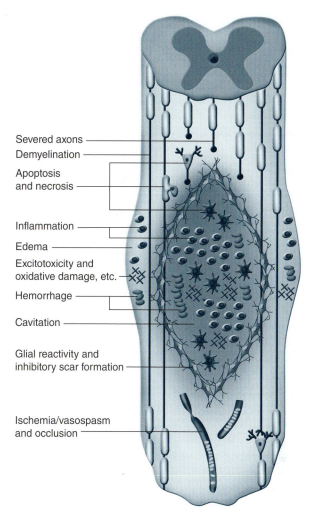

Severed axons

Demyelination

Apoptosis and necrosis

Inflammation

Edema

Excitotoxicity and oxidative damage, etc.

Hemorrhage

Cavitation

Glial reactivity and inhibitory scar formation

Ischemia/vasospasm and occlusion

Figure 25-4. Pathophysiology of spinal cord injury. (From Mothe AJ, Tator CH. Advances in stem cell therapy for spinal cord injury. *J Clin Invest.* 2012; 122(11):3824-3834. Reproduced with permission of the American Society for Clinical Investigation.)

ANESTHETIC CONSIDERATIONS

Acute SCI above C4 may require immediate intubation for respiratory support, because innervation to the diaphragm is likely to be compromised. A hard cervical collar should be used to limit neck movement. Intubation may be accomplished by awake fiber optic intubation or by direct laryngoscopy with "in line stabilization" of the head and neck. In parturients at 24 weeks' gestation or beyond, a small wedge placed to achieve 10 degrees or more of lateral uterine tilt to prevent aortocaval compression by the gravid uterus is recommended.

Immediate volume resuscitation and pressor support is needed in the acute phase of spinal shock. Signs of internal hemorrhage can be masked by spinal shock symptoms, and proper evaluation of the abdomen to exclude hemorrhage may also be difficult due to the gravid uterus. Serial hematocrit measurements, diagnostic peritoneal lavage, and a high index of suspicion for internal hemorrhage are necessary. Cardiotocography can be useful in the setting of acute SCI for fetal heart rate tracing and uterine contraction monitoring. After initial stabilization, management includes measures to prevent pulmonary infections, urinary tract infections, decubitus ulcers, constipation, anemia and respiratory failure, and prophylactic anticoagulation treatment, as there is increased risk of deep vein thrombosis and pulmonary embolism. These parturients have a higher risk of spontaneous abortion, congenital fetal malformation, preterm labor, placental abruption[21] and also increased risk for unattended delivery, secondary to unrecognized uterine contractions.

General anesthesia may be preferred over regional anesthesia for surgery in acute SCI parturients, because optimal positioning of the patient may limit placement of neuraxial techniques. The time frame for the upregulation of acetylcholine receptors can be variable; thus, succinylcholine should not be administered after SCI because of the potential for uncontrolled hyperkalemia. Accordingly, high-dose nondepolarizing muscle relaxants or fiberoptic awake intubation should be utilized for intubation. A deep plane of anesthesia is needed to limit ADR with vigilant monitoring for hypotension, dysrhythmia, and uterine atony.[28] Regional anesthesia, if positioning is possible, has also been used. Proper hydration and monitoring are required to prevent hypotension. The sensory level must definitively reach a T6 level to prevent ADR.

Patients with a previous SCI should have prenatal anesthesia consultation to establish an anesthetic management plan for labor and delivery, including multidisciplinary management in a high-risk obstetric unit. Regional anesthetic techniques with a continuous intrathecal catheter are preferred for incremental dosing because these avoid the risk of major hypotension and limit the chance of a high spinal. To prevent hypotension, adequate prehydration is crucial before initiating regional anesthesia and any manifestation of hypertension after regional placement can be indicative of an inadequate block and activation of ADR. Epidural anesthesia using a combination of a local anesthetic with an opioid, but not opioids alone, can be very effective in blocking afferent impulses below the level of SCI and preventing ADR. Epidural anesthesia is preferred but may be difficult to place in parturients with previous spinal surgery/instrumentation, and so continuous spinal is also another option to consider. Epidural placement should be considered prior to the onset of labor for parturients with a high risk of developing ADR. Continuous hemodynamic monitoring by electrocardiogram, pulse oximetry, or arterial line may be necessary during labor, depending on hemodynamic stability. The rate of spontaneous vaginal delivery is higher in parturients with SCI below the T6 level, whereas the rate of assisted vaginal and caesarean delivery is higher in patients with spinal cord lesions at or above the T6 level. The latter are more likely to develop ADR.

Acute onset of ADR during labor can be difficult to distinguish from preeclampsia, but delay in diagnosis can result in decreased uteroplacental blood flow, fetal hypoxemia, and fetal bradycardia. Antihypertensive medications should be readily available for use. Both spinal and epidural anesthesia can provide protection against ADR during cesarean delivery. For emergent cesarean delivery, general anesthesia may be required, with the same considerations as in acute SCI parturients, although succinylcholine may not be as problematic 1 year after the SCI.[28]

POSTPARTUM CARE

Parturients with chronic SCI should be carefully monitored postdelivery for any signs of ADR. Epidural catheters may be left in situ for longer than usual depending on the SCI, for the prevention and treatment of ADR, which can be triggered by postdelivery contractions. Breastfeeding may be challenging due to SCI disability, ADR, inhibition of the milk ejection reflex due to an underlying neurologic defect, and problems with holding the infant.

Brain Tumors

EPIDEMIOLOGY

The incidence of brain tumor is similar in both pregnant and nonpregnant women, occurring at approximately 3 to 6 per 100,000 live births. The tumor histologic types are also similar between nonpregnant and pregnant women, with the exception that tumors may be larger in pregnant women due to increased hormone levels, blood volume, and fluid retention.[29]

ETIOLOGY/RISK FACTORS

Brain tumors are classified by their location and whether they are benign or malignant. In parturients, there can be a delay in diagnosis because symptoms associated with brain tumors such as headache, nausea, vomiting, and visual symptoms are often attributed to common obstetric syndromes such as hyperemesis gravidarum or preeclampsia. Diagnosis is usually confirmed by MRI.

MANAGEMENT

Clinical management depends on the type of tumor and whether there is the potential for increased ICP or herniation/compression effects. Increases in ICP are initially managed with dexamethasone 4 mg every 6 hours. Long-term high-dose use of steroids may lead to in utero fetal adrenal suppression.

ANESTHETIC CONSIDERATIONS

The anesthetic goals are to maintain hemodynamic stability, eliminate fluctuations in intracranial pressure, and provide adequate pain control. If the patient is neurologically stable, the pregnancy may progress to term with the option of normal vaginal delivery or an elective cesarean delivery. If the patient is neurologically unstable, an emergent cesarean delivery and craniotomy may be considered. Labor pain and bearing down during the second stage of labor often leads to worsening of increased ICP.[30] Epidural anesthesia will effectively decrease labor pain, bearing down, and mitigate wide fluctuations in blood pressure. Epidural medications should be administered in small boluses of 3 to 5 mL incrementally because administration of large volumes of drug may transiently worsen increased ICP by transmitted mechanical effect. Epidural placement by an experienced anesthesiologist is suggested, to avoid the risk of accidental dural puncture, which may result in cerebral herniation especially if a large-bore (17-gauge) epidural needle is used. Spinal anesthesia is not recommended because of the potential adverse effects of hypotension causing vomiting and increased ICP.

General anesthesia may be required in neurologically unstable parturients, having the advantage of having control of the airway and maintaining hypocapnia during surgery (which also reduces ICP). Disadvantages include the risk of aspiration, unexpected difficult airway, and inability to assess maternal level of consciousness as a surrogate neurologic monitor. A smoothly controlled anesthetic induction is important in patients with intracranial pathology, to avoid the possibility of elevating ICP during stressful periods such as with laryngoscopy and intubation. Hemodynamic stress during induction, intubation, and extubation may be reduced by using appropriate anesthetic agents and adjuvants such as remifentanil, lidocaine, and propofol. There is the potential risk of a slight transient increase in ICP with succinylcholine use, however it can be used for rapid sequence induction. Maternal hypoxia, hypercapnia, and hypertension are to be avoided. Prostaglandin and ergotamine may cause hypertension and raise ICP, however, a synthetic oxytocin has been successfully used in patients with intracranial tumors.[31]

Neurosurgery is usually avoided during pregnancy unless the brain tumor jeopardizes the life of the mother. In addition to routine monitoring, central venous catheter, invasive arterial monitoring, and Doppler ultrasound to detect venous air emboli should be considered. If the fetus is viable and close to term, an obstetrician and neonatologist should be available in the operating room with all the necessary surgical instruments in case of serious nonreassuring fetal status requiring urgent cesarean section. Hyperventilation to improve ICP may affect the fetus by reducing maternal cardiac output from decreased venous return and decreasing the blood flow to the uterus. Hyperventilation leading to hypocapnia can also cause uterine and umbilical artery vasoconstriction and a left shift of the oxygen dissociation curve. This may also reduce oxygen delivery to the fetus and create potential fetal myocardial depression.[32] Studies in animals and humans have suggested that osmotic diuretics such as mannitol may cause fetal hypovolemia and dehydration from redistribution of vascular volume from the fetus to the mother. Furosemide is an appropriate alternative to mannitol for this purpose. Steroids in pregnant neurosurgical patients reduce peritumor edema while increasing surfactant production to accelerate fetal lung maturity. Multidisciplinary discussion should also include the advisability of continuous or intermittent fetal heart rate monitoring for detection of intraoperative fetal hypoxia, which may result from decreased uterine blood flow during periods of relative maternal hypotension and hyperventilation. Adequate arterial pressure should be maintained during surgery to avoid uterine hypoperfusion and fetal hypoxia. It is also important to minimize the risk of aortocaval compression by tilting the operating table laterally or by placing a wedge under the patient's right hip.

POSTPARTUM CARE

Postpartum management of these patients is not significantly different than with other parturients. A multimodal analgesic approach to pain control with preincisional skin infiltration, intraperitoneal use of local anesthetic, and use of acetaminophen and nonsteroidal anti-inflammatory drugs (NSAIDs) may assist in pain control.

Cerebral Hemorrhage

EPIDEMIOLOGY

Cerebral hemorrhage is rare during pregnancy, occurring in 6 of 100,000 deliveries. However, it is the most common nonobstetric cause of maternal death.[33] Approximately 65% of cerebral hemorrhages are related to a ruptured aneurysm and the remaining 35% from arteriovenous malformations. Pregnancy alone does not increase the incidence of hemorrhage but can increase the risk of rebleeding (3%-6% versus 25% in pregnant women), with the circle of Willis being the most common location for rupture (specifically the anterior portion).[34]

ETIOLOGY/RISK FACTORS/PATHOPHYSIOLOGY

Symptoms of cerebral hemorrhage include sudden onset of frontal or suboccipital headache associated with nausea, vomiting, photophobia, neck stiffness, blurring of vision, and neurologic impairment, all of which can mimic other neurologic diseases (eg, meningitis, eclampsia). Thus, care must be taken to distinguish these conditions as early diagnosis and surgery improve outcomes. Cerebral MRI and angiography are commonly used to diagnose cerebral hemorrhage.[35] The risk of rupture may be increased during pregnancy due to the increased circulating blood volume, cardiac output, and hormone-related vascular changes. Following cerebral hemorrhage, there is the risk of rebleeding (4% in the first 24 hours increasing to approximately 10%-20% in the first month) and cerebral vasospasm leading to cerebral ischemia.[34]

MANAGEMENT

Cerebral hemorrhage is managed by either clipping or endovascular coiling techniques depending on the pathology. If an aneurysm or arteriovenous malformation is diagnosed prior to conception, an elective obliteration technique should be undertaken prior to pregnancy. If an aneurysm is diagnosed late in pregnancy, the pregnancy may be allowed to progress to term, with close monitoring, depending on the characteristics of the aneurysm. Aneurysms less than 1 cm in size, in patients with no history of prior subarachnoid hemorrhage, can be managed conservatively as the risk of rupture is very low (approximately 0.05% per year).[34] The risk of rupture decreases significantly by shortening the second stage of labor, with instrument-assisted and pain-free delivery under epidural analgesia. Patients with symptomatic aneurysms, history of prior aneurysm rupture, aneurysms greater than 1 cm, and those with serial increase in size of the aneurysm must be treated immediately because the risk of hemorrhage increases as the pregnancy advances.

ANESTHETIC CONSIDERATIONS

During neurosurgical procedures in parturients, maintaining uteroplacental blood flow, ensuring adequate fetal oxygenation, and preventing preterm delivery are critical. In addition, neurologic considerations such as decreasing ICP by reducing cerebral blood flow with hyperventilation, reducing brain swelling by diuresis, reducing the chance of cerebral bleeding with deliberate hypotension, and decreasing cerebral metabolism with hypothermia; are manipulations that are necessary to preserve maternal health, but may compromise fetal well-being.

Deliberate hypotension can be induced by using a volatile anesthetic or using a nitroglycerine/nitroprusside infusion, all of which have their own inherent risks, and will result in decreased uteroplacental blood flow. Reduction in systolic blood pressure by 25% to 30%, or a mean arterial pressure less than 70 mm Hg, can result in decreased uteroplacental blood flow[36] and hypotension in the fetus. In the event of deliberate hypotension, fetal heart rate monitoring should be used to establish the lower limits at which fetal well-being is preserved. Earlier studies suggested that nitroprusside use was contraindicated due to the risk of cyanide toxicity to the fetus. However, the doses used in these animal studies were large, and there is no evidence to suggest that nitroprusside, as used in clinical practice for short periods, results in adverse fetal effects. Hyperventilation, with a target goal of $PaCO_2$ at approximately 30 mm Hg, is frequently used to reduce cerebral flow and ICP. Osmotic agents and loop diuretics are often used to produces diuresis and cause shrinkage of the brain parenchyma perioperatively. The use of diuresis may cause dehydration and hypotension, uterine hypoperfusion, and fetal hypoxia. Mannitol should be used cautiously as it crosses the placenta and can result in fetal hypotension.[36]

The use of corticosteroids for long periods may cause fetal adrenal suppression and hypoadrenalism. Hemodynamic stability is important to preserve both cerebral and uteroplacental perfusion and is achieved by administering fluids, monitoring intra-arterial blood pressure, prophylactic use of vasopressor drugs, and avoiding aortocaval compression by effectively displacing the gravid uterus to the left. Central venous access assists in monitoring central venous pressure, air emboli, and allows administration of vasoactive drugs. Blood pressure should be closely monitored and regulated to maintain baseline values.

For anesthetic management during a cesarean section, the main objective is to maintain stable transmural pressure (mean arterial pressure minus ICP) across the aneurysm so as to prevent its rupture. Choice of anesthetic technique varies based on the individual patient, weighing the risk versus benefit. In emergent cases, general anesthesia may be necessary. Hemodynamic stress during induction should be reduced by using nitroglycerine, propofol, lidocaine, and/or remifentanil/fentanyl. Preinduction intra-arterial line placement may allow earlier intervention to prevent hypertension and also maintain uteroplacental perfusion. A smooth controlled induction and extubation is essential to avoid further bleeding in cases of ruptured aneurysm.

POSTPARTUM CARE

Postoperative care is not different from nonparturients having neurosurgical procedures. Analgesia considerations for postcraniotomy pain as well as postpartum pain management will depend on the type of surgery as well as whether the patient is still pregnant (fetal toxicity issues) or breastfeeding (drug safety profile for lactation).

Cerebral Venous Thrombosis

EPIDEMIOLOGY

Cerebral venous thrombosis (CVT) is a rare but potentially life-threatening condition, caused by clot formation in a cerebral vein that impairs venous flow and leads to venous stasis and hypertension. Women between 20 and 35 years of age are more commonly affected. They are particularly vulnerable prior to delivery or in the postpartum period because of pregnancy associated hypercoagulability and hormonal changes. The incidence of CVT is 7 per 1,000,000 in general population.[37]

ETIOLOGY/RISK FACTORS

CVT is a life-threatening condition if undiagnosed, and it should be considered as a potential diagnosis in all parturients presenting with either new-onset seizures or signs of intracranial hypertension. Bacterial meningitis and frontal sinusitis, dehydration, polycythemia, anemia, acquired clotting disorders such as the factor V Leiden or antiphospholipid syndrome in addition to pregnancy, cesarean section, and traumatic delivery are potential risk factors for CVT.[38] CVT symptoms include severe headache, vomiting, mental status changes, photophobia, aphasia, ataxia, seizures, lethargy, and coma. CVT is most often mistaken for eclampsia, ruptured aneurysm, and postdural puncture headache. Magnetic resonance venography is the preferred diagnostic imaging method for the direct visualization of the dural venous sinuses and the large cerebral veins.[38] Treatment options include anticoagulation, thrombolytic therapy, and surgical thrombectomy.

PATHOPHYSIOLOGY

The cerebral venous system is comprised of a network of sinuses, which facilitate venous drainage from the cranium. The sagittal and cavernous sinuses are most commonly affected with CVT. The resulting intracranial hypertension from obstructed venous drainage leads to cerebral edema, infarction, hemorrhage, and stroke.

MANAGEMENT AND ANESTHETIC CONSIDERATIONS

If symptomatic CVT is diagnosed during labor, an urgent cesarean delivery may be required. General anesthesia with a controlled rapid-sequence induction is preferable in patients with CVT to avoid the possibility of elevating ICP and worsening the symptoms. Hemodynamic stress during induction, intubation, and extubation can be reduced by using remifentanil, lidocaine, and short-acting β-blockers. Isoflurane may be a preferable inhalation agent for anesthetic maintenance because ICP is reported to be stable at concentrations below 1% without increasing CSF production.[39]

POSTPARTUM CARE

Most CVT cases (75%) occur in the postpartum period. The recurrent risk of CVT in future pregnancies is low. It should be noted the use of estroprogestogen contraceptive medications is contraindicated in patients who have had CVT.[40]

Pseudotumor Cerebri/Benign Intracranial Hypertension

EPIDEMIOLOGY

Pseudotumor cerebri, or benign intracranial hypertension (BIH), is defined by increased CSF pressure in the absence of intracranial pathology. It is more common in young women with obesity. The reported incidence of BIH is 0.9 per 100,000 per year in the general population but 19.3 per 100,000 for obese women between the ages of 20 to 44 years.[41]

ETIOLOGY/RISK FACTORS

The most frequent symptom of BIH is headache with photophobia (90% of patients). Other symptoms include neck pain, tinnitus, nausea and vomiting, and visual disturbances including visual field loss, and loss of visual acuity, as well as diplopia. Papilledema (swelling of the optic disk), occurs in most BIH patients; however, not all are symptomatic. Untreated, BIH can lead to permanent blindness in as many as 10% of patients.[42]

MRI is the diagnostic test of choice in patients suffering from BIH, and imaging studies should be performed prior to lumbar puncture. Medical management consists of diuretics (acetazolamide), corticosteroids, control of excessive weight gain, and surgical management, such as CSF diversion using lumbar-peritoneal shunt (LP shunt) and optic nerve sheath fenestration for restoration of vision.

PATHOPHYSIOLOGY

Although the pathogenesis of BIH is still unclear, the most accepted etiology is the impaired absorption of CSF in the arachnoid villi, due to raised venous pressure from venous outflow obstruction in the brain.

MANAGEMENT

Symptoms may worsen during pregnancy in 50% of patients but usually resolve postpartum. The course of labor and delivery is expected to be normal in pregnant women with BIH. The second stage of labor can significantly increase ICP, which may worsen the symptoms in parturients with BIH. Therefore, shortening the second stage of labor with an instrumental vaginal delivery may be considered.

ANESTHETIC CONSIDERATIONS

Epidural analgesia during labor may attenuate increases in ICP related to pain during uterine contractions and bearing-down efforts. Continuous epidural infusion techniques are recommended over intermittent boluses of large volumes of local anesthetic, which may transiently increase ICP in patients with preexisting intracranial hypertension. Care should be taken to avoid accidental dural puncture with large (18-gauge) epidural needles, which may lead to intracranial hypotension and postdural puncture headache, often confused with the symptoms of BIH. Spinal anesthesia has been used successfully for cesarean delivery in parturients with BIH, as lumbar puncture is considered therapeutic in these patients by decreasing CSF pressure and improving symptoms. Because ICP is uniformly elevated, the risk of herniation is small.[43] Parturients with BIH do not require general anesthesia because of their disease. If general anesthesia is chosen, a smooth controlled induction is important in patients with BIH to avoid the possibility of elevating ICP and worsening the symptoms.

If there is an LP shunt present, the shunt should be evaluated for its placement and function before proceeding with a regional technique. There are conflicting recommendations for the use of neuraxial anesthesia in parturients with functioning LP shunts. The concerns are possible damage to the shunt by the epidural needle, risk of shunt entanglement by the epidural catheter, leaking of local anesthetic into shunt and infection of the shunt. Because the rate of shunt infection is very low, there are insufficient data available for the use of prophylactic antibiotics in patients with LP shunt before placing regional anesthesia.

POSTPARTUM CARE

Postdural puncture headache is a very rare complication in parturients with BIH and has been successfully managed using epidural blood patch.[44]

NEUROMUSCULAR DISORDERS

Myasthenia Gravis

EPIDEMIOLOGY

Myasthenia gravis (MG) is an autoimmune disorder resulting in fatigue and progressive muscle weakness, which worsens with activity and improves with rest. Diagnosis is based on clinical history, physical examination, improvement of muscle strength following anticholinesterase drug treatment (eg, edrophonium), electrophysiology findings, and detection of autoantibodies to neuromuscular junction proteins. The incidence of MG is reported to be approximately 3 to 4 per million per year, with a prevalence of about 60 per million. The disease occurs twice as frequently in women compared to men. In women, the onset of symptoms peaks in the third decade, and therefore there is potential for women of childbearing age to have MG. MG does not affect fertility in women with the disease.[45] The clinical course of MG is variable, ranging from complete remission after a single episode to repeated acute exacerbations. The effects of pregnancy on MG are variable as well.

ETIOLOGY/RISK FACTORS

The progression of muscle weakness is usually in the cranial to caudal direction, with ocular or pharyngeal muscle weakness being the most common initial presentation. In approximately two-thirds of cases, the maximal intensity of weakness occurs within the first year after onset. For this reason alone, it is recommended to delay pregnancy until after the first year of diagnosis.[21] Polymorphisms have been associated with increased susceptibility to MG, including genes in the major histocompatibility complex (*HLA-DQ, HLA-DQ, HLA-A*), the master autoimmune regulator (*AIRE*), and the α subunit of acetylcholine receptor (*CHRNA1*).[46]

PATHOPHYSIOLOGY

MG is an autoimmune disease. There is the elaboration of autoantibodies aimed against proteins involved in neuromuscular junction function, such as nicotinic acetylcholine receptors (nAChR) (Figure 25-5). Anti-nAChR antibodies can be detected in 80% to 85% of patients with MG. In those patients who are

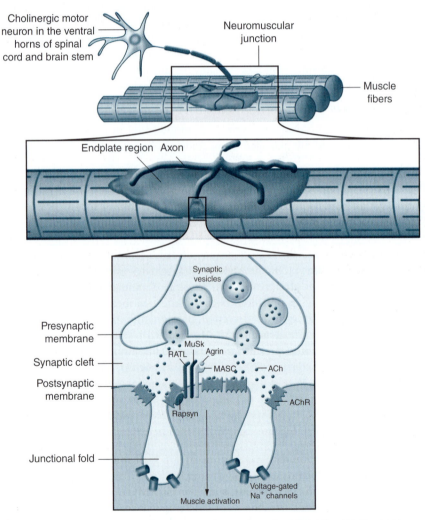

Figure 25-5. The neuromuscular junction. (From Conti-Fine BM, Milani M, Kaminski HJ. Myasthenia gravis: past, present, and future. *J Clin Invest.* 2006;116(11):2843-2854. Reproduced with permission of the American Society for Clinical Investigation.)

nAChR seronegative, other autoantibodies affecting the neuromuscular junction are present, such as autoantibodies to muscle-specific receptor tyrosine kinases (MuSK) or to muscle proteins. MuSK-seropositive disease is associated with more severe ocular-bulbar defects and often requires immunosuppressant treatment.[46] Most cases of early-onset MG also have associated abnormal thymus function. Thus, patients should be screened for possible thymoma or abnormal formation of thymus. If thymoma is present, thymectomy is associated with improvement and possible remission of MG and may also have a protective effect against neonatal MG.[47]

MANAGEMENT

MG is a disease with fluctuating symptoms characterized by periods of relapse and remission.

MG patients are at risk for developing myasthenic and cholinergic crises. In myasthenic crisis, respiration is impaired due to paralysis of respiratory muscles, and mechanical ventilation may be required. Triggers for myasthenia crisis include pregnancy, medications (noncompliance or adverse effects), infection, and stress. Cholinergic crisis is due to administration of an excess cholinesterase inhibitor medication, which can cause cholinergic symptoms such as miosis, diarrhea, urinary incontinence, bradycardia, emesis, lacrimation, or salivation in addition to muscle weakness and respiratory failure. An edrophonium test can differentiate these two types of crisis. When prescribing a clinical regimen, it is important to intermittently monitor the levels of cholinesterase inhibitors, especially during pregnancy which has the potential to affect pharmacokinetics.[45]

Depending on the underlying cause of MG, treatment options include generalized immunosuppressive therapy with steroids, azathioprine, cyclosporine, methotrexate, immunotherapy such as plasma exchange and intravenous immunoglobulins, acetylcholinesterase inhibitors, and thymectomy. Treatment options may be modified during pregnancy due to potential risks to the mother and the fetus.[48]

For many women, MG symptoms may improve during the second and third trimesters due to pregnancy-related immunosuppression. In contrast, there may be exacerbations during the first trimester and the postpartum period. There may be also fewer exacerbations of MG during pregnancy in women who have had a thymectomy.

The risk of mortality to the woman with MG during pregnancy is inversely correlated to the duration of the disease, the highest risk being in the first year. The risk decreases to a nadir at about 7 years after the onset of the disease. Pregnancy complicated by preeclampsia may be problematic because magnesium sulfate worsens MG muscle weakness. Indeed, maternal deaths have been reported in myasthenic women who have received magnesium sulfate for the treatment of preeclampsia. Maternal MG is also a rare cause of fetal arthrogryposis multiplex congenita, a congenital disorder characterized by multiple joint contractures and other anomalies, probably resulting from lack of movement in utero.[49] Frequent sonographic examinations are necessary to detect signs of fetal akinesia.

ANESTHETIC CONSIDERATIONS

All MG patients should be seen by an anesthesiologist early in the course of pregnancy. The use of tranquilizers, narcotics, and magnesium sulfate should be avoided or used judiciously due to their potential negative effects on the neuromuscular junction. Epidural anesthesia can be safely used during vaginal delivery to decrease the requirements of narcotics, reduce fatigue, and provide anesthesia for forceps or vacuum procedures. Combined spinal-epidural technique is another alternative to labor epidural, as it offers the advantage of effective analgesia with minimal motor block. For all patients, caution must be exercised with the use of neuraxial opioids because of the risk of respiratory depression. The half-life of ester local anesthetic agents may be prolonged, due to decreased plasma cholinesterase activity in patients taking anticholinesterase drugs. An amide local anesthetic agent may be preferable.

Vaginal delivery is the preferred method of delivery, and cesarean section should be performed for obstetric indications. The first stage of labor is not compromised by MG because the uterus consists of smooth muscle. However, the second stage of labor involves striated muscles, which are at risk for easy fatigue. Accordingly, a forceps or vacuum delivery is recommended. During labor, oral anticholinesterase agents should be replaced with parenteral administration because of unpredictable gastric absorption (2.0 mg of pyridostigmine intramuscularly is recommended every 3-4 hours or neostigmine 0.5 mg intravenously every 3-4 hours). Prednisone can also administered parentally to help muscle strength.

Continuous monitoring during pregnancy is recommended. In cases of severe deterioration or extensive MG-related weakness, elective section should be considered. For cesarean delivery, both spinal and epidural anesthetic techniques have been used successfully.

General anesthesia should be considered in patients with severe bulbar involvement or respiratory compromise in order to secure the airway before surgery. Because of the reduced number of normal nAChRs, MG patients have an unpredictable response to neuromuscular-blocking agents. When depolarizing muscle relaxants (eg, succinylcholine) are used, patients have a prolonged block if they are treated with cholinesterase inhibitors, which inhibits plasma cholinesterase, causing delayed inactivation of succinylcholine than usual. Those who are not taking cholinesterase inhibitors are relatively resistant to succinylcholine because they have reduced numbers of normal nAChRs and cannot cause a depolarization.

On the other hand, myasthenic patients are extremely sensitive to nondepolarizing muscle relaxants because of the reduced number of receptors. If a nondepolarizing muscle relaxant has to be used, shorter acting agents in reduced doses should be used. Volatile anesthetic agents also potentiate muscle relaxation. Neuromuscular blockade should be monitored before the paralysis and continually during the entire case with a nerve stimulator.

POSTPARTUM CARE

The main risk during the postoperative period is progressive central weakness and the need for postoperative ventilation. The following predictors of the need for postoperative ventilation have been identified in the nonparturient surgical population: (1) female gender (2) forced expiratory flow 25% to 75%, less than 3.3 L/s and less than 78% of predicted; (3) forced vital capacity less than 2.6 L; and (4) maximum expiratory flow 50% less than 0.9 L/s and less than 80% of predicted.[50]

Transitory neonatal myasthenia gravis (TNMG) is a temporary (lasting up to 3 weeks) form of myasthenia occurring in 12% to 20% of infants born to myasthenic mothers.[51] TNMG is caused by the placental transfer of the nicotinic acetylcholine receptor antibodies from mother to the fetus. It develops during the first 4 days of life, with two-thirds of the cases manifesting within a few hours after birth. The varied onset of TNMG in the infant is due to the anticholinesterase drug also passing through the placenta and neonatal myasthenia manifesting only after the drug is metabolized and excreted by the infant. Symptoms of TNMG include lethargy, faint cry, slow respiration, and muscle weakness. The diagnosis can be made using the edrophonium chloride challenge test and there is spontaneous recovery by 4 weeks.

Women with MG must be monitored carefully during the first 3 weeks postpartum, since sudden and severe exacerbations may occur in one-third of these patients.[47] Regardless of the mode of delivery, careful monitoring and continued medication, in addition to plasmapheresis and high-dose steroids, are the most successful management options in preventing myasthenic crisis. Breastfeeding is contraindicated in women taking azathioprine, methotrexate, mycophenolate mofetil, or cyclophosphamide treatment, as well as with neonatal MG.

Muscular Dystrophies

EPIDEMIOLOGY

Muscular dystrophies are inherited myogenic disorders characterized by progressive muscle wasting and weakness of variable distribution and severity. Duchenne muscular dystrophy (DMD) and Becker's muscular dystrophy (BMD) are X-linked recessive diseases of skeletal and cardiac muscle. DMD usually affects males; females who carry the abnormal X chromosome are mostly asymptomatic.[52] Limb-girdle muscular dystrophies (LGMD) are a group of genetic skeletal muscle disorders with predominant involvement of the pelvic and shoulder girdle muscles and have variable inheritance patterns. The incidence of LGMD is estimated at 1 to 6.5 per 100,000. Facioscapulohumeral dystrophy is an autosomal dominant disease, with progressive muscle weakness of the shoulders and face that affects either gender, though symptoms may be less severe in women.

ETIOLOGY/RISK FACTORS

For DMD, symptoms begin between the ages of 2 and 5 years, and patients may be wheelchair-bound at very young ages. Manifestations include kyphoscoliosis, delayed gastric emptying, cardiac dysrhythmias, mitral valve regurgitation, restrictive lung disease, ineffective cough leading to pneumonia, and eventually death, most commonly due to pneumonia or congestive heart failure. These patients usually manifest with delayed motor milestones, waddling gait, frequent falls, and Gowers sign (using hands when rising from the floor).[52] Suspicion of

DMD/BMD is usually related to incidental elevated creatine phosphokinase levels detected before onset of symptoms. Newer molecular diagnostic techniques have allowed for further differentiation of muscular dystrophy types characterized by specific genetic mutations.

PATHOPHYSIOLOGY

Muscular dystrophies are caused by genetic mutations in specific genes that affect muscle development or function. The conditions are characterized by impaired muscle strength and progressive muscle weakness due primarily to muscle fiber degeneration. Fibrosis and inflammation may also occur as the disease progresses. The genetic locus, Xp21, is affected in both DMD and BMD. Most patients with DMD have a congenital absence of dystrophin and thus have a more severe clinical phenotype. In contrast, BMD has a more indolent course because dystrophin is usually present, albeit in an altered form and in reduced amounts.

MANAGEMENT

There are no treatment options currently available to cure muscular dystrophy, although much research is focused on gene therapy techniques to correct/replace the defective or absent protein. Symptomatic treatment and prevention of cardiac and respiratory complications are the mainstay of therapy. Parturients with history of DMD have delayed gastric emptying due to gastric hypomotility and pulmonary dysfunction due to smooth muscle dystrophy. To date, there is no evidence regarding uterine smooth muscle function or adverse effects on labor progression.

ANESTHETIC CONSIDERATIONS

The major concerns related to the administration of general anesthesia in patients with DMD and BMD are the potential for prolonged impaired respiratory function and cardiac issues. General anesthesia should be avoided if possible because there is respiratory weakness; decreased ability to cough; sleep apnea, which may be present contributing to the development of pulmonary hypertension; increased skeletal muscle permeability leading to decreased cardiopulmonary reserve; and hypomotility of the gastrointestinal tract, leading to increased risk of pulmonary aspiration. Regional anesthesia is preferred over general anesthesia, which can be associated with life-threatening complications, including cardiac dysrhythmias, cardiac arrest, and malignant hyperthermia.[53] Epidural anesthesia is favorable to spinal, because epidurals can be titrated slowly, to prevent respiratory failure from an inadvertently high block. Epidural analgesia should be placed early in labor and if necessary can be used for cesarean delivery, if needed, thus avoiding the administration of general anesthesia.

In emergent situations where general anesthesia is unavoidable, the risk of malignant hyperthermia–like syndrome is increased in parturients with muscular dystrophies. Therefore, nontriggering precautions should be utilized, which include using a new breathing circuit, flushing the anesthesia machine with fresh gas for at least 15 minutes prior to induction, and having dantrolene available to promptly treat any signs of malignant hyperthermia.

POSTPARTUM CARE

Patients appear to be particularly vulnerable during the postpartum period and should be closely monitored for exacerbations, particularly affecting bulbar and respiratory function. Neuraxial analgesia may facilitate chest physiotherapy in the postoperative period. Muscular dystrophy patients have an increased risk of recurring pneumonia. Neonatal screening and counseling may also be necessary.

Myotonia and Periodic Paralysis

EPIDEMIOLOGY

Myotonic syndromes are a spectrum of ion channel disorders causing skeletal muscle degeneration, where there is persistent contracture after voluntary muscle activity (myotonia) or muscle electrical stimulation. Myotonia dystrophica, the most common and most severe form, is autosomal dominant, with symptoms presenting usually during the 1920s to 1930s. It is estimated to occur in 2.4 to 5.05 per 100,000 population. In contrast, myotonia congenita, usually presents at birth or in early childhood, and also can be inherited as an autosomal dominant (Thomsen type) or as an autosomal recessive (Becker type) disorder. Other rare forms of myotonic dystrophy include paramyotonia congenita and Schwartz-Jampel syndrome. Periodic paralysis involves sodium channel (hyperkalemic periodic paralysis) and calcium channel disorders (hypokalemic periodic paralysis).

ETIOLOGY/RISK FACTORS

Myotonia dystrophica usually presents with facial weakness, dysphagia, and myotonia. There may also be associated mental retardation, frontal baldness, cataracts, endocrine gland impairment, and increased serum creatine kinase levels. Treatment is supportive, usually with phenytoin. There is progressive involvement of skeletal, cardiac, and smooth muscle, and symptoms are exacerbated by pregnancy. Obstetric complications related to the disease include uterine atony and retained placenta following vaginal delivery, increased risk of fetal loss, preterm delivery, placenta previa, and polyhydramnios.

Myotonia congenita is generally not a progressive disease and varies in severity. Phenytoin and quinine may be used to treat the disease. Periodic paralysis diagnosis includes muscle weakness induction after glucose infusion for hypokalemic periodic paralysis or from oral potassium for hyperkalemic periodic paralysis. Treatment with acetazolamide is used for both types.

PATHOPHYSIOLOGY

The underlying pathophysiology is determined by the genetic mutation affecting the muscle membrane voltage-sensitive channel. Myotonic dystrophies are due to extra nucleotide repeats—type 1 due to CTG repeats in the 3' untranslated region of *DMPK* gene and type 2 to CCTC repeat in the first intron of the *ZNF9* gene.[54] Myotonia congenita is due to mutations in the chloride channel *CLCN1* gene. Sodium channel disorders, including hyperperiodic paralysis, involve mutations in the voltage-gated sodium channel, *SCN4A* gene. Calcium channel disorders, including hypoperiodic paralysis, involve mutations in the L-type voltage-dependent calcium channel, *CACNA1S* gene.[55]

MANAGEMENT

There is no cure for myotonic disorders and treatment is supportive. Some patients may be asymptomatic prior to pregnancy but then develop muscle weakness during pregnancy. For periodic paralysis, treatment is both symptomatic using carbonic anhydrase inhibitors, such as acetazolamide or dichlorphenamide, and behavioral, with avoidance of triggers such as eating frequent small meals to avoid large carbohydrate loads, avoidance of sodium or potassium-rich foods, fasting, and medications that increase serum potassium to prevent hyperkalemic attacks in hyperperiodic patients. During pregnancy acetazolamide is contraindicated due to teratogenic effects; salbutamol is a substitute therapy.[56]

ANESTHETIC CONSIDERATIONS

For all parturients with myotonic dystrophy or periodic paralysis, succinylcholine (a potassium-releasing drug) needs to be avoided due to the risk of prolonged skeletal muscle contraction and potential for malignant hyperthermia–like syndromes. Relatively short-acting nondepolarizing muscle relaxants, such as rocuronium, may be used but always with monitoring of neuromuscular function. Total intravenous anesthesia may circumvent the need for paralysis altogether.[56] Maintaining normothermia is critical to avoid shivering and hypothermia, which may precipitate myotonia.

For parturients with myotonia dystrophica, there may be cardiomyopathy (even in asymptomatic patients) and respiratory muscle weakness. Myocardial depression can occur with use of volatile anesthesia, and cardiac dysrhythmias may occur severe enough to require treatment. Anesthesia complications are more common with type 1 myotonic dystrophy as compared to type 2. Parturients with periodic paralysis may also have the potential for cardiac rhythm abnormalities.[56] Patients with myotonias have increased sensitivity to the respiratory depressant effects of barbiturates, opioids, benzodiazepines, and propofol. In addition, they may be susceptible to develop hypersomnolence and central sleep apnea. In periodic paralysis parturients, serum potassium levels should be monitored throughout anesthetic management and the adequate restoration of neuromuscular function achieved before extubation.

POSTPARTUM CARE

There is no evidence to suggest that pregnancy worsens the lifetime course of the myotonias. Periodic paralysis may be associated with postoperative paralysis. NSAIDS should also be used with caution because they potentially can cause hyperkalemia, especially if renal disease is also present. Perinatal mortality is reported as high 15%, mainly due to congenitally affected offspring.

Polio

EPIDEMIOLOGY

There are approximately 300,000 survivors of poliomyelitis in the United States. After recovery from the acute phase of the disease, some patients continue to suffer from chronic neurologic and respiratory complications. Kyphoscoliosis may be seen in 12% of patients with poliomyelitis necessitating corrective spinal surgery.[57]

ETIOLOGY/RISK FACTORS/PATHOPHYSIOLOGY

Poliomyelitis is an infection caused by a single-stranded RNA enterovirus transmitted by the fecal-oral route. It presents with neurologic symptoms such as asymmetric flaccid paralysis. Major risk factors for contracting polio are lack of polio vaccination or living in polio-prevalent regions in the world without vaccination. The estimated risk of paralysis after infection approximates to 1% to 2%, with 50% of those presenting with muscle weakness progressing to permanent motor function loss, affecting the lower limbs and respiratory muscles. There is an increased risk of pregnancy-related complications in females affected by polio, resulting in adverse operative and perinatal outcomes, as well as increased risk of developing preeclampsia irrespective of maternal parity or age.[58]

MANAGEMENT AND ANESTHETIC CONSIDERATIONS

There are no reported adverse effects of regional anesthesia in patients with polio; both spinal and epidural have been safely used for analgesia during normal labor and cesarean delivery without significant complications.[57] General anesthesia poses a potential risk in this group of parturients, because they have a limited respiratory reserve. There are two reported cases of postpolio syndrome, where unanticipated respiratory failure occurred postoperatively and resulted in cardiorespiratory arrest and brain injury.[59] In both cases, the respiratory failure was attributed to oversedation with opioid medications. The response to neuromuscular blockers such as succinylcholine is unpredictable and may result in hyperkalemia from damaged motor neuron end plates and should be avoided. Nondepolarizing muscle relaxants also have a variable effect in patients with poliomyelitis and postpolio syndrome, so heightened vigilance and neuromuscular function monitoring is required when they are used.

POSTPARTUM CARE

Postpartum care is dependent on patient history and delivery method. There is also an increased risk of lower birth weight and perinatal complications, including renal issues.

CONCLUSION

Neurologic and neuromuscular comorbidities in parturients require careful multidisciplinary preparation during pregnancy and the puerperium. In some cases, planning can occur prenatally, but for some patients, pregnancy may precipitate neurologic or neuromuscular diseases for the first time. Individual neurologic/neuromuscular disorders have been discussed separately in this chapter; they can also occur in combination and parturients can present with several comorbidities. Anesthetic management should to be tailored to each unique situation—for example, the avoidance of succinylcholine to prevent hyperkalemia when there may be damaged motor neuron end plates, or anesthetic techniques modified such as the use of low-dose and gently dosed epidural analgesia regimen. Anesthetic considerations also include balancing of different requirements, ranging from neurologic function to obstetric and fetal indications. Even following delivery, each comorbidity presents unique challenges and concerns with the need for vigilance and monitoring, particularly in the postpartum period. However, with careful planning and involvement of a multidisciplinary team throughout, it is possible to achieve a successful clinical outcome.

CASE STUDY

A 33-year-old white woman with a history of new-onset (3 months) MS presents to the preoperative holding area for her assessment prior to her scheduled primary cesarean section at 38 weeks' gestation. Past medical history includes asthma. Her medications currently are azathioprine, oral steroids, albuterol (inhaler), and steroids (inhaler). She has no known drug allergies. Her brain MRI (Figure 25-6) shows multiple pericallosal hyperintense lesions. Her MS presented clinically with paresthesias and balance difficulties and unilateral visual loss; all of these symptoms have since resolved.

Questions

1. Is it appropriate that this patient is seen for the first time by the anesthesiology team on the day of her cesarean section?

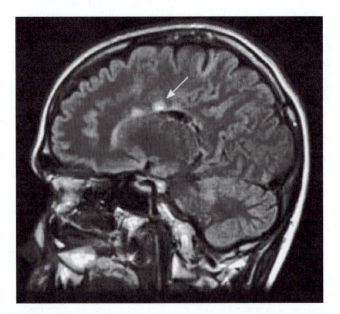

Figure 25-6. Magnetic resonance image from case study. Sagittal view of the brain, showing multiple pericallosal hypertense lesions (arrow) on fluid attenuation inversion recovery (FLAIR). (Reproduced with permission from The Royal Australian College of General Practitioners from Tsang B, Macdonell R. Multiple sclerosis. Diagnosis, management and prognosis. *Aust Fam Physician* 2011;40(12):948-955.)

2. Are all the medications that she is receiving appropriate for her current condition?

3. Is regional anesthesia a good choice for her cesarean section?

4. What additional investigations would you suggest for her complete preoperative assessment?

5. Would there be any difference in her intraoperative management compared to other parturients?

Answers

1. As with all significant neurologic disorders, a multidisciplinary approach to assessment and management of the patient would be ideal. This should involve a maternal and fetal medicine specialist and a neurologist. In addition, early consultation with an obstetric anesthesiologist for planning of perioperative and peripartum care of this patient is essential.

2. Her medications include azathioprine, which although appropriate for MS therapy in nonpregnant patients, may not be a good choice for use during pregnancy.[60]

3. If general anesthesia were considered, it is not clear if there is a preferable general anesthetic agent to use; however, in terms of muscle relaxation, succinylcholine should be avoided as it may cause hyperkalemia if there is muscle loss and subsequent up-regulation of extrajunctional acetylcholine receptors. Recovery from nondepolarizing muscle relaxants, on the other hand, may be prolonged,[61] so dosing may need to be reduced and accurate neuromuscular twitch monitoring utilized. Regional anesthesia is not contraindicated in MS patients as it has not been shown to interfere with the MS progression, the concern of a single reported retrospective study of higher levels of epidural local anesthesia concentration and MS relapse, particularly with autonomic nervous system lesions, may require careful thought. Whichever technique is chosen, it is important to have careful monitoring of this patient both intraoperatively and in the immediate postpartum, with heightened vigilance on her body temperature compared to other parturients.

4. Pulmonary function tests may be indicated in some patients with MS; however, they are not likely needed in this patient with such an early presentation and no pulmonary symptoms with well controlled asthma. Accurate body temperature management is very important in these patients with a concerted effort to avoid the patient becoming too warm; as there is some evidence that increased temperature worsens the progression of the disease.[61]

5. The clinical pattern of relapsing and remitting symptoms are typical, which progress slowly over time. With a complete remission in the symptoms of the first MS presentation in this patient, it argues for a slow progression course of her disease. Pregnancy does not seem to have a negative effect on MS progression, and actually many pregnant patients report an improvement in their symptoms,[6] which may be evident here.

REFERENCES

1. Tsang BK, Macdonell R. Multiple sclerosis—diagnosis, management and prognosis. *Aust Fam Physician.* 2011;40(12):948-955.
2. Lövblad KO, Anzalone N, Dörfler A, et al. MR imaging in multiple sclerosis: review and recommendations for current practice. *AJNR Am J Neuroradiol.* 2010;31(6):983-989.
3. Young CA. Factors predisposing to the development of multiple sclerosis. *QJM.* 2011;104(5):383-386.
4. Ferrero S, Pretta S, Ragni N. Multiple sclerosis: management issues during pregnancy. *Eur J Obstet Gynecol Reprod Biol.* 2004;115(1):3-9.
5. Tsui A, Lee MA. Multiple sclerosis and pregnancy. *Curr Opin Obstet Gynecol.* 2011;23(6):435-439.
6. Vukusic S, Hutchinson M, Hours M, et al. Pregnancy and multiple sclerosis (the PRIMS study): clinical predictors of post-partum relapse. *Brain.* 2004;127(Pt 6):1353-1360.
7. Brooks H, Christian AS, May AE. Pregnancy, anaesthesia and Guillain Barre syndrome. *Anaesthesia.* 2000;55(9):894-898.
8. Uncini A. A common mechanism and a new categorization for anti-ganglioside antibody-mediated neuropathies. *Exp Neurol.* 2012;235(2):513-516.
9. Chan LY, Tsui MH, Leung TN. Guillain-Barré syndrome in pregnancy. *Acta Obstet Gynecol Scand.* 2004;83(4):319-325.
10. Chiapparini L, Saletti V, Solero CL, Bruzzone MG, Valentini LG. Neuroradiological diagnosis of Chiari malformations. *Neurol Sci.* 2011;32(suppl 3):S283-S286.
11. Ramón C, Gonzáles-Mandly A, Pascual J. What differences exist in the appropriate treatment of congenital versus acquired adult Chiari type I malformation? *Curr Pain Headache Rep.* 2011;15(3):157-163.
12. Hullander RM, Bogard TD, Leivers D, et al. Chiari I malformation presenting as recurrent spinal headache. *Anesth Analg.* 1992;75(6):1025-1026.
13. Chantigian RC, Koehn MA, Ramin KD, et al. Chiari I malformation in parturients. *J Clin Anesth.* 2002;14(3):201-205.
14. Ghaly RF, Candido KD, Sauer R, et al. Anesthetic management during Cesarean section in a woman with residual Arnold-Chiari malformation Type I, cervical kyphosis, and syringomyelia. *Surg Neurol Int.* 2012;3:26.
15. Mueller DM, Oro' J. Chiari I malformation with or without syringomyelia and pregnancy: case studies and review of the literature. *Am J Perinatol.* 2005;22(2):67-70.
16. Borthen I, Gilhus NE. Pregnancy complications in patients with epilepsy. *Curr Opin Obstet Gynecol.* 2012;24(2):78-83.
17. Devinsky O, Vezzani A, Najjar S, et al. Glia and epilepsy: excitability and inflammation. *Trends Neurosci.* 2013. pii: S0166-2236(12)00205-6. doi: 10.1016/j.tins.2012.11.008.
18. Vajda FJ, Hitchcock A, Graham J, et al. Seizure control in antiepileptic drug-treated pregnancy. *Epilepsia.* 2008;49(1):172-176.
19. Kjaer D, Horvath-Puhó E, Christensen J, et al. Antiepileptic drug use, folic acid supplementation, and congenital abnormalities: a population-based case-control study. *BJOG.* 2008;115(1):98-103.
20. American Academy of Pediatrics, 2003.
21. Kuczkowski KM. Labor analgesia for the parturient with neurological disease: what does an obstetrician need to know? *Arch Gynecol Obstet.* 2006;274(1):41-46.
22. Iijima T, Nakamura Z, Iwao Y, Sankawa H. The epileptogenic properties of the volatile anesthetics sevoflurane and isoflurane in patients with epilepsy. *Anesth Analg.* 2000;91(4):989-995.
23. Shih CJ, Doufas AG, Chang HC, et al. Recurrent seizure activity after epidural morphine in a post-partum woman. *Can J Anaesth.* 2005;52(7):727-729.
24. Lateef TM, Nelson KB. In utero exposure to antiepileptic drugs: teratogenicity and neonatal morbidity. *Curr Neurol Neurosci Rep.* 2007;7(2):133-138.
25. Pereira L. Obstetric management of the patient with spinal cord injury. *Obstet Gynecol Surv.* 2003; 58(10):678-687.
26. Mothe AJ, Tator CH. Advances in stem cell therapy for spinal cord injury. *J Clin Invest.* 2012; 122(11):3824-3834.
27. Karlsson AK. Autonomic dysfunction in spinal cord injury: clinical presentation of symptoms and signs. *Prog Brain Res.* 2006;152:1-8.

28. Vercauteren M, Waets P, Pitkänen M, et al. Neuraxial techniques in patients with pre-existing back impairment or prior spine interventions: a topical review with special reference to obstetrics. *Acta Anaesthesiol Scand.* 2011;55(8):910-917.

29. Swensen R, Kirsch W. Brain neoplasms in women: a review. *Clin Obstet Gynecol.* 2002;45(3):904-927.

30. Imarengiaye C, Littleford J, Davies S, et al. Goal oriented general anesthesia for Cesarean section in a parturient with a large intracranial epidermoid cyst. *Can J Anaesth.* 2001;48(9):884-889.

31. Chang L, Looi-Lyons L, Bartosik L, et al. Anesthesia for cesarean section in two patients with brain tumours. *Can J Anaesth.* 1999;46(1):61-65.

32. Balki M, Manninen PH. Craniotomy for suprasellar meningioma in a 28-week pregnant woman without fetal heart rate monitoring. *Can J Anaesth.* 2004 Jun-Jul;51(6):573-576.

33. Bateman BT, Schumacher HC, Bushnell CD, et al. Intracerebral hemorrhage in pregnancy: frequency, risk factors, and outcome. *Neurology.* 2006;67(3):424-429.

34. Selo-Ojeme DO, Marshman LA, Ikomi A, et al. Aneurysmal subarachnoid haemorrhage in pregnancy. *Eur J Obstet Gynecol Reprod Biol.* 2004;116(2):131-143.

35. Kizilkilic O, Albayram S, Adaletli I, et al. Endovascular treatment of ruptured intracranial aneurysms during pregnancy: report of three cases. *Arch Gynecol Obstet.* 2003;268:325-328.

36. Wang LP, Paech MJ. Neuroanesthesia for the pregnant woman. *Anesth Analg.* 2008;107(1):193-200.

37. Acheson J, Malik A. Cerebral venous sinus thrombosis presenting in the puerperium. *Emerg Med J.* 2006;23(7):e44.

38. Edlow JA, Caplan LR, O'Brien K, et al. Diagnosis of acute neurological emergencies in pregnant and post-partum women. *Lancet Neurol.* 2013;12(2):175-185.

39. Younker D, Jones MM, Adenwala J, et al. Maternal cortical vein thrombosis and the obstetric anesthesiologist. *Anesth Analg.* 1986;65(10):1007-1012.

40. Bousser MG, Crassard I. Cerebral venous thrombosis, pregnancy and oral contraceptives. *Thromb Res.* 2012;130 (suppl 1):S19-S22.

41. Karmaniolou I, Petropoulos G, Theodoraki K. Management of idiopathic intracranial hypertension in parturients: anesthetic considerations. *Can J Anaesth.* 2011;58(7):650-657.

42. Zamecki KJ, Frohman LP, Turbin RE. Severe visual loss associated with idiopathic intracranial hypertension (IIH) in pregnancy. *Clin Ophthalmol.* 2007;1:99-103.

43. Paruchuri SR, Lawlor M, Kleinhomer K, et al. Risk of cerebellar tonsillar herniation after diagnostic lumbar puncture in pseudotumor cerebri. *Anesth Analg.* 1993;77(2):403-404.

44. Lussos SA, Loeffler C. Epidural blood patch improves postdural puncture headache in a patient with benign intracranial hypertension. *Reg Anesth.* 1993;18(5):315-317.

45. Angelini C. Diagnosis and management of autoimmune myasthenia gravis. *Clin Drug Investig.* 2011;31(1):1-14.

46. Mays J, Butts CL. Intercommunication between the neuroendocrine and immune systems: focus on myasthenia gravis. *Neuroimmunomodulation.* 2011;18(5):320-327.

47. Hoff JM, Daltveit AK, Gilhus NE. Myasthenia gravis in pregnancy and birth: identifying risk factors, optimizing care. *Eur J Neurol.* 2007;14(1):38-43.

48. Ferrero S, Pretta S, Nicoletti A, et al. Myasthenia gravis: management issues during pregnancy. *Eur J Obstet Gynecol Reprod Biol.* 2005;121(2):129-138.

49. Hoff JM, Daltveit AK, Gilhus NE. Artrogryposis multiplex congenita—a rare fetal condition caused by maternal myasthenia gravis. *Acta Neurol Scand Suppl.* 2006;183:26-27.

50. Naguib M, el Dawlatly AA, Ashour M, Bamgboye EA. Multivariate determinants of the need for postoperative ventilation in myasthenia gravis. *Can J Anaesth.* 1996 Oct;43(10):1006-1013.

51. Djelmis J, Sostarko M, Mayer D, et al. Myasthenia gravis in pregnancy: report on 69 cases. *Eur J Obstet Gynecol Reprod Biol.* 2002;104(1):21-25.

52. Molyneux MK. Anaesthetic management during labour of a manifesting carrier of Duchenne muscular dystrophy. *Int J Obstet Anesth.* 2005;14(1):58-61.

53. Gurnaney H, Brown A, Litman RS. Malignant hyperthermia and muscular dystrophies. *Anesth Analg.* 2009;109(4):1043-1048.

54. Turner C, Hilton-Jones D. The myotonic dystrophies: diagnosis and management. *J Neurol Neurosurg Psychiatry.* 2010;81(4):358-367.

55. Burge JA, Hanna MG. Novel insights into the pathomechanisms of skeletal muscle channelopathies. *Curr Neurol Neurosci Rep.* 2012;12(1):62-69.

56. Mackenzie MJ, Pickering E, Yentis SM. Anaesthetic management of labour and caesarean delivery of a patient with hyperkalaemic periodic paralysis. *Int J Obstet Anesth.* 2006;15(4):329-331.

57. Costello JF, Balki M. Cesarean delivery under ultrasound-guided spinal anesthesia [corrected] in a parturient with poliomyelitis and Harrington instrumentation. *Can J Anaesth.* 2008 Sep;55(9):606-611.

58. Veiby G, Daltveit AK, Gilhus NE. Pregnancy, delivery and perinatal outcome in female survivors of polio. *J Neurol Sci.* 2007 Jul 15;258(1-2):27-32.

59. Wernet A, Bougeois B, Merckx P, et al. Successful use of succinylcholine for cesarean delivery in a patient with postpolio syndrome. *Anesthesiology.* 2007;107(4):680-681.

60. Houtchens MK. Pregnancy and multiple sclerosis. *Semin Neurol.* 2007;27(5):434-441.

61. Dorotta IR, Schubert A. Multiple sclerosis and anesthetic implications. *Curr Opin Anaesthesiol.* 2002; 15(3):365-370.

Anesthetic Management of the Parturient With Respiratory Disease

26

Ashley M. Tonidandel and Jessica L. Booth

INTRODUCTION

A majority of women experience subjective breathlessness during pregnancy. This complicates the diagnosis of true respiratory pathology. "Dyspnea of pregnancy" is likely related to normal physiologic alterations, summarized in Table 26-1, that serve to maintain the fetus and prepare the mother for labor and delivery.[1] The dyspnea associated with pregnancy does not interfere with activities of daily living and is not related to exertion, coughing, or wheezing. Physiologic dyspnea usually improves as pregnancy progresses, particularly with "quickening," which is defined as the maternal perception of initial fetal movement. In contrast, pathologic dyspnea from cardiac or pulmonary origins may have an abrupt onset, be progressive in its severity, occur even at rest, or be associated with cough, chest pain, fever, or hemoptysis. Dyspnea due to cardiac or respiratory pathology worsens as the pregnancy reaches the third trimester. Pregnant women with a respiratory rate greater than 20 breaths/min, increased work of breathing, or the presence of rales, wheezing, or murmurs deserve prompt evaluation for potential cardiopulmonary pathology.[2]

ACUTE RESPIRATORY FAILURE

Epidemiology

Acute respiratory failure (ARF) is defined by the inability to maintain adequate oxygenation or ventilation. Although ARF is rare (occurring in less than 0.1% of pregnancies), it remains one of the most common indications for intensive care

Table 26-1. Physiologic Changes During Pregnancy

Organ System	Change During Pregnancy
Respiratory	
Tidal volume	Increased 40%
Minute ventilation	Increased 40%-50%
Respiratory rate	Increased 10%
Oxygen consumption	Increased 40%
Expiratory reserve volume	Decreased 20%
Functional residual capacity	Decreased 12%-25%
Arterial PCO_2	Decreased ~10%
Chest wall compliance	Decreased 45%
Cardiovascular	
Cardiac output	Increased 20%-50%
Stroke volume	Increased 30%
Systemic vascular resistance	Decreased 30%
Heart rate	Increased 20%
Hematologic	
Plasma volume	Increased 55%
Blood volume	Increased 45%
Hematocrit	Decreased (physiologic anemia)
Gastrointestinal	
Gastrointestinal motility	Decreased
Lower esophageal sphincter tone	Decreased
Intragastric pressure	Increased

Data from Dean LS, D'Angelo R.[1]

unit admission in pregnant women.[3] The etiology of ARF in pregnancy is diverse and may or may not be directly related to pregnancy (Table 26-2). Acute respiratory distress syndrome (ARDS) has been defined by the American-European Consensus Conference with the following criteria: lung injury of an acute onset, bilateral infiltrates present on chest x-ray, PaO_2-to-FiO_2 ratio less than or equal to 200, and pulmonary artery wedge pressure less than 18 mm Hg or the absence of clinical evidence of left atrial hypertension.[3] The estimated maternal mortality rate due to ARF is reported to be 30% to 35% and, in the setting of ARDS, regardless of the inciting etiology, the mortality rate can be as great as 70%.[4] Fetal mortality is also high, most commonly reported at 20% to 30%, and it is usually due to complications from premature delivery or perinatal hypoxia.[3]

Pathophysiology

A respiratory insult during pregnancy may be more likely to lead to ARF. Increased oxygen consumption and decreased functional residual capacity (FRC) render pregnant women, particularly in the latter half of pregnancy, more susceptible to hypoxia, hypercarbia, and acidosis during short periods of apnea or hypoventilation. Chronic mild respiratory alkalosis during pregnancy helps promote

Table 26-2. Differential Diagnosis of Acute Respiratory Failure in Pregnancy

Exacerbation of Preexisting Lung Disease
  Asthma
  Cystic fibrosis
  Chronic obstructive pulmonary disease/emphysema
Embolism
  Amniotic fluid embolism
  Pulmonary embolism
  Venous air embolism
Pneumonia
  Community-acquired
  Influenza
  Aspiration
  Nosocomial
Pulmonary Edema
  Preeclampsia
  Tocolytic-induced (eg, terbutaline)
  Cardiogenic
Trauma
  Pulmonary contusion
  Pulmonary hemorrhage
  Rib fractures, sternal injuries
Sepsis
  Chorioamnionitis
  Systemic infections
  Pneumonia
Cardiomyopathy
Acute respiratory distress syndrome
Transfusion-related acute lung injury
Drug overdose

elimination of fetal waste but limits buffering capacity during periods of maternal acidosis.[3] Maternal mortality with ARF is found to be associated with low pH, initial loss of consciousness, which is probably related to hypoxia, disseminated intravascular syndrome (DIC), and sepsis.[4]

Management and Anesthetic Considerations

Obstetric patients admitted to the hospital with ARF should be followed closely in an intensive care unit. Some hospitals have obstetric critical care units to meet the special demands of caring for sick parturients and planning for delivery.

The primary management goals for patients with ARF include identification and treatment of the underlying cause of lung injury, optimizing adequate oxygen delivery, and maintaining fluid homeostasis. Additional goals include nutritional support, monitoring of fetal status, and planning for delivery.

Low alveolar closing pressure, due to a decreased FRC, increases the risk of alveolar collapse and atelectasis, especially in the supine position.[3] Fetal hemoglobin has a higher affinity for oxygen than adult hemoglobin (see Figure 26-1). However, oxygenation needs of the fetus require higher maternal oxygen saturation compared to nonpregnant women. Maternal oxygen saturation greater than 90% and/or maternal PaO_2 greater than 65 mm Hg are reasonable goals to ensure adequate fetal oxygenation.[5,6] Hyperventilation should be avoided because hypocarbia can lead to uterine artery vasoconstriction, and alkalosis can diminish oxygen unloading to the fetus. Adequate oxygen delivery may be achieved by supplying higher inspired concentration of oxygen by face mask, noninvasive positive pressure ventilation, or by mechanical ventilation. Vigorous mechanical ventilation should be avoided because it can result in reduced placental perfusion as a result of low maternal cardiac output and venous return to the heart, augmented by aortocaval compression. Bronchodilator therapy and vasopressors might be useful adjuncts.[7]

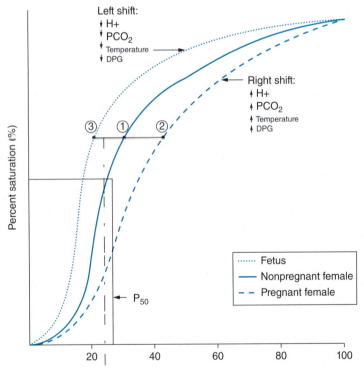

Figure 26-1. Theoretical oxyhemoglobin dissociation curves. Curve 1: Normal oxyhemoglobin dissociation curve in a nonpregnant adult. Curve 2: Oxyhemoglobin dissociation curve of a pregnant female at term gestation. Note that the curve is shifted to the right due to a 30% increase in erythrocyte 2,3–DPG to improve oxygen delivery to the fetus. Curve 3: Oxyhemoglobin dissociation curve of a fetus. Note that the curve is shifted to the left.

Goals of mechanical ventilation are to provide adequate oxygenation and to optimize ventilation with avoidance of barotrauma and increased transpulmonary pressure. Indications for intubation and mechanical ventilation for pregnant women are the same as for nonpregnant women and include the need for airway protection or failure to maintain adequate oxygenation and ventilation. Extra equipment and/or personnel should be available during endotracheal intubation in near-term pregnant women because of the potential for difficult airway management. Uterine displacement, either manually or with adequate pelvic tilt, is recommended to prevent aortocaval compression and improve preload in the supine position. Pregnant women should generally be considered as "full stomach aspiration risk" regardless of nothing-by-mouth status. Except in the most life-threatening emergencies, they should receive a nonparticulate antacid and a rapid-sequence induction with cricoid pressure. Preoxygenation is critical due to the potential to rapidly develop worsening hypoxia with apnea. Gentle manipulation of the upper airway is required during laryngoscopy to prevent trauma and bleeding, and a smaller endotracheal tube should be used because of a smaller glottic opening. A nasal airway should be avoided to prevent epistaxis.

Fetal monitoring, if appropriate for gestational age, should be performed, and a multidisciplinary plan for rapid delivery should be agreed on in the event of maternal or fetal deterioration. Cesarean delivery should be reserved primarily for obstetric indications, because optimizing the maternal cardiorespiratory status should promote fetal well-being and growth. Such delivery should be reserved for maternal indications or when the fetus is near term if labor and vaginal delivery are not attainable due to maternal condition.[3,5]

Extreme mechanical hyperventilation (end-tidal CO_2 less than 24 mm Hg) may cause uterine vasoconstriction and a decrease in maternal cardiac output.[1] Invasive hemodynamic monitoring, such as an arterial line or pulmonary artery catheter, may be required to optimize fluid homeostasis and thus prevent pulmonary edema while maintaining adequate organ perfusion. The head of the bed should also be elevated to decrease aspiration risk, and appropriate oral hygiene care should be performed to decrease nosocomial infections.[3] Analgesia or even sedation may be necessary for maternal comfort and reduction of oxygen demands during positive pressure ventilation.[3] The impact of maternal sedation on fetal heart tracings will need to be considered in making decisions about fetal health and indications for delivery. Prophylactic measures to prevent the development of deep venous thromboses is particularly important for pregnant or postpartum women due to their hypercoagulable state.[1]

PNEUMONIA

Epidemiology

Pneumonia complicates an estimated 0.4 to 2.7 per 1000 deliveries and is the most common cause of maternal mortality resulting from nonobstetric infection. The overall maternal mortality rate from pneumonia has improved to less than 4% over the past 50 years because of targeted treatment with more effective antibiotics and better critical care management.[6,8] Community-acquired pneumonia (CAP) is a common but serious cause of hospital admission for hypoxia, fever, shortness of breath, cough, and pleuritic chest pain. Nonpregnant and pregnant women are susceptible to similar pathogens. The most common bacterial agents for CAP are *Streptococcus pneumoniae* and *Haemophilus influenzae*. Atypical agents such as *Legionella* species and *Mycoplasma pneumoniae* are seen rarely, and specific serologic testing for these organisms is usually not performed.[5,8]

Viral pathogens responsible for pneumonia in pregnancy include influenza A and B (including swine flu, H1N1 virus), varicella zoster virus, and coronavirus (severe acute respiratory syndrome). The novel H1N1 strain of the 2009-2010 influenza season created a historic epidemic that resulted in severe illness in pregnant women. Parturients infected with the H1N1 virus were at increased risk for complications, including hospitalization, respiratory failure, premature delivery, nonreassuring fetal status, and even death. Data collected by the Centers for Disease Control and Prevention (CDC) from August to December 2009 indicated an alarming 5% maternal mortality rate among 509 hospitalized pregnant women with H1N1.[9] Regardless of H1N1, influenza during pregnancy in general has a high complication rate even during normal influenza seasons. For instance, parturients experience a near 10-fold increase in influenza-related morbidity as compared to nonpregnant women afflicted with the disease (10.5 versus 1.9 per 10,000 women).[5] The CDC recommends that all pregnant women receive the influenza vaccine. Also recommended is the use of pneumococcal vaccine for high-risk parturients with chronic diseases, such as asplenia, immunocompromise, sickle cell disease, and so on.[5]

Etiology/Risk Factors

Women with asthma or anemia, which is defined as hematocrit less than or equal to 30%, also have a five-fold increase of developing pneumonia during pregnancy. Additionally, substance abuse, smoking, chronic medical conditions, preexisting pulmonary disease, and human immunodeficiency virus (HIV) infection are also associated with higher rates of pneumonia in pregnancy.[10] The mode of delivery may also affect the incidence of pneumonia. For instance, during the postpartum period, women having a cesarean delivery have a greater incidence of pneumonia than those having a vaginal delivery.[10]

Pathophysiology

The physiologic changes that occur during pregnancy render parturients more susceptible to developing pneumonia. The decreased FRC and increased oxygen requirement associated with pregnancy compromise respiratory functions. Delayed gastric emptying, increased intragastric pressure, and a relaxed gastroesophageal sphincter predispose to aspiration. In addition, multiple immunologic changes occur that decrease the maternal immune response to infection.[10] For instance, the activity of natural killer cells, helper T-type 1 cells, and T-cytotoxic 1 cells are reduced, thereby reducing the production of interleukin-2, interferon, and tumor necrosis factor.

Pneumonia may also be associated with several pregnancy-related complications. The incidence of preterm labor in women with CAP has been reported to be as high as 44%, and one-third of women may deliver prematurely.[5,6,8-10] The incidence of premature rupture of membranes is increased in women with pneumonia as compared to those without pneumonia. In addition, women with pneumonia during pregnancy are nearly twice as likely to have intrauterine growth restriction with lower birth weights.[5]

Management and Anesthetic Considerations

Monotherapy with macrolides (erythromycin, azithromycin) is the mainstay of treatment in bacterial pneumonia and is successful in 99% of patients. In cases of drug-resistant *Streptococcus* pneumonia, ceftriaxone or cefotaxime should be added. Current CDC guidelines recommend that all pregnant women and women who are less than or equal to 2 weeks' postpartum with documented exposure to the influenza virus or symptoms in the first 48 hours of illness should receive treatment with oseltamivir (Tamiflu) or zanamivir (Relenza) to reduce perinatal morbidity and mortality. Patients with varicella pneumonia had high mortality rate (35%-40%) before the introduction of antiviral therapy; with the advent of antiviral therapy, this is reduced to approximately 15%. These patients should be hospitalized early, and antiviral treatment with intravenous acyclovir should be initiated to reduce respiratory complications.[6] As described in Table 26-3, American Thoracic Society guidelines can be adapted and applied during pregnancy with a 96% success rate at predicting a complicated pneumonia course requiring critical care support.[5] Given the rapidity of complications that can occur, some obstetricians choose to hospitalize all pregnant women with pneumonia for overnight observation to complete a full workup, including chest x-ray, complete blood count, electrolyte panel, blood cultures if clinically warranted, and oxygen assessment of both the mother and fetus.[6]

Patients admitted to the hospital for severe symptoms of pneumonia should be treated in a supportive manner by a multidisciplinary team. A collaborative effort from infectious disease physicians, critical care physicians, respiratory therapists, obstetricians, neonatal staff, labor and delivery nurses, and anesthesiologists is

Table 26-3. Possible Risk Factors for a Complicated Course of Community-Acquired Pneumonia During Pregnancy[a]

Presence of coexisting chronic disease
Altered mental status
Respiratory rate ≥ 30 breaths/min
Temperature > 38.3°C
White blood cell count < 4×10^9/L or > 30×10^9/L
PaO_2 < 60 mm Hg or $PaCO_2$ > 50 mm Hg
Creatinine > 1.2 mg/dL
Unfavorable chest radiograph findings (eg, multilobar involvement)

[a]Data from The American Thoracic Society.

required to optimally care for the parturient and her fetus. A chest radiograph, with an abdominal shield, should be performed early to avoid a delay in diagnosis. Other potential diagnoses, including pulmonary embolism, amniotic fluid embolism, pulmonary edema, sepsis, or cardiomyopathy should be considered. Antimicrobial or antiviral therapy should be started according to the appropriate infectious disease guidelines. Supportive treatment with hydration, antipyretic therapy, and supplemental oxygen are important for both maternal and fetal well-being. The use of mechanical ventilation for severe respiratory failure should be utilized if needed. Prevention of aspiration with a nonparticulate antacid and elevation of the head of the bed are important measures. The patient should also be monitored in a setting that is prepared for potential preterm labor or fetal distress.[6]

If a parturient with systemic infection goes into labor or requires a cesarean delivery, the decision to perform a regional anesthetic technique should be individual and based on the patient's risk of central nervous system infection versus the benefit of regional anesthesia. Although most experts agree that central neuraxial blocks should not be performed in untreated bacteremic patients, patients with systemic infection on appropriate antibiotic therapy may safely undergo subarachnoid anesthesia. However, patients should be followed closely afterward for signs or symptoms of central nervous system infection.[11]

ASTHMA AND REACTIVE AIRWAY DISEASE

Epidemiology

Asthma affects approximately 8% of pregnant women, making it one of the most common medical diseases encountered in pregnancy.[12] The course of asthma during pregnancy is variable, with approximately 23% of women showing improvement and 30% worsening of symptoms.[13] Poorly controlled asthma is associated with higher rates of preeclampsia, intrauterine growth restriction, preterm delivery, congenital malformations, and perinatal death.[14] Due to the variable effects of pregnancy on asthma symptoms and the serious maternal and fetal implications, the American College of Obstetricians and Gynecologists (ACOG) recommends that all pregnant women with asthma undergo clinical evaluation to assess disease severity and optimize symptom control.[13]

Pathophysiology

Asthma is defined as a chronic disease of airway inflammation with increased reactivity to a variety of stimuli that result in partially or completely reversible airway obstruction. The immune-mediated inflammatory response involves a complex cascade of T and B lymphocytes, mast cells, eosinophils, and neutrophils that are triggered by allergens, infections, or exercise. Patients typically experience wheezing, shortness of breath, coughing, and chest tightness during exacerbations.[15] Although exact mechanisms are not known, pregnancy may improve asthma symptoms in some patients due to progesterone-mediated bronchodilation and increased serum free cortisol levels. In contrast, deterioration of symptoms may be caused by stress, increased reflux, bronchitis, or medication noncompliance due to fetal safety concerns.[15] Pregnancy complications in asthma patients may be related to severity of disease, fetal oxygenation problems, or medication side effects.[12]

Management and Anesthetic Considerations

The primary goal of management is to provide adequate oxygenation to mother and thus to fetus during asthma attacks. The comprehensive management plan includes objective assessment, avoidance of triggers (exposure to allergens such as dust, mold, animal dander, tobacco smoke, infection), monitoring of respiratory functions, optimization of pharmacologic management, and education.

Diagnostic criteria of asthma in pregnant patients are similar to those in non-pregnant patients. Wheezing, cough, and shortness of breath associated with triggers (allergen, infection, exercise) are common symptoms. During a severe asthma attack, wheezing may be absent due to absence of air entry. Spirometry should reveal improvement (at least more than 12%) in FEV_1 (forced expiratory volume in 1 second) after a bronchodilator.[13] Patients with asthma should undergo a full clinical evaluation early in pregnancy to determine baseline pulmonary function and asthma severity. Education about asthma control, including avoidance of triggering factors (especially tobacco smoke), possible effect of asthma attacks on fetus, self-monitoring, and correct use of inhalers should be provided to mothers. Because asthma severity may vary throughout pregnancy, patients should be reassessed if symptom frequency changes. Measurement of FEV_1 and peak expiratory flow rate are useful parameters for periodic assessment. Table 26-4 shows

Table 26-4. Asthma Classification and Treatment During Pregnancy

Asthma Severity	Frequency of Symptoms	FEV_1	First-line Therapy	Add-on Controller Therapy (if needed)
Mild intermittent	≤ 2 d/wk	> 80% predicted	Albuterol inhaler as needed	None
Mild persistent	> 2 d/wk but not daily	> 80% predicted	Low-dose inhaled corticosteroid	Cromolyn, leukotriene receptor antagonist or theophylline (serum level 5-12 µg/mL)
Moderate persistent	Daily	60%-80% predicted	Low-dose inhaled corticosteroid and salmeterol	Medium-dose inhaled corticosteroid and leukotriene receptor antagonist or theophylline (serum level 5-12 µg/mL)
Severe persistent	Continuous	< 60% predicted	High-dose inhaled corticosteroid and salmeterol	Theophylline (serum level 5-12 µg/mL) and oral corticosteroid

Abbreviation: FEV_1, forced expiratory volume in 1 second. (Data from Dombrowski MP, Schatz M.[13,14])

the recommended treatment approaches based on asthma classification.[13,14] The National Asthma Education and Prevention Program has stated that "it is safer for pregnant women with asthma to be treated with asthma medications than it is for them to have asthma symptoms and exacerbations."[13]

ACOG emphasizes the importance of continuing asthma medication during labor and delivery.[13] Insufficient pain control and dehydration are potential triggers for bronchospasm.[13] During asthma exacerbations, the combination of dehydration and increased intrathoracic pressure from airway obstruction causes a decrease in maternal cardiac output that can adversely affect the fetus.[15] Patients receiving narcotic medications for pain control should be monitored closely for respiratory depression. Drugs associated with histamine release, such as high-dose morphine, should be used with caution. Providing adequate labor analgesia with regional techniques can reduce oxygen consumption and minute ventilation. Maternal hyperventilation during painful uterine contractions or asthma exacerbations can result in uterine artery vasoconstriction with associated fetal bradycardia.[1] Parturients taking systemic corticosteroids should receive stress-dose intravenous corticosteroids during labor and the 24 hours after delivery to prevent adrenal crisis.[13] Maternal bronchospasm and hypoxia should be promptly treated to avoid fetal distress. Due to the respiratory changes associated with pregnancy, patients with severe or unstable asthma may become hypoxic when laying flat because closing capacity will exceed FRC.[1] Also, the use of accessory muscles to breathe may indicate impending respiratory failure. Cesarean delivery will only rarely be indicated for unstable asthma.[13,14]

If general anesthesia is required for surgery, the patient is at highest risk for bronchospasm during intubation and extubation. Drugs with bronchodilatory actions, such as propofol, ketamine, and thiopental, may be helpful during rapid-sequence induction of general anesthesia. Intravenous lidocaine may also be a useful adjunct to blunt airway reflexes. Maintenance of anesthesia with halogenated agents is typically used for the added bronchodilatory effects. Patients should also be given intravenous corticosteroids and β_2-agonists, such as albuterol, before extubation. The risk of aspiration is high in the parturient; therefore, patients should generally not be extubated until fully awake with appropriate airway reflexes.[15]

Postpartum Care

Several studies have demonstrated that asthmatics have a higher incidence of postpartum hemorrhage than those without asthma. Oxytocin is the recommended drug for treating postpartum hemorrhage. Ergot alkaloids (Methergine) and prostaglandins (Hemabate) are relatively contraindicated because they can cause bronchospasm. However, clinicians may need to balance the risk-benefit ratio of bronchospasm versus uncontrolled hemorrhage to determine the most appropriate treatment.[15]

Patients should continue their asthma medications in the postpartum period. Asthma medications, such as prednisone, theophylline, cromolyn, antihistamines, inhaled corticosteroids, and β_2-agonists, are not contraindicated while breastfeeding. Patients may be able to cautiously decrease their medication needs after delivery if their asthma symptoms improve.[13]

OBSTRUCTIVE SLEEP APNEA

Epidemiology

Obstructive sleep apnea (OSA) is a sleep-related respiratory disorder characterized by recurrent episodes of apnea and hypopnea associated with intermittent hypoxia. OSA is defined by the apnea-hypopnea index (AHI), which is the total number of episodes of apnea and hypopnea during 1 hour of sleep. These are recorded by overnight polysomnogram. An AHI of greater than 5 with associated symptoms (excessive daytime sleepiness, fatigue) or an AHI greater than 15 irrespective of symptoms constitutes the definition of OSA.[16,17] The prevalence of OSA in women aged 30 to 40 years is reported to be 6.5%.[18] The exact prevalence of OSA during pregnancy is unknown because of a lack of large prospective studies. In a prospective trial with a cohort of 100 pregnant patients in the second and third trimesters, the prevalence of OSA, as diagnosed by polysomnography, was reported to be 20%.[19] Several studies have demonstrated a 10% to 25% self-reported incidence of snoring during the second and third trimesters of pregnancy.[20] The increased incidence of snoring during pregnancy combined with the obesity epidemic suggests that OSA will become a more common diagnosis.

Etiology/Risk Factors

Pregnancy may worsen OSA or represent a new diagnosis. Physiologic alterations that occur during pregnancy increase the likelihood of abnormal breathing during sleep. These alterations include elevation of diaphragm by an enlarging gravid uterus, an increase in body mass index, upper airway narrowing due to pharyngeal edema, sleep fragmentation, and reduced FRC.[20]

Pathophysiology

Early identification of OSA during pregnancy is very important for both maternal and fetal outcomes. In a retrospective review of national data, women with polysomnography-confirmed OSA during pregnancy had higher rates of preeclampsia, gestational diabetes, and gestational hypertension. These patients were also at higher risk of having preterm, low-birth-weight, and small-for-gestational age infants compared to pregnant women without OSA.[21] Snoring without formal sleep testing during pregnancy has also been linked to arterial hypertension and an increased incidence of preeclampsia. Intermittent maternal hypoxemia during apneic episodes can lead to fetal heart decelerations as described in case reports.[20] Theoretically, repetitive obstruction can lead to cyclic maternal hypoxemia, which causes subsequent hypertension and peripheral vasoconstriction, both of which are associated with reduced placental delivery to the fetus. This mechanism may explain the increased incidence of intrauterine growth restriction from placental ischemia in parturients with OSA.[20,22] Recurrent hypoxic episodes may also initiate release of inflammatory mediators and lead to oxidative stress and endothelial cell injury; the cascade of events may play a role in development of preeclampsia.[23]

Management and Anesthetic Considerations

The parturient with known or suspected OSA is at increased risk of perioperative complications if cesarean delivery is required. Currently, ACOG has no formal recommendations for screening for OSA during pregnancy. However, there are several preoperative screening tools, such as the STOP questionnaire, the American Society of Anesthesiologists (ASA) checklist, and the Berlin questionnaire, that may be helpful to identify patients at high risk for developing OSA.[24,25] Early placement of epidural or CSE may be helpful in avoiding general anesthesia during emergency cesarean section and avoidance of opioids for labor pain.[23] These patients are also at higher risk for postoperative hypoxemia and sudden death following general anesthesia. The practice guidelines released by the ASA Task Force on Perioperative Management of Patients with Obstructive Sleep Apnea provide useful recommendations that can be adapted to the management of the obese parturient with suspected OSA scheduled for cesarean delivery. These recommendations include the use of a regional anesthetic technique if possible, the early use of continuous positive airway pressure, preparation for a potential difficult airway, cautious use of systemic opioids, and continuous pulse oximetry monitoring postoperatively.[25]

CASE STUDY

A 30-year-old white female (G7, P5) presents to labor and delivery triage at 36 weeks' gestation with contractions, cough, and shortness of breath. She is a poor historian but reports cough and increasing dyspnea for the past several days. She has been out of her routine asthma medications for the past week. She denies fever, hemoptysis, or chest pain. Her past medical history is significant for tobacco use and multiple term pregnancies with small-for-gestational age infants. In addition, her previous two pregnancies were complicated by exacerbations of asthma requiring hospitalization during the third trimester. She has had limited prenatal care with this pregnancy.

Her contractions are 5 minutes apart, and her cervical examination shows 5-cm dilation, 70% effacement, and negative 3 station. Fetal heart tones are currently in the 130 beats/min range, but the strip is nonreactive. Vital signs are blood pressure 110/73 mm Hg, heart rate 117 beats/min, respiratory rate 20 breaths/min, oxygen saturation 99%, and temperature 99.5°F. Physical examination shows a thin pregnant female, with slightly labored breathing, audible wheezing, and bilateral rhonchi. Lower extremities are symmetric with no apparent edema.

Questions

1. As you decide on management strategies, what is your differential diagnosis and what additional studies would you like?

2. The patient does not want an epidural. What are your anesthetic recommendations for labor?

3. Will you plan regional or general anesthesia? Why?

4. What is your plan for induction of anesthesia? Do you need invasive monitoring?

5. The obstetrician has proceeded with cesarean delivery after induction of general anesthesia and now expresses concern about atony after delivery. What uterotonic agents do you recommend?

Answers

1. Your brief differential diagnosis includes asthma exacerbation, respiratory infection/pneumonia, pulmonary edema or cardiomyopathy, and pulmonary embolism. She should be started on oxygen therapy and intravenous (IV) fluids while awaiting further tests. A white blood cell count with differential and portable chest x-ray would assist with ruling out infection. Bronchodilator therapy and possibly IV steroids would be reasonable to initiate. Given that the patient is in active labor, a computed tomography scan is probably not logistically possible at this time. Portable chest x-ray, bedside echocardiogram, and venous Doppler could all be accomplished at bedside while providing continuous fetal monitoring. Arterial blood gas results may be helpful in determining severity of pathology and need for respiratory intervention.

> The patient initially becomes less tachypneic with albuterol therapy. Chest x-ray reveals diffuse bilateral infiltrates. Complete blood count shows white blood cell count 22,500/μL with 11% band, hemoglobin 9.1 g/dL, hematocrit 27.5%, and platelets 361,000/μL. An infectious disease consult is pending, and the patient is started on broad-spectrum antibiotic coverage. She continues to be in labor, with contractions every 3 minutes. An arterial blood gas has been ordered. Continuous pulse oximetry values range from 97% to 99% on 4 L/min via nasal cannula.

2. Many experts believe that central neuraxial blocks should not be performed in patients with untreated systemic infection.[11] This patient has signs and symptoms of severe infection, but whether she is bacteremic is up for debate. Prior to consideration of regional anesthesia, she would need to be hydrated well and able to tolerate a sympathectomy hemodynamically. Evidence suggests that regional anesthesia is likely safe in the setting of systemic infection if antibiotic therapy is initiated before possible dural puncture and the patient has shown a response to therapy, such as a decrease in fever.[11]

Adequate hydration and analgesia are important goals for labor for this patient. Inadequate pain control could trigger further bronchospasm. Lumbar anesthesia with an epidural could reduce oxygen consumption and minute ventilation during labor and should be strongly considered for this patient given that her respiratory status is improved with bronchodilator therapy and she continues to labor.[12] A dilute local anesthetic should be titrated to avoid motor blockade and thoracic sensory levels above T10.

> *Before an epidural can be placed, the patient develops worsening respiratory distress with an SpO_2 of 90%, improved to 98% on 10 L/min via face mask. Her respiratory rate is now in the 30-beat/min range. Her fetal heart tracing shows repetitive late decelerations with return to baseline, and the obstetrician calls an urgent cesarean section. Arterial blood gas results now show pH of 7.33, PCO_2 of 22 mm Hg, and PO_2 of 91 mm Hg.*

3. This patient has decompensated with impending respiratory failure. Probably she would not tolerate ablation of accessory muscles of respiration as would occur with dense spinal anesthesia necessary for surgery. She would also be unlikely to tolerate lying flat for the procedure under a regional technique. She needs intubation and ventilatory support. The status of her fetus may improve with improvement in oxygenation and ventilation because fetal compromise usually responds well to aggressive medical management.[13] However, delivery of a fetus may improve respiratory status and oxygen consumption for women with a mature fetus. Obstetric input will be necessary to make this decision.

4. This patient would benefit from a nonparticulate antacid, adequate preoxygenation, and uterine displacement to prevent aortocaval compression. She does not have predictors for difficult intubation. Mask ventilation is undesirable given her risk of aspiration. A rapid sequence induction is indicated. Ketamine would provide additional bronchodilation and should be considered as an adjunct or primary agent for induction along with succinylcholine. Arterial line placement may provide a means to closely monitor hemodynamics and assist with ventilator management. Arterial monitoring should not delay necessary surgical or respiratory interventions. Central monitoring may be a consideration to guide fluid replacement if volume status cannot be readily assessed by other means, such as urine output.

5. If high concentrations of volatile anesthetics have been used for bronchodilation, these agents should be reduced to less than 1 minimum alveolar concentration. Oxytocin should be used as first-line therapy in this setting. Undiluted rapid oxytocin IV infusion causes hypotension. Carboprost (15-methyl-prostaglandin-2α) and methylergonovine (Methergine) can both cause bronchospasm and should ideally be reserved for use as last resorts in this case.[13]

REFERENCES

1. Dean LS, D'Angelo R. Anatomic and physiologic changes of pregnancy. In: Palmer CM, D'Angelo R, Paech MJ. *Obstetric Anesthesia.* New York, NY: Oxford University Press; 2011:19-30.
2. Bobrowski RA. Pulmonary physiology in pregnancy. *Clin Obstet Gynecol.* 2010;53(2):285-300.
3. Mighty HE. Acute respiratory failure in pregnancy. *Clin Obstet Gynecol.* 2010;53(2):360-368.
4. Chen CY, Chen C, Wang K et al. Factors implicated in the outcome of pregnancies complicated by acute respiratory failure. *J Reprod Med.* 2003;48:641-648.
5. Graves CR. Pneumonia in pregnancy. *Clin Obstet Gynecol.* 2010;53(2):329-336.
6. Sheffield JS, Cunningham FG. Community-acquired pneumonia in pregnancy. *Obstet Gynecol.* 2009; 114(4):915-922.

7. Lindeman KS. Respiratory disease in pregnancy. In: Chestnut DH, Polley LS, Tsen LC, Wong CA. *Chestnut's Obstetric Anesthesia: Principles and Practice.* 4th ed. Philadelphia, PA: Mosby Elsevier; 2009: 1109-1123.

   Cunningham GF, Leveno KJ, Bloom SL, Hauth JC, Gilstrap LC, Wenstrom KD, eds. *Williams Obstetrics.* 22nd ed. 130-131.

8. Brito V, Niederman MS. Pneumonia complicating pregnancy. *Clin Chest Med.* 2011;32(1):121-132.

9. Jamieson DJ, Honein MA, Rasmussen SA, et al. H1N1 2009 influenza virus infection during pregnancy in the USA. *Lancet.* 2009;374(9688):451-458.

10. Munn MB, Groome LJ, Atterbury JL, Baker SL, Hoff C. Pneumonia as a complication of pregnancy. *J Matern Fetal Med.* 1999;8(4):151-154.

11. Wedel DJ, Horlocker TT. Regional anesthesia in the febrile or infected patient. *Reg Anesth Pain Med.* 2006;31(4):324-33.

12. Schatz M, Dombrowski MP. Clinical practice. Asthma in pregnancy. *N Engl J Med.* 2009;360(18): 1862-1869.

13. Dombrowski MP, Schatz M. Asthma in pregnancy. American College of Obstetricians and Gynecologists Practice Bulletin No. 90. *Obstet Gynecol.* 2008;111(2 pt 1):457-464.

14. Dombrowski MP, Schatz M. Asthma in pregnancy. *Clin Obstet Gynecol.* 2010;53(2):301-310.

15. Carlisle AS. The pregnant patient with asthma. In: Hughes SC, Levinson G, Rosen MA. *Schnider and Levinson's Anesthesia for Obstetrics.* 4th ed. Philadelphia, PA: Lippincott Williams & Wilkins; 2002: 487-495.

16. Park JG, Ramar K, Olson EJ. Updates on definition, consequences, and management of obstructive sleep apnea. *Mayo Clin Proc.* 2011;86(6):549-555.

17. Facco FL. Sleep-disordered breathing and pregnancy. *Semin Perinatol.* 2011;35:335-339.

18. Young T, Palta M, Dempsey J, Skatrud J, Weber S, Badr S. The occurrence of sleep-disordered breathing among middle aged adults. *N Engl J Med.* 1993;328:1230-1235.

19. Olivarez SA, Maheswari B, McCarthy M, et al. Prospective trial on obstructive sleep apnea in pregnancy and fetal heart rate monitoring. *Am J Obstet Gynecol.* 2010;202:552 e1-e7.

20. Kapsimalis F, Kryger M. Obstructive sleep apnea in pregnancy. *Sleep Med Clin.* 2007;2(4):603-613.

21. Chen YH, Kang JH, Lin CC, et al. Obstructive sleep apnea and the risk of adverse pregnancy outcomes. *Am J Obstet Gynecol.* 2012;206:136.e1-e5.

22. Edwards N, Middleton PG, Blyton DM, Sullivan CE. Sleep disordered breathing and pregnancy. *Thorax.* 2002;57(6):555-558.

23. Louis J, Auckley D, Bolden N. Management of obstructive sleep apnea in pregnant women. *Obstet Gynecol.* 2012;119(4):864-868.

24. Chung F, Yegneswaran B, Liao P, et al. Validation of the Berlin questionnaire and American Society of Anesthesiologists checklist as screening tools for obstructive sleep apnea in surgical patients. *Anesthesiology.* 2008;108(5):822-830.

25. American Society of Anesthesiologists Task Force on Perioperative Management. Practice guidelines for the perioperative management of patients with obstructive sleep apnea: a report by the American Society of Anesthesiologists Task Force on Perioperative Management of patients with obstructive sleep apnea. *Anesthesiology.* 2006;104(5):1081-1093.

Managing the Obese Parturient

27

Melissa Russo, Allison Clark, and Stuart Hart

EPIDEMIOLOGY

Obesity is a growing epidemic in the United States and throughout the developed world. According to the Centers for Disease Control and Prevention (CDC), only 13% of Americans were considered obese in 1962. This number significantly increased to 35% by 2013. Today, every state in the country has at least a 20% prevalence of obesity, with two states now over 35%.[1] This trend extends to parturients, with over half of all pregnant patients being overweight and obese, and 8% reaching extreme obesity.[2]

Definition

The classification of obesity has been standardized with the use of the body mass index (BMI, kg/m^2), with a value of 30 or greater being considered obese. While the World Health Organization (WHO) has subdivided obesity into three classes (Table 27-1), the Institute of Medicine guidelines regarding gestational weight gain do not discriminate based on this classification (Table 27-2).[3,4]

ETIOLOGY

Obesity results from an imbalance of caloric intake and physical activity. While it is recommended to perform at least 30 minutes of exercise daily during pregnancy, most parturients do not meet this goal.[5,6]

Table 27-1. Body Mass Index (BMI) Classification System

Classification	BMI (kg/m^2)
Underweight	< 18.5
Normal	18.5-24.99
Overweight	25-29.9
Obese class I	30-34.99
Obese class II	35-39.99
Obese class III	> 40

From World Health Organization (WHO).[2]

Obesity is an independent risk factor for maternal and neonatal morbidity.[7] Therefore, preconception counseling should occur for all obese women of childbearing age to 1) educate these patients about their risk and 2) enable weight reduction strategies to occur prior to pregnancy. When pregnancy occurs, patients should be educated about the effects of obesity on the course of pregnancy, labor and delivery.[2] Nutritional consultation and exercise goals should be established early and evaluated throughout pregnancy. Despite adequate consultation, only 19% of obese parturients believe their weight affects pregnancy risk.

EFFECTS OF OBESITY ON THE FETUS

Maternal obesity, has been implicated as a risk factor for structural defects in the fetus, including congenital heart defects, facial clefting, hydrocephalus, limb reduction and most commonly neural tube defects.[9]

These congenital anomalies may be poorly visualized during prenatal ultrasound due to decreased image resolution and quality related to abdominal wall adiposity. For this reason, it is advised to delay evaluation of fetal anatomy until after the 18th week of pregnancy.[7]

The incidence of intrauterine fetal demise and stillbirth is increased more than two-fold in obese parturients.[10] Although the exact etiology is unclear, placental insufficiency secondary to associated maternal comorbidities may play a role.

Both preterm delivery (possibly due to maternal medical indications) and postterm deliveries are more prevalent. Offspring of obese mothers are more likely to be large for gestational age (LGA) and to suffer from childhood obesity.[9,11,12,13]

Table 27-2. Institute of Medicine Recommendations for Total Weight Gain During Pregnancy, Based on Prepregnancy Body Mass Index (BMI)

Prepregnancy BMI	BMI (kg/m^2)	Total Weight Gain (lb)
Underweight	< 18.5	28-40
Normal weight	18.5-24.9	25-35
Overweight	25.0-29.9	15-25
Obese (includes all classes)	≥ 30.0	11-20

PATHOPHYSIOLOGY

During pregnancy, physiologic changes occur that affect nearly every organ system. Obesity can exacerbate these altered states, increasing the risk to both mother and fetus. The 2006-2008 data collected by the Centre for Maternal and Child Enquiries (CEMACE) reported that 49% of the maternal deaths occurred in women who were either overweight or obese. Seventy-eight percent of mothers who died from thromboembolism and 61% of mothers who died from cardiac disease were overweight or obese.[14]

Cardiovascular

During normal pregnancy, there is an increase in cardiac output which peaks immediately postpartum. Obesity further increases cardiac output by 30 to 50 mL/min for every 100-g increase in adipose tissue weight, which leads to a relative increase in heart rate, decreased diastolic interval, and resultant diastolic dysfunction.[15] Plasma volume expansion is increased further with obesity, which results in further left ventricular hypertrophy.

The decrease in systemic vascular resistance is attenuated as a result of increased levels of plasma leptin, insulin, and inflammatory mediators resulting in an increase in sympathetic activity.[16] This pressure overload may result in dilation of the myocardium and systolic dysfunction.

Obese parturients are more likely to enter pregnancy with chronic hypertension. Furthermore, endothelial dysfunction from an elevation in C-reactive protein, interleukin-6, and tumor necrosis factor-α leads to an increased incidence of pregnancy-induced hypertension in obese parturients, with over two times the risk for class I obesity and triple the risk for class II obese parturients. The incidence of preeclampsia is 10% to 25% greater in the obese than the nonobese, with a two-fold increase in risk for every 5- to 7-unit increase in BMI.[17]

Respiratory

The plasma expansion of pregnancy results in capillary engorgement of the upper airway and resultant tissue edema and friability. Obesity compounds these changes with relative increase in tissue mass, neck circumference, and enlarged breasts, making airway management especially challenging in the obese parturient.

Obstructive sleep apnea (OSA) is often underdiagnosed in pregnancy. Hormonal changes lead to an increased sensitivity of the respiratory center to apneic episodes that in theory should decrease the incidence of OSA. However, this condition may lead to pulmonary hypertension, intrauterine growth restriction, and preeclampsia and should be addressed.[18]

There is a decrease in parturients' functional residual capacity (FRC) due to diaphragmatic elevation from the enlarging uterus and increased chest wall resistance. Although some studies show an improvement in FRC when obese women become pregnant, these results were obtained from women in the sitting position. However, the effects of a general anesthetic in obese women in the supine position are unknown. Furthermore, FRC may fall below closing capacity in obese parturients, leading to shunting. Oxygen consumption increases with increasing weight, as does the work of breathing proportionally related to the degree of obesity.

Gastrointestinal

Decreased lower esophageal sphincter tone and increased intragastric pressure are normal physiologic changes seen during pregnancy that place parturients at an increased risk for aspiration. Although studies have shown no decrease in gastric emptying in nonlaboring patients that are either of normal weight or obese, one should still be concerned for aspiration due to the decreased barrier pressure and the increased incidence of hiatal hernia observed in obese parturients.[17]

Furthermore, patients may become pregnant following bariatric surgery. Decrease in the rates of diabetes, hypertensive disorders, OSA, and fetal macrosomia are benefits; however, serious complications can occur. Band slippage, gastrointestinal bleeding, internal intestinal herniation, and maternal death have all been reported. For this reason, ACOG recommends that a bariatric surgeon jointly monitor postbariatric surgery patients during their pregnancy. Vitamin supplementation may be required for patients who have undergone procedures causing a malabsorption syndrome, and, in others, adjustment of lap bands may be required to allow for adequate maternal weight gain.[2,19] Early anesthetic consultation is advised, and potential gastrointestinal obstruction or severe reflux disease should be considered when developing an anesthetic plan.

Metabolic

Obese parturients have a greater risk of beginning pregnancy with diabetes mellitus and of developing gestational diabetes during pregnancy. Patients with a history of previous gestational diabetes mellitus, macrosomia, or a family history of diabetes should be considered to be at risk. Screening for diabetes should be undertaken early in the first trimester for obese parturients and may be repeated as necessary. Although gestational diabetes mellitus is observed in 1% to 3% of normal weight parturients, 17% of obese parturients will develop the condition.[17] Gastroparesis due to autonomic dysfunction may complicate obesity, leading to a decrease in gastric emptying and therefore increased risk of aspiration.

MANAGEMENT AND ANESTHETIC CONSIDERATIONS

Obstetric Complications: Peripartum

The serum concentration of leptin, an oxytocin antagonist, is elevated in obese parturients and may be implicated in the higher rate of postdates pregnancy, dysfunctional labor, and slower cervical dilation observed in the obese population as compared to normal-weight parturients. Thus, obese parturients have a greater risk of requiring induction of labor and augmentation with oxytocin. Early amniotomy is also performed more frequently in these patients.

Maternal obesity is an independent risk factor for fetal macrosomia. When these patients do succeed at vaginal delivery, the risk of shoulder dystocia is increased by more than a factor of three as compared to nonobese women, and maneuvers to deliver the infant are less successful. Instrumented vaginal delivery, including the use of forceps and vacuum, occurs in 17.3% of obese women versus 8.4% in nonobese parturients. The incidence of third-degree and fourth-degree tears is also greater.[17]

Induction of labor is more likely to fail and progress to cesarean delivery in obese parturients (14.9% versus 7.9%).[17] Risk of progressing to cesarean delivery may be greatest during the first stage of labor.[20] Potential factors include primary uterine inertia and inadequate uterine contractions, cephalopelvic disproportion from soft tissue dystocia and fetal macrosomia, and challenging fetal heart rate and contraction monitoring due to technical difficulties in monitoring. Obese parturients are also twice more likely to fail at vaginal birth after cesarean when compared to normal-weight parturients.[17]

The rate of cesarean delivery is increased two to four times in obese women proportional to BMI. If the accepted ACOG rate of cesarean delivery is 20.7% in parturients of normal weight, it increases to 33.8% in class I obese women and 47.4% in class II obese women.[2] Many factors contribute to the increased risk of cesarean delivery, including higher rates of failed labor, inaccurate estimations of fetal weight by prenatal ultrasound, emergency cesarean section from complications related to diabetes or hypertensive disorders, and prior cesarean deliveries.

Obesity is an independent risk factor for uterine atony and postpartum hemorrhage. Abdominal wall adiposity can make surgery more challenging and operative times longer.[21] Adequate surgical exposure often requires retraction of the panniculus, which may lead to cardiorespiratory compromise.

Anesthetic Considerations

PREOPERATIVE EVALUATION

A mere 13% of obstetricians routinely discuss the additional anesthetic risks of obesity with their patients.[22] To best educate patients and coordinate plans for their delivery, ACOG encourages early anesthesiology consultation for all obese parturients, prior to delivery if possible, but definitely on arrival on the labor floor for those who have not received earlier evaluation.[2] A comprehensive assessment of end-organ function and comorbidities is essential. There should be a multidisciplinary plan for not only labor but also for cesarean delivery and postpartum care. Risks of complications from anesthesia and logistics of the delivery should be discussed. Education may be presented in a clinic visit with an anesthesiologist or another anesthesia provider, along with videos, pamphlets, or other media.

ANALGESIA FOR LABOR AND VAGINAL DELIVERY

Adequate intravenous access should be attained early in labor. Intravenous cannulation can prove difficult in obese parturients because of poor visualization and palpation of peripheral veins. Ultrasound has been utilized to secure peripheral venous access when blind techniques fail, and central access should be attained early in labor if peripheral cannulation is unsuccessful. Consideration should be given to an arterial line if conical deformation of the upper extremity related to obesity interferes with accurate blood pressure measurement.

Obese parturients should undergo epidural placement early in labor for several reasons. These patients are more likely to require cesarean delivery.[23] The epidural can be reinforced quickly, thus avoiding the need for a general anesthetic and potentially difficult airway management. A neuraxial technique may prove challenging and thus it is preferable to perform the epidural early in labor when the patient is more comfortable and able to cooperate with positioning. The incidence of failed epidural analgesia is greater in obese parturients (17% vs. 3%).[24] Up to 75% of class III obese parturients will require multiple attempts, with 14% requiring greater than three attempts at placement.[25] The inability to palpate bony landmarks and to have the patient flex the back have been noted as the two most significant factors in determining number of passes and procedure time for epidural placement in obese parturients. BMI has positively correlated with both of these objectives.[26] For each unit increase in BMI, the distance from the skin to the epidural space increases by 11% (Table 27-3).[27] It has been reported that the epidural space is encountered at a depth of about 5 cm in normal-weight women; however, up to 17% of obese parturients may have an epidural space depth greater than 8 cm.[28]

The excess subcutaneous fat may also result in false loss of resistance. More importantly, the excess subcutaneous tissue may cause outward migration of the catheter as the patient is turned from a compressed sitting position to a looser supine position. For this reason, it is recommended that the patient return to a neutral position prior to fixating the catheter to the back. Initially threading the catheter 5 to 6 cm into the epidural space is advised to prevent subsequent dislodgement, because the catheter may draw back up to 2 cm.[25] A catheter fixation device, adhesive solution, large sterile dressing, ample tape, and placement of the catheter directly up the midline are useful in preventing migration and kinking of the catheter. Several manipulations can improve the likelihood of successful epidural placement in the obese parturient if using a blind technique. Optimal patient positioning is of utmost importance when attempting neuraxial techniques in the obese parturient. The sitting position is preferred for the obese parturient because this helps identify the midline in those who have no palpable bony landmarks.[17]

Table 27-3. Body Mass Index (BMI) and Corresponding Distance From Skin to Epidural Space

BMI (kg/m²)	Depth (cm)
30	5.3
35	6.2
40	6.6
45	7.2
> 50	7.5

Data from Clinkscales CP, Greenfield ML, Vanarase M, Polley LS.[20]

The patient should be seated at 90 degrees to the anesthesia provider with the feet resting comfortably on a raised surface for stabilization. Discussion of the importance of positioning with the patient is vital prior to beginning the procedure, and the nursing staff should assist the patient in maintaining correct posture. Attempts to contact spinous processes during skin and subcutaneous tissue infiltration of local anesthetic may guide the anesthesia provider to an open interspace. A thirteen centimeter Tuohy needle may be required in some patients and should be made available. Right versus left discrimination by the patient may be helpful when maternal landmarks are lacking.[29] A dural puncture technique may be preferred as cerebrospinal fluid (CSF) flow confirms midline positioning and thus may increase the likelihood of successful epidural analgesia and anesthesia.[30,31] Intrathecal dosing may be safely administered for maternal indications, although potential for fetal bradycardia in conjunction with suboptimal fetal monitoring is of concern.[32] In those women at greatest risk for airway complications, the epidural component of combined spinal-epidural anesthesia must be tested and be reliably functioning in case of an emergency cesarean delivery or shoulder dystocia (see Figure 27-1).

Obese parturients are more likely to have complications from epidural placement. Procedure time may be longer.[24] Discomfort during placement and soft tissue trauma from multiple attempts at epidural space localization are more frequent. Accidental dural puncture is more likely, although data regarding the frequency of postdural puncture headache is conflicting.[17,33] (see Figure 27-2).

Ultrasound guidance may help identify the midline and intervertebral foramina. However, ultrasound guidance may be more challenging in obese parturients because image quality is compromised with increasing depth. Despite this, preprocedure scanning appears promising in this population. Ultrasound has been shown

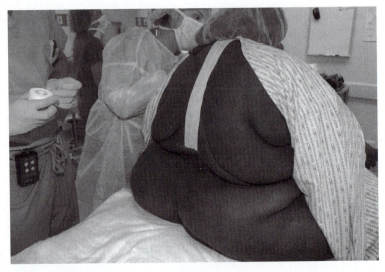

Figure 27-1. Tape epidural catheter along midline of back in obese parturient to avoid kinking once supine.

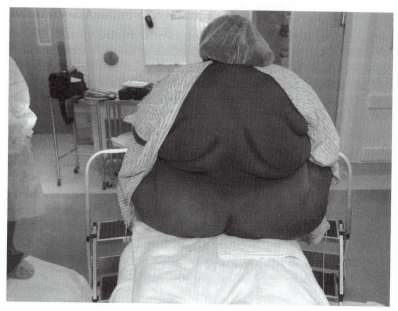

Figure 27-2. A 5-ft 2-in, 486-lb parturient (body mass index 88.9 kg/m²) with twin gestation, who required two stools for stabilization because she was unable to rest both feet on one stool due to leg circumference.

superior to the blind technique in determining the exact interspace being traversed, which has been quoted as having anywhere from 50% to 70% inaccuracy rate. Ultrasound has been reported to improve the learning curve for providing neuraxial anesthesia, decrease the incidence of side effects such as dural puncture, and decrease the incidence of failed neuraxial blocks.[34] In the obese population, which is at greater risk for requiring emergent cesarean delivery, this last point is significant. In light of the numerous reported benefits and the ever increasing obesity epidemic, anesthesia providers would be well advised to become adept at ultrasound utilization for neuraxial anesthesia placement.

ANESTHESIA FOR CESAREAN DELIVERY

The need for operative delivery—either instrumental vaginal or more often cesarean delivery—should be anticipated because the incidence of cesarean delivery is almost three times greater in obese women as compared to their normal-weight counterparts. In almost two-thirds of patients requiring intrapartum cesarean delivery, it is performed as an urgent or emergent procedure.[24]

Patient Preparation

As mentioned earlier, adequate intravenous access should be obtained prior to entering the operating room. At times, a large, funnel-shaped arm makes blood pressure monitoring questionable or inaccurate; therefore, materials for arterial cannulation should be available.

All obese parturients should receive aspiration prophylaxis prior to entering the operating suite. This may include nonparticulate antacids, H_2-receptor antagonists, and/or metoclopramide.[35]

Operating Room Preparation

The weight capacity of the operating room table must be checked prior to transport. If the patient's weight exceeds this limit, consideration should be given to performing the cesarean delivery on the labor bed itself. Bed extenders may be necessary and should be immediately available.

A variety of airway equipment should be ready for use, including a short-handled laryngoscope, oral airways and endotracheal tubes of various sizes, difficult airway cart, and laryngeal mask airways (LMAs) of various sizes. If general endotracheal anesthesia is required, a video laryngoscope may be preferable to direct laryngoscopy due to superior view.[36] Experienced staff should perform laryngoscopy after a rapid-sequence induction maintaining cricoid pressure. An awake fiberoptic intubation should be considered when significant concern about the patient's airway is present or standard induction is deemed unsafe. The LMA should not be utilized outside of the difficult airway algorithm in the obese parturient.

Patient Arrival to Operating Room

Transport into the operating room can take substantially longer with obese parturients. Transfers should be made with the patient's cooperation to decrease risk to the patient or cause injury to the provider. Particular care should be taken if an epidural catheter is in place to prevent dislodgement. The patient should be positioned supine with careful attention to left uterine displacement. The weight of the panniculus may exacerbate uterine compression of the great vessels, leading to further decreases in cardiac output and reduced placental perfusion. Maternal death has occured, due to exaggerated supine hypotensive syndrome upon assuming the supine position after neuraxial placement for cesarean delivery.[25,37] Cephalad retraction of the panniculus facilitates operative exposure but may cause further respiratory and hemodynamic compromise. The patient should be placed in a ramped position to inhibit cephalad spread of local anesthetic and to aid in laryngoscopy if conversion to general anesthesia becomes necessary.

EPIDURAL ANESTHESIA

Preexisting epidural catheters should be dosed incrementally in obese patients, with close attention to maternal blood pressure until an adequate level is obtained. Problems with epidural anesthesia for cesarean delivery include a high incidence of failed block in this population, as well as inferior anesthesia when compared to subarachnoid block.[24,25] Caution should be exercised in supplementation of an inadequate block with nitrous oxide or intravenous medications because airway obstruction and hypoxemia can occur more frequently,[25] especially in those women with preexisting obstructive sleep apnea or excessive upper airway adiposity.

SPINAL ANESTHESIA

Spinal anesthesia is an acceptable technique offering a dense, bilateral block and low risk of postdural puncture headache. A larger bore (22G) spinal needle may be helpful when landmarks are difficult to discern. Although routine intrathecal dosing is generally recommended for the obese parturient,[38] patient stature should be assessed and intrathecal dose should be chosen accordingly.[39]

COMBINED SPINAL-EPIDURAL ANESTHESIA

Combined spinal-epidural is likely the ideal anesthetic for cesarean delivery in obese parturients. This technique offers the dense, reliable block offered by spinal anesthesia, with the potential for extending the anesthetic in case of failed spinal or prolonged surgical duration.

CONTINUOUS SPINAL ANESTHESIA

Continuous spinal anesthesia may be a useful technique in the obese parturient when rapid neuraxial anesthesia needs to be obtained for delivery. Landmarks are more easily determined with the larger Tuohy needle and a catheter can be thread quickly to allow for spinal dosing and prolonged anesthesia if required. Although risk of PDPH is increased with this technique, this complication is acceptable when weighed against a difficult maternal airway and GETA.

GENERAL ANESTHESIA

Despite early evaluation and planning, the need for emergency cesarean delivery persists in obese parturients. Although some believe the fear of general anesthesia may be unnecessarily exaggerated in obese parturients, statistics of maternal morbidity and mortality prove otherwise. Whenever possible, regional anesthesia is strongly encouraged due to the inherent risks of administering general anesthesia, particularly the risk of difficult airway management and rapid desaturation in obese women. Anesthesia is the 11th leading cause of maternal mortality, with a significant proportion of deaths attributed to general anesthesia, failed intubation, or pulmonary aspiration.[14] Even in emergent situations, the mother's life should never be jeopardized to save the compromised fetus. Maternal safety should always remain the primary concern.

The incidence of difficult airway is increased sevenfold in parturients. One in 280 to 750 obstetric intubations fail, and up to one-third of these failures may be caused by an unexpected difficult airway.[24] For this reason, all obese parturients should be treated as having a potentially difficult airway regardless of airway examination. Increased neck circumference predicts difficulty more reliably than BMI, and therefore the distribution of the patient's adipose tissue must be taken into consideration.

When regional anesthesia is contraindicated, one should proceed with general anesthesia with caution. The patient should be placed in a ramped position on the operative bed, aligning the sternal notch and external auditory meatus to improve visualization of the glottic opening. Careful attention to left uterine displacement should be maintained. Because these patients will desaturate more rapidly, the bed should be placed in reverse Trendelenburg to improve FRC. Preoxygenation should be provided for an extended period prior to induction. There should be additional trained personnel to apply cricoid pressure and help with the difficult airway algorithm should difficulties be encountered.

Postpartum Care

Postpartum care is as essential as intrapartum care. Obese parturients are at greater risk for postpartum complications including infection, venous thromboembolism, and respiratory compromise. Infectious complications, including cystitis, wound infection, pneumonia, and endometritis, are more common in obese as compared to nonobese patients, with an incidence of 7% to 20%. The increased infection rate may in part be due to inadequate tissue concentrations of antibiotics following standard dosing prophylaxis with cefazolin therefore adequate weight-based dosing should be administered.[40]

The increased risk of developing venous thromboembolism in obese parturients applies throughout pregnancy and into the postpartum period, with obesity and cesarean deliveries being major risk factors. Although the Royal College of Obstetricians and Gynaecologists (RCOG) of the United Kingdom has affirmed guidelines regarding anticoagulation of the obese parturient, ACOG has not yet made recommendations regarding anticoagulation of these patients. Graduated compression stockings, adequate hydration, and early mobilization are universally recommended.[2,17]

BMI inversely correlates with postoperative respiratory function following spinal anesthesia. These parturients double their risk of pulmonary complications including hypoxemia, atelectasis, and pulmonary edema. This increased risk remains for up to 2 days postoperatively.[17,24] Supplemental oxygen to correct hypoxemia, semiupright position to optimize FRC, and incentive spirometry to minimize atelectasis may be required.

Pain relief is essential for early mobilization. In this regard, neuraxial opioids provide the most effective postoperative analgesia. However, adequacy of respiration monitoring is essential because the risk of delayed respiratory depression is increased among obese patients given intraspinal morphine, especially in those parturients with preexisting obstructive sleep apnea. The risk of obtundation and hypoventilation is also increased in obese patients receiving intravenous patient-controlled analgesia. American Society of Anesthesiologists guidelines for monitoring patients after neuraxial opioids should be strictly observed and pulse oximetry may be advised.[41]

Multimodal therapy, including a mix of transverse abdominis plane (TAP) blocks or local infiltration, intravenous acetaminophen and nonsteroidal anti-inflammatory drugs, and narcotic supplementation for breakthrough pain control, is likely ideal for obese parturients.[17] TAP blocks are gaining popularity in obstetric anesthesia, and when performed under ultrasound guidance may allow for omission of intrathecal morphine in those patients at highest risk for airway obstruction and respiratory depression.

Obese mothers are up to four times less likely to breastfeed their newborns.[42] This choice contributes to the difficulty attaining postpartum weight loss and a higher likelihood of entering a subsequent pregnancy at a higher BMI. Preconception counseling at the first postpartum visit regarding proper nutrition, activity, and lifestyle changes is recommended.

SUMMARY

Obesity in parturients remains a significant comorbidity, with increased risk of hypertension, diabetes, operative delivery, and death. The anesthesia provider should be well aware of the obstetric and anesthetic risks associated with obese parturients and should anticipate these issues when assuming their care.

REFERENCES

1. Centers for Disease Control and Prevention. Overweight and obesity. http://www.cdc.gov/obesity. Accessed October 2014.
2. American College of Obstetricians and Gynecologists (ACOG). Obesity in pregnancy. ACOG Committee Opinion No. 549. *Obstet Gynecol* 2013;121:213-217.
3. World Health Organization (WHO). Obesity: preventing and managing the global epidemic. Report on a WHO consultation. Technical Report Series 894. Geneva: World Health Organization; 2000.
4. Artal R, Lockwood CJ, Brown HL. Weight gain recommendations in pregnancy and the obesity epidemic. *Obstet Gynecol.* 2010;115:152-154.
5. Poudevigne MS, O'Connor PJ. A review of physical activity patterns in pregnant women and their relationship to psychological health. *Sports Med.* 2006;36(1):19-38.
6. American College of Obstetricians and Gynecologists (ACOG). Exercise during pregnancy and the postpartum period. ACOG Committee Opinion No. 267. *Obstet Gynecol.* 2002;99:171-173.
7. Catalano PM. Management of obesity in pregnancy. *Obstet Gynecol.* 2007;109:419-433.
8. Eley VA, Donovan K, Walters E, Brijball R, Eley DS. The effect of antenatal anaesthetic consultation on maternal decision making, anxiety level, and risk perception in obese pregnant women. *Int J Obstet Anesth.* 2014; 23(2):118-124.
9. Sothard KJ, Tennant PW, Bell R, et al. Maternal overweight and obesity and the risk of congenital anomalies: a systematic review and meta-analysis. *JAMA.* 2009;301:636-650.
10. Cnattingius S, Bergstrom R, Lipworth L, Kramer MS. Prepregnancy weight and the risk of adverse pregnancy outcomes. *N Engl J Med.* 1998;338:147-152.
11. Rode L, Nilas L, Wojdemann K, Tabor A. Obesity-related complications in Danish single cephalic term pregnancies. *Obstet Gynecol.* 2005;105:537-42.
12. Stephansson O, Dickman PW, Johansson A, Cnattingius S. Maternal weight, pregnancy weight gain, and the risk of antepartum stillbirth. *Am J Obstet Gynecol.* 2001;184:463-469.
13. Watkins ML, Rasmussen SA, Honein MA, Botto LD, Moore CA. Maternal obesity and risk for birth defects. *Pediatrics.* 2003;111:1152-1158.
14. Centre for Maternal and Child Enquiries (CMACE). Saving Mothers' Lives: reviewing maternal deaths to make motherhood safer: 2006-2008. The Eighth Report on Confidential Enquiries into Maternal Deaths in the United Kingdom. *BJOG.* 2011;118(suppl 1):1-201.
15. Veille JC, Hanson R. Obesity, pregnancy and left ventricular functioning during the third trimester. *Am J Obstet Gynecol.* 1994;171:980-983.
16. Saravanakumar K, Rao SG, Cooper GM. Obesity and obstetric anaesthesia. *Anaesthesia.* 2006;61:36-48.
17. Mace HS, Paech MJ, McDonnell NJ. Obesity and obstetric anaesthesia. *Anaesth Intensive Care.* 2011;39:559-570.
18. Roush SF, Bell L. Obstructive sleep apnea in pregnancy. *J Am Board Fam Med.* 2004;17:292-294.
19. American College of Obstetricians and Gynecologists (ACOG). Bariatric surgery and pregnancy. ACOG Practice Bulletin No. 105. *Obstet Gynecol.* 2009;113:1405-1413.
20. Fyfe EM, Anderson NH, North RA, et al. Risk of first-stage and second-stage cesarean delivery by maternal body mass index among nulliparous women in labor at term. *Obstet Gynecol.* 2011;117:1315-1322.
21. Perlow JH, Morgan MA. Massive maternal obesity and perioperative cesarean morbidity. *Am J Obstet Gynecol.* 1994;170:560-565.
22. Mhyre JM, Greenfield ML, Polley LS. Survey of obstetric providers' views on the anesthetic risks of maternal obesity. *Int J Obstet Anesth.* 2007;16:316-322.

23. Weiss JL, Malone FD, Emig D, Ball RH, Nyberg DA, Comstock CH, et al. Obesity, obstetric complications and cesarean delivery rate-a population-based screening study. FASTER Research Consortium. *Am J Obstet Gynecol.* 2004;190:1091-1097.

24. Tonidandel A, Booth J, D'Angelo R, Harris L, Tonidandel S. Anesthetic and obstetric outcomes in morbidly obese parturients: a 20-year follow-up retrospective cohort study. *Int J Obstet Anesth.* 2004;23(4):357-364.

25. Roofthooft E. Anesthesia for the morbidly obese parturient. *Curr Opin Anesthesiol.* 2009;341-346.

26. Ellinas EH, Eastwood DC, Patel SN, et al. The effect of obesity on neuraxial technique difficulty in pregnant patients: a prospective, observational study. *Anesth Analg.* 2009;109:1225-1231.

27. Clinkscales CP, Greenfield ML, Vanarase M, Polley LS. An observational study of the relationship between lumbar epidural space depth and body mass index in Michigan parturients. *Int J Obstet Anesth.* 2007;16:323-327.

28. Balki M, Halpern S, Carvalho J. Ultrasound imaging of the lumbar spine in the transverse plane: the correlation between estimated and actual depth to the epidural space in obese parturients. *Anesth Analg.* 2009;108:1876-1881.

29. Marroquin BM, Fecho K, Salo-Coombs V, Spielman FJ. Can parturients identify the midline during neuraxial block placement? *J Clin Anesth.* 2011;23(1):3-6.

30. Gambling D, Berkowitz J, Farrell TR, Pue A, Shay D. A randomized controlled comparison of epidural analgesia and combined spinal-epidural analgesia in a private practice setting: pain scores during first and second stages of labor and at delivery. *Anesth Analg.* 2013;116(3):636-643.

31. Gupta D, Srirajakalidindi A, Soskin V. Dural puncture epidural analgesia is not superior to continuous labor epidural analgesia. *Middle East J Anaesthesiol.* 2013;22(3):309-316.

32. Simmons SW, Taghizadeh N, Dennis AT, Hughes D, Cyna AM. Combined spinal-epidural versus epidural analgesia in labour. *Cochrane Database Syst Rev.* 2012;10:CD003401.

33. Miu M, Paech MJ, Nathan E. The relationship between body mass index and post-dural puncture headache in obstetric patients. *Int J Obstet Anesth.* 2014; 23(4):371-375.

34. Carvalho JC. Ultrasound-facilitated epidurals and spinals in obstetrics. *Anesthesiol Clin.* 2008;26:145-158.

35. American Society of Anesthesiologists Task Force on Obstetric Anesthesia. *Anesthesiology.* 2007;106(4):843-863.

36. Turkstra TP, Armstrong PM, Jones PM, et al. Glidescope use in the obstetric patient. *Int J Obstet Anesth.* 2009;123-124.

37. De-Giorgio F, Grassi VM, Vetrugno G, d'Aloja E, Pascali VL, Arena V. Supine hypotensive syndrome as the probable cause of both maternal and fetal death. *J Forensic Sci.* 2012;57(6):1646-1649.

38. Carvalho B, Collins J, Drover D, Ralls L, Riley E. ED50 and ED95 of intrathecal bupivacaine in morbidly obese patients undergoing cesarean delivery. *Anesthesiology.* 2011;114:529-535.

39. Zhou Q, Xiao W, Shen Y. Abdominal girth, vertebral column length, and spread of spinal anesthesia in 30 minutes after plain bupivacaine 5 mg/mL. *Anesth Analg.* 2014;119:203-206.

40. Pevzner L, Swank M, Krepel C, et al. Effects of maternal obesity on tissue concentrations of prophylactic cefazolin during cesarean delivery. *Obstet Gynecol.* 2011;117:877-882.

41. Horlocker TT, Burton AW, Connis RT, et al; American Society of Anesthesiologists Task Force on Neuraxial Opioids. Practice guidelines for the prevention, detection, and management of respiratory depression associated with neuraxial opioid administration. *Anesthesiology.* 2009;110:218-230.

42. Mehta UJ, Siega-Riz AM, Herring AH, et al. Maternal obesity, psychological factors, and breastfeeding initiation. *Breastfeed Med.* 2011;6:1-8.

Substance Abuse and the Human Immunodeficiency Virus

28

Alan Santos and Migdalia Saloum

INTRODUCTION

The prevalence of substance abuse in women of reproductive age has increased markedly over the past 20 years. Thus, it is likely that an anesthesiologist will encounter a pregnant woman who abuses illicit drugs.[1] A combination of drug abuse and related social ills can lead to poor fetal outcomes and serious maternal morbidity or even mortality.[2] Anesthesiologists are likely to first meet drug-abusing parturients in an acute setting, either when labor analgesia is requested or in an emergency situation such as fetal distress, placental abruption, uterine rupture, or sudden onset of maternal dysrhythmias. These women often have not had the benefit of prenatal care. Risk factors associated with drug abuse include lack of prenatal care, history of premature labor, and cigarette smoking.[3] The possibility of drug abuse should also be considered if there is an unanticipated untoward reaction to an otherwise routine anesthetic.

Polysubstance abuse is common among drug abusers. It has been estimated that 50% of unregistered patients admitted to labor and delivery test positive for cocaine and that 25% of these patients also test positive for other drugs.[4] Complication rates are significantly higher when drugs are used in concert than when one drug is used alone.[5] When interviewed by anesthesiologists or obstetricians, drug-abusing parturients will most likely not be forthcoming about their addiction. However, the most common cause of failure to diagnose drug abuse is a failure to ask. The American College of Obstetricians and Gynecologists (ACOG) recommends that a drug history be obtained from all patients. In addition, ACOG advocates that support, aid, and counseling be made available to all women who acknowledge substance abuse. The role of caregivers should be to focus on prevention and treatment rather than punitive measures against the mother. Routine drug testing in patients with a history of drug abuse should be considered as a method to encourage abstinence.[1]

COCAINE

Cocaine abuse continues to be a major problem affecting society. Although it is difficult to estimate the prevalence of cocaine use in parturients, its use appears to be on the rise. In 2008, 772,000 adolescents and adults reported first-time cocaine use.

Diagnosing the cocaine-abusing parturient poses unique challenges because the hallmarks associated with cocaine use—tachycardia, hypertension, and dysrhythmias—may also be confused with cardiac responses to normal labor. In addition to the cardiovascular symptoms, other signs of cocaine use are seizures, hyperreflexia, fever, dilated pupils, emotional instability, proteinuria, and edema. Cocaine-induced hypertension, seizures, and proteinuria can be mistakenly diagnosed as preeclampsia-eclampsia. The differential diagnosis is usually aided by toxicology screening. Most commonly, cocaine metabolites are tested for in maternal urine and can be detected for up to 60 hours after use. A rapid latex agglutination test can detect urine cocaine metabolites within a few minutes, and this test can be performed easily at the bedside in labor and delivery or in an emergent situation. Otherwise, maternal urine can be sent for analysis by the hospital laboratory. Cocaine can be detected in neonatal urine, meconium, and maternal hair over longer time periods.[1]

Maternal Effects

Cocaine is highly lipid soluble and has a low molecular weight, which allows for easy diffusion through lipid membranes. It produces prolonged adrenergic stimulation by blocking the presynaptic uptake of sympathomimetic neurotransmitters, including norepinephrine, serotonin, and dopamine. The euphoric effects arise from prolongation of dopaminergic activity in the cerebral cortex and limbic system. Additionally, adrenergic stimulation is prolonged by blockade of catecholamine-binding mechanisms, allowing free catecholamines to continue to stimulate the sympathoadrenal axis.[4]

Complications of cocaine use in parturients include hypertension, tachycardia, malignant cardiac dysrhythmias, cardiac ischemia, premature rupture of membranes, placental abruption, uterine rupture, hepatic rupture, cerebral ischemia and hemorrhage, and death. By increasing the three major determinants of myocardial oxygen demand—heart rate, arterial blood pressure, and left ventricular contractility—cocaine increases the risk of myocardial ischemia and infarction. Parturients are at particular risk for myocardial ischemia because of the underlying increase in oxygen demand from the normal physiology of pregnancy.[1] Some data suggest that pregnancy may be associated with an increased sensitivity of the cardiovascular system to cocaine. This is believed to be secondary to an increased sensitivity of α-adrenergic receptors or an increased metabolism to the biologically active metabolite *nor*-cocaine, mediated by increased levels of progesterone.[6]

Fetal Effects

The unique pharmacologic properties of cocaine may cause deleterious effects in the fetus. A low molecular weight and high lipophilicity, coupled with the fact that it exists primarily in the unionized form, allows cocaine to readily cross the placenta, leading to rapid accumulation in fetal tissue and blood. Fetal anomalies associated with cocaine use in early pregnancy include urogenital tract abnormalities, gastroschisis, microcephaly, growth restriction, central nervous system (CNS) defects, and musculoskeletal derangements. Chronic maternal cocaine use has been associated with postnatal learning deficiencies and low IQ scores. Preterm delivery is four times more likely with cocaine-exposed fetuses as compared to non–cocaine-exposed ones. With acute cocaine use, there is a significantly increased risk of fetal distress and intrauterine fetal demise.[6] The fetus is at particular risk for uteroplacental insufficiency, hypoxia, and acidosis from the concomitant decrease in uteroplacental blood flow, as a result of maternal hypertension associated with the vasoconstrictive effects of cocaine.

Anesthetic Management

The use of neuraxial anesthesia may be beneficial to cocaine-abusing parturients, by reducing the level of circulating catecholamines and diminishing the systemic effects of cocaine, particularly during labor. However, an individualized anesthetic plan should be established based on the clinical presentation. Concerns regarding the use of regional anesthesia may include hypotension, altered pain perception, combative behavior, and cocaine-induced thrombocytopenia. A well-documented phenomenon is that cocaine and opioid users frequently complain of pain, even with a demonstrable adequate level of neuraxial anesthesia. This seems to be particularly true during regional anesthesia for a cesarean section. It has been suggested that abnormalities in endorphin levels and chronic changes in both μ and κ opioid receptor densities likely to play a role.[4,7]

When general anesthesia is indicated, it is important to remember that surges in catecholamines during periods of light anesthesia, such as laryngoscopy, can produce dysrhythmias in the presence of cocaine. Hypertension and myocardial ischemia have also been reported. Ketamine should be used with caution, if at all, because its CNS-stimulating properties and increasing catecholamine levels may potentiate the cardiac effects of cocaine.

Care must be taken to minimize the severe hypertension and tachycardia that can accompany stimulation from laryngoscopy in cocaine-intoxicated patients. It is recommended that pharmacologic control be exerted before induction. Several approaches have been suggested to lower the risk of severe hypertension, but the optimal sequence remains to be determined. Nonselective β-blockers such as propranolol are relatively contraindicated because of the potential for unopposed α-adrenergic stimulation that can occur in the face of cocaine intoxication. In addition, nonselective β-blockers have also been implicated in enhancing cocaine-induced coronary vasoconstriction. It is clear that administration of a pure β-blocker can worsen cardiac perfusion and/or produce paradoxical hypertension. If a nonselective β-blocker must be used, esmolol may provide effective short-term on-and-off control of tachycardia and hypertension because of its short elimination half-life. Labetalol, with its 7:1 ratio of β- and α-blocker action, has also been used with success even though predominantly, it is a β-blocker. A combination of labetalol with nitroglycerin has been recommended as an effective treatment of cocaine-induced severe hypertension. Incremental small doses of nitroglycerin are safe and effective for lowering blood pressure acutely and can also be given to relieve coronary artery spasm pain caused by acute cocaine ingestion. Hydralazine is a direct vasodilator that also has been used in the treatment of cocaine-induced hypertension, even though it may produce a reflex tachycardia that can be problematic in an already tachycardic patient.[1]

Pregnant cocaine abusers may also present to the labor and delivery unit with hypertension and chest discomfort related to acute cocaine ingestion. Most patients with cocaine-induced myocardial ischemia develop chest pain within 1 hour of ingestion of cocaine, when the blood level is highest. The pathogenesis of the myocardial ischemia involves an increase in myocardial oxygen demand with a concomitant low oxygen supply resulting from coronary artery vasoconstriction and enhanced platelet aggregation and thrombus formation. The electrocardiogram may be abnormal in about 50% of these patients.[8] Guidelines from the American Heart Association recommend the administration of benzodiazepines and nitroglycerin as first-line agents.

AMPHETAMINES

Amphetamines, like cocaine, are a group of noncatecholamine indirect-acting sympathomimetics that increase the release of norepinephrine, serotonin, and dopamine from presynaptic neurons and inhibit their breakdown. They are powerful stimulants of the CNS with an ability to produce profound euphoria, wakefulness, alertness, and decreased appetite. Methamphetamine (N-methyl-1-phenyl-propan-2-amine) is methylated amphetamine, and it is the most commonly abused form of amphetamine. More powerful than amphetamine, methamphetamine is the only illicit drug that can be produced from legally obtained ingredients such as decongestants and cold medications. Because methamphetamine is easy to produce, has a low cost, and is highly addictive, it has become a major drug of abuse. Historically, in the United States, the most prevalent regions for methamphetamine abuse have been in the West and Southwest; however, its use has been spreading steadily to include the rest of the country. It has been estimated that where methamphetamine abuse is most prevalent in the United States, 5.2% of women have used methamphetamine at some point during their pregnancy.

Clinically, amphetamine intoxication is indistinguishable from that of cocaine. Hypertension, tachycardia, dilated pupils, cardiac dysrhythmias, and cardiac ischemia are all presenting signs of acute methamphetamine use. Coexistence of seizures, hyperreflexia, and proteinuria with acute cocaine or amphetamine use has been mistaken for eclampsia. Chronic use of amphetamines depletes body stores of catecholamines and may manifest clinically with anxiety, somnolence, or psychosis.[2]

Anesthetic management of amphetamine-intoxicated parturients is similar to that of cocaine-affected parturients. Emergent cesarean section may be likely secondary to fetal jeopardy, placental abruption, or other obstetrical emergencies. Reports of cardiac decompensation and even death during cesarean section using either regional or general anesthesia have been described. There is no apparent contraindication to regional anesthesia, but clinicians should be prepared to treat hypotension related to sympathectomy, and these women may have unpredictable responses to vasopressors. Indeed, due to depleted body stores of catecholamines, indirect-acting pressors (ie, ephedrine) may not be effective in treating hypotension and direct-acting pressors such as phenylephrine should be considered. Acute intake of amphetamines can increase the minimum alveolar concentration (MAC) of potent inhaled anesthetics, whereas chronic ingestion may decrease the dose requirements of general anesthetics. Inhaled volatile anesthetics may sensitize the myocardium to endogenous catecholamines, and it is recommended that halothane be avoided.[1]

ETHANOL

Alcohol consumption by pregnant women remains a major problem in society. More than 15 million people in the United States are addicted to alcohol, and women account for 25% of these individuals.[9] The 2006 national survey on drug use and health found that 11.8% of pregnant women reported current alcohol use and 2.9% reported binge drinking (five drinks or more on one occasion).[10] Because alcoholism is more subtle and more difficult to diagnose than other drug addictions, it is frequently overlooked.

Stigma, shame, fear of legal repercussions, and fear of mandatory placement into detoxification programs may lead pregnant alcohol users to underreport alcohol use and avoid consistent prenatal care. Simple, sensitive, and effective evidence-based screening tools have been developed to help physicians detect problem drinking in patients. There is good evidence overall for the effectiveness of screening and behavioral interventions in reducing the amount of drinking in pregnant patients. Various four to five question surveys have been widely validated. The TWEAK questionnaire is preferred because it takes into tolerance (Tolerance: how many drinks does it take to make you high?, Worried, Eye-opener, Amnesia [blackouts], Cut[K] down) into account. The tolerance question assumes that the patient is drinking and avoids patient denial.[11]

Maternal Effects

Alcohol has numerous effects on the CNS and acts as both a depressant and a stimulant. With acute intoxication, patients may be unable to adequately protect their airway and risk pulmonary aspiration. With chronic use, ethanol can lead to liver disease, malnutrition, altered drug metabolism, coagulopathy, pancreatitis, esophageal varices, neuropathies, and cardiomyopathy. Hypoglycemia and electrolyte imbalances may also be present when heavy alcohol consumption is coupled with poor nutritional intake.

Alcohol withdrawal symptoms can be encountered in patients 6 to 18 hours after cessation of consumption, although delays of up to 10 days have been reported. Symptoms of withdrawal include nausea/vomiting, tachycardia, dysrhythmias, hypertension, delirium, hallucinations, seizures, and cardiac failure. Delirium tremens is a rare, although life-threatening medical emergency. Symptoms of withdrawal can be treated with benzodiazepines, α-adrenergic agonists (eg, clonidine), or ethanol.[12]

Fetal Effects

Alcohol and its metabolites (eg, acetaldehyde) freely cross the placenta and can cause structural and behavioral teratogenicity. No safe level of consumption has been established during pregnancy. Therefore, abstinence appears to be the safest choice for pregnant women.[2]

Spontaneous abortion, prenatal and postnatal growth restriction, low birth weight, birth defects, and neurodevelopmental deficits are all increased in pregnant women who abuse alcohol. Fetal alcohol syndrome is the best known disorder, and it is associated with characteristic facial features; growth retardation; physical anomalies; and developmental abnormalities, including mental retardation.[13]

Anesthetic Management

Depending on the degree of dependence and the timing of most recent intake, patients can present to labor and delivery with a variety of clinical manifestations. Acutely intoxicated patients may present to labor and delivery with the fetus in "nonreassuring" status and/or be at a higher risk for pulmonary aspiration.

Regional anesthesia can be safely administered to cooperative patients. Contraindications to neuraxial anesthesia are usually encountered in chronic abusers with end-stage liver failure and coagulopathy. Patients may have neuropathy, usually as a result of vitamin deficiency, but this should not pose a contraindication to a regional technique. However, the extent of the neuropathy should be determined and documented prior to proceeding with regional anesthesia. In addition, intravascular fluid status should be assessed and corrected to avoid excessive hypotension as a consequence of the sympathetic blockade.

In case of emergency delivery or if patients are too sedated or uncooperative to protect their airway, general anesthesia is warranted. Acute alcohol consumption can decrease the MAC for anesthetics due to the additive effects of CNS depressants. The notion that chronic alcohol abusers have a higher MAC for inhaled or hypnotic anesthetics has not been substantiated.[12] Anesthesia providers should avoid arbitrarily administering high doses of inhaled anesthetics to pregnant patients with a history of chronic alcohol abuse, because these women, in addition to requiring lower MAC as a result of their pregnancy, can also be at risk for intra-vascular volume depletion, cardiomyopathy, and hypoalbuminemia. A bispectral index monitor may be useful in guiding anesthetic depth. High concentrations of inhaled volatile anesthetics can also depress uterine tone and may increase blood loss at cesarean delivery.

OPIOIDS

Opioids include the opiates, which are natural or semisynthetic morphine-like substances, as well as the fully synthetic opioid compounds. The opiates include morphine, codeine, hydromorphone, and heroin. Synthetic opioids include meperidine, fentanyl, and methadone. Opioids can be abused orally, subcutane-ously, or intravenously. Most of the information on the effects of opioids on the mother and fetus derives from studies involving heroin or methadone. More recently, there has been an increase in the use of prescription opioids such as hydromorphone and codeine.

Maternal Effects

Pregnant women who use heroin can expect a sixfold increase in obstetric com-plications such as intrauterine growth restriction (IUGR), third-trimester vaginal bleeding, malpresentation, preterm delivery, and nonreassuring fetal status.[14] In addition to the chemical effects of heroin, the drug can pose additional risks because it is injected intravenously. Patients who use intravenous drugs are at increased risk for developing cellulitis, skin abscesses, sepsis, thrombophlebitis, hepatitis, human immunodeficiency virus (HIV), endocarditis, and malnutrition. Patients should be counseled regarding the benefits of a methadone maintenance program. Methadone maintenance treatment provides a steady concentration of opiates in pregnant women's circulation and therefore prevents acute withdrawal, which can be detrimental to both mothers and their fetuses. Women who use methadone have decreased use of other illicit drugs, better compliance with pre-natal care, better obstetric outcomes, and improved infant birth weights. Maternal methadone, however, is also associated with neonatal abstinence syndrome.[15]

Fetal Effects

All opioids freely cross the placenta. There are no specific congenital abnormali-ties associated with chronic opioid abuse, but there is a higher risk of stillbirth, meconium staining, decreased head circumference, and depressed Apgar scores in fetuses of opioid-abusing parturients. Neonatal abstinence syndrome can be observed in 50% to 95% of infants exposed to heroin and is manifested by signs and symptoms withdrawal from an addictive substance. Neonatal withdrawal symptoms are similar to those encountered in adults, with the addition of irritabil-ity, poorly coordinated sucking, and in the most severe cases, seizures and death. Infants born to mothers who abuse hydromorphone or oxycodone have also been shown to develop neonatal withdrawal syndrome.[1,15] The use of opioid antagonist may precipitate withdrawal.

Anesthetic Management

Opioid-addicted parturients present several challenges to the anesthesiologist. In addition to concerns regarding acute opioid overdose or withdrawal, difficulties with placement of vascular access, and management of labor analgesia and postoperative pain may also occur.

Opioid-abusing parturients may present with symptoms of overdose or acute opioid withdrawal. Opioid overdose can be characterized by a slow respiratory rate, increased tidal volumes, and miotic pupils. Acute withdrawal is manifested by increased sympathetic nervous system activity (ie, restlessness, lacrimation, sweating, diarrhea, insomnia, mydriasis, tachycardia, tachypnea, and hypertension). CNS manifestations of acute withdrawal can range from dysphoria to unconsciousness. Withdrawal symptoms can occur 4 to 6 hours following the last dose of opioids and peak at 48 to 72 hours. Symptoms of opioid withdrawal can be treated with nonopioid medications such as clonidine, doxepin, or diphenhydramine. Clonidine attenuates withdrawal symptoms by replacing opioid-mediated inhibition with α_2-agonist–mediated inhibition of the CNS. Administration of opioid antagonists or agonist-antagonists must be avoided in these patients because they can precipitate acute withdrawal syndrome. Opioid withdrawal syndrome may develop within minutes of naloxone administration.

Methadone maintenance has been an acceptable form of therapy for opiate-addicted pregnant women since the late 1960s. More recently, buprenorphine has also been used; it has less placental transfer to the fetus than methadone, reducing the incidence of neonatal abstinence syndrome. Patients who have previously been on methadone maintenance therapy should continue with their regular dosing during labor and throughout the postpartum period. It is recommended that patients recovering from opioid addiction have a clear plan in place for pain management before labor. A multidisciplinary approach involving the obstetrician, anesthesiologist, and drug addiction treatment service is best.[16]

Regional anesthesia may be safely administered to opioid-addicted parturients. However, increased tendency for hypotension following spinal or epidural anesthesia should be anticipated. Extra-analgesic requirements during regional anesthesia for cesarean section have been reported, which is consistent with the theory of opioid-induced abnormal pain sensitivity.[17] An increased incidence of spinal, epidural, and disk space infections has also been reported in these patients, regardless of the type of anesthesia used; any symptoms and signs of neuraxial infection should be evaluated immediately. Acute opioid ingestion reduces anesthetic requirements and may also cause respiratory depression and loss of airway reflexes. Chronic opioid-abusing parturients may have decreased production of endogenous peptides, which may be responsible for the degree of exaggerated pain they can experience postoperatively.

MARIJUANA

Marijuana is used by 3% to 16% of parturients. Although the most important and potent chemical from the cannabis plant is delta 9-tetrahydrocannabinol

(THC), more than 400 chemical impurities can be found mixed into a marijuana cigarette. Marijuana is highly lipophilic and rapidly accumulates in adipose tissue. Complete elimination of a single dose may take up to 30 days. The presenting signs of patients intoxicated with marijuana can include euphoria, tachycardia, conjunctival congestion, and anxiety.

Even though THC readily crosses the placenta, there is no known increase in risk of serious congenital abnormalities in the fetus. The evidence regarding fetal effects of marijuana is inconclusive, but it is suggested that chronic use of marijuana results in decreased uteroplacental perfusion and IUGR.[18]

Anesthetic concerns related to marijuana use are mainly due to potential depression of the myocardium. During general anesthesia, the additive effects marijuana and potent inhaled anesthetics can result in pronounced myocardial depression. Marijuana can also have additive effects with other CNS depressants. Acute marijuana use may also produce tachycardia, and sympathomimetic drugs such as ketamine, pancuronium, atropine, and epinephrine should be avoided. Emphysema, bronchitis, and squamous metaplasia can result from chronic cannabis use, as they do in tobacco smoking. It has been reported that airway obstruction from uvular edema and oropharyngitis may result from recent preoperative marijuana smoking.[13]

HUMAN IMMUNODEFICIENCY VIRUS

Women, often of reproductive age, are the fastest growing population infected with human immunodeficiency virus (HIV) in the United States. In 2000, almost 30% of new HIV infections were in women. The prevalence of seropositivity in pregnant women in the United States has been estimated to be as high as 1.7 per 1000.[19]

HIV is an RNA virus that belongs to the lentivirus family, a subtype of human retroviruses. The virus is characterized by its cytopathic action on CD4+ lymphocytes. It is transmitted (1) via contact with sexual fluids or blood and blood products or (2) by vertical transmission from an infected mother to her fetus. Te greatest risk factor for HIV transmission in women is heterosexual at-risk activity with high-risk partners. Other risk factors include substance abuse (intravenous drug abuse and crack/cocaine use), sexually transmitted disease, and tattoo of body surfaces. Screening women with risk factors detects only about 50% of the patients who are seropositive, but if screening is applied to all pregnant women, the detection rate increases to approximately 87%.

Given that chemoprophylaxis can dramatically improve perinatal outcome, ACOG recommends that voluntary HIV screening be included in the comprehensive antenatal laboratory testing. Most women test positive within 1 month of primary infection. However, in rare circumstances, seroconversion may not occur for 6 months. Therefore, a second screening test is recommended once again at the beginning of the third trimester. If high-risk parturients present with undocumented HIV status on labor and delivery, a rapid test can be performed. Viral load levels (cells/mL) usually correlate with the CD4+ T-lymphocyte count. The goal of successful anti-HIV therapy should be viral load suppression to an undetectable level.

Among newborns with perinatally acquired HIV, 60% to 70% are infected with HIV during the intrapartum period, with the remainder infected before the onset of labor. The vertical transmission rate is estimated to be 20% to 30%. Intrapartum transmission is thought to be the result of maternal-fetal microtransfusion during uterine contractions, fetal exposure to maternal blood, and vaginal secretions during delivery. Breastfeeding significantly increases the risk of HIV transmission to infants and is contraindicated in infected women. Breastfeeding adds a 12% to 26% risk of vertical infection over and above the risk of transmission at delivery or in utero.[20] HIV-infected infants have the same frequency of congenital abnormalities as those not infected, and there is no consistent pattern of defects.

A significant reduction in the vertical transmission of HIV can be achieved with treatment of HIV-infected women with highly active antiretroviral therapy (HAART), regardless of their CD4+ count or viral load. Using this regimen, mother-to-child transmission can be decreased to less than 2% as long as breastfeeding is not undertaken. Risk factors for intrapartum transmission of HIV include severity of disease (maternal viral load), prolonged rupture of membranes, chorioamnionitis, vaginal delivery, and invasive fetal monitoring.[21] A cesarean section has the advantage of decreasing the time of contact between maternal blood and the neonate, and studies have shown a significant reduction in vertical transmission when it is combined with preoperative intravenous zidovudine infusion. Current ACOG guidelines recommend that women who have an HIV RNA level greater than 1000 copies/mL near term should undergo elective cesarean section at 38 weeks' gestation, before the onset of labor and rupture of membranes. Intravenous zidovudine should be administered 3 hours before the cesarean section. For those women with viral loads less than 1000 copies/mL, studies have not shown that cesarean section further decreases the rate of HIV transmission to the infant. In the absence of other obstetric indications, ACOG recommends that patients with viral loads less than 1000 copies/mL may deliver vaginally with a loading dose of zidovudine followed by a continuous infusion throughout labor.[22,23] Viral load testing should be performed every 3 months during pregnancy.

Clinical Manifestations

The clinical manifestation of HIV and acquired immunodeficiency syndrome (AIDS) can be that of the viral infection itself, opportunistic infections, neoplasms, or by the antiretroviral drugs or antiopportunistic drugs used for therapy. In the early stages of the AIDS epidemic, the predominant symptoms were those of immune suppression (eg, opportunistic infections, unusual malignancies). As improvements in prophylaxis and treatment of opportunistic infections have increased longevity, it has become apparent that HIV eventually affects multiple organ systems.

CENTRAL AND PERIPHERAL NERVOUS SYSTEM ABNORMALITIES

The manifestations of neurologic involvement vary depending on the stage of the disease. In the early stages of infection, headache, photophobia, meningoencephalitis, depression, irritability, Guillain-Barré–like syndromes, or cranial and peripheral neuropathies can be observed. Viral particles can be isolated from cerebrospinal fluid at the time of primary infection. During the latent phase of infection, some patients may remain neurologically asymptomatic. The late stage of HIV infection is rare in obstetric patients. In the late stage, intracranial masses, meningitis, or opportunistic infections may cause cerebral edema and increase intracranial pressure (ICP). In this case, anesthetic management would include measures to decrease ICP and in general would preclude the use of neuraxial anesthesia. Autonomic dysfunction, such as orthostatic syncope, hypotension, and diarrhea may also appear in people infected with late-stage HIV. Peripheral neuropathy is the most frequent neurologic complication, affecting nearly 35% of AIDS patients, and manifests as a polyneuropathy and/or myopathy.

PULMONARY ABNORMALITIES

Pulmonary manifestations of HIV infection are primarily a result of opportunistic infections. The most common, *Pneumocystis carinii* infection, has become rarer with the use of HAART. A person with a CD4+ lymphocyte count less than 200 cells/mm^3 is at increased risk for developing *P carinii* pneumonia (PCP). The disease may present as acute respiratory distress syndrome (ARDS), consisting of severe hypoxemia and a pattern of diffuse interstitial infiltrates on chest radiography. The mortality rate of patients who develops PCP and requires intubation is as high as 75%. Those who survive PCP are at risk for developing chronic airway disease. Reactivation of latent tuberculosis is common in HIV patients, as is bacterial pneumonia caused by encapsulated organisms (eg, *Streptococcus pneumoniae*, *Haemophilus influenzae*), and fungal pneumonia (eg, *Aspergillus*, *Cryptococcus*, *Coccidioides*).

CARDIAC ABNORMALITIES

Pericarditis has been reported to be the most common cardiac disorder in HIV patients. The most common offending agents are cytomegalovirus (CMV), herpes simplex virus, Kaposi's sarcoma, malignant lymphoma, and HIV itself. Accelerated coronary arteriosclerosis can result from elevations in serum cholesterol and triglycerides related to antiretroviral agents. Pulmonary hypertension can also develop from repeated PCP episodes or from cytokine-mediated endothelial injury. Decreased left ventricular contractility from focal myocarditis can also occur but is rare.

HEMATOLOGIC ABNORMALITIES

A wide spectrum of hematologic abnormalities can occur at any stage of infection in HIV patients. Idiopathic thrombocytopenic purpura is common and typically is caused by serum platelet immunoglobulins or direct HIV infection of megakaryocytes. Thrombocytopenia can also be a result of antiviral therapy. Leukopenia is a hallmark of the disease and results from direct CD4+ lymphocyte infection. Anemia is common and may be due to neoplastic or infectious bone marrow infiltration, poor nutrition, and occult gastrointestinal bleeding. Thromboembolic events have also been noted as a result of a hypercoagulable state that can result from HIV-related illnesses, malignancies, and antiretroviral drug therapy.

RENAL ABNORMALITIES

HIV-infected patients are at risk for acute renal failure secondary to sepsis, dehydration, and drug toxicity. Chronic renal failure can result from deposition of HIV antigen-immune complexes within the renal glomeruli, causing a proliferative glomerulonephritis. HIV-associated nephropathy, seen almost exclusively in African-American patients, is a focal segmental glomerulosclerosis that is characterized by extremely rapid deterioration of renal function and has a worse prognosis than other causes of renal failure.

GASTROINTESTINAL ABNORMALITIES

Gastrointestinal disturbances are common during all stages of HIV infection. Dysphagia is common, and typically results from CMV, herpes, or candidal esophagitis. Abnormal liver function tests are also common and reflect the decreased secretory and metabolic function of the liver in addition to coagulation abnormalities.

ENDOCRINOLOGIC AND METABOLIC ABNORMALITIES

Endocrinologic disorders can result from HIV effects on various glands by opportunistic infections, neoplasm, or antiretroviral drugs. Primary or secondary adrenal insufficiency is the most serious endocrinologic complication in HIV patients. Thyroid function tests in AIDS patients may be abnormal, although clinical hypothyroidism is rare.[20,21]

Anesthetic Considerations

HIV seropositivity alone should not influence the anesthetic management of parturients. The presence of clinical manifestations of HIV/AIDS infection, coexisting diseases, urgency of delivery, and obstetric indications should dictate the method of anesthesia. HIV infection alone does not preclude the use of regional anesthesia. In the past, there was concern that introduction of a spinal needle in HIV-positive patients could facilitate spread of the virus from the blood into the CNS and increase the risk of developing accelerated neurologic complications. However, HIV is a neurotrophic virus that infects the CNS early in the course of the disease process, and there is no evidence that neuraxial anesthesia produces any adverse neurologic sequelae. The neurotrophic predisposition of the HIV virus is responsible for symptoms of neurologic dysfunction in 30% to 40% of patients initially diagnosed with the disease. Therefore, a detailed neurologic history and documentation is important prior to neuraxial anesthesia. Systemic effects of HIV/AIDS infection that could preclude regional anesthesia include increased intracranial pressure, CNS infection, sepsis, and clotting abnormalities. Although data are limited, there is no evidence that performing a blood patch on an HIV-infected patient who has a postdural puncture headache accelerates the disease.

The multiorgan effects of HIV/AIDS infection and concomitant antiretroviral drug therapy should be considered when general anesthesia is administered. Increased sensitivity to opioids and benzodiazepines has been reported, especially when HIV-associated mental status changes such as dementia are present. There have been concerns about general anesthesia's transiently decreasing immune function; however, studies have shown that no anesthetic technique accelerates the disease. In addition, there is insufficient evidence to suggest that HIV or antiretroviral drugs increase the rate of pregnancy complications or that pregnancy alters the course of HIV infection.[20,24]

SUMMARY

Women of reproductive age may use illicit drugs, often multiple drugs, which can have a deleterious effect on pregnancy outcome. It is important for anesthesiologists to understand that social stigma often prevents women from being fully frank about their history. In addition, social and lifestyle conditions may also predispose to developing HIV infection. In approaching these women, care and compassion will often gain trust so that the full extent of their disease is appreciated and an appropriate delivery and anesthetic care plan can be created.

REFERENCES

1. Saloum M, Epstein JN. Drugs, alcohol, and pregnant women: anesthetic implications for mother and newborn. In: Bryson EO, Frost E. *Perioperative Addiction*. New York, NY: Springer; 2012.
2. Kuczkowski K. Anesthetic implications of drug abuse in pregnancy. *J Clin Anesth*. 2003;15:382-394.
3. McCalla S, Minkoff HL, Feldman J, et al. Predictors of cocaine use in pregnancy. *Obstet Gynecol*. 1992;79:641-644.
4. Kuczkowski KM. Cocaine abuse in pregnancy—anesthetic implications. *Int J Obstet Anesth*. 2002;11:204-210.
5. Birnbach DJ, Browne IM, Kim A, et al. Identification of polysubstance abuse in the parturient. *Br J Anesth*. 2001;87:488-490.
6. Plessinger MA, Woods JR. Maternal, fetal, and placental pathophysiology of cocaine exposure during pregnancy. *Clin Obstet Gynecol*. 1993;36:267-278.
7. Kreek MJ. Cocaine dopamine, and the endogenous opioid system. *J Addict Dis*. 1996;15:73-96.
8. Lange RA, Hilis LD. Cardiovascular complications of cocaine use. *N Engl J Med*. 2001;345:351-358.
9. Ebrahim SH, Luman ET, Floyd RL, et al. Alcohol consumption by pregnant women in the United States during 1988-1995. *Obstet Gynecol*. 1998;92:187-192.
10. Kilmer G, Roberts H, Hughes E, et al. Surveillance of certain health behaviors and conditions among states and selected local areas—behavioral risk factor surveillance system, United States 2006. *MMWR Surveill Summ*. 2008;57(7):1-188.
11. Burns E, Gray R, Smith LA. Brief screening questionnaires to identify problem drinking during pregnancy: a systematic review. *Addiction*. 2010;105:601-614.
12. chapter authors. Chapter title. In: Chestnut DH, Polley LS, Tsen LC, et al. *Obstetric Anesthesia: Principles and Practice*. 4th ed. Philadelphia, PA: Elsevier Mosby; 2009.
13. Keegan J, Parva M, Finnegan M, Gerson A, Belden M. Addiction in pregnancy. *J Addict Dis*. 2010;29:175-191.
14. Minozzi S, Amato L, Vecchi S, Davoli M. Maintenance agonist treatment for opiate dependent pregnant women. *Cochrane Database Syst Rev*. 2008:CD006318.
15. Lim S, Prasad MR, Samuels P, Gardner DK, Cordero L. High dose methadone in pregnant women and effect on duration of neonatal abstinence syndrome. *Am J Obstet Gynecol*. 2009;200:70, el-e5.
16. Rayburn W, Bogenschutz MP. Pharmacotherapy for pregnant women with addiction. *Am J Obstet Gynecol*. 2004;191:1885-1897.
17. Cassidy B, Cyna AM. Challenges that opioid-dependent women present.
18. Van Gelder M, Reefhius J, Caton A, et al. Characteristics of pregnant illicit drug users and associations between cannabis use and perinatal outcome in a population based study. *Drug Alcohol Depend*. 2010;109:243-247.

19. Centers for Disease Control and Prevention. Twenty-five years of HIV/AIDS—United States, 1981-2006. *MMWR Morb Mortal Wkly Rep.* 2006;55:585-589.

20. Evron S, Glezerman M, Harow E, Sadan O, Ezri T. Human immunodeficiency virus: anesthetic and obstetric considerations. *Anesth Analg.* 2004;98:503-511.

21. Chestnut DH, Polley LS, Tsen LC, et al. *Obstetric Anesthesia: Principles and Practice.* 4th ed. Philadelphia, PA: Elsevier Mosby; 2009.

22. Read JS, Tuomala R, Kpamegan E, et al. Mode of delivery and postpartum morbidity among HIV infected women: the women and infants transmission study. *J Acquir Immune Defic Syndr.* 2001;26(3):236-245.

23. European Mode of Delivery Collaboration. Elective cesarean section versus vaginal delivery in prevention of vertical HIV-1 transmission: a randomized clinical trial. *Lancet.* 1999;353(9158):1035-1039.

24. Kuczkowski M. Human immunodeficiency virus in the parturient. *J Clin Anesth.* 2003;15:224-233.

Section 6

Trauma During Pregnancy

Trauma During Pregnancy

29

Erica N. Grant, Oren Guttman, and Weike Tao

The authors have no financial interests to disclose.

INCIDENCE

The risk of maternal death in the United States has decreased nearly 99% during the twentieth century—from 850 maternal deaths per 100,000 live births in 1900 to 7.5 in 1982. However, since the 1980s, this rate has remained relatively unchanged.[1] Trauma is the leading cause of nonobstetric maternal death,[2] comprising 6% to 7% of all fatalities.[3] Motor vehicle accidents are the most common cause of injury, followed by falls and assaults.[2] Young maternal age, nonwhite ethnicity, substance and alcohol abuse, and domestic violence have been identified as risk factors for obstetric trauma.[4,5]

HEMORRHAGIC SHOCK IN PREGNANCY

During pregnancy, hemorrhage is difficult to reliably assess by conventional clinical parameters. Normal indicators of early shock, such as narrowed pulse pressure typically seen with 15% to 25% blood volume loss, are diminished due to progesterone-induced peripheral vasodilation. Additionally, classic signs such as tachycardia that are commonly seen with a 25% to 40% loss of blood volume may already exist during normal pregnancy; healthy parturients may exhibit a 40% increase in heart rate above prepregnancy baseline.

Plasma volume expansion begins as early as the sixth week of pregnancy,[6] peaking at 48% above baseline during the third trimester,[7] thereby causing a dilutional anemia. This could lead to a misinterpretation if a low hemoglobin or hematocrit was to be assessed as a lone value. For this reason, hemoglobin or hematocrit should be followed only as a trend during assessment and treatment of maternal trauma and injuries.[8] Pregnancy is associated with a hypercoagulable state, characterized by an elevation of certain coagulation factors, accelerated coagulation, and fibrinolysis.[9] However, the substantial blood loss along with further dilution of coagulation factors and platelets that can occur with aggressive fluid resuscitation and transfusion of packed red blood cells (PRBCs) may disrupt clotting activities, resulting in coagulopathy. Even in the absence of obstetric complications, such as uterine hypotonia, abruptio placentae, and placenta previa, parturients have an increased background incidence of hypofibrinogenemia and elevated fibrin split products (FSPs).[8] In the setting of trauma, rapid degradation of fibrin results in hypofibrinogenemia and elevated FSP levels, which can disrupt platelet function and further exacerbate coagulopathy during trauma resuscitation. This has been defined as "acute trauma coagulopathy."[10] Finally, the underlying coagulation abnormalities and tissue injuries that may occur during trauma and/or delivery predispose parturients to develop disseminated intravascular coagulation (DIC), a consumptive process of coagulation factors and platelets.[11]

Healthy pregnant women typically have good cardiovascular reserve and may not need full resuscitative measures until an excess of 30% blood volume is lost.[12] When a blood transfusion is warranted during pregnancy, there are some unique considerations. Fetal-maternal hemorrhage occurs in up to 30% of traumas; therefore, most experts recommend that all Rh-negative women receive Rho(D) immune globulin.[13] Uterine blood flow ranges from 500 mL/min in early pregnancy to just under 1000 mL/min at term gestation,[14] and thus the entire blood volume of a woman passes through the uterus in just under 8 minutes. With an expanded pelvic floor space, the parturient can "hide" a significant amount of blood in the intrauterine cavity.[15] Accordingly, during resuscitation, two large-bore (14- or 16-gauge) peripheral intravenous lines in the upper extremities or neck are preferred for optimal resuscitation. Lower extremity access is discouraged because of diminished venous return as a result of inferior vena cava compression from the gravid uterus.

Intraoperative cell salvage is controversial secondary to concern for maternal exposure to amniotic fluid, fetal squamous cells, tissue factors, or meconium, all of which have been implicated in amniotic fluid embolism pathophysiology and cardiovascular collapse. During life-threatening situations, the use of cell saver is warranted because the washing process reduces activated tissue factors, leukocytes, and fetal squamous cells to safe levels.[16]

The choice of blood products for resuscitation should follow standard massive transfusion protocol but with a few important exceptions. A 1:1 ratio of PRBC to fresh frozen plasma (FFP) is recommended with early and aggressive use of cryoprecipitate. Early and appropriate use of cryoprecipitate has been shown to decrease overall requirements for PRBCs, FFP, and platelets during massive obstetric hemorrhage.[17]

The use of recombinant activated factor VIIa (rFVIIa) is controversial. Although not approved for obstetric use and relatively contraindicated in thrombotic states such as DIC, it has been used successfully, with improved coagulation status, fewer PRBC transfusions, and lower mortality rates.[18] For improved efficacy, rFVIIa should be given early and after correction of the "lethal trauma triad" of hypothermia, coagulopathy (particularly platelets and fibrinogen), and acidosis. Finally, it should be noted that randomized control trials are needed to demonstrate its safety and confirm efficacy in the obstetrical population.

CARDIOPULMONARY RESUSCITATION

Effective cardiopulmonary resuscitation (CPR) in nonpregnant women leads to approximately 30% of normal cardiac output.[19] This is impossible to achieve in pregnant patients without adequate displacement of the uterus. Beginning at 16 to 18 weeks' gestation, the gravid uterus exerts a mass effect, causing aortocaval compression, thereby diminishing preload, stroke volume, cardiac output, and blood pressure. During CPR in near-term pregnant women, to achieve effective chest compressions, supine hypotension must be prevented with pelvic tilt. Special monitoring, such as an arterial line, may be useful, because the uterine vasculature is maximally dilated in pregnancy and autoregulation is diminished, leaving uterine blood flow close to completely dependent on maternal mean arterial pressure (MAP).[20] If resumption of spontaneous circulation does not occur after CPR and other measures, the standard of 5-minute "arrest to delivery" of the fetus should be followed to maximize maternal and fetal outcomes.[21] Assuming the fetus is viable (usually at 24 weeks or greater gestation), the resuscitation team leader should initiate a perimortem cesarean delivery. This requires early mobilization and delegation of responsibilities, including surgical preparation of the abdomen, availability of necessary surgical instruments and massive suction capacity, and prompt notification and arrival of the neonatal resuscitation team.[11]

AIRWAY MANAGEMENT IN OBSTETRICAL TRAUMA

In some circumstances, pregnancy may render women susceptible to aspiration. By 12 weeks, the lower esophageal sphincter is mechanically displaced by the gravid uterus. This displacement, along with increased gastric acidity and production, may place parturients at increased risk for aspiration pneumonitis and/or pneumonia. Trauma and pregnancy are both situations presenting with a full stomach and securing the airway with an endotracheal tube is the rule not the exception, particularly if patients are obtunded or severely hypotensive. Direct laryngoscopy can be challenging in pregnant women for several reasons. First, anatomic changes during pregnancy, such as enlarged breast tissue, may interfere with introduction of the laryngoscope into the oral cavity. Edema of the oral and nasopharynx, tongue enlargement, mouth floor rigidity secondary to elevated estrogen levels, and tissue friability distort airway anatomy. Also, there is approximately a 35% decrease in functional residual capacity and 20% increase in oxygen consumption that predisposes parturients to hypoxia during periods of apnea and hypoventilation, necessitating rapid securing of the airway or ventilation with cricoid pressure as a salvage maneuver. Finally, obstetric trauma patients may present with a confirmed or unconfirmed injury to the neck, limiting optimal positioning of the head during intubation. Although laryngeal mask airway has been used for elective cesarean delivery in noncomplicated patients with appropriate nothing-by-mouth status,[22] this is best left for dire emergencies and used primarily as a conduit to intubation in the case of a difficult airway. Video laryngoscopy and awake fiberoptic intubation may be indicated in select patients with a complex airway or neck injury.

ANESTHETIC MANAGEMENT

Regardless of the mechanism of injury, the mother's stability and survival is a priority.[23] A collaborative effort must be maintained between trauma surgeons, obstetricians, anesthesiologists, and neonatologists, and other consultant specialties may be included. Standard American Society of Anesthesiologists (ASA) monitors should be placed. If patients require induction of anesthesia, a rapid-sequence induction following preoxygenation is preferable using a cardiovascular stable induction agent such as etomidate (0.2-0.3 mg/kg). Ketamine (1-2 mg/kg), possessing sympathomimetic properties, can be used but with caution. In trauma patients, catecholamines may be depleted, and the use of ketamine may cause myocardial depression, especially in large doses. Further, large doses of ketamine (greater than 1-2 mg/kg) have been associated with increase in basal uttering tone, which may decrease placental perfusion. Following the standard technique of rapid-sequence induction with cricoid pressure, succinylcholine (1-1.5 mg/kg) should be used to facilitate tracheal intubation unless contraindicated. An alternative is to use rocuronium (1.2 mg/kg) for muscle relaxation. Narcotics should be used judiciously, especially in cases where delivery may be imminent. Parturients have decreased minimum alveolar concentration requirements; therefore, volatile agents should be used at a decreased dose based on the patient's tolerance. Nitrous oxide is routinely avoided in trauma anesthesia.

Maintenance of anesthesia should consist of a multimodal based technique. The combined use of narcotics, volatiles, and muscle relaxants can be used to achieve surgical anesthesia and prevent awareness.

Fluid resuscitation should be guided by clinical indicators, acid-base balance, and signs of organ perfusion. The use of crystalloids, colloids, and blood products should be used to maintain MAP within 20% of baseline.

NEONATAL RESUSCITATION

Neonatal injuries related to maternal trauma continue to increase and carry a 40% to 50% risk of fetal death.[24] Adverse fetal outcome ranges from spontaneous abortion to direct fetal injury, such as fractures and intracranial hemorrhage[12] Anticipation, adequate preparation, accurate evaluation, and prompt initiation of resuscitative measures are crucial for survival.[25]

OTHER CONSIDERATIONS

Fetal heart rate (FHR) monitoring is essential where possible because placental abruption, uterine rupture, or hypovolemia from trauma may manifest as nonreassuring FHRs and prompt immediate delivery. If delivery is not imminent and the fetus is viable, FHR monitoring should be performed on a continuous basis, if feasible. If nonviable or impractical in the case of abdominal surgery, fetal heart tones should be documented before (time permitting) and after surgery. Trauma, surgery, and/or analgesics may predispose parturients to preterm labor, necessitating uterine contraction monitoring to help guide management and possible need for tocolytic therapy in the perioperative period.

Intraoperative awareness more frequently occurs during obstetric surgery,[26] which could be exacerbated by the potential inadequate anesthesia due to hemodynamic instability. Anesthesia providers should be vigilant about end-tidal anesthetic gas concentrations and other objective signs of intraoperative awareness. Proper use of medications with amnestic properties that are least likely to alter hemodynamics may aid in the prevention of intraoperative awareness.

General and regional anesthesia inhibits the body's ability to thermoregulate.[27] Surgical procedures, especially those involving open cavities, hasten hypothermia due to rapid blood loss with massive amounts of fluids and blood product replacement. Active warming has been shown to reduce maternal shivering and improve fetal blood pH.[28] Further, prevention of hypothermia will decrease the risk of coagulopathy. Forced air blankets, warm intravenous fluids, and warming mattresses should be utilized for parturients. Although efforts in the perioperative period may be aimed at preventing and treating hypothermia, if the resumption of spontaneous circulation occurs after CPR, there is a role for therapeutic hypothermia to 32°C to 34°C for 12 to 24 hours in the parturient.[29]

In treating pregnant trauma patients, management should be based on clinical findings, because laboratory results usually serve only to confirm the clinical diagnosis; they are time consuming, and there is a lack of specificity during pregnancy. Effective treatment includes rapid correction of the underlying cause and replacement of volume and blood products, including fibrinogen from cryoprecipitate to maintain levels above 100 mg/mL.[30]

Expertise from obstetricians or maternal-fetal medicine specialists is useful in performing vaginal examinations, assessing uterine tone, and monitoring transvaginal fetal heart tones. Assessment of fetal well-being should be sought early during trauma and surgery. Other consultants may include trauma, neurologic, cardiovascular, vascular, and burn surgeons, as well as critical care specialists.

SUMMARY

Trauma remains an important cause of maternal and fetal morbidity and mortality. Maternal changes occurring during pregnancy may underestimate the extent of hemorrhage and also affect resuscitation. Successful therapy involves a multidisciplinary team approach.

REFERENCES

1. Centers for Disease Control and Prevention. Pregnancy-related mortality surveillance—United States, 1991-1999. *MMWR.* 2003;52(SS02);1-8.

2. El-Kady D, Gilbert WM, Anderson J, Danielsen B, Towner D, Smith LH. Trauma during pregnancy: an analysis of maternal and fetal outcomes in a large population. *Am J Obstet Gynecol.* 2004;190(6):1661-1668.

3. Fildes J, Reed L, Jones N, Martin M, Barrett J. Trauma: the leading cause of maternal death. *J Trauma.* 1992 May;32(5):643-645.

4. Weiss HB. Pregnancy-associated injury hospitalizations in Pennsylvania, 1995. *Ann Emerg Med.* 1999;34(5):626-636.

5. Stewart DE, Cecutti A. Physical abuse in pregnancy. *CMAJ.* 1993;149(9):1257-1263.

6. Bernstein IM, Ziegler W, Badger GJ. Plasma volume expansion in early pregnancy. *Obstet Gynecol.* 2001;97(5 pt 1):669-672.

7. Pritchard JA. Changes in the blood volume during pregnancy and delivery. *Anesthesiology.* 1965;26:393-399.

8. Ickx BE. Fluid and blood transfusion management in obstetrics. *Eur J Anaesthesiol.* 2010;27(12):1031-1035.

9. Chestnut D, Polley L, Tsen L, Wong C. *Chestnut's Obstetric Anesthesia: Principles and Practice.* 4th ed. (Expert Consult—Online and Print). Philadelphia, PA: Mosby Elsevier; 2009.

10. Brohi K, Singh J, Heron M, Coats T. Acute traumatic coagulopathy. *J Trauma.* 2003;54(6):1127-1130.

11. Suresh MS, LaToya Mason C, Munnur U. Cardiopulmonary resuscitation and the parturient. *Best Pract Res Clin Obstet Gynaecol.* 2010;24(3):383-400; E-pub April 24, 2010.

12. El Kady D. Perinatal outcomes of traumatic injuries during pregnancy. *Clin Obstet Gynecol.* 2007;50(3):582-591.

13. Hill CC, Pickinpaugh J. Trauma and surgical emergencies in the obstetric patient. *Surg Clin North Am.* 2008;88(2):421-440, viii.

14. Konje JC, Kaufmann P, Bell SC, Taylor DJ. A longitudinal study of quantitative uterine blood flow with the use of color power angiography in appropriate for gestational age pregnancies. *Am J Obstet Gynecol.* 2001;185(3):608-613.

15. Oxford CM, Ludmir J. Trauma in pregnancy. *Clin Obstet Gynecol.* 2009;52(4):611-629.

16. Allam J, Cox M, Yentis SM. Cell salvage in obstetrics. *Int J Obstet Anesth.* 2008;17(1):37-45.

17. Arendt KW, Segal S. Present and emerging strategies for reducing anesthesia-related maternal morbidity and mortality. *Curr Opin Anaesthesiol.* 2009;22(3):330-335.

18. Hossain N, Shamsi T, Haider S, et al. Use of recombinant activated factor VII for massive postpartum hemorrhage. *Acta Obstet Gynecol Scand.* 2007;29:1-7.

19. Basic Life Support Working Group of the European Resuscitation Council. The 1998 European Resuscitation Council guidelines for adult single rescuer basic life support. *BMJ.* 1998;316(7148):1870-1876.

20. Nelson TW, Kuczkowski KM. Trauma in pregnancy: anesthetic management of a parturient with hypotensive shock and trauma to the gravid uterus. *Acta Anaesthesiol Scand.* 2004;48(5):662.

21. Katz VL, Dotters DJ, Droegemueller W. Perimortem cesarean delivery. *Obstet Gynecol.* 1986;68(4):571-576.

22. Han TH, Brimacombe J, Lee EJ, Yang HS. The laryngeal mask airway is effective (and probably safe) in selected healthy parturients for elective Cesarean section: a prospective study of 1067 cases. *Can J Anaesth.* 2001;48(11):1117-1121.

23. Mirza FG, Devine PC, Gaddipati S. Trauma in pregnancy: a systematic approach. *Am J Perinatol.* 2010;27(7):579-586.

24. Weiss HB, Lawrence BA, Miller TR. Pregnancy-associated assault hospitalizations. *Obstet Gynecol.* 2002;100(4):773-780.

25. Kattwinkel J, Perlman JM, Aziz K, et al. American Heart Association. Neonatal resuscitation: 2010 American Heart Association Guidelines for Cardiopulmonary Resuscitation and Emergency Cardiovascular Care. *Pediatrics.* 2010;126(5):e1400-13; E-pub October 18, 2010.

26. Ghoneim MM, Block RI, Haffarnan M, Mathews MJ. Awareness during anesthesia: risk factors, causes and sequelae: a review of reported cases in the literature. *Anesth Analg.* 2009;108(2):527-535.

27. Sessler DI. Mild perioperative hypothermia. *N Engl J Med*. 1997;336(24):1730-1737.

28. Horn EP, Schroeder F, Gottschalk A, et al. Active warming during cesarean delivery. *Anesth Analg*. 2002;94(2):409-414.

29. Rittenberger JC, Kelly E, Jang D, Greer K, Heffner A. Successful outcome utilizing hypothermia after cardiac arrest in pregnancy: a case report. *Crit Care Med*. 2008;36(4):1354-1356.

30. Lee RH. Postpartum hemorrhage. In: Goodwin TM, Montoro MN, Muderspach L, Paulson R, Roy S, eds. *Management of Common Problems in Obstetrics and Gynecology*. 5th ed. Oxford, England: Wiley-Blackwell; 2010:67-70.

Cardiopulmonary Resuscitation in Pregnancy

30

Andi McCown and Robert S.F. McKay

INTRODUCTION

Pregnancy poses anatomic and physiologic impediments to cardiopulmonary resuscitation. Recent studies have shown that nearly 40% of obstetric providers are unaware of the pronounced differences between the resuscitation of pregnant women versus nonpregnant women.[1] This chapter will review physiologic changes that occur in pregnancy, as well as causes of maternal arrest, which will form a foundation for understanding the modifications that must take place when resuscitating pregnant women.

PERTINENT PHYSIOLOGIC CHANGES OF PREGNANCY

The cardiovascular system changes dramatically throughout pregnancy. By 32 weeks' gestation, cardiac output has increased 30% to 50% above baseline because of an increase in circulating blood volume (increased preload). Progesterone-induced smooth muscle relaxation decreases systemic vascular resistance, leading to reduced afterload and up to a 15% to 20% increase in heart rate. During labor, cardiac output will increase an additional 10% to 15% above baseline.[2] It is imperative to understand that uterine blood flow is at its maximum by late pregnancy and cannot be further increased during hypoxic or low-flow states; thus, during cardiopulmonary arrest, there will be vasoconstriction of the uteroplacental bed, further compromising the fetus.[3]

A dilutional anemia occurs secondary to a 50% increase in plasma volume and only a 30% increase in red blood cell mass. Because of the increase in plasma volume, a substantial amount of hemorrhage can take place before signs of hypovolemia become apparent.[1] This physiologic anemia may have an impact on oxygen delivery to vital organ systems, especially during cardiopulmonary arrest.[3]

By 20 weeks' gestation, the uterus reaches the level of the inferior vena cava. With a pregnant woman in the supine position, the uterus may cause compression of the inferior vena cava and decrease cardiac output.[2] Quantitative cardiovascular magnetic resonance imaging has shown a 24% decrease in cardiac output at 32 weeks' gestation in the supine position as compared to the lateral position.[4] By the third trimester, the uterus may completely obstruct the inferior vena cava, leading to syncope, hypotension, and bradycardia.[5,6] Compression of pelvic veins is also a concern in the pregnant patient. Signs and symptoms of compression in the pelvis are dependent edema, venous stasis, varicose veins, and hemorrhoids.[5] This increased venous pressure may lead to rapid blood loss in cases of injuries to the pelvis and lower extremities; therefore, it is best to avoid intravenous lines in lower extremities, especially for resuscitation efforts, because venous return from the lower extremities to the central circulation is not assured.[1,5] Most importantly, in addition to compression of major vessels, the gravid uterus exerts pressure on the diaphragm, which may limit forward blood flow during chest compressions (Figure 30-1).[3]

The gravid uterus affects not only the cardiovascular system but the respiratory system as well. As stated previously, the diaphragm will be displaced cephalad as a result of the gravid uterus.[1,5] This leads to a 10% to 25% reduction in residual volume and functional residual capacity.[2,3,5] Concurrently, maternal oxygen requirements increase 15% to 20%.[1,5] The decrease in function residual capacity along with an increase in maternal oxygen demand causes hypoxia to occur quickly with respiratory arrest.[2,3] The chronic respiratory alkalosis in pregnancy leads to a decrease in bicarbonate and thus a loss of blood-buffering capacity. The fetus is able to adapt to the chronic alkalosis by adjusting its carbon dioxide level and diffusing carbon dioxide from its higher fetal concentration to the lower maternal carbon dioxide concentration. Acute changes are more difficult for the fetus; when maternal hypercapnia occurs, as during cardiopulmonary arrest, the pressure gradient is altered, and the fetus cannot transfer as much carbon dioxide

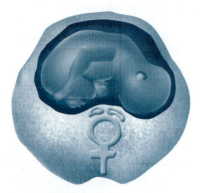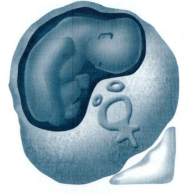

Figure 30-1. Aortocaval compression in the supine position and its alleviation with uterine displacement.

to the mother.[7] Fortunately, the fetus is protected from asphyxia by several mechanisms. First, fetal hemoglobin carries 20% to 50% more oxygen than maternal hemoglobin, leading to a leftward shift of the fetal oxyhemoglobin dissociation curve. Second, fetal acidosis relative to the mother enhances oxygen uptake by fetal blood in the placental bed (Bohr effect). Third, fetal circulation during hypoxia causes increased blood flow to the fetal brain, heart, and adrenal glands. Theoretically, the fetus can survive hypoxia for greater than 10 minutes, although reports of intact fetal neurologic status and recovery from maternal arrest beyond 10 minutes are rare.[8]

The pregnant woman is at increased risk of aspiration secondary to a decrease in gastric motility and reduced gastric sphincter response.[3,5] In addition, there is increased gastric acid production, which will theoretically increase pulmonary damage if aspiration occurs.[5] These physiologic changes will mandate rapid airway management during cardiopulmonary resuscitation (CPR). Upper gastrointestinal changes that occur include edema and fragility of the pharynx and larynx secondary to an increase in estrogen and subsequent increase in interstitial water. A narrower airway lumen may be encountered secondary to pharyngeal and vocal cord edema, hindering the passage of the endotracheal tube; therefore, the use of a smaller than usual endotracheal tube may be prudent. A pregnant woman may have an increase in nasal mucosal congestion, especially after high blocks and/or labor; therefore, care should be taken when placing a nasogastric or nasotracheal tube, and these tubes should only be used when absolutely necessary.[1]

Pregnancy leads to an increase in volume of distribution. As a result, resuscitation drugs may be less effective, although dose adjustments are not generally recommended during initial resuscitative efforts. Although they are necessary for resuscitation, endogenous and exogenous catecholamines can vasoconstrict the uterine artery; this leads to a decrease in fetal oxygenation and fetal carbon dioxide exchange during resuscitation.[3]

CAUSES OF MATERNAL ARREST

Cardiopulmonary arrest in pregnant women is rare (incidence: 1 in 30,000 pregnancies).[1] Having a thorough understanding of the physiologic changes that occur in pregnancy will help in determining the underlying cause of maternal arrest. This is important for improving maternal and fetal outcomes after cardiopulmonary arrest. The causes of arrest may be obstetric or nonobstetric (Table 30-1).

Hemorrhage is responsible for 25% of maternal deaths in pregnancy.[5] Peripartum hemorrhage is frequently seen in cases of abruptio placentae, placenta previa, uterine rupture, and uterine atony, with atony being the most common cause of maternal hemorrhage. Massive hemorrhage and subsequent blood transfusion can result in acute respiratory distress syndrome (ARDS), which itself is associated with cardiac arrest and maternal death.[3]

Preeclampsia and the complications of preeclampsia (pulmonary edema, cardiac dysfunction, stroke, cerebral edema, and the hemolysis, elevated liver enzymes, low platelets [HELLP] syndrome) have also been implicated in cases of cardiac arrest.[3] Although hypertension is observed in preeclampsia, these patients are often

Table 30-1. Causes of Maternal Cardiac Arrest

Obstetric	Nonobstetric
Hemorrhage	Trauma
Venous air embolism	Pulmonary embolism
Peripartum cardiomyopathy	Infection and/or sepsis
Amniotic fluid embolism	Stroke
Pregnancy-induced hypertension/preeclampsia/HELLP syndrome	Myocardial infarction
Eclampsia	Aortic dissection
Local anesthetic toxicity (eg, intravenous injection)	Heart failure
Magnesium toxicity	Hyperthyroidism and thyroid storm
High or total spinal	Status asthmaticus
Hypoxia/anoxia from airway loss (multiple causes) or failed intubation	Acute respiratory distress syndrome
	Homicide
	Suicide

Abbreviation: HELLP, hemolysis, elevated liver enzymes, low platelets.

severely intravascularly volume depleted with significant third spacing of fluid, both of which increase the degree of difficulty in resuscitative efforts (including venous access, intubation, and response to hemodynamic support).

Abrupt cardiovascular collapse and coagulopathy during labor or immediately postpartum may be related to amniotic fluid embolism.[5,9] Unfortunately, the mortality rate can be as high as 50%.[3] This syndrome, sometimes called the "anaphylactoid syndrome of pregnancy," may require the use of cardiopulmonary bypass. Bypass has been efficacious in managing cardiovascular collapse from severe pulmonary vasoconstriction.[10,11]

Anesthetic complications include anoxia and hypoxia from difficult intubation or aspiration, hemodynamic and respiratory collapse from a high or total spinal, and drug toxicity.[12] Local anesthetic toxicity is an important concern in the pregnant woman. The American Society of Regional Anesthesia and Pain Medicine calls for specific guidelines, including immediate airway management, lower than normal doses of epinephrine (less than 1 μg/kg), avoidance of vasopressin, use of lipid emulsion, and notification of facilities having cardiopulmonary bypass capability when epinephrine and other therapies have failed.[13]

Idiopathic peripartum cardiomyopathy is rare. Typically seen during the last month of pregnancy through 6 months after delivery, it is cardiac failure in the absence of preexisting cardiac disease.[2,3] Because symptoms of peripartum cardiomyopathy mirror those of pregnancy itself, the diagnosis is often overlooked, with cardiac arrest or sudden death being unfortunate presentations.

The nonobstetric causes of cardiopulmonary arrest are also numerous, as listed in Table 30-1. The pregnant patient presenting as a trauma warrants a careful examination of the abdomen, because the uterus displaces intra-abdominal organs and makes localization of injuries challenging. Due to desensitization of the abdominal wall, masking of abdominal pain and tenderness may occur. The patient should be assessed for the presence or absence of uterine contractions, uterine tenderness, or vaginal bleeding.[5]

The number one cause of nonobstetric maternal arrest is pulmonary thromboembolism. Thromboembolism occurs secondary to stasis and pregnancy-induced hypercoagulability. During uncomplicated pregnancies, women are hypercoagulable secondary to a net increase in clotting factors and prolonged bed rest during labor. Coexisting conditions, including factor V Leiden, antiphospholipid syndrome, and lupus erythematosus also contribute to hypercoagulability. Venous stasis, hypercoagulability, and vascular damage (Virchow triad) combine to make thromboembolism the leading cause of maternal death in developed countries.[3,9]

Pregnant women are particularly susceptible to infections such as chorioamnionitis, pneumonia, and urinary tract infections.[3] In fact, urinary tract infections are the most common site of infection for critically ill obstetric patients.[9] Septic shock, requiring fluid resuscitation and inotropic support, may occur as frequently as 1 in 5000 gestations.[3]

As women are waiting later in life to have children, the incidence of myocardial infarction during pregnancy has increased. The demands that pregnancy place on the cardiovascular system are great; this affects patients with preexisting cardiac disease.[5] Risk factors for myocardial infarction during pregnancy include hypercholesterolemia, hypertension, diabetes mellitus, left ventricular hypertrophy, and smoking.[3] Pregnant women are also at increased risk for spontaneous aortic dissection during pregnancy.[5,10] This occurs because of hormonal changes on smooth muscle and connective tissue.[5] Preexisting heart failure will affect management of the pregnant woman. Those with New York Heart Association class III or IV may require a pulmonary artery catheter to assess intravascular volume, cardiac output, and oxygen delivery.[3]

Poor control of asthma has been related to poor maternal and fetal outcomes, including preeclampsia, uterine hemorrhage, preterm delivery, and low birth weight.[9] Other respiratory complications such as ARDS can occur secondary to pneumonia, sepsis, and/or amniotic fluid embolism.[9]

Pregnant women are often victims of domestic violence, making it imperative to consider attempted homicide and suicide when presented with an unexplained cardiopulmonary arrest. These are significant causes of mortality during pregnancy.[10]

As with any patient presenting in cardiopulmonary arrest, it is important to remember reversible causes of cardiac arrest (Table 30-2).[10,14]

Table 30-2. Possible Causes of Cardiac Arrest

Causes Beginning With "H"	Causes Beginning With "T"
Hypoxia	Thromboembolism (pulmonary embolism)
Hypovolemia (hemorrhage or sepsis)	Tablets or toxins (eg, magnesium, local anesthetics)
Hyperkalemia/hypokalemia or other metabolic disorders	Tension pneumothorax
Hypothermia	(Cardiac) tamponade
Hydrogen ions (acidosis)	Thrombosis (myocardial infarction)
Hypoglycemia/hyperglycemia	Trauma

RESUSCITATION OF THE PREGNANT PATIENT IN CARDIOPULMONARY ARREST

Basic Life Support (BLS) and Advanced Cardiac Life Support (ACLS) will not be reviewed here. Rather, the following is a guide to the modifications that must occur specific for the resuscitation of a pregnant woman to be successful. The treatment goal is to maintain adequate blood flow to optimize both maternal and fetal oxygenation (Table 30-3).[15]

Recently, the American Heart Association has introduced five evidence-based changes to promote more effective CPR.[1] These include effective chest compression, creation of a universal compression-to-ventilation ratio for lone rescuers, the recommendation of 1-second breaths during CPR, restructuring defibrillation methods, and endorsing automated external defibrillator (AED) usage.

Because cardiac output during optimally effective CPR is only 30% of normal, effective chest compressions are key to a successful resuscitation. Uninterrupted chest compressions allow for adequate blood flow and perfusion to vital organ systems. Compressions must allow for the chest to fully recoil in order to maximize filling of the heart.[1]

The new compression-to-ventilation ratio is 30:2. This ensures less interruption of compressions. Whereas previously it was recommended to perform CPR with chest compressions only, this has been abandoned because ventilation is crucial to ensure optimal outcome of both mother and baby.

During the first few minutes of CPR after an acute arrest, oxygen content in the bloodstream may remain adequate. However, cardiac output decreases as resuscitation continues, and less blood flows through the heart and lungs. Therefore, shorter ventilation efforts can still provide adequate oxygenation and effective carbon dioxide elimination. It is important to avoid hyperventilation after intubation, because this has been associated with poor outcome. In addition, positive pressure ventilation may inhibit cardiac output further.

Current energy requirements for adult defibrillation are appropriate for the pregnant woman. When using an AED, one shock should be delivered, with CPR and chest compressions immediately following. Delays of more than 30 seconds may occur if waiting to analyze cardiac rhythm. In addition, if the AED is not effective initially in controlling ventricular fibrillation, resumption of CPR is more valuable than performing a second shock. Finally, even if the AED eliminates ventricular fibrillation, the normal heart rhythm may not return for several minutes.[1]

Table 30-3. Modifications for Resuscitation of Pregnant Patients

Uterine displacement: place patient 15-30 degrees left lateral
Airway: secure immediately using continuous cricoid pressure
Intravenous access: place in upper extremity, if possible
Chest compressions: perform 1-2 cm higher on sternum than in nonpregnant patients
Vasopressor agents: may require increased doses secondary to increased volume of distribution
"4-minute rule:" cesarean section should begin 4 minutes after cardiac arrest

The modifications for resuscitation of pregnant women are very closely tied to the anatomic and physiologic changes that occur during pregnancy. As stated previously, the gravid uterus may compromise venous return from the inferior vena cava and limit effectiveness of chest compressions in restoring cardiac output.[10] Because optimal CPR produces cardiac output that is 30% of normal, uterine displacement is critical.[8] The uterus needs to be shifted away from the inferior vena cava and the aorta by placing the patient 15 to 30 degrees left lateral, although recent theoretical analysis suggests that 15 degrees may be inadequate to prevent aortocaval compression.[16] However, beyond an angle of 30 degrees, chest compressions are not as effective.[9,14] Therefore, the Cardiff wedge, which produces a tilt of 27 degrees, has been suggested as the best compromise for cardiopulmonary resuscitation.[1,5] Tilt can also be accomplished manually or by placing a rolled blanket or other object under the right hip, or preferably lumbar area.[2,10,11] In the left lateral position, it is important to remember that blood pressure cuff readings will be higher in the left arm.[7]

Aspiration is increased during pregnancy for reasons mentioned above. The pregnant airway should be secured immediately, because this maximizes oxygenation, protects the airway, and decreases the risk of aspiration.[9,10,14] Continuous cricoid pressure should be applied during mask positive pressure ventilation and maintained until the airway is definitively secured.[10] Because hypoxemia may occur rapidly during management of the airway, it is important to be prepared to support oxygenation and ventilation.[10] Smaller endotracheal tubes may be needed secondary to airway edema. Correct placement should be verified by an exhaled CO_2 monitor.[10]

Intravenous (IV) access is obviously essential. Due to vena caval compression, IV medications delivered through IV access below the uterus may not reach the heart or arterial circulation.[5] Therefore, IV access is preferably started in an upper extremity. When IV access is unattainable, an intraosseous needle should be placed in the humerus for rapid access to the central circulation.

Chest compressions should be performed 1 to 2 cm higher on the sternum in pregnant women than in nonpregnant patients due to the elevation of the diaphragm and abdominal contents by the gravid uterus.[10,17]

Vasopressor agents will decrease blood flow to the uterus; however, there are no recommended changes to the usual doses of indicated medications.[10] Because volume of distribution is increased during pregnancy and cardiac output is decreased during CPR, higher doses of vasopressor agents should be administered if there is no response to standard doses.[3]

There are no modifications to ACLS defibrillation doses.[10] However, any internal fetal monitoring equipment that might conduct electricity to the fetus should be removed before delivering shocks.[1,10]

Despite these modifications, BLS and ACLS may not immediately reverse cardiopulmonary arrest. It is difficult to perform effective closed chest cardiac massage in the face of significant aortocaval compression due to impeded venous return. Any time a pregnant woman arrests, consideration for rapid emergency cesarean section should take place.[10] Katz et al. have described the "4-minute rule," stating that the best survival rate for infants at greater than 24 to 25 weeks occurs when the delivery of the infant is achieved no more than 5 minutes after the mother's heart stops beating; therefore, cesarean section should begin 4 minutes after cardiac arrest unresponsive to resuscitation. This time interval considers oxygen consumption, prevention of neurologic injury, and the fact that fetal viability begins about 24 to 25 weeks' gestation.[1,10] Although portable ultrasonography may be helpful in determining the gestational age of the fetus, this should not delay the decision for emergency cesarean section.[10] Gestational age can be estimated by palpation of the abdomen; by 20 weeks, the uterine fundus is at the level of the umbilicus.[5] At a gestational age less than 20 weeks, urgent cesarean section is generally not considered unless improved maternal outcomes are anticipated, because the size of the uterus is unlikely to compromise venous return and maternal cardiac output.[15] Between 20 and 23 weeks' gestation, an emergency hysterotomy should be performed strictly to allow for successful resuscitation of the mother, not the survival of the delivered infant. If a pregnant woman is apparently dead, and the gestational age of the fetus is approximately 24 weeks, a cesarean section should be performed.[3]

The emergency cesarean section should be performed by the most skilled provider who is available and should ideally take place at a medical center with a neonatal intensive care unit.[1,10] The procedure should ideally take no more than a few minutes. There has been much debate over the ideal location for cesarean section. Moving the patient to an operating room is usually not necessary and may lead to worse outcomes.[5,14] Indeed, recent simulation studies have demonstrated that even in the best of circumstances, delivery within 5 minutes cannot be achieved with movement of the patient to the operating room suite.[1] An important consideration is that little blood loss will occur with decreased cardiac output from the mother.[5,14] Emergency equipment must be readily available in emergency departments and labor wards. This includes antiseptic solution, scalpels, and sterile packs for the uterus and abdomen.[6]

Emergency cesarean section will facilitate resuscitation by relieving venous obstruction and aortic compression.[1,10] Cardiac output has been shown to increase 25% to 56% secondary to the emptying of the uterus and due to autotransfusion with uterine involution.[3] In addition, cesarean section allows for more effective chest compressions.[9] Open cardiac massage through the diaphragm has been proposed as an alternative.[14] Displacement of abdominal contents will be relieved, thus decreasing intrathoracic pressure. This allows for increased venous return to the heart, increased cardiac output, and increased tissue perfusion.[7] Functional residual capacity will increase, leading to improved oxygenation during resuscitation.[3] During and after cesarean section, CPR must be maintained. This will maximize cardiac output, perfusion of maternal organ systems, and uteroplacental perfusion.[3,9]

The delivered infant has an increased survival if the interval between maternal arrest and delivery is short. In addition, survival is increased when maternal hypoxia was not sustained before arrest. Finally, minimal or no signs of fetal distress before maternal cardiac arrest lead to greater survival.[10]

CONCLUSION

Recent Confidential Enquiry into Maternal and Child Health (CEMACH) reports have suggested substandard care in more than 50% of maternal deaths.[1] An understanding of the physiologic changes of pregnancy, the causes of maternal arrest, and modifications of CPR are crucial to successful resuscitation in pregnant women.

REFERENCES

1. Suresh MS, LaToya Mason C, Munnur U. Cardiopulmonary resuscitation and the parturient. *Best Pract Res Clin Obstet Gynaecol.* 2010;24:383-400.

2. Dellinger RP. Cardiopulmonary complications of pregnancy. *Crit Care Med.* 2005;33:1616-1622.

3. Whitty JE. Maternal cardiac arrest in pregnancy. *Clin Obstet Gynecol.* 2002;45:377-392.

4. Rossi A, Cornette J, Johnson MR, et al. Quantitative cardiovascular magnetic resonance in pregnant women: cross-sectional analysis of physiologic parameters throughout pregnancy and the impact of the supine position. *J Cardiov Magn Reson.* 2011;13:31.

5. Campbell TA. Cardiac arrest and pregnancy. *J Emerg Trauma Shock.* 2009;1:34-42.

6. Catling-Paull C, McDonnell N, Moores A, Homer CS. Maternal mortality in Australia: learning from maternal cardiac arrest. *Nurs Health Sci.* 2011;13:10-15.

7. Fillion DN. Being prepared for a pregnant code blue. *Am J Matern Child Nurs.* 1998;23:240-245.

8. Nelissen EC, de Zwaan C, Marcus MA, et al. Maternal cardiac arrest in early pregnancy. *Int J Obstet Anesth.* 2009;18:60-63.

9. Shapiro JM. Critical care of the obstetric patient. *J Intensive Care Med.* 2006;21:278-286.

10. 2005 American Heart Association Guidelines for Cardiopulmonary Resuscitation and Emergency Cardiovascular Care. Part 10.8: Cardiac Arrest Associated With Pregnancy. *Circulation.* 2005;112: IV150-153.

11. Zhou ZQ, Shao Q, Zeng Q, Song J, Yang JJ. Lumbar wedge versus pelvic wedge in preventing hypotension following combined spinal epidural anesthesia for caesarean delivery. *Anesth Intensive Care.* 2008;36:835-839. Einav S, Matot I, Berkenstadt H, Bromiker R, Weiniger CF. A survey of labour ward clinicians' knowledge of maternal cardiac arrest and resuscitation. *Int J Obstet Anesth.* 2008;17:238-242.

12. Ezri T, Lurie S, Weiniger CF, Golan A, Evron S. Cardiopulmonary resuscitation in the pregnant patient—an update. *Israel Med Assoc J.* 2011;13:306-310.

13. Neal JM, Bernards CM, Butterworth JF IV. ASRA practice advisory on local anesthetic systemic toxicity. *Reg Anesth Pain Med.* 2010;35:152-161.

14. Grady K, Howell C, Cox C, editors. *The MOET Course Manual: Managing Obstetric Emergencies and Trauma.* 2nd ed. (Chapter 4, Cardiopulmonary resuscitation in the non-pregnant and pregnant patient.) London, England: RCOG Press; 2011. (ILCOR update.)

15. Stringer M, Brooks PM, King K, Biesecker B. New guidelines for maternal and neonatal resuscitation. *J Obstet Gynecol Neonatal Nurs.* 2007;34:624-635.

16. Summers RL, Harrison JM, Thompson JR, Porter J, Coleman TG. Theoretical analysis of the effect of positioning on hemodynamic stability during pregnancy. *Acad Emerg Med.* 2011;18:1094-1098.

17. Cohen SE, Andes LC, Carvalho B. Assessment of knowledge regarding cardiopulmonary resuscitation of pregnant women. *Int J Obstet Anesth.* 2008;17:20-25.

Index

NOTE: Page numbers followed by *f* and *t* denotes figures and tables, respectively.